Gastrointestinal Health: Clinical Research and Therapeutic Innovations

Gastrointestinal Health: Clinical Research and Therapeutic Innovations

Guest Editor

Ludovico Abenavoli

MDPI

Basel • Beijing • Wuhan • Barcelona • Belgrade • Novi Sad • Cluj • Manchester

Guest Editor
Ludovico Abenavoli
Department of Health
Sciences
University "Magna Græcia"
Catanzaro
Italy

Editorial Office
MDPI AG
Grosspeteranlage 5
4052 Basel, Switzerland

This is a reprint of the Special Issue, published open access by the journal *Life* (ISSN 2075-1729), freely accessible at: https://www.mdpi.com/journal/life/special_issues/2AC14SSMJ6.

For citation purposes, cite each article independently as indicated on the article page online and as indicated below:

Lastname, A.A.; Lastname, B.B. Article Title. *Journal Name* **Year**, *Volume Number*, Page Range.

ISBN 978-3-7258-7867-3 (Hbk)
ISBN 978-3-7258-7868-0 (PDF)
https://doi.org/10.3390/books978-3-7258-7868-0

Cover image courtesy of Ludovico Abenavoli

Contents

About the Editor

Ludovico Abenavoli

Ludovico Abenavoli earned his MD from the Sacred Heart Catholic University in 2002. He completed a postgraduate Master's degree in Alcohol-Related Diseases at the University of Florence in 2003, followed by residency training in Internal Medicine at the Sacred Heart Catholic University in 2007. In 2009, he obtained a Master's degree in Diagnostic Ultrasonography. In 2010, he earned a PhD in Nutrition from the University of Rome Tor Vergata. He has held international clinical and research positions, including a fellowship at the Pierre et Marie Curie University in 2005 and an appointment as an invited researcher at Paris XIII University in 2011. From 2008 to 2016, he served as a researcher at the University "Magna Graecia" of Catanzaro, where he was promoted to associate professor from 2016 to 2024. Since 2024, he has been a full professor of Gastroenterology at Department of Health Sciences of the same institution. He is also a Visiting Professor at several international universities, including Batna (Algeria), Novi Sad (Serbia), Cluj-Napoca and Timișoara (Romania), and the Taras Shevchenko National University of Kyiv (Ukraine). Since 2020, he has served as Director of the Post-Graduate School of Digestive Diseases at the University "Magna Graecia" of Catanzaro, and since 2019, he has been included in the Top 2% of Scientists Worldwide ranking by Stanford University.

life

MDPI

Editorial

Gastrointestinal Health: Clinical Research and Therapeutic Innovations

Giuseppe Guido Maria Scarlata [1,2] and Ludovico Abenavoli [1,2,*]

1 Department of Health Sciences, University "Magna Graecia", 88100 Catanzaro, Italy; giuseppeguidomaria.scarlata@unicz.it
2 Center for Chronic Liver Diseases, "Renato Dulbecco" University Hospital, 88100 Catanzaro, Italy
* Correspondence: l.abenavoli@unicz.it; Tel.: +39-09-6136-94387

The gastrointestinal system is one of the most complex and dynamic biological interfaces between the human body and the external environment. Beyond its primary role in digestion and nutrient absorption, the gastrointestinal system is increasingly recognized as a central regulator of systemic physiology, integrating metabolic, immune, microbial, and inflammatory signals that influence multiple organs and biological pathways. Advances in clinical and translational research have significantly increased our understanding of digestive diseases, highlighting their multifactorial nature and close relationship with systemic health. This Special Issue, "Gastrointestinal Health: Clinical Research and Therapeutic Innovations", published in *Life*, gathers a multidisciplinary collection of studies that address the key aspects of modern gastroenterology. The contributions span a wide range of topics, including gastrointestinal oncology, inflammatory bowel diseases (IBDs), hepatobiliary disorders, microbiome research, surgical management, and emerging diagnostic and therapeutic approaches. Several studies focus on gastrointestinal malignancies and tumor biology. Real-world clinical data on total neoadjuvant therapy in rectal cancer provide insights into gastrointestinal toxicity and the predictors of treatment outcomes [1]. In addition, the COVID-2019 pandemic seriously affected cancer care worldwide, and its impact on gastric cancer management highlights the need for adaptive clinical strategies during global health crises [2]. Additionally, tumor biology and diagnostic biomarkers remain central topics in gastrointestinal oncology. An exploratory immunohistochemical study evaluated Ki-67 expression and tumor size, contributing to our understanding of proliferative activity in small bowel tumors [3]. Other studies addressed rare and complex oncological scenarios, including synchronous ileal metastasis from pancreatic ductal adenocarcinoma and diagnostic challenges related to neuroendocrine tumors in liver transplant recipients [4,5]. Together, these investigations underline the importance of integrating molecular, pathological, and clinical perspectives in gastrointestinal oncology.

The gut microbiota plays a fundamental role in maintaining host homeostasis and influencing metabolic and immune pathways. Advances in metagenomic technologies have enabled deeper characterizations of microbial communities. Specifically, a shotgun analysis of gut microflora in healthy older adult individuals produced valuable insights into microbial diversity and community structure across populations [6]. These findings contribute to establishing reference microbial profiles that may help interpret the microbiome alterations associated with gastrointestinal and systemic diseases. Acute gastrointestinal conditions remain a major cause of morbidity and hospitalization worldwide. Several studies provided updated clinical insights into the management of gastrointestinal bleeding. In this context, retrospective analyses of variceal and non-variceal upper gastrointestinal bleeding provide valuable epidemiological data, and the researchers proposed updated management algorithms to improve patient outcomes [7,8]. In addition, hepatobiliary and pancreatic diseases were addressed in studies focusing on surgical and clinical management. A study on bile duct injuries following cholecystectomy shed light onto surgical repair strategies and outcomes in specialized referral centers [9]. Similarly, an epidemiological investigation of biliary acute pancreatitis contributes to a better understanding of disease patterns and risk factors in tertiary care settings [10]. Surgical advances are further highlighted in studies comparing laparoscopic and open distal pancreatectomy, emphasizing the importance of minimally invasive approaches in pancreatic surgery [11].

IBDs represent a central area of research in gastroenterology. Several articles address different aspects of disease pathophysiology and clinical management. Psychological factors such as depression may seriously affect health-related quality of life in patients with ulcerative colitis (UC), highlighting the need for integrated multidisciplinary care [12]. Other contributions explored the specific pathological mechanisms associated with intestinal inflammation [13]. Additionally, lifestyle and nutritional factors are increasingly recognized as modulators of intestinal inflammation. In this context, a case–control study examining fruit and vegetable consumption highlighted the influences of diet on IBD risk [14]. Nutritional status assessment is also an important aspect of IBD management, as illustrated in a study evaluating phase angle as a complementary tool for assessing nutritional status in patients with UC [15].

Gastrointestinal diseases are increasingly recognized as part of broader systemic networks involving metabolic and inflammatory pathways. A growing body of evidence highlights the concept of inter-organ communication axes. In this Special Issue, the gut–kidney axis is explored through a review examining the relationship between IBDs and nephropathies, emphasizing the role of immune activation and metabolic pathways linking intestinal and renal disorders [16]. Moreover, case studies and pilot investigations evaluated metabolic-dysfunction-associated steatotic liver disease in rare genetic conditions and in patients with IBDs [17,18]. These findings underscore the complex interplay among intestinal inflammation, metabolic dysregulation, and hepatic pathology.

Another important theme in this Special Issue concerns innovative therapeutic approaches and clinical management strategies. A systematic review evaluated the efficacy of biologic therapies, such as dupilumab, yielding additional insight into emerging treatment options for eosinophilic esophagitis [19]. Novel perioperative management strategies were also investigated, including regional anesthesia techniques aimed at facilitating early extubation following liver transplantation [20]. Additional clinical innovations focused on alternative therapeutic approaches in complex medical cases. For example, the rectal administration of rifampicin and isoniazid suppositories represents a novel strategy for treating tuberculosis in patients with multiple comorbidities and gastrointestinal limitations [21]. Case reports and translational investigations further enrich this research field by addressing rare clinical conditions and emerging diagnostic approaches. These include the management of a superior mesenteric artery aneurysm associated with pancreatic cyst rupture and the use of inflammatory indices as potential biomarkers for evaluating the neoplastic potential of colon polyps [22,23]. Furthermore, experimental and translational studies also contributed to the understanding of hepatic injury and protective mechanisms. Researchers evaluated the hepatoprotective effects of *Camellia sinensis* in experimental models of cisplatin-induced liver injury, highlighting the potential therapeutic applications of natural compounds [24]. Finally, innovative clinical approaches were explored in a case study investigating functional neurology therapy in a patient with lactose intolerance [25]. Future research will increasingly rely on integrating clinical investigations, molecular biology, microbiome science, and pathophysiology to further elucidate the complex mechanisms underlying digestive diseases. Such interdisciplinary efforts will be essential for

https://doi.org/10.3390/life16040548

developing personalized diagnostic strategies and innovative therapeutic interventions to improve patient outcomes. In conclusion, this Special Issue, "Gastrointestinal Health: Clinical Research and Therapeutic Innovations", provides a comprehensive overview of the current progress in the field of gastroenterology. The presented articles not only deepen our understanding of digestive diseases but also open new perspectives to developing innovative diagnostic and therapeutic strategies oriented to improve human health.

Author Contributions: Conceptualization, G.G.M.S. and L.A.; visualization, G.G.M.S. and L.A. All authors have read and agreed to the published version of this manuscript.

Funding: This research received no external funding.

Institutional Review Board Statement: Not applicable.

Informed Consent Statement: Not applicable.

Data Availability Statement: No new data were created or analyzed in this study. Data sharing is not applicable to this article.

Conflicts of Interest: The authors declare no conflicts of interest.

Abbreviations

The following abbreviations are used in this manuscript:

IBD	Inflammatory Bowel Disease
UC	Ulcerative Colitis

References

1. Bratu, L.D.; Stovicek, P.O.; Ciurea, A.-M.; Mehedințeanu, A.M.; Berisha, T.C.; Schenker, R.A.; Dicianu, A.M.; Stamulescu, C.; Paitici, Ș.; Mogoantă, S.Ș.; et al. Gastrointestinal Toxicity and Clinical Predictors of Total Neoadjuvant Therapy in Rectal Cancer: A Real-World Retrospective Study. *Life* **2026**, *16*, 422. [CrossRef]
2. Vieru, A.M.; Radulescu, D.; Streba, L.; Trasca, E.T.; Cazacu, S.M.; Statie, R.-C.; Popa, P.; Ciurea, T. Learning from an Emerging Infection: How the COVID-19 Pandemic Reshaped Gastric Cancer Care. *Life* **2026**, *16*, 161. [CrossRef]
3. Barbu, L.A.; Cercelaru, L.; Șurlin, V.; Mogoantă, S.-S.; Țenea Cojan, T.S.; Marinescu, D.; Mărgăritescu, N.-D.; Vasile, L. Ki-67 and Tumor Size in Small Bowel Tumors: Findings from an Exploratory Immunohistochemical Analysis. *Life* **2025**, *15*, 1894. [CrossRef]
4. Țenea Cojan, T.S.; Șurlin, V.; Mogoantă, S.-S.; Mărgăritescu, N.-D.; Caragea, D.-C.; Țenea Cojan, I.-A.; Căluianu, V.; Marinaș, M.C.; Mogoș, G.F.R.; Vasile, L.; et al. Synchronous Ileal Metastasis from Pancreatic Ductal Adenocarcinoma: Case Report and Narrative Review with Practical Diagnostic and Management Points. *Life* **2025**, *15*, 1684. [CrossRef]
5. Colaci, C.; Mercuri, C.; Corea, A.; Spagnuolo, R.; Doldo, P. A Case of a Neuroendocrine Tumor in a Liver Transplant Patient: Diagnostic and Management Difficulties. *Life* **2025**, *15*, 421. [CrossRef]
6. Mahbub, M.H.; Hase, R.; Yamaguchi, N.; Asai, Y.; Harada, M.; Ichimura, N.; Hayakawa, Y.; Inohana, Y.; Umakoshi, Y.; Yamaguchi, R.; et al. Gut Microbial Diversity and Community Structure Are Largely Similar Between Apparently Healthy Elderly Japanese Males and Females: A Shotgun Metagenomic Study. *Life* **2026**, *16*, 297. [CrossRef]
7. Barbu, L.A.; Cercelaru, L.; Vîlcea, I.-D.; Șurlin, V.; Mogoantă, S.-S.; Țenea Cojan, T.S.; Mărgăritescu, N.-D.; Țenea Cojan, A.-M.; Căluianu, V.; Marinescu, D.; et al. Variceal Upper Gastrointestinal Bleeding: A Retrospective Cohort of 98 Cases, Historical Comparison, and Updated Management Algorithm. *Life* **2025**, *15*, 1626. [CrossRef] [PubMed]
8. Barbu, L.A.; Vasile, L.; Cercelaru, L.; Șurlin, V.; Mogoantă, S.-S.; Mogoș, G.F.R.; Țenea Cojan, T.S.; Mărgăritescu, N.-D.; Buliman, A. Non-Variceal Upper Gastrointestinal Bleeding: A Retrospective Cohort of 364 Cases, Historical Comparison, and Updated Management Algorithm. *Life* **2025**, *15*, 1320. [CrossRef]
9. Plahuta, I.; Turk, Š.; Lovrenčič Petreski, B.; Magdalenić, T.; Potrč, S.; Ivanecz, A. Surgical Repair of Bile Duct Injuries Due to Cholecystectomy—An Experience from a Referral Center in Slovenia. *Life* **2025**, *15*, 874. [CrossRef] [PubMed]
10. Edu, A.V.; Pahomeanu, M.R.; Olăreanu, A.; Corbu, D.G.; Treteanu, A.R.; Constantinescu, A.; Șandru, V.; Zărnescu, N.O.; Negreanu, L. Epidemiology of Biliary Acute Pancreatitis—A Seven-Year Experience of a Large Tertiary Center. *Life* **2025**, *15*, 139. [CrossRef] [PubMed]
11. Plahuta, I.; Šarenac, Ž.; Golob, M.; Turk, Š.; Ilijevec, B.; Magdalenić, T.; Potrč, S.; Ivanecz, A. Laparoscopic and Open Distal Pancreatectomy—An Initial Single-Institution Experience with a Propensity Score Matching Analysis. *Life* **2025**, *15*, 97. [CrossRef]

https://doi.org/10.3390/life16040548

12. Jaksic, D.; Vuksanovic, S.; Toplicanin, A.; Spiric-Milovancevic, J.; Maric, G.; Sokic-Milutinovic, A. Impact of Depression on Health-Related Quality of Life in Ulcerative Colitis Patients—Are We Doing Enough? A Single Tertiary Center Experience. *Life* **2025**, *15*, 612. [CrossRef] [PubMed]
13. Jucan, A.-E.; Nedelciuc, O.; Mihai, V.-C.; Dranga, M.; Andronic, M.-C.; Juncu, S.-S.; Sarbu, G.-E.; Mihai, I.-R.; Andronic, A.; Ciortescu, I.; et al. Backwash Ileitis—From Pathogenesis to Clinical Significance: Literature Review. *Life* **2025**, *15*, 567. [CrossRef]
14. Almofarreh, A.M.; Sheerah, H.A.; Arafa, A.; Algori, F.A.; Almutairi, G.R.; Alenzi, K.A.; Al-Alsehemi, M.M.; Mekwar, B.H.; Alzeer, O.; Molla, H.N. Fruit and Vegetable Consumption and Inflammatory Bowel Disease: A Case-Control Study. *Life* **2024**, *14*, 1524. [CrossRef]
15. Mendoza-Martínez, V.M.; Baños-Vázquez, R.; Melendez-Mier, G.; Carrillo-Rojas, J.I.; Santoyo-Chávez, M.A.; Ontiveros-López, S.; Gómez-Coello, A.; Escobedo, G.; de León-Rendón, J.L.; Bueno-Hernández, N. Phase Angle (PhA) Is an Easy and Complementary Tool for Assessing Nutritional Status in Ulcerative Colitis (UC) Patients: A Cross-Sectional Study. *Life* **2024**, *14*, 1511. [CrossRef]
16. de Sire, R.; La Mantia, A.; Bonacci, L.; Testa, A.; Guarino, A.D.; Rispo, A.; Nardone, O.M.; Castiglione, F. Inflammatory Bowel Diseases and Nephropathies: Exploring the Gut-Kidney Axis. *Life* **2024**, *14*, 1541. [CrossRef]
17. Boccuto, L.; Scarlata, G.G.M.; Moffitt, B.A.; Sarasua, S.M.; Phelan, K.; Rogers, C.; Abenavoli, L. Metabolic Dysfunction-Associated Steatotic Liver Disease in a Patient with Phelan–McDermid Syndrome. *Life* **2025**, *15*, 1586. [CrossRef] [PubMed]
18. Abenavoli, L.; Spagnuolo, R.; Scarlata, G.G.M.; Gambardella, M.L.; Boccuto, L.; Méndez-Sánchez, N.; Luzza, F. Metabolic Dysfunction-Associated Steatotic Liver Disease in Patients with Inflammatory Bowel Diseases: A Pilot Study. *Life* **2024**, *14*, 1226. [CrossRef] [PubMed]
19. Chu, S.-H.; Chen, J.-J.; Chen, C.-C.; Lei, W.-T.; Lien, C.-H.; Weng, S.-L.; Yeung, C.-Y.; Liu, L.Y.-M.; Tai, Y.-L.; Huang, Y.-N.; et al. Efficacy of Dupilumab in the Treatment of Eosinophilic Esophagitis: A Systematic Review and Network Meta-Analysis of Randomized Controlled Trials. *Life* **2025**, *15*, 307. [CrossRef]
20. Huh, J.; Chae, M.S. The Role of the Subcostal Transversus Abdominis Plane Block in Facilitating Operating Room Extubation After Living Donor Liver Transplantation for Hepatocellular Carcinoma: A Propensity Score-Matching Analysis. *Life* **2025**, *15*, 297. [CrossRef]
21. Munteanu, I.; Burdușel, B.; Coca, C.C.; Zisu, D.; Gheorghevici, C.; Diaconu, G.A.; Stan, D.G.; Feraru, N.; Tivda, A.; Popa, C.G.; et al. Rectal Administration of Rifampicin and Isoniazid Suppositories: An Alternative Approach for the Treatment of Tuberculosis in a Patient with Multiple Comorbidities. *Life* **2025**, *15*, 773. [CrossRef] [PubMed]
22. Dragulescu, P.R.; Geana, R.C.; Robu, M.; Nayyerani, R.; Dumitrescu, C.; Dragan, A.; Vasilescu, C.; Iliescu, V.A.; Stiru, O. Management of a Rare Case of Superior Mesenteric Artery Aneurysm Associated with a Pancreatic Cyst Complicated by Acute Rupture: A Case Report and Review of Literature. *Life* **2024**, *14*, 1348. [CrossRef] [PubMed]
23. Ciftel, S.; Ciftel, S.; Klisic, A.; Mercantepe, F. New Approaches Based on Inflammatory Indexes in the Evaluation of the Neoplastic Potential of Colon Polyps. *Life* **2024**, *14*, 1259. [CrossRef]
24. Yilmaz, A.; Dizman, F.; Akyildiz, K.; Mataraci Karakas, S.; Mercantepe, T.; Uydu, H.A.; Tumkaya, L.; Ozturk, K. The Hepatoprotective Effects of *Camellia sinensis* on Cisplatin-Induced Acute Liver Injury. *Life* **2024**, *14*, 1077. [CrossRef]
25. Rey-Mota, J.; Escribano-Colmena, G.; Álvarez, D.M.-C.; Vasquez Perez, J.; Navarro-Jimenez, E.; Clemente-Suárez, V.J. Application of Functional Neurology Therapy in a Lactose-Intolerant Patient. *Life* **2024**, *14*, 978. [CrossRef] [PubMed]

https://doi.org/10.3390/life16040548

life

MDPI

Article

Gastrointestinal Toxicity and Clinical Predictors of Total Neoadjuvant Therapy in Rectal Cancer: A Real-World Retrospective Study

Lucian Dragoș Bratu [1,2], Puiu Olivian Stovicek [2,3,*], Ana-Maria Ciurea [2,4], Alina Maria Mehedințeanu [2], Tradian Ciprian Berisha [1,2], Ramona Adriana Schenker [2], Andrei Mircea Dicianu [2], Carmen Stamulescu [2], Ștefan Paitici [5], Stelian Ștefăniță Mogoantă [5,6,*] and Michael Schenker [2,4]

1 Doctoral School, University of Medicine and Pharmacy of Craiova, 200349 Craiova, Romania; lucian.bratu@gmail.com (L.D.B.); berishatc.sfn@gmail.com (T.C.B.)
2 Sf. Nectarie Oncology Center, 200347 Craiova, Romania; amciurea14@gmail.com (A.-M.C.); alina.maria591@gmail.com (A.M.M.); ramona_schenker@yahoo.com (R.A.S.); dicianuandrei@yahoo.com (A.M.D.); carmen_stamulescu@yahoo.com (C.S.); michael.schenker@umfcv.ro (M.S.)
3 Department of Pharmacology, Faculty of Nursing, Târgu Jiu Subsidiary, Titu Maiorescu University, 040441 Bucharest, Romania
4 Department of Oncology, University of Medicine and Pharmacy of Craiova, 200349 Craiova, Romania
5 Department of Surgery, University of Medicine and Pharmacy of Craiova, 200349 Craiova, Romania; stefan.paitici@umfcv.ro
6 3rd General Surgery Clinic, Emergency County Hospital, 200642 Craiova, Romania
* Correspondence: puiuolivian@yahoo.com (P.O.S.); stelian.mogoanta@umfcv.ro (S.Ș.M.)

Abstract

Background: Total neoadjuvant therapy (TNT) is increasingly administered in rectal cancer, but compared with concurrent chemoradiotherapy (CRT), data regarding the gastrointestinal (GI) toxicity profile and clinical predictors remain limited. **Objectives:** To evaluate GI toxicity associated with TNT compared with CRT and to explore clinical predictors of these adverse events (AEs). **Methods:** This retrospective study included 201 patients with rectal cancer treated with TNT (n = 157) and CRT (n = 44). GI AEs (nausea, vomiting, diarrhea) were graded according to CTCAE v5.0. In the analysis of factors associated with GI AEs, multiple clinical and pathological variables were included using multivariable logistic regression. **Results:** The composite endpoint "any GI AEs grade $\geq$ 1" was more frequent in the TNT group compared with the CRT group (33.1% vs. 15.9%; RR = 2.08; 95% CI 1.02–4.25; p = 0.038). Nausea was significantly more frequent in the TNT group (28.7% vs. 9.1%; RR = 3.15; 95% CI 1.20–8.30; p = 0.012), whereas vomiting (9.6% vs. 2.3%; p = 0.203) and diarrhea (17.8% vs. 9.1%; p = 0.242) did not reach statistical significance. In multivariable logistic regression, TNT (OR = 2.65; 95% CI 1.08–6.53; p = 0.032) and female sex (OR = 2.03; 95% CI 1.05–3.77; p = 0.033) were identified as independent predictors of grade $\geq$ 1 GI AEs. For nausea, TNT remained significant (OR = 4.37; 95% CI 1.45–13.20; p = 0.0089). Upper rectal tumor location was significantly associated with vomiting (p = 0.0054). No grade 3–4 GI AEs were observed in either treatment group. **Conclusions:** TNT was associated with a higher incidence of mild GI AEs, predominantly driven by nausea, without an increase in severe toxicities. TNT and female sex were identified as independent clinical predictors of an increased risk of GI AEs, while tumor location in the upper third of the rectum was associated with a higher occurrence of vomiting.

https://doi.org/10.3390/life16030422

Keywords: rectal cancer; total neoadjuvant therapy; chemoradiotherapy; gastrointestinal adverse events; treatment-related toxicity

1. Introduction

Colorectal cancer remains a major oncological disease, with a significant impact on healthcare systems due to its high incidence and the substantial burden associated with cancer-related morbidity and mortality [1,2]. Among these malignancies, rectal cancer represents a distinct clinical subgroup, accounting for approximately 30–35% of all colorectal cancer cases, and is characterized by a complex therapeutic approach requiring the integration of multimodal treatments to optimize both local and systemic disease control [3]. The anatomical particularities of the rectum, together with its close relationship to adjacent pelvic structures, require carefully sequenced treatment strategies, in which radiotherapy and neoadjuvant chemotherapy play a central role [4,5]. In this context, treatment evaluation extends beyond traditional oncological outcomes to include the assessment of treatment-related toxicity profiles [6]. Furthermore, recent epidemiological trends indicate a shift in the age distribution of patients diagnosed with rectal cancer, with an estimated annual increase of 1–3% in incidence among adults younger than 50 years, underscoring the need for a better understanding of treatment tolerability and short to medium-term quality of life outcomes [7,8].

Radiotherapy constitutes an integral part of rectal cancer management and is used with both curative and palliative intent, depending on disease stage and clinical objectives. Technological advances over recent decades have strengthened the role of radiotherapy through optimization of dose distribution and adaptation to the anatomical and clinical characteristics of each disease stage. The introduction of advanced irradiation techniques, such as intensity-modulated radiotherapy (IMRT) and volumetric modulated arc therapy (VMAT), has improved dose conformity to target volumes and reduced irradiation of adjacent pelvic structures, thereby contributing to a reduction in gastrointestinal (GI) toxicities associated with treatment [3,4,6,9,10].

Rectal cancer treatment relies on a multimodal approach integrating surgery, systemic therapy, and radiotherapy in different sequences and combinations, depending on tumor stage and individual patient characteristics. The selection of the therapeutic strategy and treatment sequencing is determined within a multidisciplinary team, with the aim of maximizing oncological control while minimizing the risk of treatment-related adverse events (AEs).

An important role of radiotherapy in rectal cancer is its integration with chemotherapy in the neoadjuvant setting for patients with locally advanced disease, including T3–T4 tumors and/or regional lymph node involvement (N+) [4]. In the absence of contraindications, radiotherapy is combined with chemotherapy either as concurrent chemoradiotherapy (CRT) or within the more comprehensive strategy of total neoadjuvant therapy (TNT).

The efficacy of neoadjuvant treatment is primarily assessed by postoperative pathological staging, tumor regression grade, particularly by the achievement of a pathological complete response, which is recognized as an important prognostic factor [11]. In recent years, TNT has increasingly been adopted as the preferred therapeutic strategy compared with CRT, owing to superior outcomes reported in terms of disease control and oncological outcomes [5,12,13].

Within the TNT framework, systemic therapy may be administered either as induction chemotherapy followed by CRT or as consolidation chemotherapy following CRT, most commonly using oxaliplatin-based regimens such as CAPEOX (capecitabine and oxaliplatin) or FOLFOX (5-fluorouracil, oxaliplatin, and leucovorin). Radiotherapy is administered concurrently with capecitabine or 5-fluorouracil.

https://doi.org/10.3390/life16030422

GI AEs associated with radiotherapy in rectal cancer are related to radiation-induced inflammatory processes affecting the small bowel and rectum, clinically manifesting as radiation enteritis and radiation proctitis [6,14,15]. Radiation enteritis is frequently associated with nausea, vomiting, abdominal cramping, and diarrhea, whereas radiation proctitis is characterized by tenesmus, fecal urgency, and rectal bleeding [6,14].

The primary mechanism of radiotherapy-induced GI toxicity involves damage to the intestinal epithelium, leading to impairment of absorptive function, disruption of the mucosal barrier, and inflammatory activation, clinically manifesting as diarrhea, nausea, and vomiting [6,14–16].

The incidence and severity of GI AEs vary according to individual anatomical characteristics, the volume of irradiated bowel, administered radiation doses, and the irradiation technique used [14–17]. This highlights the need for systematic evaluation of GI AEs in the context of modern neoadjuvant strategies.

GI AEs are common during neoadjuvant treatment of rectal cancer, particularly when radiotherapy is combined with chemotherapy. The incidence is typically reported to range between 20% and 40%, with diarrhea, nausea, and vomiting being the most frequent symptoms [18–20]. Diarrhea represents the most common toxicity, with reported rates generally between 10 and 25%, whereas nausea and vomiting occur less frequently, usually in fewer than 10–15% of patients, depending on the intensity of systemic treatment [4,18–20].

Dose distribution at the intestinal level is an important determinant of GI toxicity, particularly for diarrhea. Exposure of intestinal volumes to doses exceeding 15 Gy has been associated with an increased risk of GI AEs [21–24]. Modern radiotherapy techniques have reduced bowel irradiation compared with conventional approaches, contributing to improved treatment tolerability [25–27]. These findings support the dose–volume relationship as a central mechanism underlying GI toxicity induced by pelvic radiotherapy [28–30].

Despite technological advances and optimization of therapeutic regimens, data on GI AEs associated with neoadjuvant treatment of rectal cancer remain heterogeneous and incompletely characterized. Most studies primarily focus on oncological outcomes, while comparative data between TNT and CRT and the role of individual clinical predictors of GI toxicity remain limited.

In this context, a more detailed characterization of GI toxicities may optimize therapeutic planning and help identify patients who could benefit from early supportive measures, including guideline-based prophylaxis for radiotherapy- and chemotherapy-induced nausea, vomiting [31,32], and diarrhea [33]. These data may also inform multidisciplinary supportive interventions aimed at maintaining treatment tolerability and continuity.

The aim of this study was to evaluate the incidence and pattern of GI toxicities and to explore clinical predictors of these events in patients with rectal cancer treated with neoadjuvant therapy, with a focus on nausea, vomiting, and diarrhea. Specifically, we aimed to compare the GI toxicity profile of TNT with CRT and to analyze the association between the occurrence of GI AEs and a selected set of clinical and therapeutic factors. In clinical practice, the results may be useful in identifying patients at higher risk of GI toxicity who may benefit from closer clinical monitoring and the implementation of tailored supportive measures.

2. Materials and Methods

In this retrospective study, we analyzed the incidence of GI AEs associated with neoadjuvant radiotherapy in the treatment of rectal cancer. A total of 201 patients treated at Sf. Nectarie Oncology Center, Craiova, between 2020 and 2023, was included. Inclusion criteria were: age $\geq$ 18 years; histopathologically confirmed rectal adenocarcinoma; indication for neoadjuvant treatment established by a multidisciplinary oncology board; treatment with either total neoadjuvant therapy (TNT) or concurrent chemoradiotherapy (CRT); and

https://doi.org/10.3390/life16030422

complete documentation regarding the occurrence and severity of GI AEs during neoadjuvant treatment. Exclusion criteria were: incomplete toxicity documentation and absence of post-therapeutic evaluation. Of the 201 patients, 157 received TNT with either FOLFOX or CAPEOX regimens, while 44 patients underwent CRT with capecitabine. Clinical, pathological, and therapeutic data were extracted from medical records and institutional databases. GI AEs were recorded throughout the course of neoadjuvant treatment.

The inclusion and exclusion criteria were defined to ensure the homogeneity of the analyzed cohorts and to allow a comparable evaluation of GI toxicities associated with standard neoadjuvant treatment. Only patients treated with conventional CRT or TNT regimens were included, in order to avoid heterogeneity related to alternative protocols (e.g., short-course radiotherapy). Exclusion of patients who did not complete treatment or who lacked post-therapeutic imaging evaluation was necessary to allow appropriate analysis of postoperative staging and stage modification, variables subsequently incorporated into the statistical models.

In the analyzed cohort, no surgical interventions or diverting procedures were performed as a result of acute GI complications occurring during neoadjuvant treatment.

The indication for neoadjuvant treatment was established by the multidisciplinary oncology board based on clinical staging and tumor characteristics, in accordance with international guidelines and institutional protocols. Neoadjuvant treatment was primarily recommended for patients with locally advanced rectal tumors, defined by T3–T4 tumor invasion and/or the presence of regional lymph node involvement, as well as in selected cases of oligometastatic disease amenable to surgical resection. Patients were treated either with CRT or with TNT, according to the institutional protocols in use at the time of treatment. Standard chemoradiotherapy consisted of conventionally fractionated long-course radiotherapy administered concurrently with oral capecitabine. Total neoadjuvant therapy included the administration of oxaliplatin-based systemic chemotherapy prior to chemoradiotherapy, using standard regimens, followed by conventionally fractionated radiotherapy. The choice of therapeutic regimen was made on an individual basis within the multidisciplinary team, according to the patient's clinical status and the overall therapeutic strategy.

A dedicated dosimetric–volumetric analysis was not performed, as the primary objective of the study was to evaluate the clinical incidence and predictors of GI toxicities, and detailed dosimetric parameters were not uniformly available for all patients due to the retrospective design.

GI AEs were monitored throughout the course of neoadjuvant treatment and were classified according to the Common Terminology Criteria for Adverse Events (CTCAE v5.0), thus ensuring standardized grading of symptom severity [34]. GI AEs were evaluated and documented during the course of treatment in accordance with routine clinical practice, and the data were subsequently retrospectively extracted from medical records for statistical analysis.

Management of GI AEs was performed using symptomatic treatment, in accordance with current clinical practice and international guideline recommendations. Nausea and vomiting were treated with hydration and the administration of antiemetic medication, including metoclopramide or granisetron, depending on symptom severity and clinical response. Diarrhea was managed with the administration of loperamide, in association with supportive measures such as dietary adjustments, probiotic treatment, and oral or intravenous hydration, as clinically indicated. The choice and intensity of symptomatic treatment were individually adapted according to the grade of the AEs and the patient's clinical status.

The analysis focused on the incidence of GI AEs (nausea, vomiting, and diarrhea), and a composite endpoint was defined, representing the occurrence of any GI AEs of grade ≥ 1

https://doi.org/10.3390/life16030422

(ANY_GE1) during neoadjuvant treatment. For the analysis of factors associated with GI AEs, relevant clinical and pathological variables were considered, including patient age and sex, tumor differentiation grade, initial tumor stage, rectal tumor location, postoperative stage, stage modification after neoadjuvant treatment, and the type of neoadjuvant treatment administered.

The study was conducted in accordance with the principles of the Declaration of Helsinki. All included patients provided written informed consent for the use of clinical and therapeutic data for research purposes. The study protocol and the use of medical data were approved by the institutional ethics committee, in accordance with applicable local and national regulations.

Statistical Analysis

Statistical analyses were performed on a complete dataset, as patients with incomplete clinical or toxicity documentation were excluded at the eligibility stage, prior to analysis.

Descriptive methods, univariate and multivariable inferential tests, as well as advanced adjustment models and exploratory analyses of relationships between variables, were applied. Categorical variables were presented as frequencies and percentages, while continuous variables were expressed as mean ± standard deviation. Comparisons of characteristics between therapeutic groups (TNT vs. CRT) and across categories of clinical variables were performed using the Chi-square test or Fisher's exact test, depending on sample size and frequency distribution. To assess differences in the distribution of AEs grades (grade 0–grade 2) across ordinal variables (age: <50, 50–69, ≥70 years; tumor grade: G1-G3; postoperative stage), Cochran–Armitage trend tests were applied to identify potential linear trends in the risk of AEs. For multicategorical variables that showed a significant global effect (e.g., rectal tumor location: upper, middle, lower), the analysis was complemented by pairwise post hoc comparisons using Fisher's exact test to identify specific differences between categories.

To estimate the probability of GI AEs, binary logistic regression models were constructed, including relevant clinical variables (age, sex, rectal tumor location, and treatment type). The maximum severity of GI AEs (grade 0–grade 2) was evaluated using an ordinal cumulative logit regression model (proportional odds model), which is appropriate for modeling incremental severity of AEs. Model validity was assessed by examining coefficient significance, confidence intervals, and the proportional odds assumption. Multicollinearity among the predictors included in the multivariable models was assessed by calculating variance inflation factors (VIF). All VIF values were below the threshold of 5 (range 1.43–4.87), supporting the stability of the estimated effects.

Given the marked imbalance in sample size between the TNT and CRT groups, a propensity score–based method using inverse probability of treatment weighting (IPTW) was applied to adjust for baseline differences between treatment groups. Propensity scores were estimated using logistic regression, including baseline clinical variables (age, sex, tumor location, tumor grade, and initial stage). The weighted model was subsequently used in a logistic regression analysis to estimate the adjusted treatment effect on the binary composite endpoints: occurrence of ANY_GE1 and occurrence of grade 2 GI AEs.

The co-occurrence of different types of GI AEs (nausea, vomiting, and diarrhea) was assessed using the phi (φ) coefficient, which quantifies the association between two binary variables. To synthesize estimates obtained using different statistical approaches (logistic regression, ordinal regression, and IPTW), a forest plot was constructed to graphically display odds ratios (ORs) and 95% confidence intervals, allowing comparison of the effects of TNT and female sex on the risk of GI AEs. All statistical tests were two-tailed, and p values < 0.05 were considered statistically significant.

https://doi.org/10.3390/life16030422

3. Results

The study cohort included 116 male (57.7%) and 85 female (42.3%) patients, with the majority aged between 50 and 69 years ($n = 106$).

The distribution of GI AEs according to demographic and clinicopathological characteristics is presented in Table 1. Nausea was the most frequent GI AE of grade ≥ 1, with incidences ranging between 20.7% and 29.4% according to sex and between 20.7% and 35.9% according to rectal tumor location, with the highest values observed in stage IVA (60.0%). Diarrhea was less frequent in most subgroups (13.6–18.5%) but increased substantially in advanced stages, particularly stage IVA (40.0%). Vomiting of grade ≥ 1 was rare, with incidences generally below 10%, reaching higher values only in subgroups with a small number of patients. Grade 2 GI AEs were infrequent across all analyzed categories, and no grade 3 or 4 events were reported.

Table 1. Descriptive distribution of gastrointestinal adverse events according to baseline demographic and tumor characteristics.

Variable	Category	N	Nausea (Grade) n (%)			Vomiting (Grade) n (%)			Diarrhea (Grade) n (%)		
			0	1	2	0	1	2	0	1	2
Age	<50	22	16 (72.7)	5 (22.7)	1 (4.6)	19 (86.4)	1 (4.5)	2 (9.1)	19 (86.4)	1 (4.5)	2 (9.1)
	50–69	106	80 (75.5)	18 (17.0)	8 (7.5)	97 (91.5)	8 (7.5)	1 (0.9)	87 (82.1)	11 (10.4)	8 (7.5)
	≥70	73	56 (76.7)	15 (20.5)	2 (2.8)	69 (94.5)	3 (4.1)	1 (1.4)	63 (86.3)	8 (11.0)	2 (2.7)
Sex	M	116	92 (79.3)	17 (14.7)	7 (6.0)	106 (91.4)	7 (6.0)	3 (2.6)	99 (85.3)	9 (7.8)	8 (6.9)
	F	85	60 (70.6)	21 (24.7)	4 (4.7)	79 (92.9)	5 (5.9)	1 (1.2)	70 (82.4)	11 (12.9)	4 (4.7)
Tumor location	S	39	25 (64.1)	12 (30.8)	2 (5.1)	36 (92.3)	2 (5.1)	1 (2.6)	32 (82.1)	3 (7.7)	4 (10.2)
	I	75	58 (77.3)	12 (16.0)	5 (6.7)	71 (94.7)	2 (2.7)	2 (2.7)	64 (85.3)	7 (9.3)	4 (5.4)
	M	87	69 (79.3)	14 (16.1)	4 (4.6)	83 (95.4)	3 (3.4)	1 (1.2)	73 (83.9)	10 (11.5)	4 (4.6)
Tumor grade	G1	65	50 (76.9)	11 (16.9)	4 (6.2)	59 (90.8)	4 (6.2)	2 (3.1)	53 (81.5)	9 (13.8)	3 (4.7)
	G2	90	67 (74.4)	19 (21.1)	4 (4.5)	82 (91.1)	6 (6.7)	2 (2.2)	77 (85.6)	6 (6.7)	7 (7.7)
	G3	46	35 (76.1)	8 (17.4)	3 (6.5)	44 (95.7)	2 (4.3)	0 (0.0)	40 (87.0)	2 (4.3)	4 (8.7)
Initial stage	IIA	18	14 (77.8)	1 (5.6)	3 (16.7)	16 (88.9)	1 (5.6)	1 (5.6)	15 (83.3)	3 (16.7)	0 (0.0)
	IIB	5	4 (80.0)	1 (20.0)	0 (0.0)	5 (100)	0 (0.0)	0 (0.0)	5 (100)	0 (0.0)	0 (0.0)
	IIIA	28	22 (78.6)	5 (17.9)	1 (3.6)	25 (89.3)	1 (3.6)	2 (7.1)	26 (92.9)	2 (7.1)	0 (0.0)
	IIIB	108	85 (78.7)	19 (17.6)	4 (3.7)	100 (92.6)	7 (6.5)	1 (0.9)	93 (86.1)	9 (8.3)	6 (5.6)
	IIIC	32	23 (71.9)	7 (21.9)	2 (6.3)	31 (96.9)	1 (3.1)	0 (0.0)	24 (75.0)	5 (15.6)	3 (9.4)
	IVA	10	4 (40.0)	5 (50.0)	1 (10.0)	8 (80.0)	2 (20.0)	0 (0.0)	6 (60.0)	1 (10.0)	3 (30.0)

S = upper rectum; I = middle rectum; M = lower rectum.

Table 2 allows the correlation of postoperative stage and type of tumor evolution (downstaging, complete response, stable disease, or upstaging) with the distribution of GI AEs, without demonstrating a consistent pattern of AEs according to stage evolution.

Grade ≥ 1 nausea ranged from 23.7% in postoperative stage I to 36.4% in stage IIIB, without a clear progressive pattern. Grade ≥ 1 diarrhea was observed in 16.3% of patients with stage I and 24.3% in stage IIA. Grade ≥ 1 vomiting was generally below 10% across most categories. According to stage modification, grade ≥ 1 nausea was reported in 23.8% of patients with downstaging, 24.3% in those with complete response, and 23.5% in stable disease, while grade ≥ 1 diarrhea ranged between 13.5% and 18.2% in these groups. Grade 2 events were rare, and no grade 3 or 4 events were reported.

Advanced statistical analyses were subsequently performed to evaluate treatment-related differences and identify clinical predictors of GI AEs. Comparative analyses between treatment groups are presented in Table 3, univariate and trend analyses in Table 4, multivariable regression models in Tables 5 and 6, and sensitivity analyses in Table 7.

https://doi.org/10.3390/life16030422

Table 2. Descriptive distribution of gastrointestinal adverse events according to postoperative stage and stage evolution.

Variable	Category	*N*	Nausea (Grade) *n* (%)			Vomiting (Grade) *n* (%)			Diarrhea (Grade) *n* (%)		
			0	1	2	0	1	2	0	1	2
Post-operative stage	I	80	61 (76.3)	14 (17.5)	5 (6.2)	73 (91.3)	7 (8.7)	0 (0.0)	67 (83.8)	7 (8.8)	6 (7.5)
	IIA	37	25 (67.6)	10 (27.0)	2 (5.4)	34 (91.9)	2 (5.4)	1 (2.7)	28 (75.7)	7 (18.9)	2 (5.4)
	IIB	4	1 (25.0)	2 (50.0)	1 (25.0)	1 (25.0)	2 (50.0)	1 (25.0)	1 (25.0)	1 (25.0)	2 (50.0)
	IIC	1	0 (0.0)	1 (100)	0 (0.0)	0 (0.0)	1 (100)	0 (0.0)	0 (0.0)	0 (0.0)	1 (100)
	IIIA	14	9 (64.3)	4 (28.6)	1 (7.1)	11 (78.6)	3 (21.4)	0 (0.0)	12 (85.7)	1 (7.1)	1 (7.1)
	IIIB	22	14 (63.6)	6 (27.3)	2 (9.1)	18 (81.8)	3 (13.6)	1 (4.5)	19 (86.4)	2 (9.1)	1 (4.5)
	IIIC	6	4 (66.7)	1 (16.7)	1 (16.7)	6 (100)	0 (0.0)	0 (0.0)	4 (66.7)	0 (0.0)	2 (33.3)
	pCR	37	28 (75.7)	6 (16.2)	3 (8.1)	35 (94.6)	1 (2.7)	1 (2.7)	32 (86.5)	3 (8.1)	2 (5.4)
Stage modification	D	143	109 (76.2)	26 (18.2)	8 (5.6)	134 (93.7)	8 (5.6)	1 (0.7)	117 (81.8)	15 (10.5)	11 (7.7)
	C	37	28 (75.7)	7 (18.9)	2 (5.4)	34 (91.9)	1 (2.7)	2 (5.4)	32 (86.5)	5 (13.5)	0 (0.0)
	U	4	2 (50.0)	2 (50.0)	0 (0.0)	3 (75.0)	1 (25.0)	0 (0.0)	4 (100)	0 (0.0)	0 (0.0)
	S	17	13 (76.5)	3 (17.6)	1 (5.9)	14 (82.4)	2 (11.8)	1 (5.9)	16 (94.1)	0 (0.0)	1 (5.9)

D = Downstaging; C = Complete; U = Upstaging; S = Stable.

Table 3. Comparative analysis of gastrointestinal adverse events by treatment arm (TNT vs. CRT) with risk ratio estimates.

Adverse Event	Arm	Grade 0 *n* (%)	Grade 1 *n* (%)	Grade 2 *n* (%)	≥Grade 1 *n* (%)	RR (95% CI)	*p* Value (Fisher)
Nausea	TNT ($n = 157$)	112 (71.3)	35 (22.3)	10 (6.4)	45 (28.7)	3.15 (1.20–8.30)	0.012
	CRT ($n = 44$)	40 (90.9)	3 (6.8)	1 (2.3)	4 (9.1)	—	—
Vomiting	TNT ($n = 157$)	142 (90.4)	11 (7.0)	4 (2.5)	15 (9.6)	4.20 (0.57–30.95)	0.203
	CRT ($n = 44$)	43 (97.7)	1 (2.3)	0 (0.0)	1 (2.3)	—	—
Diarrhea	TNT ($n = 157$)	129 (82.2)	18 (11.5)	10 (6.4)	28 (17.8)	1.96 (0.73–5.29)	0.242
	CRT ($n = 44$)	40 (90.9)	2 (4.5)	2 (4.5)	4 (9.1)	—	—
ANY_GE1	TNT ($n = 157$)	—	—	—	52 (33.1)	2.08 (1.02–4.25)	0.038
	CRT ($n = 44$)	—	—	—	7 (15.9)	—	—

RR, risk ratio; CI, confidence interval. *p*-values were calculated using Fisher's test.

Table 4. Univariate and trend analyses of clinical factors associated with grade ≥ 1 gastrointestinal adverse events.

Variable	Nausea ≥ Grade 1		Vomiting ≥ Grade 1		Diarrhea ≥ Grade 1	
	p (Global)	*p* (Trend)	*p* (Global)	*p* (Trend)	*p* (Global)	*p* (Trend)
Age	0.604	0.71	0.886	0.21	0.853	0.74
Sex	0.184	—	1.000	—	0.241	—
Tumor location	0.168	—	0.0054	—	0.9	—
Tumor grade	0.936	0.379	0.586	0.888	0.788	0.605
Initial stage	0.161	—	0.5478	—	0.1013	—
Postoperative stage	0.099	0.13	0.336	0.31	0.952	0.86
Stage modification	0.692	—	0.23	—	0.433	—

https://doi.org/10.3390/life16030422

Table 5. Multivariable logistic and ordinal regression models for the composite endpoint (ANY_GE1).

Variable	Logistic Regression (ANY_GE1) OR (95% CI)	*p* Value	Ordinal Regression (Grade 0 → Grade 2) OR (95% CI)	*p* Value
Age (years)	1.01 (0.98–1.03)	0.50	1.01 (0.98–1.03)	0.47
Sex (F vs. M)	2.03 (1.05–3.77)	0.033	1.92 (1.03–3.59)	0.04
TNT (vs. CRT)	2.65 (1.08–6.53)	0.032	2.62 (1.04–6.60)	0.038
Upper tumor (vs. lower)	2.09 (0.91–4.88)	0.081	2.12 (0.93–4.86)	0.075
Middle tumor (vs. lower)	0.92 (0.42–2.01)	0.83	0.89 (0.41–1.95)	0.78

Table 6. Multivariable logistic models for gastrointestinal adverse events ≥ grade 1 (composite and individual endpoints).

Endpoint	Predictor	OR	95% CI	*p*-Value
ANY_GE1 (composite)	Age (per year)	1.007	0.977–1.037	0.6454
	Female (vs. Male)	1.913	1.021–3.584	0.043
	TNT (vs. CRT)	2.841	1.157–6.974	0.0227
Nausea ≥ grade 1	Age (per year)	1.009	0.978–1.042	0.5728
	Female (vs. Male)	1.718	0.882–3.349	0.1119
	TNT (vs. CRT)	4.373	1.449–13.202	0.0089
Vomiting ≥ grade 1	Age (per year)	0.978	0.932–1.025	0.3484
	Female (vs. Male)	1.036	0.364–2.954	0.9468
	TNT (vs. CRT)	4.051	0.511–32.085	0.1852
Diarrhea ≥ grade 1	Age (per year)	1.002	0.966–1.039	0.9334
	Female (vs. Male)	1.732	0.803–3.737	0.1614
	TNT (vs. CRT)	2.253	0.729–6.963	0.1581

The incidence and grade distribution of GI AEs according to treatment regimen (TNT vs. CRT), together with risk ratios (RRs), are presented in Table 3. Grade ≥ 1 nausea was significantly more frequent in the TNT arm compared with CRT (28.7% vs. 9.1%; RR = 3.15, 95% CI 1.20–8.30; $p = 0.012$), indicating a 3.15-fold higher risk associated with TNT. For grade ≥ 1 vomiting, the incidence was higher in the TNT arm (9.6%) compared with CRT (2.3%); however, the difference did not reach statistical significance (RR = 4.20, 95% CI 0.57–30.95; $p = 0.203$), possibly due to the small number of events. Grade ≥ 1 diarrhea also showed a higher frequency in the TNT group (17.8% vs. 9.1%), without statistical significance (RR = 1.96, 95% CI 0.73–5.29; $p = 0.242$). The composite endpoint ANY_GE1 was significantly more frequent in the TNT arm (33.1% vs. 15.9%; RR = 2.08, 95% CI 1.02–4.25; $p = 0.038$), corresponding to an approximately two-fold higher probability of GI AEs in the TNT arm. Grade 2 GI AEs were rare in both groups and did not show statistically significant differences between treatments.

Univariate and trend analyses of clinical factors associated with grade ≥ 1 GI AEs are presented in Table 4. Univariate analysis did not identify significant associations between age, sex, tumor differentiation grade, initial tumor stage, postoperative stage, or stage modification and the occurrence of grade ≥ 1 nausea or diarrhea (all p values > 0.05). Values close to the threshold of statistical significance were observed for the postoperative stage in the case of nausea ($p = 0.099$) and for the initial stage in the case of diarrhea ($p = 0.101$), without reaching statistical significance. Rectal tumor location was the only clinical variable significantly associated with the occurrence of grade ≥ 1 vomiting in the

https://doi.org/10.3390/life16030422

global analysis ($p = 0.0054$), with patients presenting tumors located in the upper third of the rectum showing a higher frequency compared with middle and lower locations. For nausea and diarrhea, tumor location did not show significant differences. Trend analysis applied to the included ordinal variables (age, tumor grade, and postoperative stage) did not identify significant linear relationships between category order and the incidence of grade $\geq$ 1 GI AEs. Rates of nausea, vomiting, and diarrhea varied across subgroups without a consistent gradient, and trend tests were non-significant for all types of AEs analyzed (all p values > 0.05).

Table 7. Sensitivity analyses of multivariable models for gastrointestinal adverse events.

Type of Analysis	Endpoint	Variable	Category	OR (If Applicable)	p-Value
A. Adverse events grade 2	Nausea grade 2	Sex	M/F	—	0.7628
		Tumor location	S/I/M	—	0.8418
		Tumor grade	G1–G3	—	0.8436
		Initial stage	IIA–IVA	—	0.3129
		Postoperative stage	I–pCR	—	0.989
		Stage modification	Down/Stable/Up/Complete	—	0.9706
	Vomiting grade 2	Sex	M/F	—	0.6392
		Tumor location	S/I/M	—	0.7569
		Tumor grade	G1–G3	—	0.5085
		Initial stage	IIA–IVA	—	0.255
		Postoperative stage	I–pCR	—	0.4284
		Stage modification	Down/Stable/Up/Complete	—	0.1842
	Diarrhea grade 2	Sex	M/F	—	0.7645
		Tumor location	S/I/M	—	0.4443
		Tumor grade	G1–G3	—	0.6213
		Initial stage	IIA–IVA	—	0.0143
		Postoperative stage	I–pCR	—	0.704
		Stage modification	Down/Stable/Up/Complete	—	0.3395
B. Multivariable logistic regression (AE $\geq$ grade 1)	AE $\geq$ grade 1	TNT vs. CRT	—	2.62	0.05
		Female vs. Male	—	1.87	0.073
		Tumor location (upper vs. lower)	—	2.25	0.09
		Age (per year)	—	1.01	0.73
C. Grade 2 TNT vs. CRT	Total grade 2	Treatment	TNT vs. CRT	2.72	0.256
D. Subgroup 50–80 years	AE $\geq$ grade 1	TNT vs. CRT	—	2.62	0.05
		Female vs. Male	—	1.87	0.073
		Tumor location (upper vs. lower)	—	2.25	0.09
		Age (per year)	—	1.01	0.73

The results of the multivariable analyses (logistic and ordinal) are presented in Table 5. In the logistic regression model, with the occurrence of ANY_GE1 as the endpoint, female sex and TNT treatment remained significant independent predictors. Female sex was independently associated with an approximately twofold increased risk of GI AEs

https://doi.org/10.3390/life16030422

(OR = 2.03; 95% CI 1.05–3.77; p = 0.033), while TNT treatment was associated with an approximately 2.6-fold increase in the odds of developing at least one grade ≥ 1 GI AE compared with CRT (OR = 2.65; 95% CI 1.08–6.53; p = 0.032). Tumor location in the upper third of the rectum showed a borderline association with the risk of GI AEs (OR = 2.09 vs. lower rectum; p = 0.081), without reaching statistical significance, whereas age did not significantly influence the probability of GI AEs (OR = 1.01 per year; p = 0.50). The results of the ordinal regression were concordant with those of the logistic model, both in terms of effect direction and magnitude of the estimates. Female sex (OR = 1.92; 95% CI 1.03–3.59; p = 0.04) and TNT treatment (OR = 2.62; 95% CI 1.04–6.60; p = 0.038) were associated with an increased probability of belonging to a higher severity level. Upper rectal tumor location again showed a borderline association (OR = 2.12; p = 0.075), whereas age and middle rectal tumor location did not have a significant independent contribution.

Multivariable logistic regression models for GI AEs ≥ grade 1, analyzed separately and as a composite endpoint, are presented in Table 6. For the composite endpoint ANY_GE1, TNT treatment and female sex remained independently associated with the risk of GI AEs. TNT treatment was associated with a significant increase in risk (OR = 2.84; 95% CI 1.16–6.97; p = 0.0227), while female sex was associated with an approximately twofold increased risk (OR = 1.91; 95% CI 1.02–3.58; p = 0.043). Age did not have a significant effect on this endpoint (p = 0.6454).

In the separate analysis by type of GI AEs, only grade ≥ 1 nausea was significantly associated with TNT treatment. Patients treated with TNT had a more than fourfold higher risk of grade ≥ 1 nausea compared with those treated with CRT (OR = 4.37; 95% CI 1.45–13.20; p = 0.0089). Female sex and age were not significantly associated with the risk of nausea. For grade ≥ 1 vomiting and grade ≥ 1 diarrhea, none of the predictors included in the models (age, sex, and treatment type) showed statistically significant associations (all p values > 0.05). Overall, the difference observed for the composite endpoint ANY_GE1 is mainly driven by the increased incidence of grade ≥ 1 nausea in the TNT arm, while vomiting and diarrhea had limited and non-significant contributions to the overall differences in GI AEs.

Sensitivity analyses were performed to assess the consistency of the main results regarding GI AEs, as shown in Table 7. Evaluation of grade 2 AEs according to clinical characteristics did not reveal significant associations for nausea or vomiting (all p values > 0.25). In contrast, grade 2 diarrhea was significantly associated with initial tumor stage (p = 0.0143), with more severe episodes predominantly observed in advanced stages, suggesting a possible impact of disease extent on diarrhea severity.

Repeating the multivariable logistic analysis for the endpoint AE ≥ grade 1 confirmed the stability of the predictors identified in the main models. TNT treatment and female sex remained associated with an increased risk of GI AEs, with p values within the range of statistical significance or borderline significance, while age did not demonstrate an independent effect.

Analysis of grade 2 AEs according to treatment type showed a low number of events, particularly in the CRT arm. Although the odds ratio suggested a higher risk in the TNT group (OR = 2.72), the difference did not reach statistical significance (p = 0.256), limiting the ability to draw firm conclusions regarding AEs of this grade.

Subgroup analysis for patients aged between 50 and 80 years confirmed the consistency of the main results. TNT treatment remained associated with the occurrence of ANY_GE1, with a borderline result (p = 0.050), while female sex and upper rectal tumor location showed statistically non-significant trends. Overall, these sensitivity analyses support the direction of the associations observed in the main analyses, indicating that TNT treatment

https://doi.org/10.3390/life16030422

remains associated with more GI AEs in comparison to CRT, and that influence of female gender is maintained in the same direction across sensitivity analyses.

The estimates of the independent effect of TNT treatment and female sex on the risk of grade ≥ 1 GI AEs were evaluated using three complementary statistical models: binary logistic regression, ordinal regression, and inverse probability of treatment weighting (IPTW) analysis (Figure 1). Estimates derived from the ordinal regression models are presented to compare the direction of associations and are not directly comparable with the risk estimates obtained from binary logistic models. For the logistic regression and IPTW models, odds ratios (ORs) with 95% confidence intervals are shown. For the ordinal model, exponentiated coefficients are displayed to indicate the direction and relative magnitude of the association. The vertical dashed line indicates the neutrality value (OR = 1). Across all applied models, TNT treatment was associated with an increased risk of ANY_GE1 (ORs 2.57–2.65), and female sex showed a consistent association with a higher risk of GI AEs (ORs 1.90–2.03). Confidence intervals are not reported for the ordinal model because the estimates are derived from proportional log-odds coefficients and are not directly comparable with those from binary logistic models. The convergence of OR values across methods indicates consistency of the results and stability of the effect of the estimates.

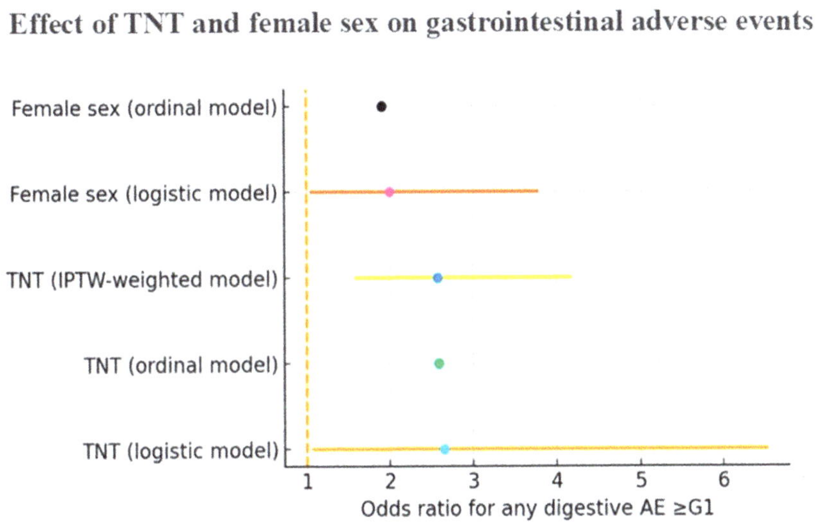

Figure 1. Forest plot of the effect of TNT treatment and female sex on the risk of GI AEs $\geq$ grade 1 based on logistic regression, ordinal regression, and IPTW analysis. Absolute numbers and corresponding percentages for the composite endpoint ANY_GE1 were 52/157 (33.1%) in the TNT group and 7/44 (15.9%) in the CRT group. Dots represent odds ratios (OR), and horizontal lines indicate 95% confidence intervals (CI). The dashed vertical line represents OR = 1 (no effect).

To assess the consistency of the observed results and to explore additional relationships between GI AEs and clinical characteristics, post hoc analyses and additional multivariable models were performed. Post hoc analyses revealed a significant difference in the distribution of grade ≥ 1 vomiting according to rectal tumor location: tumors located in the upper rectal tumor location showed significantly higher rates compared with middle and lower locations (upper vs. lower: $p = 0.0212$; upper vs. middle: $p = 0.0083$). Ordinal variables (age, grade, postoperative stage) did not show significant linear trends. Additional multivariable models confirmed the independent association of female sex and TNT treatment with the severity of GI AEs, while age and tumor location did not demonstrate

https://doi.org/10.3390/life16030422

statistically significant effects. The results were confirmed by standard logistic regression (OR for TNT = 2.65; 95% CI 1.08–6.53) and by IPTW analysis (OR = 2.57; 95% CI 1.59–4.17; $p = 0.00012$). Correlation analysis showed moderate associations between nausea and vomiting ($\varphi = 0.454$) and between nausea and diarrhea ($\varphi = 0.466$), whereas vomiting and diarrhea showed minimal correlation ($\varphi = 0.053$).

4. Discussion

The present results indicate that total neoadjuvant therapy (TNT) is associated with a higher incidence of GI AEs compared with concurrent chemoradiotherapy (CRT), predominantly driven by an increased frequency of mild symptoms, without a proportional rise in severe toxicities. This pattern suggests that TNT primarily influences short-term treatment tolerability rather than escalating overall GI toxicity severity [4,12]. Similar trends have been reported in randomized trials such as RAPIDO and PRODIGE 23, where TNT was associated with a higher rate of mostly low-grade GI AEs without compromising overall safety [5,13]. Although differences in radiotherapy techniques, chemotherapy sequencing, and toxicity reporting limit direct quantitative comparisons across studies [5,13], the present real-world data support the concept of a distinct TNT-related GI toxicity profile. In parallel, evidence indicating improved downstaging and pathological complete response rates with TNT further consolidates its role as a preferred strategy in locally advanced rectal cancer [35]. The reported clinical benefits, favorable tolerability profile, and positive impact on quality of life support the continued interest in this therapeutic approach in clinical practice [36,37].

In our study, nausea emerged as the principal contributor to the increased GI toxicity observed in the TNT group, largely accounting for the difference between TNT and CRT, while vomiting and diarrhea had a limited impact on overall between-group variation. This finding aligns with previous reports indicating that TNT-based regimens are frequently associated with a higher incidence of predominantly low-grade nausea, without consistent increases in severe GI AEs [38,39]. Although typically mild in intensity, nausea may substantially affect quality of life and treatment adherence, highlighting the importance of early recognition and guideline-based supportive management [31,32]. Prospective data using standardized quality-of-life instruments further confirm that even low-grade GI symptoms can significantly impair physical and emotional functioning during pelvic radiotherapy [40]. Recent analyses evaluating toxicity and treatment compliance during total neoadjuvant therapy have reported a predominance of low-grade GI AEs, without a significant increase in grade ≥ 3 toxicity [39,41]. These considerations support systematic symptom monitoring and timely supportive interventions in patients undergoing TNT [31–33].

Multivariable analyses identified female sex as an independent risk factor for GI AEs, irrespective of treatment strategy. Similar observations have been reported in studies evaluating pelvic radiotherapy and chemoradiotherapy toxicity profiles [26,42], suggesting increased susceptibility of female patients to GI symptoms. Although the underlying mechanisms remain incompletely defined, proposed explanations include anatomical differences potentially leading to greater small bowel exposure, as well as hormonal and functional factors influencing intestinal motility, mucosal permeability, and inflammatory response [16,17,28]. While these hypotheses are biologically plausible, further prospective research integrating anatomical and dosimetric parameters is needed to clarify this association. Clinically, female sex may therefore represent a relevant factor in risk stratification and supportive monitoring, without implying the need for modification of standard neoadjuvant regimens.

https://doi.org/10.3390/life16030422

Tumor location in the upper third of the rectum was associated with a higher occurrence of vomiting in both global and post hoc analyses. A possible explanation relates to anatomical and planning considerations, as irradiation of upper rectal tumors may involve larger volumes of small bowel, thereby increasing exposure to clinically relevant doses. The dose–volume relationship at the small bowel level is a recognized determinant of GI toxicity in pelvic radiotherapy [9,21,24], and modern techniques such as IMRT/VMAT have demonstrated reductions in bowel irradiation and GI complications [9,10,42–44].

However, in the absence of a dedicated dosimetric–volumetric analysis in the present study, this finding should be interpreted with caution. The observed association may reflect the combined influence of anatomical factors, treatment planning characteristics, and individual variability, and should be considered hypothesis-generating pending confirmation in prospective studies incorporating detailed dosimetric parameters.

Age, tumor grade, initial stage, postoperative stage, and stage modification were not significantly associated with the occurrence of GI AEs, and trend analyses did not demonstrate relationships dependent on disease severity. This pattern suggests that tumor-related clinical characteristics may play a limited role in predicting acute GI toxicity in the neoadjuvant setting. These findings are consistent with evidence indicating that treatment-related characteristics and dosimetric–volumetric factors represent the most robust predictors of pelvic radiotherapy-induced toxicity, whereas disease-related clinical variables are less consistently implicated [45]. Similar observations have been reported in rectal cancer cohorts treated with chemoradiotherapy, where irradiated bowel volumes and treatment planning parameters appear more influential than age or tumor stage in determining GI toxicity risk [42,46].

Collectively, these results reinforce the concept that GI toxicity in the neoadjuvant management of rectal cancer is primarily driven by treatment-related and individual susceptibility factors rather than by tumor burden or oncological stage.

As total neoadjuvant therapy has become increasingly adopted in routine clinical practice, the present study contributes real-world data from a relatively large and heterogeneous cohort treated with TNT or CRT. Future research should aim to clarify the biological and anatomical mechanisms underlying the increased susceptibility observed in female patients and to integrate dosimetric–volumetric parameters into prospective toxicity modeling. Additionally, prospective evaluation of tailored antiemetic and antidiarrheal strategies in the context of TNT may further optimize treatment tolerability without compromising oncological outcomes.

Several limitations inherent to the study design should be acknowledged when interpreting the present findings. The retrospective design implies that GI toxicities were assessed based on existing clinical documentation, without the use of standardized tools for prospective symptom collection. The unequal distribution of patients between the TNT and CRT groups may affect the direct comparability of results, despite the use of multivariable analyses and sensitivity analyses to control for confounding factors. In addition, the analysis focused exclusively on clinically reported GI toxicities, without integrating patient-reported outcome assessments, which could have provided a more detailed characterization of the clinical impact of mild symptoms. The absence of a dedicated dosimetric–volumetric analysis limits the exploration of anatomical and radiotherapy planning mechanisms involved in the development of GI toxicities and in the associations observed with certain clinical characteristics. Nevertheless, the cohort size and the use of complementary statistical methods support the consistency of the results and allow for the formulation of hypotheses that require validation in prospective studies incorporating dosimetric–volumetric parameters and standardized symptom assessments.

https://doi.org/10.3390/life16030422

5. Conclusions

This study highlights that total neoadjuvant therapy (TNT) is associated with a higher incidence of GI AEs compared with concurrent chemoradiotherapy (CRT). Nausea represented the dominant component of this toxicity profile. Multivariable and sensitivity analyses identified TNT and female sex as independent factors associated with an increased risk of GI toxicity, while tumor location in the upper third of the rectum was associated with a higher occurrence of vomiting. Grade 2 GI AEs were infrequent, and no severe (grade 3–4) AEs were observed, suggesting an overall favorable tolerability profile for neoadjuvant treatment strategies. These findings may contribute to improved risk stratification for GI toxicity in patients with rectal cancer treated with neoadjuvant therapy and may support the identification of patients who could benefit from closer clinical monitoring and early implementation of tailored supportive measures.

Author Contributions: Conceptualization, L.D.B., M.S. and S.Ș.M.; methodology, L.D.B., S.Ș.M., M.S., P.O.S., A.-M.C. and T.C.B.; validation, L.D.B., S.Ș.M., M.S. and A.M.D.; formal analysis and investigation, L.D.B., P.O.S., R.A.S., A.M.M., A.M.D., C.S., Ș.P. and T.C.B.; writing—original draft preparation, L.D.B., R.A.S., C.S., Ș.P., A.M.M. and A.M.D.; writing—review and editing, P.O.S., R.A.S., T.C.B. and A.-M.C.; visualization, L.D.B., M.S., P.O.S. and S.Ș.M.; supervision, L.D.B., M.S., P.O.S. and S.Ș.M. All authors have read and agreed to the published version of the manuscript.

Funding: This research received no external funding.

Institutional Review Board Statement: This study was conducted according to the guidelines of the Declaration of Helsinki and approved by the Ethics Committee of Sf. Nectarie Oncology Center, Craiova, according to Decision No. 003 of 7 February 2021.

Informed Consent Statement: Patient consent was waived due to the retrospective nature of the study. At the time of treatment, all patients signed a written consent that stated that all their medical data could be used anonymously by the medical staff of Sf. Nectarie Oncology Center for research and medical quality improvement purposes.

Data Availability Statement: Data are contained within the article. All data are available by request to the corresponding authors.

Conflicts of Interest: The authors declare no conflicts of interest.

Abbreviations

The following abbreviations are used in this manuscript:

TNT	Total neoadjuvant therapy
CRT	Concurrent chemoradiotherapy
GI	Gastrointestinal
AEs	Adverse events
IMRT	Intensity-modulated radiotherapy
VMAT	Volumetric modulated arc therapy
CTCAE	Common terminology criteria for adverse events
IPTW	Inverse probability of treatment weighting
OR	Odds ratios
CI	Confidence intervals
CAPEOX	Capecitabine and oxaliplatin
FOLFOX	5-fluorouracil, oxaliplatin, and leucovorin

https://doi.org/10.3390/life16030422

References

1. Bray, F.; Laversanne, M.; Sung, H.; Ferlay, J.; Siegel, R.L.; Soerjomataram, I.; Jemal, A. Global cancer statistics 2022: GLOBOCAN estimates of incidence and mortality worldwide for 36 cancers in 185 countries. *CA Cancer J. Clin.* **2024**, *74*, 229–263.
2. Arnold, M.; Sierra, M.S.; Laversanne, M.; Soerjomataram, I.; Jemal, A.; Bray, F. Global patterns and trends in colorectal cancer incidence and mortality. *Gut* **2017**, *66*, 683–691.
3. Glynne-Jones, R.; Wyrwicz, L.; Tiret, E.; Brown, G.; Rödel, C.; Cervantes, A.; Arnold, D.; ESMO Guidelines Committee. Rectal cancer: ESMO Clinical Practice Guidelines for diagnosis, treatment and follow-up. *Ann. Oncol.* **2017**, *28*, iv22–iv40. [CrossRef]
4. Sauer, R.; Becker, H.; Hohenberger, W.; Rödel, C.; Wittekind, C.; Fietkau, R.; Martus, P.; Tschmelitsch, J.; Hager, E.; Hess, C.F.; et al. Preoperative versus postoperative chemoradiotherapy for rectal cancer. *N. Engl. J. Med.* **2004**, *351*, 1731–1740. [PubMed]
5. Bahadoer, R.R.; Dijkstra, E.A.; van Etten, B.; Marijnen, C.A.M.; Putter, H.; Kranenbarg, E.M.; Roodvoets, A.G.H.; Nagtegaal, I.D.; Beets-Tan, R.G.H.; Blomqvist, L.K.; et al. Short-course radiotherapy followed by chemotherapy before total mesorectal excision versus preoperative chemoradiotherapy in locally advanced rectal cancer (RAPIDO): A randomised, open-label, phase 3 trial. *Lancet Oncol.* **2021**, *22*, 29–42.
6. Bentzen, S.M. Preventing or reducing late side effects of radiation therapy: Radiobiology meets molecular pathology. *Nat. Rev. Cancer* **2006**, *6*, 702–713. [CrossRef] [PubMed]
7. Siegel, R.L.; Miller, K.D.; Goding Sauer, A.; Fedewa, S.A.; Butterly, L.F.; Anderson, J.C.; Cercek, A.; Smith, R.A.; Jemal, A. Colorectal cancer statistics, 2020. *CA Cancer J. Clin.* **2020**, *70*, 145–164.
8. Vuik, F.E.; Nieuwenburg, S.A.; Bardou, M.; Lansdorp-Vogelaar, I.; Dinis-Ribeiro, M.; Bento, M.J.; Zadnik, V.; Pellisé, M.; Esteban, L.; Kaminski, M.F.; et al. Increasing incidence of colorectal cancer in young adults in Europe over the last 25 years. *Gut* **2019**, *68*, 1820–1826. [CrossRef]
9. Guerrero Urbano, M.T.; Henrys, A.J.; Adams, E.J.; Norman, A.R.; Bedford, J.L.; Harrington, K.J.; Nutting, C.M. Intensity-modulated radiotherapy in patients with locally advanced rectal cancer reduces bowel dose and acute gastrointestinal toxicity. *Int. J. Radiat. Oncol. Biol. Phys.* **2006**, *65*, 907–915. [PubMed]
10. Engels, B.; De Ridder, M.; Tournel, K.; Sermeus, A.; De Coninck, P.; Storme, G.; Van den Heuvel, F. Preoperative intensity-modulated and image-guided radiotherapy with a simultaneous integrated boost in locally advanced rectal cancer. *Int. J. Radiat. Oncol. Biol. Phys.* **2009**, *75*, 677–684.
11. Lotfollahzadeh, S.; Kashyap, S.; Tsoris, A.; Recio-Boiles, A.; Babiker, H.M. Rectal cancer. In *StatPearls*; StatPearls Publishing: Treasure Island, FL, USA, 2024.
12. Garcia-Aguilar, J.; Chow, O.S.; Smith, D.D.; Marcet, J.E.; Cataldo, P.A.; Varma, M.G.; Kumar, A.S.; Oommen, S.; Coutsoftides, T.; Hunt, S.R.; et al. Effect of adding mFOLFOX6 after neoadjuvant chemoradiation in locally advanced rectal cancer: A multicentre, phase 2 trial. *Lancet Oncol.* **2015**, *16*, 957–966. [CrossRef]
13. Conroy, T.; Bosset, J.F.; Etienne, P.L.; Rio, E.; François, É.; Mesgouez-Nebout, N.; Vendrely, V.; Artignan, X.; Bouché, O.; Gargot, D.; et al. Neoadjuvant chemotherapy with FOLFIRINOX and preoperative chemoradiotherapy for patients with locally advanced rectal cancer (UNICANCER-PRODIGE 23): A multicentre, randomised, open-label, phase 3 trial. *Lancet Oncol.* **2021**, *22*, 702–715. [CrossRef] [PubMed]
14. Andreyev, J. Gastrointestinal complications of pelvic radiotherapy: Are they of any importance? *Gut* **2005**, *54*, 1051–1054. [CrossRef]
15. Denham, J.W.; Hauer-Jensen, M. The radiotherapeutic injury—A complex "wound". *Radiother. Oncol.* **2002**, *63*, 129–145. [CrossRef] [PubMed]
16. Andreyev, J.; Davidson, S.; Gillespie, C.; Allum, W.; Swarbrick, E. Practice guidance on the management of acute and chronic gastrointestinal problems arising as a result of treatment for cancer. *Gut* **2012**, *61*, 179–192. [CrossRef]
17. Wedlake, L.; Thomas, K.; McGough, C.; Andreyev, J. Small bowel bacterial overgrowth and lactose intolerance during radical pelvic radiotherapy: An observational study. *Eur. J. Cancer* **2008**, *44*, 2212–2217. [CrossRef]
18. Roh, M.S.; Colangelo, L.H.; O'Connell, M.J.; Yothers, G.; Deutsch, M.; Allegra, C.J.; Kahlenberg, M.S.; Baez-Diaz, L.; Ursiny, C.S.; Petrelli, N.J.; et al. Preoperative multimodality therapy improves disease-free survival in patients with carcinoma of the rectum: NSABP R-03. *J. Clin. Oncol.* **2009**, *27*, 5124–5130. [CrossRef]
19. Bosset, J.F.; Collette, L.; Calais, G.; Mineur, L.; Maingon, P.; Radosevic-Jelic, L.; Daban, A.; Bardet, E.; Beny, A.; Ollier, J.C. Chemotherapy with preoperative radiotherapy in rectal cancer. *N. Engl. J. Med.* **2006**, *355*, 1114–1123. [CrossRef] [PubMed]
20. Smalley, S.R.; Benedetti, J.K.; Williamson, S.K.; Robertson, J.M.; Estes, N.C.; Maher, T.; Fisher, B.; Rich, T.A.; Martenson, J.A.; Kugler, J.W.; et al. Phase III trial of fluorouracil-based chemotherapy regimens plus radiotherapy in postoperative adjuvant rectal cancer: GI INT 0144. *J. Clin. Oncol.* **2006**, *24*, 3542–3547. [CrossRef]
21. Robertson, J.M.; Lockman, D.; Yan, D.; Wallace, M. The dose–volume relationship of small bowel irradiation and acute grade 3 diarrhea during chemoradiotherapy for rectal cancer. *Int. J. Radiat. Oncol. Biol. Phys.* **2008**, *70*, 413–418. [CrossRef]
22. Robertson, J.M.; Sohn, M.; Yan, D. Predicting grade 3 acute diarrhea during radiation therapy for rectal cancer using a cutoff-dose logistic regression normal tissue complication probability model. *Int. J. Radiat. Oncol. Biol. Phys.* **2010**, *77*, 66–72.

https://doi.org/10.3390/life16030422

23. Gunnlaugsson, A.; Kjellén, E.; Nilsson, P.; Bendahl, P.O.; Willner, J.; Johnsson, A. Dose–volume relationships between enteritis and irradiated bowel volumes during 5-fluorouracil- and oxaliplatin-based chemoradiotherapy in locally advanced rectal cancer. *Acta Oncol.* **2007**, *46*, 937–944. [CrossRef]
24. Chen, R.C.; Mamon, H.J.; Ancukiewicz, M.; Killoran, J.H.; Crowley, E.M.; Blaszkowsky, L.S.; Wo, J.Y.; Ryan, D.P.; Hong, T.S. Dose–volume effects on patient-reported acute gastrointestinal symptoms during chemoradiation therapy for rectal cancer. *Int. J. Radiat. Oncol. Biol. Phys.* **2012**, *83*, e513–e517.
25. Samuelian, J.M.; Callister, M.D.; Ashman, J.B.; Young-Fadok, T.M.; Borad, M.J.; Gunderson, L.L. Reduced acute bowel toxicity in patients treated with intensity-modulated radiotherapy for rectal cancer. *Int. J. Radiat. Oncol. Biol. Phys.* **2012**, *82*, 1981–1987.
26. Garofalo, M.; Moughan, J.; Hong, T.; Bendell, J.; Berger, A.; Lerma, F. RTOG 0822: A phase II study of preoperative chemoradiotherapy utilizing IMRT in combination with capecitabine and oxaliplatin for patients with locally advanced rectal cancer. *Int. J. Radiat. Oncol. Biol. Phys.* **2011**, *81*, S3–S4. [CrossRef]
27. Arbea, L.; Ramos, L.I.; Martinez-Monge, R.; Moreno, M.; Aristu, J. Intensity-modulated radiation therapy versus 3D conformal radiotherapy in locally advanced rectal cancer: Dosimetric comparison and clinical implications. *Radiat. Oncol.* **2010**, *5*, 17. [PubMed]
28. Simpson, D.R.; Song, W.Y.; Moiseenko, V.; Rose, B.S.; Yashar, C.M.; Mundt, A.J.; Mell, L.K. Normal tissue complication probability analysis of acute gastrointestinal toxicity in cervical cancer patients undergoing intensity-modulated radiation therapy and concurrent cisplatin. *Int. J. Radiat. Oncol. Biol. Phys.* **2012**, *83*, e81–e86. [CrossRef] [PubMed]
29. Roeske, J.C.; Bonta, D.; Mell, L.K.; Lujan, A.E.; Mundt, A.J. A dosimetric analysis of acute gastrointestinal toxicity in women receiving intensity-modulated whole-pelvic radiation therapy. *Radiother. Oncol.* **2003**, *69*, 201–207.
30. Devisetty, K.; Mell, L.K.; Salama, J.K.; Schomas, D.A.; Miller, R.C.; Jani, A.B.; Roeske, J.C.; Aydogan, B.; Chmura, S.J. A multi-institutional acute gastrointestinal toxicity analysis of anal cancer patients treated with concurrent intensity-modulated radiation therapy and chemotherapy. *Radiother. Oncol.* **2009**, *93*, 298–301. [CrossRef]
31. Herrstedt, J.; Clark-Snow, R.; Ruhlmann, C.H.; Molassiotis, A.; Olver, I.; Rapoport, B.L.; Aapro, M.; Dennis, K.; Hesketh, P.J.; Navari, R.M.; et al. 2023 MASCC and ESMO guideline update for the prevention of chemotherapy- and radiotherapy-induced nausea and vomiting. *ESMO Open* **2024**, *9*, 102195. [CrossRef]
32. Hesketh, P.J.; Kris, M.G.; Basch, E.; Bohlke, K.; Barbour, S.Y.; Clark-Snow, R.A.; Danso, M.A.; Dennis, K.; Dupuis, L.L.; Dusetzina, S.B.; et al. Antiemetics: ASCO Guideline Update. *J. Clin. Oncol.* **2020**, *38*, 2782–2797. [CrossRef]
33. Andreyev, J.; Adams, R.; Bornschein, J.; Chapman, M.; Chuter, D.; Darnborough, S.; Davies, A.; Dignan, F.; Donnellan, C.; Fernandes, D.; et al. British Society of Gastroenterology practice guidance on the management of acute and chronic gastrointestinal symptoms and complications as a result of treatment for cancer. *Gut* **2025**, *74*, 1040–1067. [CrossRef]
34. National Cancer Institute. *Common Terminology Criteria for Adverse Events (CTCAE)*; Version 5.0; U.S. Department of Health and Human Services: Bethesda, MD, USA, 2017.
35. Bratu, L.D.; Schenker, M.; Stovicek, P.O.; Schenker, R.A.; Mehedințeanu, A.M.; Berisha, T.C.; Donoiu, A.; Mogoantă, S.Ș. Retrospective Evaluation of the Efficacy of Total Neoadjuvant Therapy and Chemoradiotherapy Neoadjuvant Treatment in Relation to Surgery in Patients with Rectal Cancer. *Medicina* **2024**, *60*, 656. [CrossRef]
36. Ochiai, K.; Bhutiani, N.; Ikeda, A.; Uppal, A.; White, M.G.; Peacock, O.; Messick, C.A.; Bednarski, B.K.; You, Y.-Q.N.; Skibber, J.M.; et al. Total Neoadjuvant Therapy for Rectal Cancer: Which Regimens to Use? *Cancers* **2024**, *16*, 2093. [CrossRef] [PubMed]
37. Iwamoto, M.; Ueda, K.; Kawamura, J. Neoadjuvant Treatment for Locally Advanced Rectal Cancer: Current Status and Future Directions. *Cancers* **2025**, *17*, 2540. [CrossRef]
38. Conces, M.L.; Tursun, N.; Ozgur, I.; Yilmaz, S.; Elamin, D.; Patil, S.; Bouferraa, Y.; Gorgun, E.; Liska, D.; Weinstein, E.; et al. Total neoadjuvant therapy in early-onset versus average-onset locally advanced rectal cancer: Patient characteristics and tolerance of therapy. *ESMO Gastrointest. Oncol.* **2025**, *8*, 100170. [CrossRef] [PubMed]
39. Seow, W.; Murshed, I.; Bunjo, Z.; Bedrikovetski, S.; Stone, J.; Sammour, T. Compliance and toxicity of total neoadjuvant therapy in locally advanced rectal cancer: A systematic review and network meta-analysis. *Ann. Surg. Oncol.* **2025**, *32*, 6728–6739. [CrossRef] [PubMed]
40. Schenker, M.; Bițînă, L.C.; Schenker, R.A.; Ciurea, A.M.; Mehedințeanu, A.M.; Berisha, T.C.; Bratu, L.D.; Cara, M.L.; Dicianu, A.M.; Stovicek, P.O. Prospective Evaluation of the Influence of Chemoradiotherapy and Stoma on Functional and Symptomatic Outcomes in Rectal Cancer Patients. *Cancers* **2025**, *17*, 2052. [CrossRef]
41. Barba, M.C.; De Franco, P.; Russo, D.; Cavalera, E.; Ciurlia, E.; De Matteis, S.; Di Paola, G.; Federico, C.; Leone, A.; Papaleo, A.; et al. Total Neoadjuvant Therapy for Locally Advanced Rectal Cancer: Evaluation of Sequencing, Response, and Toxicity in a Single-Institution Cohort. *Cancers* **2025**, *17*, 2416. [CrossRef]
42. Yang, T.J.; Oh, J.H.; Son, C.H.; Apte, A.; Deasy, J.O.; Wu, A.; Goodman, K.A. Predictors of Acute Gastrointestinal Toxicity during Pelvic Chemoradiotherapy in Patients with Rectal Cancer. *Gastrointest. Cancer Res.* **2013**, *6*, 129–136.
43. Feeney, G.; Sehgal, R.; Sheehan, M.; Hogan, A.; Regan, M.; Joyce, M.; Kerin, M. Neoadjuvant Radiotherapy for Rectal Cancer Management. *World J. Gastroenterol.* **2019**, *25*, 4850–4869. [CrossRef] [PubMed]

https://doi.org/10.3390/life16030422

44. Parekh, A.; Truong, M.T.; Pashtan, I.; Qureshi, M.M.; Martin, N.E.; Nawaz, O.; Cerda, S.; Willins, J.; Hartshorn, K.L.; Kachnic, L.A. Acute Gastrointestinal Toxicity and Tumor Response with Preoperative Intensity-Modulated Radiation Therapy for Rectal Cancer. *Gastrointest. Cancer Res.* **2013**, *6*, 137–143. [PubMed]
45. Ching, J.C.; Liu, K.C.; Pang, I.K.; Nicol, A.J.; Leung, V.W.; Cai, J.; Lee, S.W. Predictive Factors for Gastrointestinal and Genitourinary Toxicity Following Radiotherapy in Pelvic Tumors: A Scoping Review. *Diagnostics* **2025**, *15*, 1331. [CrossRef] [PubMed]
46. Xu, B.; Guo, Y.; Chen, Y.; Lu, H.; Tang, T.; Yue, Z.; Guan, G.; Chi, P. Is the Irradiated Small Bowel Volume Still a Predictor for Acute Lower Gastrointestinal Toxicity during Preoperative Concurrent Chemo-Radiotherapy for Rectal Cancer? *Radiat. Oncol.* **2015**, *10*, 257. [CrossRef]

https://doi.org/10.3390/life16030422

life

MDPI

Article

Gut Microbial Diversity and Community Structure Are Largely Similar Between Apparently Healthy Elderly Japanese Males and Females: A Shotgun Metagenomic Study

M. H. Mahbub [1,2], Ryosuke Hase [1], Natsu Yamaguchi [1], Yoshiyuki Asai [2,3,4], Masanori Harada [1,5], Naoyuki Ichimura [1,5], Yoshihiro Hayakawa [6], Yusuke Inohana [6], Yutaka Umakoshi [6], Ryo Yamaguchi [6], Ren Kimura [7], Hisashi Tsujimura [7], Mitsuharu Matsumoto [8], Fumiaki Higashijima [9], Takuya Yoshimoto [9], Kazuhiro Kimura [9], Tsunahiko Hirano [10], Keiji Ohishi [10], Keiko Doi [10,11], Kazuto Matsunaga [10] and Tsuyoshi Tanabe [1,*]

1 Department of Public Health and Preventive Medicine, Graduate School of Medicine, Yamaguchi University, Ube 755-8505, Japan; hossain@yamaguchi-u.ac.jp (M.H.M.); hase@yamaguchi-u.ac.jp (R.H.); natsu@yamaguchi-u.ac.jp (N.Y.); masa.harada@mac.com (M.H.); ichimura.naoyuki.02@pref.yamaguchi.lg.jp (N.I.)

2 Division of Systems Medicine and Informatics, Research Institute for Cell Design Medical Science, Yamaguchi University, Ube 755-8505, Japan; asai@yamaguchi-u.ac.jp

3 Department of Systems Bioinformatics, Graduate School of Medicine, Yamaguchi University, Ube 755-8505, Japan

4 AI Systems Medicine Research and Training Center, Graduate School of Medicine, Yamaguchi University Hospital, Yamaguchi University, Ube 755-8505, Japan

5 Support Center for Rural Medicine, Yamaguchi Prefectural Grand Medical Center, Hofu 747-8511, Japan

6 Shimadzu Corporation, Kyoto 604-8511, Japan; yo-haya@shimadzu.co.jp (Y.H.); ino-yu@shimadzu.co.jp (Y.I.); umakoshi.yutaka.xm4@shimadzu.co.jp (Y.U.); ryama@shimadzu.co.jp (R.Y.)

7 Analytical Science Research, Kao Corporation, Sumida-ku, Tokyo 131-8501, Japan; kimura.ren@kao.com (R.K.); tsujimura.hisashi@kao.com (H.T.)

8 Research Laboratories, Kyodo Milk Industry Co., Ltd., Tokyo 190-0182, Japan; m-matumoto@meito.co.jp

9 Department of Ophthalmology, Yamaguchi University School of Medicine, Ube 755-8505, Japan; higashi@yamaguchi-u.ac.jp (F.H.); takuya-y@yamaguchi-u.ac.jp (T.Y.); k.kimura@yamaguchi-u.ac.jp (K.K.)

10 Department of Respiratory Medicine and Infectious Disease, Graduate School of Medicine, Yamaguchi University, Ube 755-8505, Japan; tsuna@yamaguchi-u.ac.jp (T.H.); ohishk@yamaguchi-u.ac.jp (K.O.); decem119@yamaguchi-u.ac.jp (K.D.)

11 Department of Pulmonology and Gerontology, Graduate School of Medicine, Yamaguchi University, Ube 755-8505, Japan

* Correspondence: tanabe@yamaguchi-u.ac.jp; Tel.: +81-836-22-2231

Abstract

Sex differences in gut microbiota may affect health and aging, but evidence in elderly populations is limited and inconsistent. This study examined sex-specific similarities and differences in gut microbiota diversity and composition among apparently healthy elderly Japanese individuals using shotgun metagenomic sequencing. A cross-sectional study was conducted in 100 community-dwelling adults aged 75–83 years (54 males, 46 females). Fecal samples underwent metagenomic sequencing. Alpha and beta diversity were assessed across six taxonomic levels, and taxonomic differences were evaluated using non-parametric tests. No significant sex differences were observed in alpha diversity indices (Shannon, Simpson, evenness, Chao1) at any taxonomic level. Beta diversity based on Bray–Curtis dissimilarity and PCoA also showed no sex-specific clustering. However, certain taxa differed in relative abundance. Males showed higher abundances of *Bacteroidota* (phylum), *Bacteroidia* and *Betaproteobacteria* (class), and *Bacteroidales* and *Burkholderiales* (order) ($p < 0.05$). No significant differences were detected at the family, genus, or species levels. Overall, gut microbial diversity and community structure were largely similar between elderly males and females, with only modest sex-associated differences at higher

 https://doi.org/10.3390/life16020297

taxonomic levels. These findings suggest that biological sex may have a limited influence on gut microbiota composition in advanced age and provide population-level reference data for future longitudinal and interventional studies in elderly cohorts.

Keywords: gut microbiota; shotgun metagenomics; sex differences; elderly; microbial diversity

1. Introduction

The world's population is rapidly aging, leading to a higher prevalence of various diseases and associated disabilities among the elderly. With aging, the gut microbiota undergoes age-related changes [1], often characterized by reduced microbial diversity [2]. In humans, the gut microbiota plays a crucial role in host homeostasis and health, by continuously contributing to metabolism, digestion, nutrition, and host immune regulation [3].

Numerous studies have demonstrated that alterations in the gut microbiota, or dysbiosis, may trigger various pathogenic processes, potentially resulting in a wide range of health disorders, including endocrine and metabolic diseases, immune-mediated conditions, cardiovascular and neurologic disorders, and various cancers [4–6]. Accordingly, studies suggest that targeted modulation of the gut microbiota could be a potential strategy to prevent or manage diseases and may promote healthy aging [7,8]. Therefore, a clearer understanding of the baseline gut microbiota composition in healthy elderly is essential, as this knowledge could inform microbiota-modulating strategies for maintaining a healthy gut microbiome and promoting healthy aging.

In the existing literature, biological sex has been recognized as a key determinant of disease susceptibility and pathogenesis, as well as disease prevention, progression, and prognosis of various adverse health outcomes [9,10]. Sex has also been associated with gut microbiome composition and circulating metabolites [11,12]. Therefore, to develop tailored microbiota-modulating interventions for the elderly, a clear understanding of their sex-specific composition is essential. Also, an important question is whether the same intervention would be applicable to both elderly males and females. However, the current literature reveals a significant gap in our knowledge regarding the sex-associated differences in gut microbiota composition among the healthy elderly population. Limited published studies on humans showing sex differences in the gut microbiome often included subjects over a broad age range, complicating interpretation for the elderly population [1]. The situation is further complicated by inconsistent and inconclusive results, with some studies reporting significant associations between sex and the gut microbiota [13,14], while others do not [11,15]. Moreover, the same microbial taxa showed opposing trends in relative abundance (increase or decrease) between studies. For example, while Hopkins et al. observed an increase in Bacteroides species in the feces of elderly subjects, Woodmansey et al. reported a decline in these species among them [16,17]. Adding to the complexity, many of these studies used 16S rRNA amplicon sequencing, which exclusively targeted bacteria [11–14]. Thus, while titles refer broadly to "gut microbiota", the analyses are limited to bacteria, potentially overlooking sex-associated variations in other microbial domains such as archaea, fungi, and viruses. Moreover, published studies vary in the taxonomic levels at which findings are reported, limiting comparability across studies.

These limitations and inconsistencies in the current literature highlight uncertainty regarding sex-associated patterns of the gut microbiota in the healthy elderly. Therefore, it is important to directly assess and characterize potential sex-specific differences within this population. Improved knowledge of sex-specific composition and sex-associated similarities and differences in gut microbiota among healthy elderly may not only con-

https://doi.org/10.3390/life16020297

tribute to the development of effective intervention strategies for healthy aging but also aid in understanding disease susceptibility and informing the progression, prevention, and management of various diseases in this vulnerable population.

In light of these considerations, this study aimed to examine sex-associated similarities and differences in gut microbiota diversity across six taxonomic levels in a cohort of apparently healthy elderly Japanese males and females, using shotgun metagenomic sequencing. Additionally, we sought to identify sex-stratified dominant microbial profiles within this cohort.

2. Materials and Methods

2.1. Participants

This study was conducted in accordance with the Declaration of Helsinki, and the study protocol was approved by the Institutional Review Board of Yamaguchi University (Approval No. 2020-183-3). Written informed consent was obtained from all participants prior to enrollment. The data presented here are based on partial baseline analyses from a cohort study examining the effects of exercise intervention and yogurt intake in elderly individuals. Participants were apparently healthy community-dwelling elderly individuals aged 75–83 years at the time informed consent was obtained. In the present study, participants were considered apparently healthy if they were community-dwelling, able to complete the study assessments, and had no severe, acute, or unstable disease requiring active medical intervention at enrollment. Common chronic conditions that were stable and medically controlled (with or without medication), such as hypertension, diabetes, and metabolic abnormalities, were not treated as exclusion criteria, as these conditions are highly prevalent in this age group. Participants were recruited from Ajisu City, Yamaguchi Prefecture, Japan, through advertisements including posters, bulletin board notices, and local newsletters. A total of 104 volunteers initially expressed interest and were invited to participate. The inclusion criteria were: ability to stand unassisted; a Mini-Mental State Examination (MMSE) score ≥ 24; not being certified as requiring long-term nursing care level 2 or higher; absence of neurological, musculoskeletal, or connective tissue disorders; no serious medical conditions such as cancer or renal failure; and no regular use of antibiotics at the time of recruitment.

The study protocol was explained in detail to potential participants at a designated location. After informed consent was obtained, the MMSE was administered and long-term nursing care certification status was confirmed. Among the 104 volunteers, two withdrew due to procedural difficulties and two were excluded due to the need for medical treatment. The remaining 100 participants (54 males, 46 females) met all eligibility criteria and were enrolled in the study.

Following enrollment, participants underwent physical examinations and clinical and laboratory testing to confirm clinical stability, including screening for conditions suggestive of anemia or frailty. In addition, personal and medical history information was collected using a self-administered questionnaire.

2.2. Collection of Blood Samples and Hematological Analyses

A total of 55 mL of venous blood was collected from the cubital vein with the participant seated after an overnight fast. This sampling volume was approved by the institutional ethics committee and was required to obtain sufficient serum/plasma and whole-blood aliquots for the comprehensive hematological, biochemical, and biomarker assessments specified in the parent intervention protocol, of which the present report represents a subset of baseline data. Hematological analyses were conducted using the Sysmex XN-1000 (Sysmex, Kobe, Japan). Biochemical analyses were performed with the LABOSPECT 006

https://doi.org/10.3390/life16020297

(Hitachi High-Technologies, Tokyo, Japan) using enzymatic methods. HbA1c was measured via high-speed ion-exchange liquid chromatography using the HLC-723 (Tosoh Co., Tokyo, Japan).

2.3. Collection of Stool Samples

Stool samples were collected using FS-0007 kits (TechnoSuruga Laboratory Co., Ltd., Shizuoka, Japan), which can preserve microbiota at room temperature for up to four weeks. Participants collected fecal samples at home and delivered them within four days. Upon receipt, the samples were stored at 4 °C, typically for an average of three days, in the cold storage facility of the Department of Public Health and Preventive Medicine, Yamaguchi University Graduate School of Medicine, until they were transported to Takara Bio Inc. (Shiga, Japan) for shotgun metagenomic analysis.

2.4. Metagenomic Library Preparation and Sequencing

From the stool samples, DNA was extracted using the NucleoSpin Soil extraction kit (Macherey-Nagel, Germany) following the manufacturer's instructions. Prior to library construction, the quality and quantity of DNA samples were verified through agarose gel electrophoresis and fluorescence quantification using the Qubit 2.0 Fluorometer (Thermo Fisher Scientific, Waltham, MA, USA), respectively. DNA samples were mechanically fragmented to the desired insert size using the Covaris acoustic DNA shearing system (Covaris, Inc., Woburn, MA, USA). AMPure XP beads (Beckman Coulter Inc., Brea, CA, USA) were then employed for DNA selection based on size. After smoothing and phosphorylating the ends of the size-selected DNA, adapters were ligated, using ThruPLEX DNA-Seq Kit (Takara Bio Inc, Shiga, Japan). The DNA with ligated adapters served as a template, and PCR amplification was conducted using primers with indexes to create a sequencing library.

The quality of the generated sequencing library was assessed using the Agilent 2100 TapeStation system (Agilent, Santa Clara, CA, USA). The DNA libraries were sequenced across four lanes of an Illumina NovaSeq 6000 system (Illumina, Inc., San Diego, CA, USA) with a read length of 150 bp (paired-end). Real-time analysis was performed using NovaSeq Control Software v1.7.5 and Real Time Analysis v3.4.4 ((Illumina, Inc., San Diego, CA, USA), both executed on the NovaSeq instrument computer. To generate the sequence data, the bcl2fastq 2.20.0.422 pipeline was employed ((Illumina, Inc., San Diego, CA, USA). Per-sample shotgun metagenomic sequencing and read-processing metrics are provided in Supplementary Table S1.

2.5. Bioinformatic Analysis

Trimmomatic (v0.39) was utilized to trim all paired-end reads in raw FASTQ files, and low-quality reads were removed. All sequence reads were mapped to the existing human reference genome using Bowtie2 v2.2.5 (Johns Hopkins University, Baltimore, MD, USA), and host reads were eliminated. Taxonomic classification of the resulting shotgun metagenomic reads was performed using Kaiju, a protein-level fast and sensitive metagenomic classifier, against the NCBI non-redundant (nr) database. Because Kaiju classifies reads against NCBI-nr, the analysis inherently included taxa from bacteria, archaea, fungi, viruses, and eukaryotes, and no microbial domains were excluded a priori. Hits matched with NCBI Taxonomy ID were converted to taxonomic names using TaxonKit, and the relative abundance of microbial communities in each sample were calculated based on the number of reads assigned to each taxon.

https://doi.org/10.3390/life16020297

2.6. Statistical Analysis

The continuous variables in this study were assessed for normal distribution using the Kolmogorov–Smirnov and Shapiro–Wilk tests. Subsequently, non-parametric tests were employed. In tables and figures (except those reporting microbial taxa abundance), continuous variables are presented as the median and interquartile range (IQR), while categorical variables are expressed as numbers and percentages. The comparison between male and female groups was performed utilizing the Mann–Whitney U-test for continuous variables and the Chi-square (χ^2) test for categorical variables. Alpha diversity metrics, including the Shannon index, Simpson index, and Chao 1 index, were measured. These analyses were based on the relative abundance at each taxonomic level. The differential distribution of the overall microbial community between males and females was assessed by measuring beta diversity. Principal coordinate analysis (PCoA) of quarter root-transformed data based on the Bray–Curtis similarity matrix was conducted for this purpose. PCoA plots were generated using the first two principal coordinates (PCs), illustrating the differences between male and female groups. Additionally, group differences were examined using permutational multivariate analysis of variance (PERMANOVA) with 999 permutations. The analyses were performed using Past version 4.03 [18].

The top ten most abundant microbial taxa at each taxonomic level were identified separately for male and female groups, excluding unclassified taxa to focus on well-defined taxonomic units. For this purpose, we calculated the average percent relative abundances and presented the data as mean $\pm$ standard error (SE), consistent with common reporting formats in gut microbiota studies. However, in line with the statistical framework of this study, differences in the relative abundances of taxonomic units between sexes were assessed using non-parametric (Mann–Whitney U-test) tests.

In addition to PAST, SPSS version 22 for Windows (SPSS Inc., Chicago, IL, USA) was employed for data analysis. All statistical tests adopted in this study were two-tailed, and the significance level was considered at $p < 0.05$. To account for multiple comparisons in taxonomic differential-abundance testing, p-values obtained from the Mann–Whitney U-test for taxa were additionally adjusted using the Benjamini–Hochberg false discovery rate (FDR) method.

3. Results

Table 1 illustrates the demographic and clinical characteristics of the study population based on sex. Both males and females exhibited a similar age and BMI (Mann–Whitney U-test, $p > 0.05$). Additionally, no statistically significant differences were observed in any clinical variables between the two groups (Mann–Whitney U-test, all $p > 0.05$).

Next, alpha diversity of the microbial community was compared between males and females (Figure 1). No significant differences in Shannon, Simpson, or Chao 1 indexes were observed between male and female populations at different taxonomic levels ($p > 0.05$).

The results of beta diversity are presented as two-dimensional plots using PCoAs (Figure 2). The analysis revealed that the gut microbiota of males and females did not cluster away from each other. This was confirmed by the one-way PERMANOVA test, which showed no statistically significant difference in beta diversity at any taxonomic level between elderly males and females (PERMANOVA: F = 1.03 to 1.61, p = 0.111 to 0.380).

https://doi.org/10.3390/life16020297

Table 1. Demographic and clinical characteristics of the study subjects. Values are expressed as median and IQR.

	Male, n = 54		Female, n = 46		p *
Variables	**Median**	**IQR**	**Median**	**IQR**	
Age (Years)	77.5	3.0	77.0	2.0	0.812
BMI (kg/m^2)	23.5	4.4	22.6	3.3	0.407
FPG (mg/dL)	101.0	16.0	97.5	17.3	0.653
AST (U/L)	25.5	7.0	23.5	9.0	0.136
ALT (U/L)	18.0	10.3	18.0	10.5	0.750
GGT (U/L)	25.5	21.0	19.5	14.0	0.114
HDLC (mg/dL)	66.4	31.9	64.4	29.3	0.917
LDLC (mg/dL)	127.5	33.0	118.0	39.5	0.675
TG (mg/dL)	89.5	53.8	102.0	54.3	0.356
UA (mg/dL)	5.6	1.1	5.5	2.4	0.263

BMI, body mass index; ALT, Alanine aminotransferase; AST, aspartate aminotransferase; FPG, fasting plasma glucose; GGT, gamma-glutamyl transpeptidase; HDLC, high-density lipoprotein cholesterol; LDLC, low-density lipoprotein cholesterol; UA, uric acid; TG, triglyceride. * Two-tailed p-values were obtained using the Mann–Whitney U-test for two independent samples.

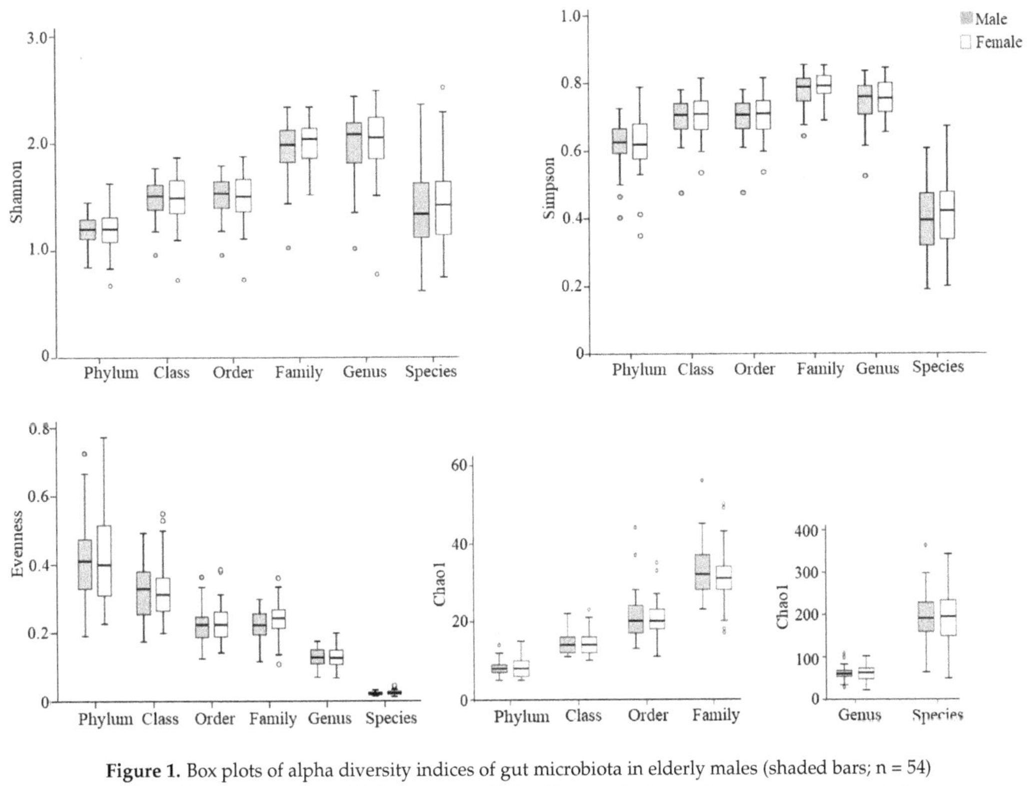

Figure 1. Box plots of alpha diversity indices of gut microbiota in elderly males (shaded bars; n = 54) and females (open bars; n = 46). The Shannon index, Simpson index, and evenness are presented as unitless values, while the Chao1 index is shown as the estimated number of taxa, reflecting species richness. Outliers are indicated by circles.

https://doi.org/10.3390/life16020297

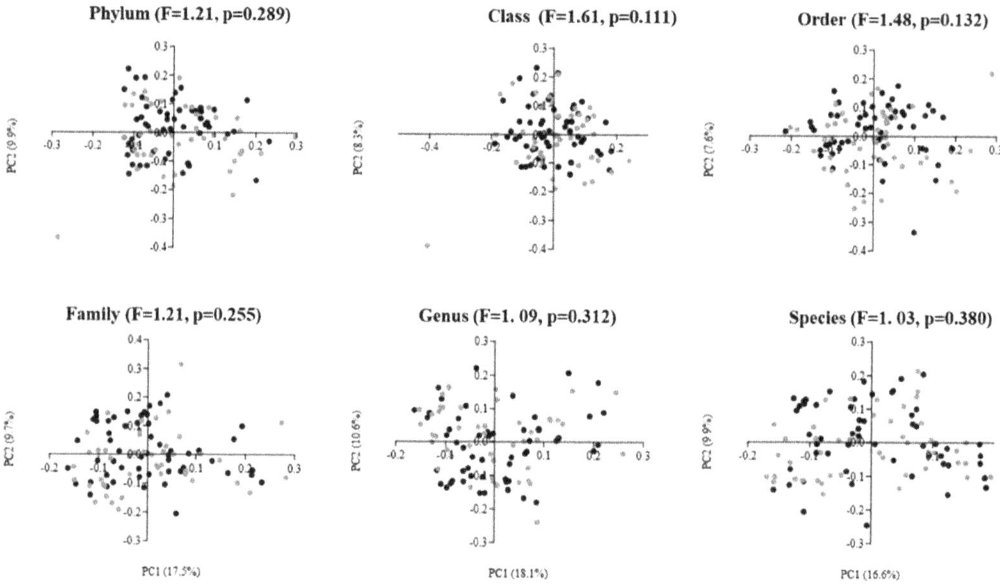

Figure 2. Principal coordinate analysis (PCoA) plots of gut microbiota in elderly males (black dots; n = 54) and females (gray dots; n = 46) using Bray–Curtis dissimilarity index at different taxonomic levels. The PCoA results are depicted as two-dimensional plots, with the axes indicating the percentage of data variance explained by the first two principal coordinate dimensions. The results of the PERMANOVA, comparing dissimilarity indices among groups, are displayed at the top of the plots for each corresponding taxonomic level.

Finally, we examined whether the relative abundance of the top ten most abundant taxa at each taxonomic level differed between male and female participants (Table 2). At the phylum level, in both male and female groups, the same taxa comprised the top ten list, with *Bacillota* (formerly *Firmicutes*) and *Bacteroidota* (formerly *Bacteroidetes*) as the core taxa making up the majority of the gut microbial community (>70% combined). At this level, no specific phyla were identified that differed significantly in relative abundance between males and females, except for *Bacteroidota*, the relative abundance of which was higher in males than in females (Mann–Whitney U-test, unadjusted $p < 0.05$; Table 2). At the class level, the most abundant microbial taxa were the same in both males and females, with Bacteroidia and Clostridia comprising the majority (>60% combined) of the gut microbiota. Compared with females, Bacteroidia and Betaproteobacteria showed a higher abundance in the male subjects (Mann–Whitney U-test, unadjusted $p < 0.05$; Table 2). When classified according to the order, OTU abundance revealed that Bacteroidales, Clostridiales, and Bifidobacteriales dominated the gut microbiota composition in both males and females (>70%). On the other hand, the relative abundance of Bacteroidales and Burkholderiales was higher in fecal samples of males compared to females (Mann–Whitney U-test, unadjusted $p < 0.05$; Table 2). However, after Benjamini–Hochberg FDR correction for multiple testing, none of the observed taxonomic differences in Table 2 remained statistically significant.

At the family and genus levels, nine, and at the species level, six of the top ten abundant taxa were common in both males and females (Table 2). However, the two groups of elderly subjects did not demonstrate any significant differences in any of the included taxa at these three (Family, Genus, Species) taxonomic levels.

https://doi.org/10.3390/life16020297

Table 2. (**a**) Percent relative abundances (mean ± SE) of the top ten most abundant taxa (ranked by overall abundance) at phylum, class and order taxonomic levels in elderly male and female participants. (**b**) Percent relative abundances (mean ± SE) of the top ten most abundant taxa (ranked by overall abundance) at family, genus and species taxonomic levels in elderly male and female participants.

(**a**)

	Male		Female	
Taxa	**Gut Microbiota**	**Mean ± SE**	**Gut Microbiota**	**Mean ± SE**
Phylum	*Bacillota*	44.01 ± 1.76	*Bacillota*	46.48 ± 2.05
	Bacteroidota *	36.07 ± 1.67	*Bacteroidota*	30.36 ± 1.75
	Actinomycetota	7.08 ± 0.99	*Actinomycetota*	10.03 ± 1.98
	Pseudomonadota	3.46 ± 0.53	*Pseudomonadota*	2.75 ± 0.48
	Verrucomicrobiota	0.51 ± 0.16	*Verrucomicrobiota*	1.48 ± 0.48
	Fusobacteriota	0.12 ± 0.08	*Euryarchaeota*	0.12 ± 0.05
	Chlamydiota	0.05 ± 0.01	*Synergistota*	0.10 ± 0.05
	Euryarchaeota	0.03 ± 0.01	*Fusobacteriota*	0.09 ± 0.05
	Synergistota	0.02 ± 0.01	*Lentisphaerota*	0.04 ± 0.02
	Lentisphaerota	0.01 ± 0.00	*Chlamydiota*	0.04 ± 0.01
Class	*Bacteroidia* *	35.77 ± 1.66	*Clostridia*	35.86 ± 1.87
	Clostridia	33.27 ± 1.47	*Bacteroidia*	29.98 ± 1.73
	Actinobacteria	5.32 ± 0.89	*Actinobacteria*	8.40 ± 1.96
	Bacilli	3.09 ± 0.53	*Bacilli*	2.89 ± 0.45
	Gammaproteobacteria	2.35 ± 0.50	*Gammaproteobacteria*	1.79 ± 0.46
	Negativicutes	1.74 ± 0.22	*Coriobacteriia*	1.59 ± 0.2
	Coriobacteriia	1.73 ± 0.17	*Verrucomicrobiae*	1.47 ± 0.48
	Betaproteobacteria *	0.51 ± 0.05	*Negativicutes*	1.27 ± 0.17
	Verrucomicrobiae	0.51 ± 0.16	*Betaproteobacteria*	0.41 ± 0.08
	Erysipelotrichia	0.40 ± 0.06	*Erysipelotrichia*	0.4 ± 0.06
Order	*Bacteroidales* *	35.74 ± 1.66	*Clostridiales*	35.47 ± 1.85
	Clostridiales	33.05 ± 1.47	*Bacteroidales*	29.96 ± 1.73
	Bifidobacteriales	5.14 ± 0.89	*Bifidobacteriales*	8.22 ± 1.96
	Lactobacillales	2.89 ± 0.53	*Lactobacillales*	2.75 ± 0.45
	Enterobacterales	2.00 ± 0.46	*Enterobacterales*	1.55 ± 0.42
	Coriobacteriales	1.53 ± 0.16	*Verrucomicrobiales*	1.47 ± 0.48
	Veillonellales	0.84 ± 0.16	*Coriobacteriales*	1.31 ± 0.20
	Acidaminococcales	0.51 ± 0.07	*Veillonellales*	0.71 ± 0.15
	Burkholderiales *	0.51 ± 0.05	*Acidaminococcales*	0.45 ± 0.08
	Verrucomicrobiales	0.51 ± 0.16	*Burkholderiales*	0.41 ± 0.08

(**b**)

	Male		Female	
Taxa	**Gut Microbiota**	**Mean ± SE**	**Gut Microbiota**	**Mean ± SE**
Family	*Bacteroidaceae*	17.13 ± 1.75	*Bacteroidaceae*	15.59 ± 1.44
	Prevotellaceae	9.91 ± 1.82	*Ruminococcaceae*	10.04 ± 0.83
	Ruminococcaceae	8.92 ± 0.84	*Bifidobacteriaceae*	7.91 ± 1.91
	Lachnospiraceae	6.43 ± 0.43	*Lachnospiraceae*	6.78 ± 0.53
	Bifidobacteriaceae	4.91 ± 0.83	*Prevotellaceae*	5.63 ± 1.63
	Rikenellaceae	3.37 ± 0.93	*Rikenellaceae*	3.29 ± 0.62
	Streptococcaceae	2.27 ± 0.51	*Eubacteriaceae*	2.08 ± 0.27
	Clostridiaceae	1.9 ± 0.18	*Clostridiaceae*	1.93 ± 0.23
	Eubacteriaceae	1.82 ± 0.17	*Streptococcaceae*	1.73 ± 0.34
	Coriobacteriaceae	1.49 ± 0.16	*Akkermansiaceae*	1.47 ± 0.48

https://doi.org/10.3390/life16020297

Table 2. *Cont.*

(b)				
	Male		**Female**	
Taxa	**Gut Microbiota**	**Mean ± SE**	**Gut Microbiota**	**Mean ± SE**
Genus	*Bacteroides*	17.04 ± 1.75	*Bacteroides*	15.51 ± 1.43
	Prevotella	9.62 ± 1.80	*Bifidobacterium*	7.85 ± 1.90
	Bifidobacterium	4.87 ± 0.83	*Prevotella*	5.26 ± 1.61
	Faecalibacterium	3.41 ± 0.36	*Ruminococcus*	3.74 ± 0.58
	Ruminococcus	3.30 ± 0.49	*Faecalibacterium*	3.41 ± 0.37
	Alistipes	3.10 ± 0.90	*Alistipes*	3.03 ± 0.58
	Streptococcus	2.22 ± 0.49	*Eubacterium*	2.01 ± 0.27
	Eubacterium	1.74 ± 0.17	*Streptococcus*	1.63 ± 0.34
	Clostridium	1.60 ± 0.17	*Clostridium*	1.63 ± 0.22
	Collinsella	1.47 ± 0.15	*Akkermansia*	1.47 ± 0.48
Species	*Prevotella copri*	3.44 ± 0.68	*Prevotella copri*	1.82 ± 0.6
	Faecalibacterium prausnitzii	1.44 ± 0.17	*Faecalibacterium prausnitzii*	1.52 ± 0.20
	Bifidobacterium adolescentis	0.64 ± 0.14	*Bifidobacterium adolescentis*	1.2 ± 0.35
	Bacteroides plebeius	0.48 ± 0.11	*Bifidobacterium longum*	0.66 ± 0.21
	Bifidobacterium longum	0.40 ± 0.10	*Bacillota bacterium CAG:124*	0.52 ± 0.20
	Bacteroides stercoris	0.38 ± 0.09	*Akkermansia muciniphila*	0.44 ± 0.14
	Bacteroides vulgatus	0.38 ± 0.06	*Bacteroides plebeius*	0.43 ± 0.16
	Ruminococcus sp. *CAG:254*	0.29 ± 0.10	*Subdoligranulum* sp. *APC924/74*	0.39 ± 0.09
	Subdoligranulum sp. *APC924/74*	0.28 ± 0.05	*Gemmiger formicilis*	0.37 ± 0.07
	Eubacterium sp. *CAG:180*	0.27 ± 0.06	*Bacteroides fragilis*	0.35 ± 0.11

* Indicates unadjusted $p < 0.05$ (Mann–Whitney U-test).

4. Discussion

In humans, studying sex-related differences in gut microbiota proves challenging due to the influence of both biological sex and socio-environmental factors [11]. Therefore, in the current study, we deliberately selected a population with similar sociodemographic and clinical characteristics (as reflected in Table 1) to enhance the robustness of our findings in elucidating sex-related differences in gut microbiota.

In this study, we did not detect any differences in the alpha diversity of gut microbial communities between males and females at any taxonomic level. In a relatively large dataset of gut microbiota analyzed at the genus level using 16S rRNA gene sequencing among Japanese adults aged 70 years and older, no significant differences in α-diversity were observed between males and females [19]. Similarly, Haro et al. did not observe any differences in alpha diversity between males and females when the average age of the participants was around 60 years [20]. In contrast, a Chinese study conducted among a cohort including both young and old adults exhibited a higher Shannon index of alpha diversity for the fecal microbiota of females [14]. Similarly, in a population-based cohort study conducted among participants from the northern provinces of the Netherlands, with an age range of 18–81 years, the authors showed that females had a greater Shannon index of diversity [21]. Consistent with these findings, in a study of male and female populations aged 48.7 ± 10.2 to 53.8 ± 7.7 years, Borgo et al. observed a decreased alpha diversity at the species level in the mucosa-associated gut microbiota of male subjects [22]. Conversely, a Korean study by Shin et al. conducted among apparently healthy subjects aged 25 to 65 years and a Japanese study by Takagi et al. among healthy subjects aged 20 to 89 years did not reveal any differences between males and females in the alpha diversity of gut microbiota [11,15].

The earlier discussion of the relevant literature indicates that sex-specific differences in gut microbial alpha diversity are inconsistent and sometimes contradictory. It is also difficult to directly compare our findings on gut microbial alpha diversity with those of other studies, as the majority of published research includes both young and older subjects or centenarians, whereas our study focused solely on the elderly. Additionally, many of these studies did not clearly report the taxonomic level at which sex-related differences in gut microbial diversity were observed, or they did not conduct analyses across all taxonomic levels. However, considering both the findings from the existing literature and the results of our study, we posit that, among the elderly, sex-related differences in gut microbial alpha diversity are likely to be fairly subtle.

In our study, PCoA for beta diversity did not reveal distinct clustering patterns for elderly males and females. This aligns with findings from five separate studies that utilized PCoA showing no separation between males and females [11,12,19,22,23]. Similarly, PCoA did not demonstrate significant grouping based on sex in the colonic microbiota among healthy participants aged 7 to 52 years across five northern European countries [24]. Therefore, it seems plausible that, regardless of subjects' age, sex does not have a significant impact on the beta diversity of gut microbiota in the elderly.

At the phylum level, we observed a higher abundance of *Bacteroidota* among elderly males compared with elderly females. Koliada et al. also studied sex differences in the phylum-level human gut microbiota composition among subjects aged 0–60+ years and reported a significant decrease in the relative abundance of *Bacteroidota* in females compared to males [25]. However, this finding contradicts those of Gao et al. (2018), Shin et al. (2019), and Haro et al. (2016), who did not identify any differences in the relative abundance of specific taxa at the phylum level between the two sex groups [11,14,20].

In our study, *Bacteroidia* and *Betaproteobacteria*, at the class level, and *Bacteroidales* and *Burkholderiales*, at the order level, showed higher abundances in the fecal samples of elderly males. However, these between-sex differences were nominal (unadjusted $p < 0.05$) and did not remain statistically significant after Benjamini–Hochberg false discovery rate correction, suggesting that any sex-associated taxonomic shifts in this cohort are subtle. On the other hand, Gao et al. (2018) did not observe any significant taxonomic differences at the class or order levels between males and females [14].

In our study, at the Family and Genus taxonomic levels, the gut microbiota composition with respect to the most abundant microbial taxa was found to be similar between elderly males and females. In the available literature, a number of published studies have reported the sex-specific composition and relevant differences in gut microbiota, especially at the genus taxonomic level, although these findings are often inconsistent. For example, Haro et al. observed a higher presence of the genera *Veillonella* and *Methanobrevibacter* in fecal samples from males compared to females, while the abundance of the genus *Bilophila* was higher in females [20]. Santos-Marcos et al. found higher levels of the genera *Ruminococcus* and *Bilophila* in healthy females, and higher levels of the genera *Clostridium* and *SMB53* in males than in their opposite-sex groups [26]. Gao et al. and Takagi et al. also observed a higher abundance of the genus *Ruminococcus* in fecal samples from females compared to males [14,15]. Moreover, Takagi et al. observed elevated numbers of the genera *Prevotella, Megamonas, Megasphaera,* and *Fusobacterium* in males, while *Bifidobacterium* and *Akkermansia* were detected at higher levels in females [14,15]. In a study of a population aged 24 to 100 years, Mueller et al. observed gender effects at the genus level for the *Bacteroides-Prevotella* group, with higher levels in males [27]. In contrast, Singh and Manning, in their study among healthy individuals including elderly people, observed that the genus *Paraprevotella* was differentially abundant in the intestinal microbial community of males, whereas the genera *Dialister, Lactobacillus,* unclassified *Lactobacillaceae,* unclassified *Comamonadaceae,* and *Comamonas* were differentially abundant in females [12].

At the species level, six taxa were found to be common in both elderly males and females in our study, and no significant gender differences were observed for any of the

https://doi.org/10.3390/life16020297

top 10 taxa. At this taxonomic level, compared with females, a higher abundance of *Bacteroides plebeius* (in subjects with BMI > 33 kg/m^2) and *Coprococcus catus* (in subjects with BMI < 30 kg/m^2) was found among males in the study by Haro et al. [20]. Meanwhile, *Bacteroides thetaiotaomicron, Eubacterium eligens, Klebsiella pneumoniae, Sutterella stercoricanis, Ruminococcus obeum* and *Ruminococcus bromii* showed higher abundances among males in the study by Li et al. [28]. In contrast, after adjusting for different confounding factors, Sinha et al. revealed that *Akkermansia muciniphila* was associated with sex, with females having a higher abundance of this species [21].

All the aforementioned findings demonstrate the existence of discrepancies in the current literature regarding the composition and abundance of dominant gut microbiota in male versus female subjects at various taxonomic levels. These variations in the reported findings may, in part, stem from the inclusion of subjects across diverse races, ages, and other demographic and socio-environmental factors, as well as differences in health status and diet [29]. However, we observed a similarity in gut microbial diversity among elderly males and females, with only small differences in the gut microbial composition at three different taxonomic levels. The current study design precludes elucidating the mechanisms responsible for the disparities observed between studies regarding gut microbiota composition and diversity between males and females. It has been mentioned that sex-specific steroid hormones, such as estradiol in females and testosterone in males, could play pivotal roles in modulating gut microbial composition and differentiation between the sexes [11,30,31]. As aging progresses, there is a gradual but robust decline in testosterone production in males and almost complete loss of estrogen at menopause in females [32–35]. Therefore, it is possible that the age-related decline in circulating levels of primary sex steroid hormones in both males and females likely contributes to the decrease or disappearance of gut microbial sex differences among the elderly.

In reporting our findings, we presented the relative abundance data as mean $\pm$ SE. This approach aligns with common reporting practices in microbiome research, where mean values are widely used to summarize relative abundance data to enhance clarity and facilitate comparison across studies [17,20,22,26]. However, as noted by Gloor et al. (2017) and Weiss et al. (2017), the compositional nature of microbiome data requires cautious interpretation of such summary statistics [36,37]. Also, interpretations of our findings should also be considered in light of several potential limitations. Firstly, detailed information on diet and lifestyle was not available for this analysis. Such factors are known to influence gut microbiota composition and may also differ between males and females. Therefore, residual confounding cannot be excluded and could have attenuated or obscured modest sex-associated differences. Nevertheless, because participants were community-dwelling elderly recruited from the same geographic area and shared broadly similar socio-demographic characteristics, large between-sex differences in these exposures were likely reduced in this cohort. Future studies incorporating standardized dietary/lifestyle assessments will be important to better distinguish biological sex effects from behavioral and environmental influences. Secondly, the cross-sectional design of our study precludes any causal inference between sex and the gut microbiome. Another potential limitation is the relatively small sample size. Although the present sample size (n = 100) is acceptable for shotgun metagenomic profiling in an elderly cohort, the study may have been underpowered to detect subtle sex-associated differences at lower taxonomic levels (e.g., genus and species). Larger cohorts or multi-center studies will be necessary to validate these findings and to determine whether more granular taxonomic or functional sex-related differences emerge in advanced age. Nevertheless, we believe that our study adds useful evidence on sex-associated patterns of the gut microbiota among the elderly. Lastly, since this study

https://doi.org/10.3390/life16020297

was conducted exclusively among a Japanese elderly population, the generalizability of the observed findings may be limited.

5. Conclusions

This study revealed that gut microbial diversity and overall community structure are largely similar between apparently healthy elderly Japanese males and females, with only modest sex-associated differences observed in the relative abundance of selected taxa at higher taxonomic levels. These results suggest that, in advanced age, biological sex has a limited influence on gut microbiota composition at the population level. Accordingly, our findings provide population-level reference data for the gut microbiota of older adults and indicate that sex alone may not be a primary stratification factor when considering microbiota-modulating strategies aimed at promoting healthy aging. Future longitudinal and interventional studies are warranted to evaluate whether responses to microbiota-targeted interventions differ meaningfully by sex in older populations and to identify host or environmental factors that may better inform stratification and personalization.

Supplementary Materials: The following supporting information can be downloaded at: https://www.mdpi.com/article/10.3390/life16020297/s1, Table S1: Per-sample shotgun metagenomic sequencing and read-processing metrics.

Author Contributions: Conceptualization: M.H.M., R.H., N.Y. and T.T.; methodology: M.H.M., R.H., N.Y., Y.A. and K.O.; formal analysis: M.H.M., N.I., M.H., F.H. and T.Y.; investigation: M.H.M., R.H., N.Y., Y.A. and T.H.; resources: Y.H., Y.I., Y.U., R.Y., R.K., H.T., M.M., K.K. and K.M.; data curation: M.H.M., R.H., N.Y., Y.A. and K.D.; writing—original draft preparation: M.H.M., R.H. and N.Y.; writing—review and editing: Y.A., Y.H., Y.I., Y.U., R.Y., R.K., H.T., M.M., K.K. and K.M.; visualization: M.H.M., R.H., N.I. and M.H.; supervision: N.Y., T.H., K.O. and T.T.; project administration: R.H., N.Y., F.H., T.Y., K.D., T.H., K.O. and T.T.; funding acquisition: T.T. and M.H.M. All authors have read and agreed to the published version of the manuscript.

Funding: This research was supported by a joint project funded by Yamaguchi Prefecture, Yamaguchi City, Shimadzu Corporation, Kao Corporation, and Kyodo Milk Industry Co., Ltd. It was also supported by a Grant-in-Aid for Scientific Research (No. 21K10397) from the Japan Society for the Promotion of Science (JSPS).

Institutional Review Board Statement: This study was conducted in accordance with the principles of the Declaration of Helsinki, and the study protocol was approved by the institutional review board of Yamaguchi University (Approval No. 2020-183-3; approval date: 25 January 2021).

Informed Consent Statement: Informed consent was obtained from all subjects involved in the study.

Data Availability Statement: The data generated in this study are not currently publicly available due to data-governance agreements with collaborating partners. De-identified, host-filtered sequencing data and/or other datasets supporting the findings are available from the corresponding author upon reasonable request, subject to approval by the relevant parties and, where applicable, execution of a data-sharing agreement.

Acknowledgments: The authors express their sincere gratitude to the participants of this study and the staff of all the organizations that collaborated on this project.

Conflicts of Interest: Y.H., Y.I., Y.U. and R.Y. are employees of Shimadzu Corporation; R.K. and H.T. are employees of Kao Corporation; and M.M. is an employee of Kyodo Milk Industry Co., Ltd. The funders had no role in the design of the study; in the analysis or interpretation of the data; in the preparation of the original draft of the manuscript; or in the decision to publish. The authors declare no financial conflicts of interest related to the results or interpretation of the reported findings.

https://doi.org/10.3390/life16020297

References

1. Badal, V.D.; Vaccariello, E.D.; Mxurray, E.R.; Yu, K.E.; Knight, R.; Jeste, D.V.; Nguyen, T.T. The Gut Microbiome, Aging, and Longevity: A Systematic Review. *Nutrients* **2020**, *12*, 3759. [CrossRef] [PubMed]
2. O'Toole, P.W.; Jeffery, I.B. Gut microbiota and aging. *Science* **2015**, *350*, 1214–1215. [CrossRef] [PubMed]
3. Schroeder, B.O.; Bäckhed, F. Signals from the gut microbiota to distant organs in physiology and disease. *Nat. Med.* **2016**, *22*, 1079–1089. [CrossRef]
4. Carding, S.; Verbeke, K.; Vipond, D.T.; Corfe, B.M.; Owen, L.J. Dysbiosis of the gut microbiota in disease. *Microb. Ecol. Health Dis.* **2015**, *26*, 26191. [CrossRef]
5. Murphy, K.; O'Donovan, A.N.; Caplice, N.M.; Ross, R.P.; Stanton, C. Exploring the Gut Microbiota and Cardiovascular Disease. *Metabolites* **2021**, *11*, 493. [CrossRef]
6. Shanahan, F. The colonic microbiota in health and disease. *Curr. Opin. Gastroenterol.* **2013**, *29*, 49–54. [CrossRef]
7. Brahe, L.K.; Astrup, A.; Larsen, L.H. Can We Prevent Obesity-Related Metabolic Diseases by Dietary Modulation of the Gut Microbiota? *Adv. Nutr.* **2016**, *7*, 90–101. [CrossRef]
8. Toward, R.; Montandon, S.; Walton, G.; Gibson, G.R. Effect of prebiotics on the human gut microbiota of elderly persons. *Gut Microbes* **2012**, *3*, 57–60. [CrossRef]
9. Annandale, E.; Hammarström, A. Constructing the 'gender-specific body': A critical discourse analysis of publications in the field of gender-specific medicine. *Health* **2011**, *15*, 571–587. [CrossRef]
10. Kim, Y.S.; Kim, N. Sex-Gender Differences in Irritable Bowel Syndrome. *J. Neurogastroenterol. Motil.* **2018**, *24*, 544–558. [CrossRef]
11. Shin, J.H.; Park, Y.H.; Sim, M.; Kim, S.A.; Joung, H.; Shin, D.M. Serum level of sex steroid hormone is associated with diversity and profiles of human gut microbiome. *Res. Microbiol.* **2019**, *170*, 192–201. [CrossRef]
12. Singh, P.; Manning, S.D. Impact of age and sex on the composition and abundance of the intestinal microbiota in individuals with and without enteric infections. *Ann. Epidemiol.* **2016**, *26*, 380–385. [CrossRef] [PubMed]
13. Dominianni, C.; Sinha, R.; Goedert, J.J.; Pei, Z.; Yang, L.; Hayes, R.B.; Ahn, J. Sex, body mass index, and dietary fiber intake influence the human gut microbiome. *PLoS ONE* **2015**, *10*, e0124599. [CrossRef]
14. Gao, X.; Zhang, M.; Xue, J.; Huang, J.; Zhuang, R.; Zhou, X.; Zhang, H.; Fu, Q.; Hao, Y. Body Mass Index Differences in the Gut Microbiota Are Gender Specific. *Front. Microbiol.* **2018**, *9*, 1250. [CrossRef]
15. Takagi, T.; Naito, Y.; Inoue, R.; Kashiwagi, S.; Uchiyama, K.; Mizushima, K.; Tsuchiya, S.; Dohi, O.; Yoshida, N.; Kamada, K.; et al. Differences in gut microbiota associated with age, sex, and stool consistency in healthy Japanese subjects. *J. Gastroenterol.* **2019**, *54*, 53–63. Erratum in *J. Gastroenterol.* **2019**, *54*, 96–98. https://doi.org/10.1007/s00535-018-1504-9. [CrossRef]
16. Hopkins, M.J.; Macfarlane, G.T. Changes in predominant bacterial populations in human faeces with age and with Clostridium difficile infection. *J. Med. Microbiol.* **2002**, *51*, 448–454. [CrossRef]
17. Woodmansey, E.J.; McMurdo, M.E.; Macfarlane, G.T.; Macfarlane, S. Comparison of compositions and metabolic activities of fecal microbiotas in young adults and in antibiotic-treated and non-antibiotic-treated elderly subjects. *Appl. Environ. Microbiol.* **2004**, *70*, 6113–6122. [CrossRef]
18. Hammer, Ø.; Harper, D.A. Past: Paleontological statistics software package for education and data analysis. *Palaeontol. Electron.* **2001**, *4*, 9.
19. Hatayama, K.; Kono, K.; Okuma, K.; Hasuko, K.; Masuyama, H.; Benno, Y. Sex Differences in Intestinal Microbiota and Their Association with Some Diseases in a Japanese Population Observed by Analysis Using a Large Dataset. *Biomedicines* **2023**, *11*, 376. [CrossRef]
20. Haro, C.; Rangel-Zúñiga, O.A.; Alcalá-Díaz, J.F.; Gómez-Delgado, F.; Pérez-Martínez, P.; Delgado-Lista, J.; Quintana-Navarro, G.M.; Landa, B.B.; Navas-Cortés, J.A.; Tena-Sempere, M.; et al. Intestinal Microbiota Is Influenced by Gender and Body Mass Index. *PLoS ONE* **2016**, *11*, e0154090. [CrossRef] [PubMed]
21. Sinha, T.; Vich Vila, A.; Garmaeva, S.; Jankipersadsing, S.A.; Imhann, F.; Collij, V.; Bonder, M.J.; Jiang, X.; Gurry, T.; Alm, E.J.; et al. Analysis of 1135 gut metagenomes identifies sex-specific resistome profiles. *Gut Microbes* **2019**, *10*, 358–366. [CrossRef]
22. Borgo, F.; Garbossa, S.; Riva, A.; Severgnini, M.; Luigiano, C.; Benetti, A.; Pontiroli, A.E.; Morace, G.; Borghi, E. Body Mass Index and Sex Affect Diverse Microbial Niches within the Gut. *Front. Microbiol.* **2018**, *9*, 213. [CrossRef] [PubMed] [PubMed Central]
23. Greenhill, A.R.; Tsuji, H.; Ogata, K.; Natsuhara, K.; Morita, A.; Soli, K.; Larkins, J.A.; Tadokoro, K.; Odani, S.; Baba, J.; et al. Characterization of the gut microbiota of Papua New Guineans using reverse transcription quantitative PCR. *PLoS ONE* **2015**, *10*, e0117427. [CrossRef]
24. Lay, C.; Rigottier-Gois, L.; Holmstrøm, K.; Rajilic, M.; Vaughan, E.E.; de Vos, W.M.; Collins, M.D.; Thiel, R.; Namsolleck, P.; Blaut, M.; et al. Colonic microbiota signatures across five northern European countries. *Appl. Environ. Microbiol.* **2005**, *71*, 4153–4155. [CrossRef] [PubMed] [PubMed Central]
25. Koliada, A.; Moseiko, V.; Romanenko, M.; Lushchak, O.; Kryzhanovska, N.; Guryanov, V.; Vaiserman, A. Sex differences in the phylum-level human gut microbiota composition. *BMC Microbiol.* **2021**, *21*, 131. [CrossRef]

https://doi.org/10.3390/life16020297

26. Santos-Marcos, J.A.; Haro, C.; Vega-Rojas, A.; Alcala-Diaz, J.F.; Molina-Abril, H.; Leon-Acuña, A.; Lopez-Moreno, J.; Landa, B.B.; Tena-Sempere, M.; Perez-Martinez, P.; et al. Sex Differences in the Gut Microbiota as Potential Determinants of Gender Predisposition to Disease. *Mol. Nutr. Food Res.* **2019**, *63*, e1800870. [CrossRef]
27. Mueller, S.; Saunier, K.; Hanisch, C.; Norin, E.; Alm, L.; Midtvedt, T.; Cresci, A.; Silvi, S.; Orpianesi, C.; Verdenelli, M.C.; et al. Differences in fecal microbiota in different European study populations in relation to age, gender, and country: A cross-sectional study. *Appl. Environ. Microbiol.* **2006**, *72*, 1027–1033. [CrossRef] [PubMed]
28. Li, M.; Wang, B.; Zhang, M.; Rantalainen, M.; Wang, S.; Zhou, H.; Zhang, Y.; Shen, J.; Pang, X.; Zhang, M.; et al. Symbiotic gut microbes modulate human metabolic phenotypes. *Proc. Natl. Acad. Sci. USA* **2008**, *105*, 2117–2122. [CrossRef] [PubMed]
29. Rinninella, E.; Raoul, P.; Cintoni, M.; Franceschi, F.; Miggiano, G.A.D.; Gasbarrini, A.; Mele, M.C. What is the Healthy Gut Microbiota Composition? A Changing Ecosystem across Age, Environment, Diet, and Diseases. *Microorganisms* **2019**, *7*, 14. [CrossRef]
30. Markle, J.G.; Frank, D.N.; Mortin-Toth, S.; Robertson, C.E.; Feazel, L.M.; Rolle-Kampczyk, U.; von Bergen, M.; McCoy, K.D.; Macpherson, A.J.; Danska, J.S. Sex differences in the gut microbiome drive hormone-dependent regulation of autoimmunity. *Science* **2013**, *339*, 1084–1088. [CrossRef] [PubMed]
31. Yurkovetskiy, L.; Burrows, M.; Khan, A.A.; Graham, L.; Volchkov, P.; Becker, L.; Antonopoulos, D.; Umesaki, Y.; Chervonsky, A.V. Gender bias in autoimmunity is influenced by microbiota. *Immunity* **2013**, *39*, 400–412. [CrossRef]
32. Manly, J.J.; Merchant, C.A.; Jacobs, D.M.; Small, S.A.; Bell, K.; Ferin, M.; Mayeux, R. Endogenous estrogen levels and Alzheimer's disease among postmenopausal women. *Neurology* **2000**, *54*, 833–837. [CrossRef] [PubMed]
33. Morley, J.E.; Kaiser, F.E.; Perry, H.M., 3rd; Patrick, P.; Morley, P.M.; Stauber, P.M.; Vellas, B.; Baumgartner, R.N.; Garry, P.J. Longitudinal changes in testosterone, luteinizing hormone, and follicle-stimulating hormone in healthy older men. *Metabolism* **1997**, *46*, 410–413. [CrossRef] [PubMed]
34. Rosario, E.R.; Chang, L.; Head, E.H.; Stanczyk, F.Z.; Pike, C.J. Brain levels of sex steroid hormones in men and women during normal aging and in Alzheimer's disease. *Neurobiol. Aging* **2011**, *32*, 604–613. [CrossRef] [PubMed]
35. Scavello, I.; Maseroli, E.; Di Stasi, V.; Vignozzi, L. Sexual Health in Menopause. *Medicina* **2019**, *55*, 559. [CrossRef]
36. Gloor, G.B.; Macklaim, J.M.; Pawlowsky-Glahn, V.; Egozcue, J.J. Microbiome Datasets Are Compositional: And This Is Not Optional. *Front. Microbiol.* **2017**, *8*, 2224. [CrossRef]
37. Weiss, S.; Xu, Z.Z.; Peddada, S.; Amir, A.; Bittinger, K.; Gonzalez, A.; Lozupone, C.; Zaneveld, J.R.; Vázquez-Baeza, Y.; Birmingham, A.; et al. Normalization and microbial differential abundance strategies depend upon data characteristics. *Microbiome* **2017**, *5*, 27. [CrossRef]

https://doi.org/10.3390/life16020297

life

MDPI

Review

Learning from an Emerging Infection: How the COVID-19 Pandemic Reshaped Gastric Cancer Care

Alexandru Marian Vieru [1,†], Dumitru Radulescu [2,†], Liliana Streba [3,*], Emil Tiberius Trasca [2,*], Sergiu Marian Cazacu [4,†], Razvan-Cristian Statie [4], Petrica Popa [4] and Tudorel Ciurea [4]

1 Doctoral School, University of Medicine and Pharmacy of Craiova, Petru Rares Street No 2-4, 200349 Craiova, Romania
2 General Surgery Department, University of Medicine and Pharmacy of Craiova, Petru Rares Street No 2-4, 200349 Craiova, Romania
3 Oncology Department, University of Medicine and Pharmacy of Craiova, Petru Rares Street No 2-4, 200349 Craiova, Romania
4 Gastroenterology Department, University of Medicine and Pharmacy of Craiova, Petru Rares Street No 2-4, 200349 Craiova, Romania
* Correspondence: liliana.streba@umfcv.ro (L.S.); etrasca@yahoo.com (E.T.T.)
† These authors contributed equally to this work.

Abstract

Background/Objectives: The COVID-19 pandemic profoundly disrupted gastric cancer care, reducing access to screening, delaying diagnosis, and altering therapeutic pathways worldwide. Beyond clinical challenges, it exposed structural weaknesses in healthcare systems but also accelerated innovation. **Methods:** We conducted a narrative review supported by a structured literature search (PubMed/MEDLINE, Scopus, Web of Science; 1 January 2014–30 November 2025), with a narrative synthesis of observational studies, registry analyses, and meta-analyses addressing COVID-19–related changes in gastric cancer epidemiology, diagnosis, treatment, vaccination, and telemedicine. A PRISMA-style flow diagram was used to illustrate study selection. **Results:** Elective endoscopy volumes fell by up to 80%, leading to diagnostic backlogs and increased proportions of advanced-stage gastric cancer. Surgical postponements, modified chemotherapy and radiotherapy schedules, and reduced molecular/genetic testing further compromised outcomes. Conversely, vaccination, telemedicine, capsule endoscopy, and adaptive triage frameworks enabled partial recovery of services. Geographical variations were observed in the recovery of gastric cancer care services, with regions that had established screening infrastructure generally resuming activity more rapidly, whereas others experienced ongoing delays and diagnostic backlogs. **Conclusions:** This review integrates epidemiological, diagnostic, and therapeutic evidence to demonstrate how COVID-19 redefined gastric cancer care. By highlighting regional disparities and outlining a conceptual model for oncologic resilience, it provides an innovative framework for future crisis preparedness. The lessons of the pandemic—digital health integration, flexible treatment protocols, and international collaboration—represent a foundation for more robust, equitable gastric cancer management in the post-pandemic era.

Keywords: gastric cancer; COVID-19; early diagnosis; endoscopy; therapeutic strategies; vaccination; telemedicine; healthcare resilience

1. Introduction

1.1. Global Context of Gastric Cancer

Gastric cancer represents a major public health challenge worldwide, with over one million new cases each year and remaining one of the leading causes of cancer-related deaths despite a downward trend in recent decades [1,2].

This decline is largely attributed to improved socioeconomic conditions, enhanced hygiene practices, and better food-preservation techniques, particularly in developed regions; however, the overall number of cases remains high due to population aging and ongoing demographic growth [3].

Geographically, the incidence is notably high in East Asia; according to recent GLOBOCAN estimates (2022), age-standardized incidence rates (ASR, world standard) are 13.7 per 100,000 in China and approximately 27 per 100,000 in Japan (27.6) and South Korea (27.0), supporting the substantial regional burden and associated mortality impact [4]. In countries such as Japan and South Korea, although the absolute number of cases is still considerable, the implementation of population-based endoscopic screening programs has led to more frequent early-stage diagnoses and improved survival [5,6].

By comparison, the incidence is lower in Western Europe and North America, with age-standardized incidence rates (ASR, world standard) of 6.4 per 100,000 in Germany and 4.1 per 100,000 in the United States (GLOBOCAN 2022). In these regions, a relative shift toward proximal/cardia tumors has been described, and proximal (cardia) gastric adenocarcinoma is linked to obesity and gastroesophageal reflux disease [4,7,8].

In resource-limited regions like parts of Africa and Latin America, inadequate epidemiological data combined with poor access to healthcare continue to contribute to high mortality rates [9,10].

Helicobacter pylori infection remains the primary etiological factor, accounting for the vast majority of non-cardia gastric cancers (≈89%) and a substantial share of overall gastric cancers globally [11].

The bacterium induces chronic inflammation and atrophic gastritis, and when coupled with smoking and a high-salt, preserved-food diet, it can trigger preneoplastic changes that progress to cancer [12–14].

Genetic predisposition also plays a role, ranging from well-defined familial syndromes (such as CDH1 mutations) to less specific family history, while dietary patterns—particularly high consumption of processed foods and low intake of fruits and vegetables—further contribute to risk [12,14,15].

Despite advances in screening and treatment, the global burden of gastric cancer remains substantial; therefore, prevention strategies—risk-factor reduction, *Helicobacter pylori* eradication, early diagnosis, and modern therapies—are critical for lowering mortality [2,3,11–15].

1.2. The Role of Upper Gastrointestinal Endoscopy in Gastric Cancer Diagnosis

Upper gastrointestinal endoscopy is the preferred method for detecting and characterizing gastric lesions with malignant potential, as it permits direct visualization of the mucosa and enables targeted biopsies of suspicious areas [16,17].

In countries like Japan and South Korea, the integration of endoscopy into national screening programs has resulted in the frequent detection of early-stage gastric cancer, which directly improves survival outcomes [5,6].

Compared to barium radiography, endoscopy offers superior sensitivity for detecting early lesions, with the added advantage of providing tissue samples for histopathological confirmation [18].

https://doi.org/10.3390/life16010161

The use of advanced imaging modalities, such as narrow-band imaging and magnifying endoscopy, further enhances visualization of subtle mucosal changes and allows more precise characterization of suspicious lesions [19].

The quality of the examination and the expertise of the endoscopist are critical factors in ensuring high detection rates for early gastric lesions, and repeat endoscopies in patients with preneoplastic conditions or under surveillance can increase the likelihood of detecting progression toward advanced disease [16,18].

Beyond diagnosis, endoscopy also facilitates minimally invasive therapeutic interventions such as endoscopic mucosal resection (EMR) and endoscopic submucosal dissection (ESD). These techniques enable en bloc removal of early lesions, which is essential for accurate histological assessment and for minimizing local recurrence [20–23].

Thus, upper gastrointestinal endoscopy represents a cornerstone in reducing gastric cancer mortality, spanning the continuum from screening and diagnosis to early therapeutic management.

1.3. Objective of the Narrative Review

This review aims to assess the impact of the COVID-19 pandemic on the diagnosis and management of gastric cancer by examining epidemiological trends and the practical consequences of mobility restrictions and healthcare system reorganization.

It highlights how reduced access to endoscopic investigations and disruptions in treatment flows have led to delays in early diagnosis and an increased proportion of advanced-stage cases.

Additionally, the review explores adaptations in chemotherapy, radiotherapy, and surgical protocols for gastric cancer patients, emphasizing the roles of vaccination and telemedicine in restoring optimal oncologic services.

Finally, it discusses future directions, including enhanced screening and *Helicobacter pylori* eradication efforts, the development of adaptable emergency plans, and the importance of international collaboration to ensure the continuity of patient care during global crises.

While previous literature has addressed the general impact of the COVID-19 pandemic on oncology and, in some instances, on gastric cancer specifically, there is a lack of comprehensive reviews that systematically integrate epidemiological data, practical diagnostic and therapeutic challenges, and adaptive strategies developed during the pandemic. This review distinguishes itself by:

- Providing an integrated analysis of epidemiological, diagnostic, and therapeutic changes in gastric cancer care during the COVID-19 pandemic;
- Comparing the impact and recovery strategies across regions with different healthcare resources;
- Identifying current knowledge gaps and proposing a conceptual framework for future crisis management in gastrointestinal oncology.

By adopting this approach, the present review offers both a critical synthesis of the available evidence and practical recommendations, aiming to inform clinical practice and guide future research in the field. An integrative overview of these objectives is summarized in Figure 1, which illustrates the conceptual framework of pandemic-related disruptions and adaptive strategies in gastric cancer care.

https://doi.org/10.3390/life16010161

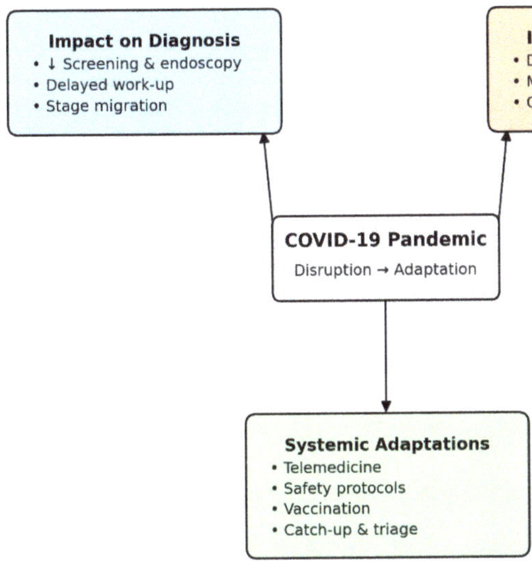

Figure 1. Conceptual framework of the impact of COVID-19 on gastric cancer care. Arrows indicate the directional influence of the COVID-19 pandemic on diagnostic and treatment pathways, and on systemic adaptations.

2. Materials and Methods

2.1. Design of the Review

This study is a narrative review supported by a structured literature search, designed to synthesize and contextualize the available evidence regarding the impact of the COVID-19 pandemic on gastric cancer care. Given the use of explicit eligibility criteria and a transparent study selection process, a PRISMA-style flow diagram was used to illustrate article identification, screening, and inclusion (Figure 2). A completed PRISMA 2020 checklist, used as a reporting and transparency aid for the selection process, is provided as Supplementary File S1. No meta-analysis was planned or performed due to substantial heterogeneity across study designs and outcomes.

2.2. Information Sources and Timeframe

The bibliographic search was performed in three major databases: PubMed/MEDLINE, Scopus, and Web of Science, covering publications from 1 January 2014 to 30 November 2025. Only full-text, peer-reviewed articles published in English and involving human subjects were considered. The inclusion of pre-pandemic studies (2014–2019) allowed the establishment of a baseline for epidemiological trends and management practices, providing context for the analysis of pandemic-related disruptions.

2.3. Search Strategy

Search queries combined controlled vocabulary and free-text terms related to gastric cancer and pandemic.

For PubMed/MEDLINE, the core search string was:

("Stomach Neoplasms"[Mesh] OR "gastric cancer" OR "stomach cancer") AND ("COVID-19"[Mesh] OR "SARS-CoV-2" OR "coronavirus disease 2019" OR pandemic) AND (screening OR endoscopy OR diagnosis OR surgery OR chemotherapy OR radiotherapy OR telemedicine OR vaccination).

https://doi.org/10.3390/life16010161

Equivalent strategies, adapted to database-specific syntax and subject headings, were used in Scopus and Web of Science, searching titles, abstracts, and keywords. No study-design filters were applied at the search stage, in order to maximize sensitivity. Keyword selection was guided by expert consensus among authors and an initial exploratory screening to ensure comprehensive coverage of epidemiology, diagnosis, treatment, vaccination, and telemedicine.

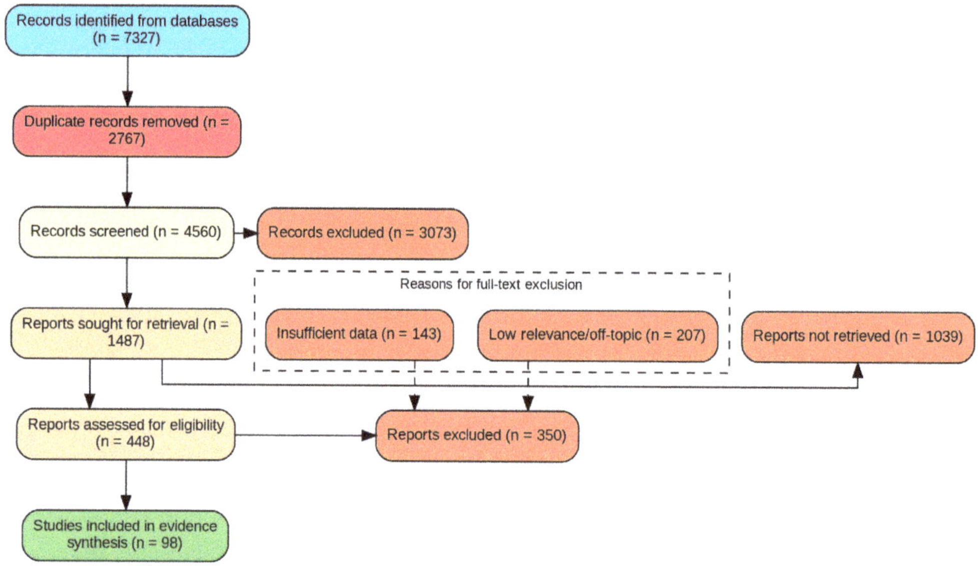

Figure 2. PRISMA flow diagram of the study selection process.

2.4. Eligibility Criteria

Inclusion: Observational studies, registry analyses, clinical series, and meta-analyses reporting data on incidence, stage distribution, diagnostic pathways (including endoscopy), treatment adaptations (surgery, systemic therapy, radiotherapy), or pandemic-specific interventions (telemedicine, vaccination).

Exclusion: Reports without clear study periods, those focusing exclusively on non-gastric neoplasms, or studies with small/ambiguous cohorts lacking interpretable outcomes.

Guidelines/consensus statements, editorials/letters, and methodological reports were included as contextual/background sources to describe practice changes, but were not treated as core evidence for quantitative statements.

2.5. Study Selection Process

The initial search yielded 7327 records. All records were exported to a reference manager and duplicates were removed prior to screening. Titles/abstracts and full texts were screened independently by two reviewers, with disagreements resolved by consensus. After screening, 1487 reports were sought for retrieval; 1039 could not be retrieved in full text. The remaining 448 reports were assessed for eligibility. Following full-text assessment, 350 reports were excluded (207 for low relevance/off-topic and 143 for insufficient data), resulting in 98 sources included in the evidence synthesis. The study selection process is summarized in the PRISMA flow diagram (Figure 2).

https://doi.org/10.3390/life16010161

2.6. Study Typology

The 98 included sources were heterogeneous in methodology. Their distribution by type is summarized in Figure 3—study typology:

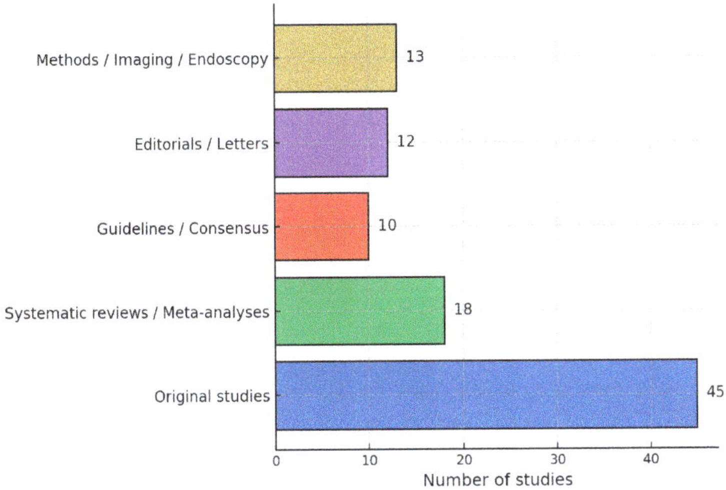

Figure 3. Distribution of the 98 Included Studies. Original studies: 45. Systematic reviews/Meta-analyses: 18. Guidelines/Consensus statements: 10. Editorials/Letters: 12. Methodological/Imaging/Endoscopy reports: 13.

2.7. Data Extraction and Synthesis

From each study we extracted design, setting, sample size, time period, key outcomes (incidence, staging, diagnostic or treatment delays, outcomes), and pandemic-related adaptations (triage, telemedicine, vaccination strategies). Data were extracted using a standardized form developed a priori; extraction was cross-checked, and any discrepancies were resolved by consensus (inter-rater statistics were not calculated). Given heterogeneity, a narrative synthesis was performed rather than a meta-analysis.

2.8. Quality and Risk of Bias Assessment

Quality appraisal was performed using criteria adapted from Joanna Briggs Institute (JBI) tools for observational research. Risk-of-bias appraisal was applied only to data-driven empirical studies (observational studies/registry analyses/clinical series and meta-analyses). Non-empirical sources (guidelines, editorials/letters, methodological reports) were not formally appraised and were used for context only.

Empirical studies providing original data (e.g., observational studies, clinical series, registry/claims analyses) were included in the core evidence synthesis and underwent quality/risk-of-bias assessment. Editorials, letters, and methodological/technical reports were included only as contextual/background sources to describe practice adaptations and emerging concepts; these were not subject to formal risk-of-bias appraisal and were not used as sole support for main conclusions. Non-empirical sources and background references were used for context and framing; therefore, the total number of references (n = 107) exceeds the number of sources included in the evidence synthesis (n = 98).

In practice, high-risk findings were not used as standalone support for key conclusions; they were reported descriptively and interpreted in light of larger/more robust datasets.

3. The COVID-19 Pandemic and the Stomach: Effects and Potential Mechanisms

3.1. Interaction Between SARS-CoV-2 and the Gastrointestinal Tract

Since the early stages of the pandemic, SARS-CoV-2 has been shown to interact with the gastrointestinal tract, supported by ACE2 receptor expression on gastric and intestinal epithelial cells and by reports of viral RNA/particles in mucosal tissue [24–27]. However, in the context of gastric oncopathology, the clinical relevance of these observations appears mainly indirect and remains incompletely defined.

Available data suggest that COVID-19 may be associated with transient mucosal injury, systemic inflammation, and (in some cohorts) gut dysbiosis and increased intestinal permeability [25,28–32]. These pathways have been proposed as potential contributors to persistent gastrointestinal symptoms and to inflammatory changes that could, in theory, influence pre-existing high-risk gastric conditions [33–37]. Importantly, the long-term impact on gastric premalignant lesions and carcinogenesis remains largely hypothetical, and current evidence does not demonstrate a direct or accelerated pathway of gastric cancer development attributable to SARS-CoV-2 [28,33,34].

From a practical standpoint, the overlap between nonspecific gastrointestinal symptoms during COVID-19 and symptoms that may also occur in gastric cancer may complicate clinical assessment and contribute to delayed investigation—particularly when routine diagnostic services are disrupted [29,33].

3.2. COVID-19 and Gastric Pathology

The COVID-19 pandemic introduced several potential biological and behavioral factors that may influence preexisting gastric conditions; however, the long-term relevance of these mechanisms to gastric carcinogenesis remains uncertain. Reports have linked COVID-19–related systemic inflammation, hypoxia, coagulopathy, and medication exposure (e.g., corticosteroids/anti-inflammatory drugs) with mucosal injury and exacerbation of ulcer-related complications, while psychological distress and lifestyle changes during lockdowns were associated with worsening gastrointestinal symptom burden in patients with functional and organic disorders [35–42].

Importantly, hypotheses suggesting that persistent inflammation or immune dysregulation after SARS-CoV-2 infection could accelerate progression of premalignant lesions (especially in the presence of *Helicobacter pylori*) remain speculative, and current evidence does not establish a direct causal link [43–45]. Therefore, in the context of gastric cancer, the most consistent and actionable impact of the pandemic is mediated through disruptions in clinical pathways and healthcare delivery, as summarized below.

Clinically, the pandemic's impact on gastric disease care has been driven primarily by disruptions in clinical pathways, including reduced diagnostic endoscopy capacity, delayed evaluation, and altered referral patterns [46–51]. For example, in South Korea, the annual number of esophagogastroduodenoscopies decreased by 6.3% in 2020 compared with 2019, and claims for advanced gastric cancer decreased by 3.6% [50]. In parallel, the gastric cancer screening rate decreased from 70.8% (2019) to 68.9% (2020), while screening within the past year dropped from 32.7% to 27.2% [51]. These healthcare-delivery effects and their downstream implications for stage at diagnosis and treatment delivery are addressed in detail in the dedicated sections on diagnostic disruption and therapeutic management.

https://doi.org/10.3390/life16010161

4. COVID-19 and Gastric Cancer: Incidence and Risk Factors

4.1. Epidemiological Changes

The COVID-19 pandemic period was associated with a higher proportion of late-stage gastric cancer diagnoses, likely reflecting disruptions in screening pathways and reduced access to elective endoscopy services [52–54].

For example, in Hiroshima (Japan), early-stage gastric cancer diagnoses decreased by more than 20% during the early COVID-19 period (e.g., stage I −23.9%) [52]. Similarly, a large single-institute cohort from Yonsei Cancer Center (South Korea) reported fewer diagnoses in 2020–2021 than in 2018–2019 (6336 vs. 4539; 264 vs. 189 cases/month; −28.4%), alongside a higher proportion of advanced-stage disease particularly in 2021 (stage IV and stage III–IV) [55]. A study-level summary of the main numerical signals of diagnostic disruption and stage migration is provided in Table 1.

Similar trends were observed in Italy and other European countries, where diagnostic rates dropped by as much as 15.9%, and in the United States, with an estimated annual decline of approximately −8.9% [46,48].

In resource-limited settings, such as parts of the Middle East and South Asia, delays in gastric cancer diagnosis were also reported due to healthcare system disruptions and reduced access to endoscopy, although specific national data remain limited [38,47].

Across multiple regions, temporary reductions in diagnostic activity and delays in referral were associated with fewer early detections and a higher proportion of locally advanced or metastatic presentations [38,46,54]. Patient hesitancy to seek medical care during surges likely compounded these effects.

Five-year survival rates for gastric cancer exceed 90% in stage I, drop to approximately 30% in stage III, and fall below 10%—with some analyses reporting rates under 3%—in stage IV, according to large-scale cohort studies and survival meta-analyses [56,57].

Moreover, the pandemic has revealed significant geographical disparities in gastric cancer care. In countries with established screening infrastructure—such as South Korea and certain regions of Japan—diagnostic volumes recovered more rapidly, which helped offset some negative outcomes [50,52]. In contrast, countries without centralized national screening policies or with underfunded public healthcare systems, including parts of Eastern Europe, Latin America, and the Middle East, experienced prolonged service disruptions and persistent diagnostic backlogs [38,46,54]. For example, South Korea saw a near-complete recovery to pre-pandemic gastric cancer screening rates within one year, whereas resource-limited settings—such as many countries in Africa—continued to experience substantial diagnostic backlogs and service disruptions months after initial pandemic waves [50]. These disparities are further exacerbated by socioeconomic inequality and unequal access to high-volume cancer centers, highlighting the need for targeted public health interventions and investment in screening programs to reduce the risk of increased gastric cancer mortality globally.

4.2. Specific Risk Factors in the Pandemic Context

Beyond disrupting healthcare systems, the pandemic has also reshaped population behaviors related to lifestyle and adherence to preventive medical care, thereby influencing risk factors associated with gastric cancer. Fears of hospital-acquired infections and hospitalization significantly hindered early diagnostic efforts. Multiple surveys and observational studies reported that patients were frequently reluctant to undergo endoscopic evaluations, even when presenting with alarming gastrointestinal symptoms—leading to delayed presentations and more advanced disease at diagnosis [37,58,59].

Additionally, lifestyle changes during lockdowns may have increased population-level vulnerability to cancer risk factors. The closure of fitness facilities and limits on outdoor

https://doi.org/10.3390/life16010161

mobility promoted sedentary behavior, while pandemic-related stress was frequently associated with higher consumption of ultra-processed foods rich in salt, sugar, and saturated fats [60].

These behavioral shifts are known to contribute to obesity and low-grade systemic inflammation—both established risk factors for gastric and other gastrointestinal cancers [15,61].

Simultaneously, collective protective measures have redirected medical equipment and staff toward COVID-19 emergencies, causing delays in testing for and eradicating *Helicobacter pylori*. For many patients, either H. pylori testing has been postponed or eradication therapies have been interrupted or shortened, potentially favoring the persistence of chronic gastritis and the progression of preneoplastic lesions in the long term [62].

Furthermore, although genetic predisposition plays a key role in gastric cancer risk, genetic counseling and molecular testing pathways were interrupted in many oncology centers due to lockdowns, staff shortages, and prioritization of urgent care. Genetic services experienced measurable declines during the first lockdown waves. For instance, at a centralized molecular diagnostics center in Serbia, overall molecular analyses fell by 38% during the state of emergency, and only 3 of 48 scheduled pre-test genetic counseling appointments were conducted; in parallel, somatic BRCA1/2 testing was temporarily suspended [63]. Similarly, a large tertiary cancer genetics clinic reported a decrease in referral volume (median 35 vs. 22 referrals/week; $p < 0.001$) and reduced genetic testing uptake (97.7% [176/180] vs. 74.1% [180/243]; $p < 0.001$), with the median time from pre-test counseling to blood draw increasing from 0 to 11 days ($p < 0.001$) [64].

These disruptions decreased access to timely risk assessments and preventive strategies, raising concerns that individuals with hereditary cancer syndromes may have missed early interventions and later received diagnoses at more advanced stages. In this way, the pandemic has not only altered healthcare delivery but also introduced new challenges in managing the global risk factors for gastric cancer—from dietary habits and lifestyle to H. pylori eradication and the proper follow-up of individuals with hereditary predispositions.

5. Gastric Cancer in COVID-19 Positive Patients

5.1. Association of COVID-19 Infection with the Progression of Gastric Cancer

The occurrence of COVID-19 infection in patients with gastric cancer has been a significant concern since the early reports on the pandemic's impact on oncology populations. In gastric cancer, tumor-induced immunosuppression—along with the clinical fragility often associated with advanced disease and multiple comorbidities—can significantly worsen the severity of SARS-CoV-2 infection, increasing the risk of respiratory failure and systemic complications [65,66].

Studies have shown that gastric cancer patients infected with COVID-19 face higher hospitalization and mortality rates compared to cancer-free individuals, with mortality estimates ranging from 20% to over 35%, depending on stage and treatment status [65–67].

Unlike many other malignancies, gastric cancers are often accompanied by poor nutritional status, with patients frequently presenting with anemia and hypoalbuminemia, conditions that further impair the body's ability to withstand severe infections [39,40].

An emerging hypothesis suggests that the interplay between chronic inflammation within the tumor microenvironment and the cytokine storm induced by SARS-CoV-2 infection may exacerbate immune dysfunction in oncology patients. This theoretical synergy could further impair antitumor immunity and contribute to disease progression [68, 69].

https://doi.org/10.3390/life16010161

Additionally, systemic cancer treatments (such as chemotherapy or targeted therapies) are known to suppress immune responses, potentially rendering SARS-CoV-2 infections more aggressive and necessitating intensified clinical monitoring [68].

Systemic hypoxia and coagulopathy seen in severe COVID-19 cases can also worsen outcomes, predisposing patients—particularly those with malignancies—to thromboembolic events such as deep vein thrombosis and pulmonary embolism [41]. Such individuals are highly susceptible to deep vein thrombosis and pulmonary embolism due to overlapping mechanisms of cancer-associated thrombosis (CAT) and COVID-associated coagulopathy (CAC), and these thrombotic complications contribute significantly to the elevated mortality observed in cancer patients with COVID-19 [41,65].

Clinically, patients with gastric cancer who contract COVID-19 face an increased risk of hemodynamic instability and acute complications such as gastrointestinal hemorrhage or ulcer perforation related to the neoplasm. This risk is compounded by recent oncologic therapies, which may deplete hematologic reserves and heighten systemic toxicity. Moreover, evolving hospitalization protocols and the need for repeated SARS-CoV-2 testing can further delay essential diagnostic or therapeutic interventions [47,49].

5.2. Diagnostic and Therapeutic Considerations

The COVID-19 pandemic has directly affected the capacity to diagnose and treat oncology patients, with this impact particularly pronounced among gastric cancer patients with active SARS-CoV-2 infection. In many centers, both endoscopic and imaging investigations have been subject to triage based on urgency, often resulting in postponed or canceled staging procedures for patients who tested positive [47,70].

To mitigate risk and manage limited resources, some institutions implemented formal triage frameworks prioritizing patients based on tumor aggressiveness, COVID-19 status, and overall prognosis [71,72]. Moreover, certain imaging modalities—such as contrast-enhanced computed tomography—were temporarily limited mainly due to staff shortages, workflow constraints, and the redirection of hospital resources toward intensive care, with infection-control considerations also contributing.

Surgical interventions (including partial or total gastrectomies) in COVID-19 positive patients carry an increased risk for both the patient and the medical team, given the aerosol-generating nature of general anesthesia and the inherent complexity of these procedures [49]. Consequently, strict preoperative testing and isolation protocols have been adopted, with surgeries often deferred until the patient recovers or achieves a negative virological status—provided the oncologic stage allows for such a delay. In cases of rapid tumor progression or complications such as acute bleeding, perforation, or obstruction, urgent surgical interventions have been carried out under enhanced protective measures and COVID-19-specific protocols [49]. For example, institutions in Italy and Iran reported increases in emergency gastric surgeries, such as subtotal gastrectomies and bleeding ulcer repairs, performed in negative-pressure operating rooms with full PPE and reduced staff to minimize exposure risk [46,53].

Chemotherapy and immunotherapy regimens have also undergone adjustments. For gastric cancer patients with active SARS-CoV-2 infection, treatment cycles are generally delayed or rescheduled until post-infection recovery to avoid the compounded risks of severe toxicity and immunosuppression [73,74]. The use of hypofractionated radiotherapy and oral treatment regimens has been employed as strategies to minimize hospital visits and reduce exposure to high-risk environments. Despite these measures, there remains concern that such delays may result in missed therapeutic opportunities—such as failure to initiate systemic chemotherapy within the optimal time window or the inability to perform timely surgical resection due to incomplete staging—particularly in patients

https://doi.org/10.3390/life16010161

with advanced disease who depend on coordinated, prompt interventions for curative or palliative outcomes [74,75].

In this challenging context, multidisciplinary teams—comprising oncology, gastroenterology, surgery, and radiotherapy—have been critical in establishing optimal management strategies, all while adhering to stringent safety protocols for healthcare providers and other patients. The inherently volatile nature of the pandemic, marked by successive waves and evolving restrictions, has necessitated continual adaptation of therapeutic plans and transparent communication with patients regarding the risks and benefits of each treatment option [37,76].

6. Gastric Cancer During the COVID-19 Pandemic

6.1. *Incidence of Endoscopic Procedures and Delayed Diagnosis*

The restrictions imposed by the COVID-19 pandemic were associated with a marked reduction in endoscopic procedures—both screening and diagnostic—which may have hampered opportunities for early detection of gastric cancer. Many centers experienced a 60–80% drop in elective endoscopies during the pandemic's peak months, a consequence of both the diversion of resources to treat SARS-CoV-2-infected patients and widespread patient apprehension about potential hospital-acquired infections [47–49]. In the United Kingdom, analysis of the National Endoscopy Database (NED) demonstrated that endoscopic activity fell to just 5% of pre-pandemic levels at the nadir, before rebounding to approximately 20% by May 2020 following targeted vetting and catch-up initiatives [58]. In the United States, data from the GI Quality Improvement Consortium (GIQuIC) registry revealed a 33.4% decrease in esophagogastroduodenoscopy (EGD) and a 38.5% decrease in colonoscopy volumes between March and September 2020, which guided the development of structured recovery plans [59]. Consequently, a substantial number of patients with early symptoms of gastric cancer have delayed seeking medical advice, often presenting at more advanced stages when clinical manifestations are more severe and treatment options are more limited.

This decline in routine investigations has created a diagnostic gap for preneoplastic or early gastric lesions, potentially leading to a higher number of cases with locoregional spread or metastases at the time of diagnosis [43,44]. The reduction in routine endoscopies has also limited opportunities for minimally invasive procedures such as EMR or ESD—interventions that are most effective when the disease is caught early. If these screening deficits are not addressed through recovery strategies, the long-term effect could be an increased mortality rate associated with gastric cancer [54].

6.2. *Relationship Between Preneoplastic and Neoplastic Lesions*

During the pandemic, the underdiagnosis of atrophic gastritis and intestinal metaplasia has raised significant concerns among gastroenterologists. Without regular consultations and periodic endoscopic surveillance, these preneoplastic conditions may progress over time to dysplasia and eventually to gastric adenocarcinoma, depriving patients of the opportunity for preventive management [43,44]. The constraints on endoscopic procedures have left many high-risk cases undetected, and cumulative delays may accelerate the progression of lesions that might otherwise have been identified and treated at an early stage.

At the same time, the pandemic has highlighted the need for additional diagnostic technologies—such as capsule endoscopy and telemedicine. However, the rapid implementation of these innovations has been uneven, and they have not yet fully replaced conventional digestive endoscopy [77,78]. It remains to be seen whether the lack of rigorous monitoring of patients with precancerous lesions will translate into a noticeable increase

https://doi.org/10.3390/life16010161

in advanced-stage disease in the coming years, and whether effective strategies can be implemented to recover the losses incurred during the pandemic.

6.3. Disruption of Oncologic Management

The pandemic has posed significant challenges to oncologic management, and in the case of gastric cancer—an already high-risk malignancy—the consequences have been particularly stark. Elective and urgent surgical interventions, such as gastrectomies, have frequently been postponed or rescheduled due to the reallocation of operating rooms and anesthesiology staff to COVID-19 units, resulting in delays that could negatively affect long-term outcomes [38,52,53]. Even when surgeries have proceeded, the preoperative process has required complex protocols for testing and isolation, leading to extended waiting times and increased hospitalization costs.

Similarly, chemotherapy and radiotherapy have faced additional obstacles related to limited outpatient scheduling, restricted access to dedicated oncology spaces, and reduced staff availability. Quantitatively, a large systematic review and meta-analysis (245 studies, 46 countries) reported an overall 28% decline in cancer treatment delivery during the pandemic, with modality-specific reductions ranging from 15% for radiotherapy to 35% for systemic treatment (including chemotherapy) compared with pre-pandemic periods [79].

Service-level radiotherapy data also demonstrate measurable disruptions. Using the National Radiotherapy Dataset in England, mean weekly radiotherapy courses decreased by 19.9% in April 2020 versus April 2019 (with attendances/fractions dropping by 29.1%), and reductions persisted in May (courses −6.2%; attendances −31.4%) and June (courses −11.6%; attendances −31.5%) [80]. To reduce hospital visits, hypofractionation was adopted more frequently; for example, ultra-hypofractionated breast regimens (26 Gy in 5 fractions) increased from 0.2% of courses in April 2019 to 60.6% in April 2020 [80].

In upper gastrointestinal oncology, registry-based data from the Netherlands further suggest shifts in multimodal treatment patterns during the first pandemic year, including a reduction in the proportion of potentially curable esophagogastric cancer patients treated with resection and neoadjuvant chemoradiotherapy (35.0% in 2017–2019 vs. 27.3% in 2020) [81]. These challenges have sometimes necessitated modifications to treatment regimens—favoring less toxic protocols or alternatives that reduce hospital visit frequency (e.g., oral therapies or hypofractionated radiotherapy)—although the long-term efficacy of these adjustments remains to be fully evaluated [73–75]. For patients with advanced gastric cancer, the need for prompt, multimodal treatment has often been in conflict with the risks of viral exposure and the limited capacity of oncology centers to maintain their standard patient throughput. The pandemic has exposed profound vulnerabilities in healthcare infrastructures and underscored the importance of inter-specialty collaboration, digitalization, and robust emergency planning to prevent critical disruptions in diagnosis and treatment.

To consolidate the quantitative findings that are discussed across Section 4.1, Section 6.1, and Section 6.3 (endoscopy volume decline, stage migration, treatment disruptions, and early recovery signals), we added two summary tables: Table 1 maps the key numerical indicators to the main supporting studies, and Table 2 provides a pre-/during-/post-COVID comparative overview.

https://doi.org/10.3390/life16010161

Table 1. Key quantitative indicators reported for endoscopy volume decline, stage migration, treatment disruption, and screening recovery in gastric cancer during COVID-19 (selected studies). Indicators and time windows differ across studies; values are therefore reported as described by each source and are not intended for direct cross-country comparison.

Domain	Setting/Data Source (as Described in Text)	Comparison Window	Key Quantitative Signal(s)	Ref.
Screening participation	South Korea (screening survey data)	2019 vs. 2020	Screening rate 70.8% → 68.9%; screening within past year 32.7% → 27.2%	[51]
Screening/claims-based signals	South Korea (claims-based analysis)	2019 vs. 2020	Esophagogastroduodenoscopies −6.3% (2020 vs. 2019); advanced gastric cancer claims −3.6%	[50]
Endoscopy volume decline	Multiple centers/multi-region reports	Peak pandemic months vs. baseline	60–80% decline in elective endoscopies	[47–49]
Endoscopy volume decline + early recovery	UK National Endoscopy Database (NED)	Nadir vs. May 2020	Endoscopic activity ~5% of pre-pandemic at nadir; ~20% by May 2020 after catch-up initiatives	[58]
Endoscopy volume decline	US GIQuIC registry	Mar–Sep 2020 vs. baseline	−ar–Sep 2020 vs. baselineoscopy	[59]
Stage migration/early-stage detection	Hiroshima (Japan)	Early COVID period vs. baseline	Early stage diagnoses decreased (e.g., stage I −23.9%)	[52]
Diagnostic volume + stage shift	South Korea (Yonsei Cancer Center cohort)	2018–2019 vs. 2020–2021	Diagnoses 6336 → 4539 (264 → 189/month; −28.4%), with higher proportion of advanced-stage disease	[55]
Diagnostic rate decline	Italy/other Europe + United States	Pandemic period vs. baseline	Diagnostic rates fell up to −15.9% (Italy/Europe); estimated annual decline ~−8.9% (US)	[46,48]
Treatment disruption (overall)	Meta-analysis across oncology care	Pandemic vs. pre-pandemic	Overall treatment delivery decline ~28%; radiotherapy ~15%; systemic therapy ~35%	[79]
Radiotherapy service impact	England (National Radiotherapy Dataset)	April 2020 vs. baseline	Mean weekly radiotherapy courses −19.9%; attendances −29.1%	[80]
Multimodal treatment pattern change	Netherlands registry-based data (upper GI oncology)	2017–2019 vs. 2020	Potentially curable esophagogastric cancer treated with resection + neoadjuvant chemoradiotherapy 35.0% → 27.3%	[81]
Screening recovery (system-level)	Systems with established screening infrastructure	Post-acute phase	Faster recovery reported; near-complete recovery to pre-pandemic screening rates within one year (South Korea)	[50,52]

https://doi.org/10.3390/life16010161

Table 2. Comparative overview of key gastric cancer pathway indicators before, during, and after the acute COVID-19 disruption (selected examples).

Care Pathway Domain	Pre-Pandemic Baseline (Illustrative)	During COVID-19 Disruption	Early Recovery/Post-Acute Phase
Screening participation/claims-based screening signals	In South Korea, screening participation was high pre-pandemic (e.g., overall screening rate 70.8% in 2019, and screening within the past year 32.7%) [51].	In 2020, screening indicators declined (e.g., overall screening rate 68.9%, screening within the past year 27.2%) [51]. Claims-based signals also changed (e.g., esophagogastroduodenoscopies decreased 6.3% in 2020 vs. 2019; advanced gastric cancer claims decreased 3.6%) [50].	Regions with established screening infrastructure tended to recover faster; South Korea showed near-complete recovery to pre-pandemic screening rates within one year [50].
Diagnostic endoscopy volume	Routine elective endoscopy capacity and organized endoscopy workflows were generally stable and supported early detection.	Many centers reported 60–80% declines in elective endoscopy during peak months [47–49]. UK NED activity fell to ~5% of pre-pandemic at the nadir, rebounding to ~20% by May 2020 after catch-up initiatives [58]. US GIQuIC: −33.4% EGD and −38.5% colonoscopy (Mar–Sep 2020) [59].	Catch-up and prioritization approaches partially restored capacity (e.g., NED rebound by May 2020) [58]. Faster recovery was reported where screening systems were already established [50,52].
Stage at diagnosis/diagnostic rates	Earlier-stage detection is clinically critical (stage-dependent outcomes are markedly different) [56,57].	Stage migration signals were reported: in Hiroshima (Japan) early-stage diagnoses fell (e.g., stage I −23.9%) [52]. In a Korean single-center cohort (Yonsei), diagnoses decreased (6336 → 4539; −28.4%) with a higher proportion of advanced-stage disease [55]. Other settings showed diagnostic reductions (Italy up to −15.9%, US approx. −8.9%) [46,48].	Where diagnostic volumes recovered more rapidly, this may have partially offset downstream harm [50,52]. (However, endpoints and follow-up remain heterogeneous across studies.)
Surgery/operative pathways	Curative-intent surgery and perioperative pathways were generally delivered on standard schedules.	Surgical interventions were frequently postponed/rescheduled due to resource reallocation and staffing constraints [38,52,53].	Gradual restoration occurred as services recovered, but the pace differed by health-system capacity and pandemic waves (described across included reports) [38,46,54].
Systemic therapy and radiotherapy delivery	Standard multimodal therapy (perioperative chemotherapy and/or chemoradiotherapy where indicated) remained the norm.	Across oncology, a meta-analysis reported an overall 28% decline in treatment delivery during the pandemic, with modality-specific reductions (~15% radiotherapy, ~35% systemic therapy) [79]. In England, radiotherapy courses fell (e.g., −19.9% in April 2020) with fewer attendances (−29.1%) [80]. Registry data from the Netherlands suggested shifts in multimodal treatment patterns (e.g., resection + neoadjuvant chemoradiotherapy 35.0% in 2017–2019 vs. 27.3% in 2020) [81].	Many centers used regimen adaptations (e.g., less toxic/oral options, hypofractionation) to reduce visits, while longer-term oncologic impact remains under evaluation [73–75].

7. COVID-19 Vaccination and Gastric Cancer

7.1. Effects of Vaccination on Oncology Patients

Widespread vaccination against SARS-CoV-2 has become a cornerstone of global efforts to control the pandemic, significantly reducing the risk of severe COVID-19 and its associated mortality [82,83]. In patients with gastric cancer, the benefits of vaccination have been demonstrated by a lower likelihood of developing serious respiratory and systemic complications, as well as by enabling the continuation or timely resumption of oncologic

https://doi.org/10.3390/life16010161

treatments under safer conditions. Vaccination has been shown to decrease the incidence of severe disease, which in turn allows hospitals to manage oncology cases more efficiently and maintain access to essential diagnostic procedures such as endoscopy and imaging for proper cancer staging [84,85].

Although the immune response in oncology patients may be somewhat diminished compared to the general population, studies indicate that most patients with solid tumors—including those with gastric cancer—develop protective antibody levels post-vaccination, even if these titers are lower than in individuals without malignancies [85,86]. This partial immunization is generally sufficient to offer significant protection, reducing both the frequency and severity of infections while supporting a more continuous delivery of oncologic therapies. In certain cases, booster doses are recommended for patients whose initial immune response is inadequate—particularly if they are undergoing chemotherapy or immunotherapy, which can alter their immune profile [82,87,88].

Vaccination has also alleviated anxiety and reduced patient hesitancy about hospital visits, where the perceived risk of infection has previously deterred individuals from undergoing endoscopic, surgical, or systemic treatments [89]. This is especially critical for patients with intermediate or advanced gastric cancer, where timely treatment initiation can markedly influence prognosis. By providing a safer environment with a lower COVID-19 risk, vaccination helps ensure adherence to chemotherapy schedules and minimizes preoperative delays. This strategy facilitates clearer treatment planning and reduces uncertainties related to the cancelation of procedures during potential surges in infections [90,91].

7.2. Implications for Endoscopic and Oncologic Practice

As vaccination campaigns have expanded among healthcare personnel and patients, many endoscopy units and surgical departments have been able to relax some of the initial restrictions and streamline diagnostic and treatment workflows [49,88,89]. This has enabled the resumption of gastric cancer screening programs—not only in regions where such programs existed prior to the pandemic but also in areas that have more recently introduced systematic endoscopic diagnosis. Vaccination of medical teams has notably reduced concerns regarding viral transmission during aerosol-generating endoscopic procedures, which were previously considered high risk for spreading the virus [49,62].

Furthermore, vaccinated patients have gained greater confidence in the safety of hospital environments, as evidenced by increased consultation rates and a higher number of scheduled endoscopies and other gastric investigations [58,59]. In several countries, the gradual easing of strict protocols has also involved reorganizing patient pathways so that COVID-19 and non-COVID-19 areas are managed separately. This reallocation of resources has shortened waiting times and allowed for an increased volume of procedures, including the reinstatement of elective surgeries for gastric cancer that had been temporarily postponed [71,72].

Nevertheless, challenges remain regarding suboptimal immune responses in certain patients with advanced gastric cancer—especially those receiving immunosuppressive treatments. In such instances, clinical guidelines recommend monitoring antibody levels and adjusting treatment plans accordingly, either by administering additional vaccine doses or by implementing enhanced protective measures in the hospital setting [85,86]. In addition, ongoing patient education remains crucial to ensure that individuals understand the benefits of vaccination, its potential side effects, and the importance of resuming oncologic procedures. The emergence of new viral variants, which may impact vaccine effectiveness, underscores the need for flexibility and continuous monitoring in the management of patients with gastric cancer [82,84,88].

https://doi.org/10.3390/life16010161

Overall, the widespread rollout of COVID-19 vaccines has been a pivotal step in safely reopening medical services, reducing morbidity and mortality among cancer patients, and enabling clinics and hospitals to better manage oncologic caseloads. In the context of gastric cancer—where early diagnosis and prompt treatment directly correlate with improved outcomes—the restoration of comprehensive screening and complex treatment protocols has been greatly facilitated by vaccination efforts and the implementation of safety protocols for both patients and healthcare providers.

8. Diagnosis and Therapeutic Approaches in Gastric Cancer Within the Pandemic Context

8.1. Endoscopic and Imaging Techniques

Health safety restrictions and the risks associated with aerosol-generating procedures have necessitated significant modifications in the conduct of endoscopic examinations and imaging studies required for the diagnosis and staging of gastric cancer. In numerous centers, mandatory pre-procedural COVID-19 testing and the use of high-level personal protective equipment (PPE) have become standard practices to safeguard both healthcare staff and patients [49,62]. These measures have led to more stringent scheduling and a reduced procedural capacity, forcing physicians to prioritize urgent cases or those with a high suspicion of advanced gastric cancer. Additionally, patient pathways have been reorganized to clearly separate those with positive COVID-19 tests from those testing negative, thereby minimizing the risk of nosocomial transmission [49,71].

For imaging services, reduced availability was driven predominantly by operational constraints (resource reallocation, workflow adjustments, and scheduling backlogs) rather than imaging-specific procedural transmission risk. [49,62,71]

To overcome the limitations imposed on conventional endoscopy, alternative or supplementary imaging modalities have increasingly been utilized. Computed tomography (CT), magnetic resonance imaging (MRI), and even PET/CT have been employed for staging and post-treatment monitoring, offering the advantage of systemic evaluation without direct contact with the gastric mucosa [92,93]. However, these methods generally do not match the diagnostic accuracy of endoscopy combined with biopsy for early gastric lesions, raising challenges in differential diagnosis and in ruling out other mimicking conditions. While innovations such as magnetic capsule endoscopy have shown promise, their widespread adoption has been limited by equipment availability, high costs, and the requisite level of expertise [77,78]. Telemedicine and virtual consultations have also been integrated as tools for remotely interpreting imaging results, reducing the need for in-person visits while providing ongoing monitoring for patients with known gastric lesions that do not require immediate intervention [64,78].

However, despite their benefits, these emerging technologies also present limitations, including reduced diagnostic accuracy compared to traditional endoscopy, cost-related barriers, and variability in clinician expertise, thus necessitating careful consideration when integrating them into standardized diagnostic workflows [64,77,78,92,93].

8.2. Therapeutic Management

The pandemic has posed major challenges in maintaining continuity in oncologic therapies, and gastric cancer—often an aggressive malignancy—has placed additional pressures on multidisciplinary teams. Minimally invasive endoscopic procedures, such as EMR and ESD, have been prioritized for patients with early lesions and high risk of progression, as these interventions offer high curative potential and typically require shorter hospital stays [20–22]. Nevertheless, diagnostic delays and backlogs limited timely

https://doi.org/10.3390/life16010161

access for some patients, increasing the likelihood that disease would be detected at a more advanced stage [54].

Regarding surgical management, many units have been forced to delay scheduled gastrectomies, particularly during peak pandemic periods when intensive care beds and surgical staff were redirected to COVID-19 care [75,94,95]. In cases where emergency surgery was unavoidable (such as for massive hemorrhage, perforation, or obstruction), physicians operated under strict isolation protocols, and the risk of perioperative complications was elevated due to reduced staffing and constrained postoperative care conditions. Chemotherapy and radiotherapy regimens have similarly been adapted—often shifting to less toxic protocols, reducing the number of hospital visits, or employing hypofractionated radiotherapy—in an effort to minimize patient exposure to healthcare settings [73,74]. Simultaneously, telemedicine has provided a framework for managing adverse treatment reactions and monitoring stable patients, allowing for timely adjustments to treatment plans without frequent hospital visits [64,78]. However, careful evaluation is needed to assess the long-term effectiveness of these modifications, as gastric cancer generally demands intensive, multidisciplinary management. Some of the adapted treatment regimens may not sustain the optimal therapeutic outcomes, underscoring the importance of clear crisis-management guidelines to ensure that oncology patients are not disadvantaged by competing medical emergencies [71,72,74].

8.3. Considerations Regarding the Safety of Medical Teams

Since endoscopic procedures and certain surgical interventions for gastric cancer are considered aerosol-generating, the healthcare teams performing these procedures are at high risk for SARS-CoV-2 exposure. The use of advanced PPE (including FFP2/FFP3 masks, face shields, and waterproof gowns) as well as negative-pressure rooms has become standard practice in many centers. However, strict adherence to these measures has inevitably slowed patient throughput due to additional preparation and disinfection time [49,62,96]. Regular COVID-19 testing of healthcare staff in high-volume endoscopy units has also been crucial for the rapid detection and isolation of asymptomatic cases, thereby preventing nosocomial outbreaks.

The vaccination of medical personnel has further enhanced safety, significantly reducing the incidence of severe disease among healthcare workers and enabling more organized operation of surgical blocks and endoscopy suites [88,90]. Despite this, variations in vaccination rates and the emergence of new viral strains with differing transmissibility have necessitated continued vigilance, meaning that stringent protective measures remain in place even after most staff have been immunized. Thus, ensuring the safety of medical teams is a multifaceted challenge that is essential not only for protecting patients but also for sustaining uninterrupted oncologic care during a public health crisis.

9. Discussion

The COVID-19 pandemic has profoundly altered the landscape of gastric cancer diagnosis and treatment, exposing long-standing weaknesses in healthcare systems while simultaneously accelerating the adoption of innovative practices. This duality—of crisis-driven disruption and rapid innovation—offers valuable insights into the resilience of oncologic care. By synthesizing the available evidence, several recurring themes and critical gaps emerge that should inform future preparedness strategies.

9.1. Synthesis of Common Themes

Because most included studies were observational, the relationships described here should be interpreted as associations and temporal trends rather than confirmed causal

https://doi.org/10.3390/life16010161

effects. Across global cohorts, pandemic-related restrictions and the pervasive fear of nosocomial SARS-CoV-2 infection led to sharp declines in elective endoscopies and routine gastroenterological consultations [46,49–51]. This reduction in procedural volume was consistently associated with diagnostic delays across multiple cohorts, with gastric cancer more often identified at advanced stages and potentially poorer outcomes. Yet, the rapid deployment of telemedicine platforms, the introduction of pre-procedural testing, and the widespread use of enhanced PPE provided a framework that allowed many regions to resume specialized oncologic services, albeit at reduced capacity [49,90]. As illustrated in Figure 1, COVID-19 has affected gastric cancer management on multiple levels—from reduced elective endoscopies and diagnostic delays to treatment adaptations and increased reliance on telemedicine.

9.2. *Critical Comparative Analysis*

9.2.1. Regional Differences and Therapeutic Strategies

Countries with mature screening infrastructures, notably Japan and South Korea, demonstrated relative resilience by implementing catch-up strategies and leveraging robust national healthcare systems [52,54]. In contrast, European and North American centers adopted structured prioritization and triage protocols, with the UK's National Endoscopy Database (NED) showing a rebound in activity from 5% to 20% within two months of lockdown [58], while the US GIQuIC registry quantified a one-third decline in both EGD and colonoscopy, guiding phased service recovery [59]. Conversely, low-resource settings faced a disproportionate reallocation of staff and infrastructure toward COVID-19 units, resulting in longer delays, higher rates of emergency presentations, and increased late-stage diagnoses [38,47]. These disparities emphasize the importance of context-specific resilience strategies and highlight how structural inequalities exacerbate oncologic outcomes during crises.

9.2.2. Limitations of Alternative Approaches

Although capsule endoscopy, telemedicine, and virtual consultations provided innovative stopgaps during the pandemic, their long-term utility remains uncertain. While these tools increased accessibility and reduced exposure risks, questions persist regarding their diagnostic precision for early-stage lesions and their cost-effectiveness compared to conventional endoscopy [77,78]. Such limitations underscore the need for rigorous comparative validation before integrating these modalities into standard gastric cancer pathways.

9.3. *Integrating an Innovative Perspective*

9.3.1. Toward a Conceptual Model for Oncologic Resilience

The pandemic has revealed the urgent need for a conceptual model of oncologic resilience in gastric cancer care. Across the studies reviewed, resilience emerged not as a single intervention, but as the capacity of health systems to preserve timely diagnosis and treatment, protect patients and staff, and learn rapidly from evolving evidence despite major disruption. To translate this into a practical framework, the elements described in previous sections can be organized into four interrelated, measurable domains: (1) tpatient safety and infection control; (2) diagnostic and treatment continuity; (3) digital and telemedicine integration; and (4) system management and monitoring.

The patient safety and infection control domain encompasses strategies that maintain access to oncologic care while minimizing infectious risk, such as standardized pre-procedural triage and testing, COVID-19 vaccination programs targeting vulnerable cancer populations, re-design of endoscopy and surgical pathways to reduce exposure, and clear communication of safety protocols to patients and staff [71,72,97,98]. In practice, this

https://doi.org/10.3390/life16010161

domain can be monitored through indicators such as nosocomial SARS-CoV-2 and other healthcare-associated infection rates, vaccination coverage among patients and healthcare workers, adherence to personal protective equipment and testing policies, and the proportion of procedures performed in designated "cold" or low-risk pathways.

The diagnostic and treatment continuity domain reflects the ability to sustain essential cancer services despite resource constraints. In gastric cancer this includes maintaining urgent endoscopy and staging procedures, safeguarding access to curative surgery and systemic therapy, and implementing prioritization algorithms that distinguish truly deferrable from non-deferrable care [72,78]. Relevant indicators include recovery of diagnostic and screening endoscopy volumes compared with pre-pandemic baselines, time intervals from symptom onset or referral to endoscopy and to gastrectomy, changes in stage distribution at diagnosis, rates of treatment interruption or modification, and the backlog clearance time after acute waves.

The digital and telemedicine integration domain captures how effectively health systems use digital tools to support continuity of care. As illustrated in the broader oncology literature, teleconsultations, remote follow-up, electronic triage pathways, and emerging technologies such as capsule endoscopy and AI-assisted imaging can help preserve access while reducing unnecessary hospital visits [98–101]. This domain can be assessed through metrics such as the proportion of outpatient visits delivered via telemedicine, use of remote pre-assessment pathways before endoscopy or surgery, implementation of structured digital symptom-tracking tools, and validation of alternative diagnostic strategies (e.g., capsule-based or AI-supported workflows) against conventional endoscopy.

Finally, the system management and monitoring domain refers to the data infrastructure and governance mechanisms that allow continuous situational awareness and rapid adaptation. Key components include national or regional registries for gastric cancer and COVID-19, real-time dashboards tracking procedure volumes and waiting times, multidisciplinary decision structures for reallocating resources, and mechanisms for international collaboration and benchmarking [71,72,99,102,103]. Indicators in this domain include the existence and coverage of population-based registries, the timeliness of data reporting, the use of regular audit cycles to adjust priorities, and participation in multicenter or international data-sharing initiatives.

Taken together, these four domains provide an operational scaffold that can be tailored to different health-system contexts. Rather than proposing a rigid scoring system, the model offers a set of measurable dimensions and example indicators that policymakers, clinicians, and hospital managers can use to audit oncologic resilience, identify vulnerabilities, and design targeted interventions before and during future crises.

In this review, 'resilience' is used conceptually to describe service capacity to absorb disruption and recover core diagnostic and treatment pathways. Because the included studies reported non-uniform endpoints, we did not apply a single predefined KPI set; however, resilience could be operationalized using service-level indicators such as endoscopy volume recovery, backlog clearance/time-to-diagnosis, stage shift, time-to-treatment, treatment completion, and cancelation/no-show rates.

9.3.2. Future Directions

Looking forward, crisis-specific guidelines must evolve to integrate digital tools, adaptive surgical strategies, and personalized oncology care. These frameworks should not only aim to restore pre-pandemic diagnostic volumes but also proactively recover the "lost cases" that went undiagnosed during the crisis through intensified post-pandemic screening programs [104–106]. Prospective studies are also needed to clarify the long-term effects of diagnostic delays, treatment interruptions, and pandemic-related lifestyle changes

https://doi.org/10.3390/life16010161

on gastric cancer progression. Only through such comprehensive recovery strategies can oncology systems mitigate the pandemic's collateral damage and emerge stronger for future global health challenges.

9.4. Identification of Knowledge Gaps

Despite significant progress, critical knowledge gaps remain. First, the comparative precision and scalability of capsule endoscopy versus conventional endoscopy remain insufficiently validated, particularly for early gastric lesions [77]. Second, the long-term impact of pandemic-induced lifestyle changes—including sedentary behavior, poor diet, and heightened psychosocial stress—on the evolution of preneoplastic conditions requires longitudinal analysis. Third, the role of AI-based diagnostic platforms in resource-limited environments remains underexplored, though these technologies hold promise for democratizing access to high-quality oncologic care [101]. Finally, the immunologic interplay between SARS-CoV-2 infection, systemic inflammation, and the gastric tumor microenvironment is poorly understood and warrants mechanistic investigation [25,29,31]. Addressing these gaps will require multinational collaborations, prospective data collection, and the integration of digital health and AI-driven approaches into routine clinical workflows.

9.5. Concluding Perspective

Ultimately, the COVID-19 pandemic should be viewed not only as a disruptive event but also as a catalyst for reimagining gastric cancer care. By fostering adaptive resilience, embracing technological innovation, and investing in international collaboration, the oncology community can transform lessons from this crisis into sustainable strategies that protect vulnerable populations against future global health threats.

9.6. Limitations

This narrative review supported by a structured literature search is limited by the heterogeneity of the included evidence (study designs, outcomes, and settings), the English-language restriction, and reliance on observational data, which precludes causal inference. We did not perform a meta-analysis or compute pooled effect sizes, and some service-level indicators were reported inconsistently across studies, limiting direct comparability.

10. Conclusions

The COVID-19 pandemic has profoundly disrupted gastric cancer care, leading to delayed diagnoses, reduced access to screening, and interruptions in surgical and systemic treatments. At the same time, it has accelerated the adoption of new practices—telemedicine, infection-control protocols, and minimally invasive interventions—that may shape future standards of care.

What distinguishes this review is its proposal of a conceptual model of oncologic resilience **structured into four measurable domains—patient safety and infection control, diagnostic and treatment continuity, digital and telemedicine integration, and system management and monitoring—**which combines structured triage, digital technologies, international registries, and harmonized safety measures into a durable framework for crisis preparedness. This integrative perspective moves beyond documenting the pandemic's damage, offering instead a strategy to transform short-term adaptations into long-term improvements in gastric cancer management.

Future priorities must include recovering undiagnosed cases through intensified screening, validating innovative tools such as capsule endoscopy and AI-based diagnostics, and addressing the long-term impact of lifestyle changes induced by the pandemic. Strengthening international collaborations will be essential to ensure equity, rapid knowledge transfer, and coordinated responses in future global health crises.

https://doi.org/10.3390/life16010161

Thus, while COVID-19 exposed vulnerabilities in oncologic care, it also provided the momentum to reimagine gastric cancer management—shifting from reactive measures toward a more resilient, patient-centered, and future-ready paradigm.

Supplementary Materials: The following supporting information can be downloaded at: https://www.mdpi.com/article/10.3390/life16010161/s1, File S1: PRISMA 2020 Checklist (location of items in the manuscript).

Author Contributions: Conceptualization, A.M.V. and L.S.; methodology, L.S. and E.T.T.; validation, D.R. and P.P.; formal analysis, D.R.; investigation, E.T.T. and R.-C.S.; resources, S.M.C. and P.P.; data curation, S.M.C. and R.-C.S.; writing—original draft preparation, L.S. and R.-C.S.; writing—review and editing, E.T.T. and D.R.; visualization, S.M.C.; supervision, A.M.V., P.P. and T.C.; project administration, A.M.V. and T.C.; funding acquisition, T.C. All authors have read and agreed to the published version of the manuscript.

Funding: The article processing charges were funded by the University of Medicine and Pharmacy of Craiova, Romania, 200349 Craiova, Romania.

Institutional Review Board Statement: Not applicable.

Informed Consent Statement: Not applicable.

Data Availability Statement: The original contributions presented in the study are included in the article/Supplementary Material, further inquiries can be directed to the corresponding author.

Conflicts of Interest: The authors declare no conflicts of interest.

References

1. Thrift, A.P.; El-Serag, H.B. Burden of gastric cancer. *Clin. Gastroenterol. Hepatol.* **2020**, *18*, 534–542. [CrossRef]
2. Sung, H.; Ferlay, J.; Siegel, R.L.; Laversanne, M.; Soerjomataram, I.; Jemal, A.; Bray, F. Global cancer statistics 2020: GLOBOCAN estimates of incidence and mortality worldwide for 36 cancers in 185 countries. *CA Cancer J. Clin.* **2021**, *71*, 209–249. [CrossRef]
3. Zhang, T.; Chen, H.; Zhang, Y.; Yin, X.; Man, J.; Yang, X.; Lu, M. Global changing trends in incidence and mortality of gastric cancer by age and sex, 1990–2019: Findings from Global Burden of Disease Study. *J. Cancer* **2021**, *12*, 6695–6705. [CrossRef] [PubMed]
4. Ferlay, J.; Ervik, M.; Lam, F.; Laversanne, M.; Colombet, M.; Mery, L.; Piñeros, M.; Znaor, A.; Soerjomataram, I.; Bray, F. *Global Cancer Observatory: Cancer Today*; International Agency for Research on Cancer: Lyon, France, 2024. Available online: https://gco.iarc.who.int/today (accessed on 3 January 2026).
5. Shin, D.W.; Cho, B.; Guallar, E. Korean National Cancer Screening Program associated with a reduction in gastric cancer mortality. *Gastroenterology* **2014**, *146*, 396–405.e1.
6. Sato, S.; Fushimi, S.; Tahata, Y.; Mizutamari, H.; Mimori, N.; Kato, Y.; Horikawa, Y. Feasibility of endoscopic screening for upper gastrointestinal malignancy in a comprehensive health checkup. *Intern. Med.* **2021**, *60*, 1493–1499. [CrossRef] [PubMed]
7. Crew, K.D.; Neugut, A.I. Epidemiology of gastric cancer. *World J. Gastroenterol.* **2006**, *12*, 354–362. [CrossRef]
8. Lagergren, J.; Bergström, R.; Nyrén, O. Association between body mass and adenocarcinoma of the oesophagus and gastric cardia. *Gut* **1999**, *44*, 153–157.
9. Arnold, M.; Ferlay, J.; van Berge Henegouwen, M.I.; Soerjomataram, I. Global burden of oesophageal and gastric cancer by histology and subsite in 2018. *Gut* **2020**, *69*, 1564–1571. [CrossRef]
10. Bray, F.; Ferlay, J.; Soerjomataram, I.; Siegel, R.L.; Torre, L.A.; Jemal, A. Global cancer statistics 2018: GLOBOCAN estimates of incidence and mortality worldwide for 36 cancers in 185 countries. *CA Cancer J. Clin.* **2018**, *68*, 394–424. [CrossRef]
11. de Martel, C.; Georges, D.; Bray, F.; Ferlay, J.; Clifford, G.M. Global burden of cancer attributable to infections in 2018: A worldwide incidence analysis. *Lancet Glob. Health* **2020**, *8*, e180–e190. [CrossRef]
12. Collatuzzo, G.; Pelucchi, C.; Negri, E.; López-Carrillo, L.; Tsugane, S.; Hidaka, A.; Hamada, G.S.; Hernández-Ramírez, R.U.; López-Cervantes, M.; Malekzadeh, R.; et al. Exploring the interactions between Helicobacter pylori infection and other risk factors of gastric cancer: A pooled analysis in the Stomach cancer Pooling (StoP) Project. *Int. J. Cancer* **2021**, *149*, 1228–1238. [CrossRef]
13. Shikata, K.; Doi, Y.; Yonemoto, K.; Arima, H.; Ninomiya, T.; Kubo, M.; Tanizaki, Y.; Matsumoto, T.; Iida, M.; Kiyohara, Y. Population-based prospective study of the combined influence of cigarette smoking and Helicobacter pylori infection on gastric cancer incidence: The Hisayama Study. *Am. J. Epidemiol.* **2008**, *168*, 1409–1415. [CrossRef]

https://doi.org/10.3390/life16010161

14. Gaddy, J.A.; Radin, J.N.; Loh, J.T.; Zhang, F.; Washington, M.K.; Peek, R.M., Jr.; Algood, H.M.S.; Cover, T.L. High dietary salt intake exacerbates Helicobacter pylori-induced gastric carcinogenesis. *Infect. Immun.* **2013**, *81*, 2258–2267. [CrossRef] [PubMed]
15. Bertuccio, P.; Rosato, V.; Andreano, A.; Ferraroni, M.; Decarli, A.; Edefonti, V.; La Vecchia, C. Dietary patterns and gastric cancer risk: A systematic review and meta-analysis. *Ann. Oncol.* **2013**, *24*, 1450–1458. [CrossRef] [PubMed]
16. Ladigan-Badura, S.; Vangala, D.B.; Engel, C.; Bucksch, K.; Hueneburg, R.; Perne, C.; Nattermann, J.; Steinke-Lange, V.; Rahner, N.; Schackert, H.K.; et al. Value of upper gastrointestinal endoscopy for gastric cancer surveillance in patients with Lynch syndrome. *Int. J. Cancer* **2021**, *148*, 106–114. [CrossRef] [PubMed]
17. Chan, W.L.; Lam, K.O.; Lee, V.H.F.; Davidson, M.; So, T.H.; Li, J.S.; Chau, I.; Kwong, D.L.W. Gastric cancer—From aetiology to management: Differences between the East and the West. *Clin. Oncol. (R. Coll. Radiol.)* **2019**, *31*, 570–577. [CrossRef]
18. Ono, H.; Yao, K.; Fujishiro, M.; Oda, I.; Uedo, N.; Nimura, S.; Yahagi, N.; Iishi, H.; Oka, M.; Ajioka, Y.; et al. Guidelines for endoscopic submucosal dissection and endoscopic mucosal resection for early gastric cancer (second edition). *Dig. Endosc.* **2021**, *33*, 4–20. [CrossRef]
19. Muto, M.; Yao, K.; Kaise, M.; Kato, M.; Uedo, N.; Yagi, K.; Tajiri, H. Magnifying endoscopy simple diagnostic algorithm for early gastric cancer (MESDA-G). *Dig. Endosc.* **2016**, *28*, 379–393. [CrossRef]
20. Gotoda, T. A large endoscopic resection by endoscopic submucosal dissection procedure for early gastric cancer. *Clin. Gastroenterol. Hepatol.* **2005**, *3*, S71–S73. [CrossRef]
21. Isomoto, H.; Shikuwa, S.; Yamaguchi, N.; Fukuda, E.; Ikeda, K.; Nishiyama, H.; Ohnita, K.; Mizuta, Y.; Shiozawa, J.; Kohno, S. Endoscopic submucosal dissection for early gastric cancer: A large-scale feasibility study. *Gut* **2009**, *58*, 331–336. [CrossRef]
22. Nishizawa, T.; Yahagi, N. Long-term outcomes of using endoscopic submucosal dissection to treat early gastric cancer. *Gut Liver* **2018**, *12*, 119–124. [CrossRef]
23. Oda, I.; Saito, D.; Tada, M.; Iishi, H.; Tanabe, S.; Oyama, T.; Doi, T.; Otani, Y.; Fujisaki, J.; Ajioka, Y.; et al. A multicenter retrospective study of endoscopic resection for early gastric cancer. *Gastric Cancer* **2006**, *9*, 262–270. [CrossRef] [PubMed]
24. Hamming, I.; Timens, W.; Bulthuis, M.L.; Lely, A.T.; Navis, G.; van Goor, H. Tissue distribution of ACE2 protein, the functional receptor for SARS coronavirus. *J. Pathol.* **2004**, *203*, 631–637. [CrossRef] [PubMed]
25. Ziegler, C.G.K.; Allon, S.J.; Nyquist, S.K.; Mbano, I.M.; Miao, V.N.; Tzouanas, C.N.; Cao, Y.; Yousif, A.S.; Bals, J.; Hauser, B.M.; et al. SARS-CoV-2 receptor ACE2 is an interferon-stimulated gene in human airway epithelial cells and is detected in specific cell subsets across tissues. *Cell* **2020**, *181*, 1016–1035.e19. [CrossRef] [PubMed]
26. Xiao, F.; Tang, M.; Zheng, X.; Liu, Y.; Li, X.; Shan, H. Evidence for gastrointestinal infection of SARS-CoV-2. *Gastroenterology* **2020**, *158*, 1831–1833.e3. [CrossRef]
27. Jin, X.; Lian, J.S.; Hu, J.H.; Gao, J.; Zheng, L.; Zhang, Y.-M.; Hao, S.-R.; Jia, H.-Y.; Cai, H.; Zhang, X.-L.; et al. Epidemiological, clinical and virological characteristics of 74 cases of COVID-19 with gastrointestinal symptoms. *Gut* **2020**, *69*, 1002–1009. [CrossRef]
28. Hussain, I.; Cher, G.L.Y.; Abid, M.A.; Abid, M.B. Role of gut microbiome in COVID-19: An insight into pathogenesis and therapeutic potential. *Front. Immunol.* **2021**, *12*, 765965. [CrossRef]
29. Mizutani, T.; Ishizaka, A.; Koga, M.; Ikeuchi, K.; Saito, M.; Adachi, E.; Yamayoshi, S.; Iwatsuki Horimoto, K.; Yasuhara, A.; Kiyono, H.; et al. Correlation analysis between gut microbiota alterations and the cytokine response in patients with coronavirus disease during hospitalization. *Microbiol. Spectr.* **2022**, *10*, e0168921. [CrossRef]
30. Giron, L.B.; Dweep, H.; Yin, X.; Wang, H.; Damra, M.; Goldman, A.R.; Gorman, N.; Palmer, C.S.; Tang, H.-Y.; Shaikh, M.W.; et al. Plasma markers of disrupted gut permeability in severe COVID-19 patients. *Front. Immunol.* **2021**, *12*, 686240.
31. Dmytriv, T.R.; Storey, K.B.; Lushchak, V.I. Intestinal barrier permeability: The influence of gut microbiota, nutrition, and exercise. *Front. Physiol.* **2024**, *15*, 1380713. [CrossRef]
32. Sandal, S.; Tanaş, Ö.; Karabulut, Ş.; Çaydere, M.; Hücümenoğlu, S. A histopathological view at the long-term effects of COVID-19 on the gastrointestinal system in children. *Turk. J. Pediatr.* **2023**, *65*, 416–424. [CrossRef] [PubMed]
33. Andrews, P.L.; Cai, W.; Rudd, J.A.; Sanger, G.J. COVID-19, nausea, and vomiting. *J. Gastroenterol. Hepatol.* **2021**, *36*, 646–656. [CrossRef] [PubMed]
34. Deb, A.; Thongtan, T.; Costilla, V. Gastric ulcerations in COVID-19: An ominous sign? *BMJ Case Rep.* **2021**, *14*, e244059. [CrossRef] [PubMed]
35. Oliviero, G.; Ruggiero, L.; D'antonio, E.; Gagliardi, M.; Nunziata, R.; Di Sarno, A.; Abbatiello, C.; Di Feo, E.; De Vivo, S.; Santonicola, A.; et al. Impact of COVID-19 lockdown on symptoms in patients with functional gastrointestinal disorders: Relationship with anxiety and perceived stress. *Neurogastroenterol. Motil.* **2021**, *33*, e14092. [CrossRef]
36. Stepanov, Y.; Demeshkina, L.; Mosiyjchuk, L.; Zyhalo, E.; Yagmur, V.; Petishko, O. Depressive disorders in gastroenterological patients during the COVID-19 period. *J. Natl. Acad. Med. Sci. Ukr.* **2021**, *27*, 263–270.
37. Omidifar, N.; Pazoki, N.; Shokripour, M.; Fattahi, M.R.; Safarpour, A.R.; Abarghooee, E.F.; Nikmanesh, N.; Shamsdin, S.A.; Akrami, H.; Saghi, S.A.; et al. The effect of COVID-19 on the quality of associated care in patients with gastric cancer. *Middle East J. Dig. Dis.* **2024**, *16*, 12–22. [CrossRef]

https://doi.org/10.3390/life16010161

38. Li, Y.-X.; He, C.-Z.; Liu, Y.-C.; Zhao, P.-Y.; Xu, X.-L.; Wang, Y.-F.; Xia, S.-Y.; Du, X.-H. The impact of COVID-19 on gastric cancer surgery: A single-center retrospective study. *BMC Surg.* **2020**, *20*, 222. [CrossRef]
39. McElvaney, O.J.; McEvoy, N.L.; McElvaney, O.F.; Carroll, T.P.; Murphy, M.P.; Dunlea, D.M.; Ní Choileáin, O.; Clarke, J.; O'Connor, E.; Hogan, G.; et al. Characterization of the inflammatory response to severe COVID-19 illness. *Am. J. Respir. Crit. Care Med.* **2020**, *202*, 812–821. [CrossRef]
40. Zeng, Z.; Yu, H.; Chen, H.; Qi, W.; Chen, L.; Chen, G.; Yan, W.; Chen, T.; Ning, Q.; Han, M.; et al. Longitudinal changes of inflammatory parameters and their correlation with disease severity and outcomes in patients with COVID-19. *Crit. Care* **2020**, *24*, 525. [CrossRef]
41. Levi, M.; van Es, N. COVID-19 associated coagulopathy and thrombosis in cancer. *Thromb. Res.* **2022**, *213*, S72–S76. [CrossRef]
42. Mehta, P.; McAuley, D.F.; Brown, M.; Sanchez, E.; Tattersall, R.S.; Manson, J.J.; on behalf of the HLH Across Speciality Collaboration, UK. COVID-19: Consider cytokine storm syndromes and immunosuppression. *Lancet* **2020**, *395*, 1033–1034. [CrossRef] [PubMed]
43. Aydın, M.; Dülger, A.C.; Özer, S.; Dirik, Y.; Keskin, S.; Demir, C. Gastric intestinal metaplasia and COVID-19 infection. *East J. Med.* **2020**, *25*, 571–575. [CrossRef]
44. Nieuwenburg, S.A.V.; Waddingham, W.W.; Graham, D.; Rodriguez-Justo, M.; Biermann, K.; Kuipers, E.J.; Banks, M.; Jansen, M.; Spaander, M.C. Accuracy of endoscopic staging and targeted biopsies for routine gastric intestinal metaplasia and gastric atrophy evaluation: The ESTIMATE study protocol. *BMJ Open* **2019**, *9*, e032013. [CrossRef] [PubMed]
45. Darif, D.; Hammi, I.; Kihel, A.; Saik, I.E.I.; Guessous, F.; Akarid, K. The pro-inflammatory cytokines in COVID-19 pathogenesis: What goes wrong? *Microb. Pathog.* **2021**, *153*, 104799. [CrossRef]
46. Buscarini, E.; Benedetti, A.; Monica, F.; Pasquale, L.; Buttitta, F.; Cameletti, M.; Ferrari, C.; Ricciardiello, L.; Massironi, S.; Bianco, M.A.; et al. Changes in digestive cancer diagnosis during the SARS CoV 2 pandemic in Italy: A nationwide survey. *Dig. Liver Dis.* **2021**, *53*, 682–688. [CrossRef]
47. Chiriac, S.; Stanciu, C.; Căruntu, F.; Cojocariu, C.; Sfarti, C.; Singeap, A.M.; Girleanu, I.; Cuciureanu, T.; Huiban, L.; David, D.; et al. The impact of the COVID-19 pandemic on gastrointestinal endoscopy activity in a tertiary care center from Romania. *Medicina* **2021**, *57*, 457.
48. Longcroft-Wheaton, G.; Tolfree, N.; Gangi, A.; Beable, R.; Bhandari, P. Data from a large Western centre exploring the impact of COVID-19 pandemic on endoscopy services and cancer diagnosis. *Frontline Gastroenterol.* **2021**, *12*, 193–199. [CrossRef]
49. Hayee, B.; Thoufeeq, M.; Rees, C.J.; Penman, I.; East, J. Safely restarting GI endoscopy in the era of COVID-19. *Gut* **2020**, *69*, 2063–2070. [CrossRef]
50. Suh, M.A.; Park, S.B.; Kwak, M.S.; Yoon, J.Y.; Cha, J.M. Impact of the COVID-19 pandemic on esophagogastroduodenoscopy and gastric cancer claims in South Korea: A nationwide, population based study. *Yonsei Med. J.* **2023**, *64*, 549–557. [CrossRef]
51. Lee, K.; Suh, M.; Jun, J.K.; Choi, K.S. Impact of the COVID-19 pandemic on gastric cancer screening in South Korea: Results from the Korean National Cancer Screening Survey (2017–2021). *J. Gastric Cancer* **2022**, *22*, 264–272. [CrossRef]
52. Kodama, M.; Miyamori, D.; Kanno, K.; Ito, M. The impact of early stage COVID-19 pandemic on the diagnosis and treatment of gastric cancer: A cross sectional study using a large scale cancer registry in Hiroshima, Japan. *DEN Open* **2022**, *3*, e180. [CrossRef]
53. Tokunaga, M.; Yoshikawa, T.; Boku, N.; Nishida, Y.; Tanahashi, T.; Yamada, T.; Haruta, S.; Etoh, T.; Hirahara, N.; Kawachi, Y.; et al. Impact of COVID-19 on gastric cancer treatment in Japanese high volume centers: A JCOG stomach cancer study group survey. *Surg. Today* **2022**, *52*, 231–238. [CrossRef] [PubMed]
54. Walker, M.J.; Meggetto, O.; Gao, J.; Espino-Hernández, G.; Jembere, N.; Bravo, C.A.; Rey, M.; Aslam, U.; Sheppard, A.J.; Lofters, A.K.; et al. Measuring the impact of the COVID-19 pandemic on organized cancer screening and diagnostic follow up care in Ontario, Canada: A provincial, population based study. *Prev. Med.* **2021**, *151*, 106586. [CrossRef] [PubMed]
55. Hong, M.; Choi, M.; Lee, J.; Kim, K.H.; Kim, H.; Lee, C.-K.; Kim, H.S.; Rha, S.Y.; Pih, G.Y.; Choi, Y.J.; et al. Impact of COVID-19 on gastric cancer diagnosis and stage: A single institute study in South Korea. *J. Gastric Cancer* **2023**, *23*, 574–583. [CrossRef] [PubMed]
56. Zhang, H.; Yang, W.; Tan, X.; He, W.; Zhao, L.; Liu, H.; Li, G. Long term relative survival of patients with gastric cancer from a large scale cohort: A period analysis. *BMC Cancer* **2024**, *24*, 1420. [CrossRef]
57. Rikhraj, N.K. Survival outcomes in patients with stages I–III gastric adenocarcinoma treated with surgery alone versus surgery plus adjuvant chemotherapy: A systematic review. *J. Biol. Methods* **2025**, *12*, e99010060. [CrossRef]
58. Rutter, M.D.; Brookes, M.; Lee, T.J.; Rogers, P.; Sharp, L. Impact of the COVID-19 pandemic on UK endoscopic activity and cancer detection: A National Endoscopy Database analysis. *Gut* **2021**, *70*, 537–543. [CrossRef]
59. Calderwood, A.H.; Calderwood, M.S.; Williams, J.L.; Dominitz, J.A. Impact of the COVID-19 pandemic on utilization of EGD and colonoscopy in the United States: An analysis of the GIQuIC registry. *Tech. Innov. Gastrointest. Endosc.* **2021**, *23*, 313–321. [CrossRef]
60. Mattioli, A.V.; Sciomer, S.; Cocchi, C.; Maffei, S.; Gallina, S. Quarantine during COVID-19 outbreak: Changes in diet and physical activity increase the risk of cardiovascular disease. *Nutr. Metab. Cardiovasc. Dis.* **2020**, *30*, 1409–1417. [CrossRef]

https://doi.org/10.3390/life16010161

61. Renehan, A.G.; Tyson, M.; Egger, M.; Heller, R.F.; Zwahlen, M. Body mass index and incidence of cancer: A systematic review and meta analysis of prospective observational studies. *Lancet* **2008**, *371*, 569–578. [CrossRef]
62. Konorev, M.R.; Tyshevich, E.N.; Pavlyukov, R.A. Application of N acetyl glucosaminyl N acetyl muramyl dipeptide during triple component anti Helicobacter pylori therapy in the period of COVID-19. *Russ. J. Gastroenterol. Hepatol. Coloproctol.* **2023**, *33*, 60–69. [CrossRef]
63. Cavic, M.; Krivokuca, A.; Boljevic, I.; Spasic, J.; Mihajlovic, M.; Pavlovic, M.; Damjanovic, A.; Radosavljevic, D.; Jankovic, R. Exploring the real world effect of the SARS CoV 2 pandemic on the molecular diagnostics for cancer patients and high risk individuals. *Expert Rev. Mol. Diagn.* **2021**, *21*, 101–107. [CrossRef] [PubMed]
64. Norman, M.L.; Malcolmson, J.; Armel, S.R.; Gillies, B.; Ou, B.; Thain, E.; McCuaig, J.M.; Kim, R.H. Stay at home: Implementation and impact of virtualising cancer genetic services during COVID-19. *J. Med. Genet.* **2022**, *59*, 23–27. [CrossRef] [PubMed]
65. Kuderer, N.M.; Choueiri, T.K.; Shah, D.P.; Shyr, Y.; Rubinstein, S.M.; Rivera, D.R.; Shete, S.; Hsu, C.-Y.; Desai, A.; de Lima Lopes, G., Jr.; et al. Clinical impact of COVID-19 on patients with cancer (CCC19): A cohort study. *Lancet* **2020**, *395*, 1907–1918. [CrossRef]
66. de Melo, A.C.; Thuler, L.C.S.; da Silva, J.L.; de Albuquerque, L.Z.; Pecego, A.C.; Rodrigues, L.D.O.; da Conceição, M.S.; Garrido, M.M.; Quintella Mendes, G.L.; Mendes Pereira, A.C.P.; et al. Cancer inpatients with COVID-19: A report from the Brazilian National Cancer Institute. *PLoS ONE* **2020**, *15*, e0241261. [CrossRef]
67. Yekedüz, E.; Utkan, G.; Ürün, Y. A systematic review and meta analysis: The effect of active cancer treatment on severity of COVID-19. *Eur. J. Cancer* **2020**, *141*, 92–104. [CrossRef]
68. Bilich, T.; Roerden, M.; Maringer, Y.; Nelde, A.; Heitmann, J.S.; Dubbelaar, M.L.; Peter, A.; Hörber, S.; Bauer, J.; Rieth, J.; et al. Preexisting and post COVID-19 immune responses to SARS CoV 2 in patients with cancer. *Cancer Discov.* **2021**, *11*, 1982–1995. [CrossRef]
69. Salvatore, M.; Hu, M.M.; Beesley, L.J.; Mondul, A.M.; Pearce, C.L.; Friese, C.R.; Fritsche, L.G.; Mukherjee, B. COVID-19 outcomes by cancer status, site, treatment, and vaccination. *Cancer Epidemiol. Biomark. Prev.* **2023**, *32*, 748–759. [CrossRef]
70. Jones, M.; Higgs, S.; Dwerryhouse, S.; Markos, V.; Mason, K.; Green, C.; Nawwar, A.; Searle, J.; Lyburn, I. Combined PET and contrast enhanced CT (PET/CeCT) as a single staging investigation for oesophagogastric cancers during the COVID-19 pandemic: Pilot single centre experience. *Ann. R. Coll. Surg. Engl.* **2024**, *106*, 576–584. [CrossRef]
71. Bouthillier, M.-E.; Lorange, M.; Legault, S.; Wade, L.; Dahine, J.; Latreille, J.; Germain, I.; Grégoire, R.; Montpetit, P.; Prady, C.; et al. Prioritizing surgery during the COVID-19 pandemic: The Quebec guidelines. *Can. J. Surg.* **2021**, *64*, E103–E107. [CrossRef]
72. Dalu, D.; Rota, S.; Cona, M.S.; Brambilla, A.M.; Ferrario, S.; Gambaro, A.; Meroni, L.; Merli, S.; Farina, G.; La Verde, N. A proposal of a "ready to use" COVID-19 control strategy in an oncology ward: Utopia or reality? *Crit. Rev. Oncol. Hematol.* **2021**, *157*, 103168. [CrossRef]
73. Fligor, S.C.; Wang, S.; Allar, B.G.; Tsikis, S.T.; Ore, A.S.; Whitlock, A.E.; Calvillo-Ortiz, R.; Arndt, K.R.; Gangadharan, S.P.; Callery, M.P. Gastrointestinal malignancies and the COVID-19 pandemic: Evidence based triage to surgery. *J. Gastrointest. Surg.* **2020**, *24*, 2357–2373. [CrossRef] [PubMed]
74. Ma, J.; Zhu, C.; Li, W.; Qiu, Z.; Yang, J.; Ge, L.; Da, M. The effect of delayed oncology surgery on survival outcomes for patients with gastric cancer during the COVID-19 pandemic: Evidence based strategies. *Front. Oncol.* **2022**, *12*, 780949. [CrossRef] [PubMed]
75. Mitra, S.; Simson, D.K.; Khurana, H.; Tandon, S.; Ahlawat, P.; Bansal, N.; Barik, S.; Sethi, J.S.; Chufal, K.S.; Gairola, M. Treatment delay during radiotherapy of cancer patients due to the COVID-19 pandemic. *Asian Pac. J. Cancer Prev.* **2022**, *23*, 2415–2420. [CrossRef] [PubMed]
76. de Joode, K.; Dumoulin, D.W.; Engelen, V.; Bloemendal, H.J.; Verheij, M.; Van Laarhoven, H.W.M.; Dingemans, I.H.; Dingemans, A.C.; Van Der Veldt, A.A.M. Impact of the COVID-19 pandemic on cancer treatment: The patients' per-spective. *Eur. J. Cancer* **2020**, *136*, 132–139. [CrossRef]
77. Zhu, J.H.; Pan, J.; Xu, X.N.; Liu, Y.W.; Qian, Y.Y.; Jiang, X.; Jiang, B.; Zhou, W.; Linghu, E.Q.; Li, Z.S.; et al. Noncontact magnetically controlled capsule endoscopy for infection free gastric examination during the COVID-19 pandemic: A pilot, open label, randomized trial. *Endosc. Int. Open* **2022**, *10*, E163–E170. [CrossRef]
78. Lukas, H.; Xu, C.; Yu, Y.; Gao, W. Emerging telemedicine tools for remote COVID-19 diagnosis, monitoring, and management. *ACS Nano* **2020**, *14*, 16180–16193. [CrossRef]
79. Shah, R.; Hanna, N.M.; Loo, C.E.; David, M.; Mafra, A.; Fink, H.; McFerran, E.; Garcia, M.; Ghodssighassemabadi, R.; Acharya, S.; et al. The global impact of the COVID-19 pandemic on delays and disruptions in cancer care services: A systematic review and meta-analysis. *Nat. Cancer* **2025**, *6*, 194–204. [CrossRef]
80. Spencer, K.; Jones, C.M.; Girdler, R.; Roe, C.; Sharpe, M.; Lawton, S.; Miller, L.; Lewis, P.; Evans, M.; Sebag-Montefiore, D.; et al. The impact of the COVID-19 pandemic on radiotherapy services in England, UK: A population-based study from the National Radiotherapy Dataset. *Lancet Oncol.* **2021**, *22*, 309–320. [CrossRef]

https://doi.org/10.3390/life16010161

81. Doeve, B.H.; Bakx, J.A.C.; Siersema, P.D.; Rosman, C.; van Grieken, N.C.T.; Henegouwen, M.I.v.B.; van Sandick, J.W.; Verheij, M.; Bijlsma, M.F.; Verhoeven, R.H.A.; et al. The impact of the COVID-19 pandemic on the diagnosis, stage, and treatment of esophagogastric cancer. *J. Gastroenterol.* **2023**, *58*, 965–977. [CrossRef]
82. Desai, A.; Gainor, J.F.; Hegde, A.; Schram, A.M.; Curigliano, G.; Pal, S.; Liu, S.V.; Halmos, B.; Groisberg, R.; Grande, E.; et al. COVID-19 vaccine guidance for patients with cancer participating in oncology clinical trials. *Nat. Rev. Clin. Oncol.* **2021**, *18*, 313–319. [CrossRef] [PubMed]
83. Grinshpun, A.; Rottenberg, Y.; Ben-Dov, I.; Djian, E.; Wolf, D.; Kadouri, L. Serologic response to COVID-19 infection and/or vaccine in cancer patients on active treatment. *ESMO Open* **2021**, *6*, 100283. [CrossRef] [PubMed]
84. Khan, Q.J.; Bivona, C.R.; Martin, G.A.; Zhang, J.; Liu, B.; He, J.; Li, K.H.; Nelson, M.; Williamson, S.; Doolittle, G.C.; et al. Evaluation of the durability of the immune humoral response to COVID-19 vaccines in patients with cancer undergoing treatment or who received a stem cell transplant. *JAMA Oncol.* **2022**, *8*, 1053–1058. [CrossRef] [PubMed]
85. Liatsou, E.; Ntanasis Stathopoulos, I.; Lykos, S.; Ntanasis-Stathopoulos, A.; Gavriatopoulou, M.; Psaltopoulou, T.; Sergentanis, T.N.; Terpos, E. Adult patients with cancer have impaired humoral responses to complete and booster COVID-19 vaccination: A systematic review and meta analysis. *Cancers* **2023**, *15*, 2266. [CrossRef]
86. Bagus, B.I. Gastrointestinal cancer and vaccination safety during the COVID-19 pandemic. *Open Access Maced. J. Med. Sci.* **2022**, *10*, 1832–1834. [CrossRef]
87. Sultan, S.; Siddique, S.M.; Singh, S.; Altayar, O.; Caliendo, A.M.; Davitkov, P.; Feuerstein, J.D.; Kaul, V.; Lim, J.K.; Mustafa, R.A.; et al. AGA rapid review and guideline for SARS CoV 2 testing and endoscopy post vaccination: 2021 update. *Gastroenterology* **2021**, *161*, 1011–1029.e11. [CrossRef]
88. Peña-Rey, I.; Almazán, R.; Rodríguez-Camacho, E.; Cubiella, J. Resumption of endoscopy in the Galician colorectal cancer screening programme after the COVID-19 lockdown: Patient safety results. *Rev. Esp. Enferm. Dig.* **2021**, *113*, 119–121.
89. Giuffrida, P.; Ewing, I.; Wood, E.; Thoua, N.; Spranger, H.; Chin, J.L.; Asilmaz, E.; Shidrawi, R.; Marelli, L. PTH-49 Successful endoscopy recovery strategy after the first wave of the COVID-19 pandemic. *Gut* **2021**, *70*, A197.
90. Achangwa, C.; Lee, T.-J.; Lee, M.-S. Acceptance of the COVID-19 vaccine by foreigners in South Korea. *Int. J. Environ. Res. Public Health* **2021**, *18*, 12035. [CrossRef]
91. Jones, M.; Higgs, S.; Dwerryhouse, S.; Markos, V.; Mason, K.; Lyburn, I. Use of a single visit combined contrast enhanced CT with PET (PET/CeCT) in staging of oesophageal and gastric cancers during the COVID-19 pandemic—Is it adequate, timely and cost effective? *Br. J. Surg.* **2021**, *108*, znab430.203. [CrossRef]
92. Borggreve, A.S.; Goense, L.; Brenkman, H.J.; Mook, S.; Meijer, G.J.; Wessels, F.J.; Verheij, M.; Jansen, E.P.; van Hillegersberg, R.; van Rossum, P.S.; et al. Imaging strategies in the management of gastric cancer: Current role and future potential of MRI. *Br. J. Radiol.* **2019**, *92*, 20181044. [CrossRef]
93. Kwee, R.M.; Kwee, T.C. Imaging in local staging of gastric cancer: A systematic review. *J. Clin. Oncol.* **2007**, *25*, 2107–2116. [CrossRef] [PubMed]
94. Mickevicius, A.; Ignatavicius, P.; Markelis, R.; Parseliunas, A.; Butkute, D.; Kiudelis, M.; Endzinas, Z.; Maleckas, A.; Dambrauskas, Z. Trends and results in treatment of gastric cancer over last two decades at single East European centre: A cohort study. *BMC Surg.* **2014**, *14*, 98. [CrossRef] [PubMed]
95. Zheng, X.; Ding, S.; Wu, M.; Sun, C.; Wu, Y.; Wang, S.; Du, Y.; Yang, L.; Xue, L.; Wang, B.; et al. Dynamic monitoring revealed a slightly prolonged waiting time for total gastrectomy during the COVID-19 pandemic without increasing the short term complications. *Front. Oncol.* **2022**, *12*, 944602. [CrossRef] [PubMed]
96. Murthy, S.; Gomersall, C.D.; Fowler, R.A. Care for critically ill patients with COVID-19. *JAMA* **2020**, *323*, 1499–1500. [CrossRef]
97. Ang, T.L. Gastrointestinal endoscopy during COVID-19 pandemic. *J. Gastroenterol. Hepatol.* **2020**, *35*, 701–702. [CrossRef]
98. Liao, Z.; He, S.; Sha, W.; Feng, Z.; Sun, X.; Wan, J.; Pan, J.; Wang, S.; Linghu, E.; Li, Z.; et al. Capsule endoscopy practice during the COVID-19 pandemic: Recommenda-tions from the Capsule Endoscopy Group of the Chinese Society of Digestive Endoscopy. *Endosc. Int. Open* **2021**, *9*, E280–E283. [CrossRef]
99. de Steur, W.; Henneman, D.; Allum, W.; Dikken, J.; van Sandick, J.; Reynolds, J.; Mariette, C.; Jensen, L.; Johansson, J.; Kolodziejczyk, P.; et al. Common data items in seven European oesophagogastric cancer surgery registries: Towards a European upper GI cancer audit (EURECCA Upper GI). *Eur. J. Surg. Oncol.* **2014**, *40*, 325–329. [CrossRef]
100. West, H. Telemedicine in oncology: Delivering on an overdue promise in the COVID-19 era. *Front. Oncol.* **2020**, *10*, 578888. [CrossRef]
101. Jin, J.; Zhang, Q.; Dong, B.; Ma, T.; Mei, X.; Wang, X.; Song, S.; Peng, J.; Wu, A.; Dong, L.; et al. Automatic detection of early gastric cancer in endoscopy based on Mask region-based convolutional neural networks (Mask R-CNN). *Front. Oncol.* **2022**, *12*, 927868. [CrossRef]
102. Lee, A.J.X.; Purshouse, K. COVID-19 and cancer registries: Learning from the first peak of the SARS-CoV-2 pandemic. *Br. J. Cancer* **2021**, *124*, 1777–1784. [CrossRef]
103. Ali, J.K.; Riches, J.C. The impact of the COVID-19 pandemic on oncology care and clinical trials. *Cancers* **2021**, *13*, 5924. [CrossRef]

104. Ma, K.; Chen, X.; Xiang, X.; Mao, X.; Zhu, N.; Wang, T.; Ye, S.; Wang, X.; Deng, M. Willingness to undergo gastroscopy for early gastric cancer screening and its associated factors during the COVID-19 pandemic: A nationwide cross sectional study in China. *Patient Prefer. Adherence* **2023**, *17*, 505–516. [CrossRef]
105. Dhada, S.; Stewart, D.; Cheema, E.; Hadi, M.A.; Paudyal, V. Cancer services during the COVID-19 pandemic: Systematic review of patients' and caregivers' experiences. *Cancer Manag. Res.* **2021**, *13*, 5875–5887. [CrossRef]
106. Cavaliere, D.; Parini, D.; Marano, L.; Cipriani, F.; Di Marzo, F.; Macrì, A.; D'Ugo, D.; Roviello, F.; Gronchi, A. Surgical management of oncologic patients during and after the COVID-19 outbreak: Practical recommendations from the Italian Society of Surgical Oncology. *Updates Surg.* **2021**, *73*, 321–329. [CrossRef]

https://doi.org/10.3390/life16010161

life

MDPI

Article

Ki-67 and Tumor Size in Small Bowel Tumors: Findings from an Exploratory Immunohistochemical Analysis

Laurențiu Augustus Barbu [1], Liliana Cercelaru [2], Valeriu Șurlin [3], Stelian-Stefaniță Mogoantă [3], Tiberiu Stefăniță Țenea Cojan [1], Daniela Marinescu [3], Nicolae-Dragoș Mărgăritescu [3,*] and Liviu Vasile [3]

[1] Department of Surgery, Railway Clinical Hospital Craiova, University of Medicine and Pharmacy of Craiova, 200349 Craiova, Romania; laurentiu.barbu@umfcv.ro (L.A.B.); tiberiu.tenea@umfcv.ro (T.S.Ț.C.)

[2] Department of Embryology and Anatomy, University of Medicine and Pharmacy of Craiova, 200349 Craiova, Romania; liliana.cercelaru@umfcv.ro

[3] Department of Surgery, Emergency County Hospital, University of Medicine and Pharmacy of Craiova, 200349 Craiova, Romania; vsurlin@gmail.com (V.Ș.); ssmogo@yahoo.com (S.-S.M.); dtmarinescu@yahoo.com (D.M.); vliviu777@yahoo.com (L.V.)

* Correspondence: dmargaritescu@yahoo.com; Tel.: +40-723-271-941

Abstract: Background: Small bowel tumors are rare and biologically diverse, and prognostic assessment remains difficult, particularly regarding proliferative markers such as Ki-67 and tumor size. Objective: To evaluate the clinicopathological and immunohistochemical characteristics of small bowel tumors and explore factors associated with malignancy. Methods: A retrospective analysis of 61 surgically treated primary small bowel tumors (2020–2024) was performed using WHO 2019/2022 and AJCC 8th criteria. Immunohistochemistry included CD117, DOG1, CD34, SMA, and Ki-67. Results: Adenocarcinomas were most frequent (52.5%), followed by GISTs (26.2%) and NETs (9.8%). CD117 and DOG1 were expressed in 93.8% of GISTs, confirming high diagnostic specificity. The median Ki-67 index was 8%, significantly higher in non-GIST tumors ($p = 0.004$). Tumor size correlated moderately with Ki-67 ($\rho = 0.42$, $p = 0.018$). In this exploratory model, tumor size > 5 cm ($p = 0.03$) and Ki-67 > 10% ($p = 0.04$) were associated with malignancy. Conclusions: Tumor size and Ki-67 were associated with malignancy in this exploratory multivariable analysis, but these findings should be interpreted with caution due to limited follow-up and sample imbalance. Combined with CD117/DOG1 profiling, they enhance diagnostic accuracy and may inform diagnostic assessment; however, prognostic implications require outcome-based studies.

Keywords: small bowel tumors; gastrointestinal stromal tumor (GIST); Ki-67; tumor size; CD117; DOG1; CD34; immunohistochemistry

1. Introduction

Primary tumors of the small intestine are rare, accounting for approximately 3% of all gastrointestinal malignancies, yet their incidence has been steadily increasing over recent decades [1]. The four predominant histological subtypes include adenocarcinomas, neuroendocrine tumors (NETs), gastrointestinal stromal tumors (GISTs), and lymphomas, each exhibiting distinct biological behaviors and therapeutic implications [1,2]. Despite technological advances, the diagnosis of small bowel tumors remains challenging due to non-specific symptoms and the limited accessibility of the small intestine to conventional endoscopy. The use of capsule endoscopy and double-balloon enteroscopy has improved detection, although most patients are still diagnosed at advanced stages [2,3].

Adenocarcinomas and NETs represent roughly 80% of small bowel malignancies, while GISTs and lymphomas account for the remainder [2]. Adenocarcinomas arise predominantly in the duodenum and are often associated with inflammatory or hereditary conditions such as Crohn's disease and Lynch syndrome [1]. NETs occur mainly in the distal ileum and currently represent the most frequent primary small bowel cancer, with an incidence of 0.67–1.2 per 100 000 and frequent nodal or hepatic metastases at presentation [3]. GISTs constitute about 20–30% of mesenchymal small bowel tumors and demonstrate site-dependent biological heterogeneity, with higher mitotic activity and risk profiles in distal locations [4]. Small bowel lymphomas, though uncommon, comprise up to 40% of extranodal lymphomas, most often of the follicular, diffuse large B-cell, or MALT subtypes [5].

Immunohistochemistry plays a pivotal role in the diagnosis and risk assessment of these tumors. CD117 (c-KIT) and DOG1 are highly specific for GISTs, while CD34 co-expression aids in differentiating stromal from smooth-muscle lesions [6]. The Ki-67 labeling index is crucial for grading NETs, with thresholds of $<3\%$, 3–20%, and $>20\%$ defining G1, G2, and G3 categories, respectively [4]. Evaluation of mismatch-repair (MMR) and microsatellite instability (MSI) status also assists in identifying hereditary adenocarcinomas and immunotherapy candidates [1].

The aim of this study was not simply to confirm established immunohistochemical phenotypes, but to explore whether tumor size and the Ki-67 proliferation index correlate with malignancy status within a homogeneous cohort of surgically treated primary small bowel tumors, and to describe subtype-specific patterns in an anatomical and histological context. Despite major advances in immunohistochemical and molecular profiling, large homogeneous surgical series focused exclusively on small bowel tumors remain scarce. Most studies combine gastric and intestinal sites, limiting the interpretation of site-specific correlations [2,4]. In this context, the present work provides exploratory data that may support risk stratification and diagnostic assessment in small intestinal malignancies.

2. Materials and Methods

2.1. Study Design and Patient Selection

This retrospective, cross-sectional cohort study included 61 consecutive patients with histologically confirmed primary small bowel tumors who underwent surgical treatment between January 2020 and December 2024 at the Clinical County Hospital of Craiova, Romania. All patients underwent surgical treatment during the study period, performed either with curative or palliative intent depending on the extent of disease and intraoperative findings.

Inclusion criteria were (1) patients with primary small bowel tumors confirmed by histopathological and immunohistochemical examination, and (2) availability of complete clinical, surgical, and pathological data during the study period.

Exclusion criteria included (1) metastatic lesions originating from extraintestinal primaries; (2) recurrent tumors; (3) incomplete clinical documentation or missing paraffin blocks; and (4) inadequate tissue preservation for immunohistochemical analysis.

Clinical data were retrieved from institutional electronic records and included demographic characteristics, presenting symptoms, type of surgical procedure, tumor localization, and postoperative outcomes.

Segmental resection and termino-terminal anastomosis were considered a single surgical procedure, as the anastomosis is inherently performed following bowel resection. Accordingly, cases were classified under "segmental resection/enterectomy", and no isolated termino-terminal anastomoses without resection occurred in this cohort.

2.2. Study Outcomes

The primary outcome was the association between the Ki-67 proliferation index and tumor malignancy, defined according to WHO 2019/2022 histopathological criteria. Secondary outcomes included (1) the correlation between tumor size and Ki-67, (2) immunohistochemical expression patterns of CD117, DOG1, CD34 and SMA across histological subtypes, and (3) clinicopathological features by tumor type. Tumor size was measured as the largest macroscopic diameter. Ki-67 was quantified as the percentage of positive nuclei among $\geq$500 counted tumor cells in hotspot areas.

2.3. Histopathological Evaluation

All specimens were fixed in 10% neutral-buffered formalin, embedded in paraffin, and sectioned at 4 μm. Hematoxylin–eosin (H&E) staining was performed for morphological assessment. Tumors were classified according to the 2019 and 2022 World Health Organization (WHO) criteria for digestive system tumors, and pathological staging followed the 8th edition of the American Joint Committee on Cancer (AJCC) TNM classification. All NETs were classified as malignant neoplasms according to ENETS and AJCC frameworks, whereas WHO grading (G1–G3) was used to capture proliferative heterogeneity. Tumor size was measured as the largest macroscopic dimension in centimeters. Mitotic index could not be systematically evaluated because mitotic count per 5 mm^2 was not consistently recorded in archival specimens, and hotspot-based recounting was not feasible for all cases. Therefore, the mitotic index was excluded from comparative and multivariable analyses.

2.4. Immunohistochemical Analysis

Immunohistochemistry was performed on formalin-fixed, paraffin-embedded (FFPE) tissue sections using an automated staining platform (Ventana BenchMark ULTRA, Roche Diagnostics, Basel, Switzerland). The following primary antibodies were used: CD117 (c-KIT, clone YR145, Dako, Glostrup, Denmark), DOG1 (clone SP31, Thermo Fisher, Waltham, MA, USA), CD34 (clone QBEnd/10, Leica, Wetzlar, Germany), SMA (smooth muscle actin, clone 1A4, Dako), and Ki-67 (clone MIB-1, Dako). Antigen retrieval was achieved using citrate buffer (pH 6.0) or EDTA (pH 8.0), depending on the antibody specifications. The EnVision detection system (Dako) with diaminobenzidine (DAB) was used for chromogenic visualization.

Staining was independently evaluated by two experienced pathologists blinded to the clinical data. Tumors were considered positive for CD117, DOG1, CD34, or SMA when at least 10% of neoplastic cells exhibited cytoplasmic or membranous staining. The Ki-67 index was calculated as the percentage of positively stained nuclei among at least 500 tumor cells in areas of highest labeling ("hot spots"). For neuroendocrine tumors, Ki-67 grading followed WHO 2019 thresholds: G1 (<3%), G2 (3–20%), and G3 (>20%). Neuroendocrine tumors were confirmed by positivity for synaptophysin and chromogranin A, although these markers were not included in the comparative immunohistochemical analysis.

2.5. Statistical Analysis

Data were initially processed using Microsoft Excel (Microsoft Corp., Redmond, WA, USA) with XLSTAT (Addinsoft SARL, Paris, France). Statistical analyses were subsequently performed using SPSS version 25.0 (IBM Corp., Armonk, NY, USA). Continuous variables were expressed as mean $\pm$ standard deviation (SD) or median and interquartile range (IQR), depending on data distribution assessed by the Shapiro–Wilk test. Categorical variables were summarized as frequencies and percentages.

Comparisons between groups were made using the χ^2 test or Fisher's exact test for categorical variables and Student's t-test or Mann–Whitney U test for continuous variables. Correlations between continuous parameters were evaluated using Spearman's rank correlation coefficient (ρ). Binary logistic regression was applied to explore factors associated with malignancy, and multivariate analysis of variance (MANOVA) was used as an exploratory method to evaluate combined associations among clinicopathological variables. Malignancy was defined according to WHO 2019/2022 criteria as any histologically confirmed adenocarcinoma, GIST, neuroendocrine tumor, lymphoma or leiomyosarcoma. Benign tumors included leiomyoma and non-neoplastic lesions. A p-value < 0.05 was considered statistically significant. Survival analysis using the Kaplan–Meier method could not be performed due to incomplete follow-up data and the limited number of recorded outcome events.

The multivariate model was designed as an exploratory analysis due to the limited sample size. Variables were selected a priori based on two criteria: (1) clinical relevance described in the literature (tumor size, Ki-67 index, CD117/DOG1 expression, age, and sex), and (2) univariate association with malignancy using a liberal significance threshold of $p < 0.10$. No automated stepwise selection procedures were applied to avoid overfitting. Therefore, the results of the multivariate analysis should be interpreted as hypothesis-generating rather than confirmatory.

2.6. Ethical Considerations

The study protocol was approved by the Ethics Committee of the Clinical County Hospital of Craiova (Approval No. 55515/18 November 2025). All procedures were performed in accordance with the Declaration of Helsinki. Patient anonymity and data confidentiality were strictly maintained throughout the study.

3. Results

3.1. Baseline Clinical Characteristics

The baseline characteristics of the 61 patients included in the study are summarized in Table 1. The mean age was 63.1 ± 10.2 years, with a slight female predominance (60.7%). Abdominal pain was the most common presenting symptom (67.2%), followed by anemia (31.1%) and intestinal obstruction (23.0%). Segmental enterectomy with termino-terminal anastomosis was the most frequent surgical procedure (57.4%), while entero-enteric bypass was performed in 23.0% of patients, mainly for palliative purposes. Adenocarcinoma was the most frequent histological type (52.5%), followed by GIST (26.2%) and NET (9.8%) (Table 1).

Table 1. Baseline characteristics of the study population (n = 61).

Parameter	Category/Description	n (%) or Mean ± SD
Age (years)	Mean ± SD (Median [IQR])	63.1 ± 10.2 (63 [56–72])
Sex	Female	37 (60.7%)
	Male	24 (39.3%)
Presenting symptoms	Abdominal pain	41 (67.2%)
	Anemia	19 (31.1%)
	Intestinal obstruction	14 (23.0%)
	Nausea/vomiting	11 (18.0%)
	Weight loss	7 (11.5%)
	Gastrointestinal bleeding (melena/hematochezia)	6 (9.8%)
	Palpable mass	4 (6.6%)
Type of surgical intervention	Segmental enterectomy with termino-terminal anastomosis	35 (57.4%)
	Entero-enteric bypass (palliative)	14 (23.0%)

Table 1. *Cont.*

Parameter	Category/Description	n (%) or Mean ± SD
	Limited resection/biopsy	5 (8.2%)
	Ileostomy/colostomy	4 (6.6%)
	Hemicolectomy	3 (4.9%)
Histopathological type	GIST	16 (26.2%)
	Adenocarcinoma	32 (52.5%)
	Neuroendocrine tumor (NET)/Carcinoid	6 (9.8%)
	Lymphoma	3 (4.9%)
	Leiomyosarcoma/Leiomyoma	2 (3.3%)
	Benign/Other	2 (3.3%)
Ki-67 proliferation index	Median [IQR]	8% [5–15] (range 1–40%)
Pathologic stage	pT2–pT4 (predominantly pT3–T4)	48 (78.7%)
	pN1 (lymph node involvement)	5 (8.2%)
	pM1 (distant metastases)	2 (3.3%)
Tumor type	**Marker**	***n*(%)**
GIST (n = 16)	CD117 positive	15 (93.8%)
	DOG1 positive	15 (93.8%)
	CD34 positive	11 (68.8%)
	SMA positive	4 (25.0%)
Neuroendocrine tumors (NET) (n = 6)	Synaptophysin positive	6 (100%)
	Chromogranin A positive	5 (83.3%)
	CD56 positive	5 (83.3%)

3.2. *Histopathological and Immunohistochemical Findings*

Adenocarcinoma was the most frequent histopathological subtype (52.5%), followed by GIST (26.2%) and NET (9.8%). Immunohistochemistry showed high expression of CD117 and DOG1 (93.8% each) and CD34 (68.8%) in GIST, while NETs were consistently positive for synaptophysin (100%) and frequently for chromogranin A and CD56 (83.3%). The median Ki-67 index was 8% (IQR 5–15). Most tumors presented at an advanced stage (78.7% pT2–pT4), with limited nodal (8.2%) and distant metastatic involvement (3.3%).

The anatomical distribution of tumors and the corresponding variation in tumor size and Ki-67 across histological types are summarized in Table 2. Ileal tumors were the most frequent, followed by jejunal and duodenal lesions. Adenocarcinomas were predominantly located in the duodenum, whereas GISTs and NETs occurred mainly in the jejunum and ileum, respectively. Both tumor size and Ki-67 showed distinct site- and subtype-related patterns, reflecting the heterogeneous biological behavior of small-bowel tumors.

Table 2. Anatomical distribution of small bowel tumors and corresponding tumor size and Ki-67 across pathological types (n = 61).

Location	n	%	Histological Type Distribution	Median Tumor Size (cm)	Median Ki-67 (%)
Duodenum	9	14.8	Predominantly adenocarcinoma	5.9	14 [8–25]
Duodenum + pancreatic extension	1	1.6	Adenocarcinoma	—	—
Jejunum	15	24.6	Mainly GIST + NET	6.8 (GIST subset)	6 [4–12] (GIST)
Ileum	35	57.4	NET + GIST predominant	3.2 (NET subset)	3 [2–5] (NET)
Jejunum + ileum	1	1.6	GIST	6.8 (GIST subset)	6 [4–12] (GIST)
Total	61	100	Adenocarcinoma 32; GIST 16; NET 6; Lymphoma 3; Other 4	—	Overall: 8 [5–15]

3.3. Surgical Outcomes and Comparative Clinicopathological Analysis

As shown in Table 3, no significant clinical differences were observed among tumor types ($p > 0.05$). Most lesions were locally advanced (pT3–pT4), with lymph node involvement mainly in adenocarcinomas. NETs and GISTs rarely showed nodal or distant spread. Ki-67 levels were highest in adenocarcinomas and lowest in NETs, reflecting distinct proliferative patterns across groups.

Table 3. Clinical, Surgical, and Pathological Overview of the Study Population ($n = 61$).

Variable	GIST ($n = 16$)	Adenocarcinoma ($n = 32$)	NET ($n = 6$)	Others ($n = 7$)	p-Value
Mean age (years)	61.8 ± 9.7	66.2 ± 8.9	59.5 ± 11.2	64.0 ± 10.1	0.22
Female sex (%)	58.3%	66.7%	50.0%	57.1%	0.64
Abdominal pain (%)	72.2%	50.0%	66.7%	57.1%	0.38
Intestinal obstruction (%)	19.4%	41.7%	16.7%	28.6%	0.33
Segmental resection (%)	63.9%	50.0%	50.0%	57.1%	0.61
Pathologic stage pT2 (%)	11.1%	8.3%	33.3%	14.3%	—
Pathologic stage pT3 (%)	44.4%	41.7%	50.0%	28.6%	—
Pathologic stage pT4 (%)	33.3%	50.0%	16.7%	57.1%	—
Lymph node involvement (pN1, %)	2.8%	33.3%	0%	14.3%	—
Distant metastasis (pM1, %)	5.6%	8.3%	0%	0%	—
Mean Ki-67 index (%)	8.7	11.2	4.5	7.3	—
Tumor size (cm) median [IQR]	6.8 [4–9.5]	5.9 [3.2–8.0]	3.2 [2–5]	4.5 [3–6]	0.035

Immunohistochemical analysis (Table 4) showed high CD117 and DOG1 expression in GISTs, with no positivity in other tumor types ($p < 0.001$). CD34 was also more frequently expressed in GISTs ($p < 0.01$), while SMA showed no significant differences between groups. Ki-67 levels were highest in adenocarcinomas and lowest in NETs ($p = 0.002$), reflecting distinct proliferative activity across tumor types. Among NETs ($n = 6$), Ki-67–based grading identified 3 G1 lesions (<3%) and 3 G2 lesions (3–5%), with no G3 tumors observed. NETs were therefore included in the malignant group in the exploratory model, while grading information was reported separately.

Table 4. Immunohistochemical Expression by Tumor Type.

Marker	GIST (%)	Adenocarcinoma (%)	NET (%)	Others (%)	p-Value
CD117	93.8	0.0	0.0	0.0	<0.001
DOG1	93.8	0.0	0.0	0.0	<0.001
CD34	68.8	0.0–20.0	0.0	0.0–28.6	<0.01
SMA	25.0	~15.0	33.3	~28.6	0.52
Ki-67 (%) median [IQR]	8 [5–15]	18 [10–25]	3 [2–5]	8 [5–10]	0.002

As shown in Table 5, R0 resection rates were similar across groups, with slightly lower values in adenocarcinomas. R1 margins and postoperative complications were also more frequent in adenocarcinomas compared with other tumors. Ki-67 levels remained lowest in GISTs and highest in non-GIST tumors, indicating differences in proliferative behavior among histological subtypes.

On univariate analysis, CD117, DOG1, and CD34 positivity were significantly associated with GIST histology ($p < 0.001$ for all), while no significant differences were found regarding sex distribution, SMA expression, or nodal/metastatic involvement (Table 6).

Table 5. Surgical Outcomes and Clinicopathological Correlations.

Parameter/Variable	GIST (*n* = 16)	Adenocarcinoma (*n* = 32)	NET (*n* = 6)	Others (*n* = 7)	Non-GIST Total (*n* = 45)	*p*-Value
Complete resection (R0)	13 (80.6%)	21 (66.7%)	5 (83.3%)	6 (85.7%)	32 (71.1%)	—
R1 margin involvement	2 (11.1%)	8 (25.0%)	0	1 (14.3%)	9 (20.0%)	—
Postoperative complications	3 (19.4%)	11 (33.3%)	1 (16.7%)	1 (14.3%)	13 (28.9%)	—
Mean age (years)	61.8	—	—	—	65.4	0.18
Female sex (%)	58.3%	—	—	—	63.0%	0.64
Tumor size (cm, mean)	6.8	—	—	—	5.3	0.11
Ki-67 median (%)	6	—	—	—	12	0.01

Table 6. Comparative analysis of categorical variables between GIST and non-GIST tumors (*n* = 61).

Variable	Statistical Test	χ^2/Fisher Value	*p*-Value	Interpretation
CD117 positivity	Chi-square test	$\chi^2 = 42.3$	**<0.001**	**Significant** (GIST strongly associated with CD117+)
DOG1 positivity	Chi-square test	$\chi^2 = 38.6$	**<0.001**	**Significant** (DOG1 highly specific for GIST)
CD34 positivity	Chi-square test	$\chi^2 = 12.7$	**0.001**	**Significant** (frequent in GIST)
SMA positivity	Fisher's Exact test	—	**0.42**	Not significant
Sex (female/male)	Chi-square test	$\chi^2 = 0.28$	**0.60**	Not significant
pN1 (yes/no)	Fisher's Exact test	—	**0.09**	Not significant trend (adenocarcinomas more likely pN1)
pM1 (yes/no)	Fisher's Exact test	—	**0.47**	Not significant
Stage pT (T2–T4)	Chi-square test for trend	$\chi^2 = 1.92$	**0.38**	Not significant (no clear trend by tumor type)

Comparative analysis of continuous variables showed no significant differences in mean age or tumor size between GIST and non-GIST tumors (Table 7). However, the Ki-67 proliferation index remained significantly higher in non-GIST tumors compared with GISTs (median 14% [8–25] vs. 6% [4–12]; $p = 0.004$). Tumor size also differed across individual tumor types in the multigroup comparison, and a moderate positive correlation was observed between tumor size and Ki-67 ($\rho = 0.42$, $p = 0.018$), indicating that larger tumors tended to have higher proliferative activity.

Table 7. Comparative analysis of continuous variables by tumor type.

Variable	Groups Compared	Statistical Test	Mean/Median Values	Test Value	*p*-Value	Interpretation
Age (years)	GIST (*n* = 16) vs. non-GIST (*n* = 45)	Independent t-test	61.8 ± 9.7 vs. 65.4 ± 8.9	t = 1.42	0.16	NS (similar age distribution)
Tumor size (cm)	GIST vs. non-GIST	Mann–Whitney U	6.8 [4.0–9.5] vs. 5.3 [3.2–7.0]	U = 324.5	0.21	NS (no size difference)
Ki-67 (%)	GIST vs. non-GIST	Mann–Whitney U	6 [4–12] vs. 14 [8–25]	U = 102.5	0.004	Significant (higher proliferation in non-GIST)
Tumor size (cm)	GIST (*n* = 16), Adenocarcinoma (*n* = 32), NET (*n* = 6), Lymphoma (*n* = 3)	Kruskal–Wallis	medians: 6.8/5.9/3.2/4.5	H = 6.72	0.035	Significant differences across groups
Ki-67 (%) vs. tumor size	All tumors (*n* = 61)	Spearman correlation	ρ = 0.42	Z = 2.43	0.018	Positive correlation (larger tumors → higher Ki-67)

3.4. Correlation Analysis and Factors Associated with Proliferation

Spearman's correlation showed a moderate positive relationship between tumor size and Ki-67 index ($\rho = 0.42$, $p = 0.018$), indicating that larger tumors tended to have higher proliferative activity. CD117 and DOG1 demonstrated a strong association with GIST histology (Cramer's V = 0.82 and 0.78, respectively; both $p < 0.001$), confirming their diagnostic specificity (Table 8).

Table 8. Correlation analysis between clinicopathological and immunohistochemical parameters.

Relationship	Statistical Test	Correlation Coefficient	*p*-Value	Interpretation
Tumor size ↔ Ki-67 index	Spearman's ρ	**0.42**	**0.018**	*Moderate positive correlation* (larger tumors show higher proliferation)
Age ↔ Tumor size	Spearman's ρ	0.12	**0.34**	*No significant correlation*
Age ↔ Ki-67 index	Spearman's ρ	−0.09	**0.48**	*No significant association between age and proliferation*
CD117 ↔ Tumor type	Cramer's V (post χ^2)	**0.82**	**<0.001**	*Strong association* (CD117 highly specific for GIST)
DOG1 ↔ Tumor type	Cramer's V	**0.78**	**<0.001**	*Strong association* (DOG1 strongly related to GIST)
CD34 ↔ Tumor type	Cramer's V	0.46	**0.008**	*Moderate association*
SMA ↔ Tumor type	Cramer's V	0.21	**0.29**	*Weak, non-significant association*

Multivariate and correlation analyses showed that tumor size >5 cm and Ki-67 >10% were associated with malignancy in this exploratory model ($p = 0.03$ and $p = 0.04$, respectively) (Table 9). In this exploratory model, Ki-67 >10% and tumor size >5 cm were associated with a histological diagnosis of malignancy (WHO criteria), rather than clinical outcomes. CD117 and DOG1 were not significantly associated with malignancy; inverse OR values reflect statistical artifact due to collinearity and sample imbalance. MANOVA showed significant overall differences between tumor types when age, size, and Ki-67 were analyzed together (Wilks' $\lambda = 0.71$, $p = 0.046$). Cluster analysis of immunohistochemical markers identified three major subgroups, corresponding to classical GIST, partial GIST/SMA+, and non-GIST tumors.

Table 9. Summary of multivariate and correlation analyses.

Analysis Type	Variables Tested	Statistical Method	Main Results/Coefficients	*p*-Value	Interpretation
Binary logistic regression	Tumor size >5 cm	OR = 3.5 [1.1–11.1]	**Significant predictor of malignancy**	**0.030**	Larger tumors associated with malignancy
	Ki-67 > 10%	OR = 2.9 [1.0–8.3]	**Significant association (exploratory)**	**0.040**	Higher proliferation → malignancy
	CD117 positivity	OR = 0.4 [0.1–1.2]	Not significant; OR < 1 reflects collinearity	0.120	Not independent
	DOG1 positivity	OR = 0.5 [0.2–1.4]	Not significant; OR < 1 reflects collinearity	0.180	-
	Age (per 10 years)	OR = 1.2 [0.8–1.9]	Not significant	0.330	—
	Sex (male)	OR = 1.1 [0.4–3.3]	Not significant	0.820	—
Multivariate analysis (MANOVA)	Age, Size, Ki-67 vs. Tumor Type	Wilks' λ = 0.71	Global model significant	**0.046**	Combined parameters differ by tumor type
	Post hoc: Ki-67 (Adeno > GIST)	—	**Significant**	**0.004**	Adenocarcinomas more proliferative
Exploratory cluster analysis	CD117, DOG1, CD34, SMA	Hierarchical (Ward/Euclidean)	3 clusters identified:	—	—
	Cluster 1	Algorithm-defined GIST-like pattern *(NOT actual CD117/DOG1 positivity)*	28 cases (45.9%)	—	Similarity-based cluster; does not reflect true IHC expression
	Cluster 2	Mixed smooth-muscle/stromal similarity profile	8 cases (13.1%)	—	Heterogeneous cluster with partial leiomyomatous features
	Cluster 3	Non-GIST-like pattern (marker-negative dominant)	25 cases (41.0%)	—	Corresponding broadly to adenocarcinoma, NET, lymphoma

Note: Cluster patterns reflect unsupervised similarity analysis and do not indicate true immunohistochemical positivity. Actual CD117 and DOG1 expression is restricted to GISTs, as shown in Table 4. OR < 1 for CD117 and DOG1 reflects collinearity with GIST histology and extreme class imbalance, not a protective effect. The model is exploratory.

4. Discussion

4.1. Comparison with Published Data

The incidence of small bowel tumors in our cohort aligns with global epidemiological data, confirming their rarity among gastrointestinal malignancies. Small bowel tumors represent less than 5% of all gastrointestinal neoplasms, with an estimated incidence of approximately 2–3 cases per 100,000 population per year [1,2]. Duodenal involvement is the most frequent site (50–60%), followed by jejunal and ileal locations [2,3]. The apparent increase in incidence reported over recent decades is largely attributable to advances in diagnostic imaging and endoscopic techniques, rather than a true rise in disease burden [7,8].

The histologic profile in our series, in which adenocarcinomas represented the most frequent subtype (52.5%), followed by GISTs (26.2%) and NETs (9.8%), reflects the spectrum reported in large international registries such as SEER and NADEGE, where adenocarcinomas and neuroendocrine tumors together comprise the majority of small bowel malignancies, while GISTs and lymphomas account for the remainder [8–10]. The predominance of duodenal adenocarcinomas and ileal NETs described in population-based cohorts supports site-specific molecular and etiologic mechanisms [3,11]. Small bowel lymphomas remain uncommon but constitute up to 30–40% of extranodal lymphomas, most frequently of follicular or diffuse large B-cell subtype [5].

Immunohistochemical findings in our cohort parallel those reported globally. GISTs demonstrated strong CD117 (c-KIT) and DOG1 expression in more than 90% of cases, with CD34 positivity in approximately two-thirds of tumors, confirming their diagnostic reliability and stromal differentiation [6,12–15]. These rates are comparable to those reported by Varshney et al. and other large multicenter series [13–15]. In contrast, NETs displayed a typical neuroendocrine phenotype, with universal synaptophysin expression and frequent chromogranin A and CD56 positivity, in line with current WHO criteria and contemporary literature [3,16–18].

For small bowel adenocarcinomas, previous studies have reported mismatch repair deficiency and microsatellite instability (MSI) in approximately 15–20% of cases [19,20]. Although MMR/MSI status was not systematically assessed in our cohort, these data underscore the need for routine MMR testing in this subtype, given its relevance for identifying hereditary cancer syndromes and for selecting patients who may benefit from immunotherapy [19,20]. For NETs, the Ki-67–based WHO classification (G1 < 3%, G2 3–20%, G3 > 20%) remains the principal prognostic determinant [16,17]. In our series, NETs showed the lowest proliferative activity among all tumor types (median Ki-67 3%, IQR 2–5), with a predominance of G1–G2 lesions, in agreement with previous reports and consistent with their generally indolent behavior [3,16,18].

Overall, our findings are consistent with current international evidence. Adenocarcinomas, GISTs, and NETs reproduced the expected clinicopathological and immunohistochemical profiles, while Ki-67 and tumor size while Ki-67 and tumor size were associated with features of higher histological grade and malignancy in this exploratory cohort. The moderate positive correlation between tumor size and Ki-67, together with their association with histological malignancy in this exploratory model, suggests that proliferative and morphological parameters may provide complementary information in the diagnostic evaluation of small bowel tumors.

In this study, malignancy reflected histological classification according to WHO criteria rather than clinical outcomes, as systematic follow-up data were not available. Therefore, the results should be interpreted as exploratory and hypothesis-generating rather than prognostic. Given the rarity of small bowel tumors, exploratory single-center data provide complementary site-specific evidence and may support hypothesis generation for future multicenter studies.

These consistent patterns support the external validity of our findings and highlight the diagnostic value of integrating CD117, DOG1, CD34, and Ki-67 in the assessment of small bowel tumors. The present study provides original data from a surgically treated cohort in an underreported population, underscoring the relevance of comprehensive histopathological and immunohistochemical characterization for improving diagnostic accuracy and supporting diagnostic work-up.

4.2. Immunohistochemical Profile of Small Bowel Mesenchymal Tumors

The diagnosis of small bowel mesenchymal tumors remains challenging because of overlapping spindle-cell morphology among gastrointestinal stromal tumors (GISTs), leiomyomas, and schwannomas [6,13,21]. Immunohistochemistry is therefore essential for accurate classification. Among the available markers, CD117 (c-KIT) and DOG1 (Discovered On GIST-1) are the most reliable and specific identifiers of GIST, and their combined use ensures near-complete diagnostic accuracy [2,22,23]. In our cohort, this canonical immunophenotype was confirmed, with CD117 and DOG1 positivity in 93.8% of GISTs and CD34 expression in 68.8% of cases, closely mirroring rates reported in large multicenter series [6,12–15].

CD117, a transmembrane tyrosine kinase encoded by the *KIT* proto-oncogene, is expressed in more than 95% of GISTs and is associated with constitutive activation of proliferative signaling through the MAPK and PI3K pathways [6]. In contrast, leiomyomas and leiomyosarcomas typically lack CD117 and DOG1 expression, but are positive for smooth-muscle markers such as SMA and desmin, while schwannomas exhibit strong S100 expression with negativity for both markers [5,13]. **DOG1**, encoded by *ANO1* on chromosome 11q13, is a calcium-dependent chloride channel expressed in interstitial cells of Cajal, the presumed progenitor cells of GIST [22]. Unlike CD117, DOG1 expression is largely independent of *KIT* or *PDGFRA* mutational status and remains detectable in CD117-negative tumors, including those harboring *PDGFRA* exon 18 mutations [9,13]. This feature makes DOG1 particularly valuable for diagnosing KIT-negative intestinal GISTs, especially in cases with atypical morphology or extensive necrosis that complicate histopathological interpretation [7].

Recent data highlight biological heterogeneity among small intestinal GISTs. Wang et al. reported increasing tumor size, mitotic activity, and CD117/DOG1 staining intensity from the duodenum to the ileum, suggesting a gradient of aggressiveness along the intestinal axis [4]. In line with these observations, most GISTs in our series presented at an advanced local stage (predominantly pT3–pT4), and their Ki-67 index, although lower than in non-GIST tumors, increased with tumor size, contributing to the overall positive correlation between size and proliferative activity ($\rho = 0.42$, $p = 0.018$).

Among the NETs in our cohort, Ki-67–based grading demonstrated an exclusively low-grade profile: three tumors were classified as G1 (<3%) and three as G2 (3–5%), with no G3 lesions identified. This distribution aligns with the typically indolent biological behavior of small-bowel NETs and corresponds to the lowest proliferation indices observed in ileal tumors.

Beyond their diagnostic value, CD117 and DOG1 also have prognostic and therapeutic implications, as their expression correlates with KIT or PDGFRA mutations predictive of response to tyrosine kinase inhibitors such as imatinib [1,19]. Co-expression of CD117 and DOG1 in duodenal and jejunal GISTs—often associated with larger size and higher mitotic rate—identifies lesions at increased risk of recurrence and guides adjuvant therapy decisions [4,24]. In a multicentric analysis, Varshney et al. reported CD117 and DOG1 positivity in 98% and 94% of cases, respectively, while CD34 expression (≈72%) correlated with intermediate-to-high-risk categories [13]. Similar findings were described by Terada, who reported concurrent CD117 and CD34 positivity in intestinal GISTs with intermediate mitotic indices [22]. Our rates of CD117, DOG1, and CD34 expression thus reinforce the external validity of these patterns in a surgically treated cohort.

Additional markers involved in apoptosis and cell-cycle regulation, such as p21^WAF1^ and Bax, have been associated with malignant potential, suggesting that CD117 and DOG1 expression may coexist with other molecular features of aggressive behavior [6]. The absence of CD117 and DOG1 expression in non-stromal small bowel neoplasms further enhances diagnostic specificity; duodenal lymphomas, typically CD20- or CD3-positive, consistently lack both markers, ensuring distinction from stromal tumors [5]. Accurate immunohistochemical characterization therefore enables limited resections for duodenal GISTs instead of radical pancreaticoduodenectomy, reducing morbidity without compromising oncologic outcomes [25].

According to the 2019 and 2022 World Health Organization (WHO) classifications, CD117 and DOG1 are mandatory diagnostic criteria for GISTs and should be included in all immunohistochemical panels for gastrointestinal mesenchymal tumors [3]. In our study, the integration of the Ki-67 proliferation index with CD117, DOG1, and CD34 expression provided additional insight into tumor grade and biological behavior, suggesting that Ki-67 and tumor size may act as complementary markers associated with histological malignancy in small bowel mesenchymal tumors [3,26].

4.3. Findings and Comparative Analysis

In our surgical cohort, adenocarcinomas represented the most frequent histological subtype (52.5%), followed by GISTs (26.2%) and NETs (9.8%), a distribution broadly consistent with large registry data for small bowel malignancies [8–11]. At the immunohistochemical level, GISTs showed the expected profile, with high CD117 and DOG1 expression (93.8% each) and CD34 positivity in approximately two-thirds of cases, in line with the diagnostic performance reported by Varshney et al. and Terada [13,22]. NETs were consistently positive for synaptophysin and frequently expressed chromogranin A and CD56, supporting their neuroendocrine lineage and the applicability of current WHO grading schemes [16,17].

As shown in Table 2, tumor location showed clear variation in both tumor size and proliferative activity. Duodenal tumors were mainly adenocarcinomas and exhibited higher Ki-67 levels, whereas jejunal lesions were predominantly GISTs and ileal lesions were enriched in well-differentiated NETs, which had the lowest proliferation indices. These site-specific patterns support the biological heterogeneity along the small intestine and help explain subtype-related differences in clinical and pathological presentation.

Statistical analyses confirmed a strong association between GIST histology and CD117/DOG1 expression (Cramer's V = 0.82 and 0.78, respectively; both $p < 0.001$), whereas SMA showed only a weak, non-significant relationship with tumor type. The Ki-67 index was significantly lower in GISTs than in non-GIST tumors (median 6% vs. 14%; $p = 0.004$), and a moderate positive correlation between tumor size and Ki-67 ($\rho = 0.42$, $p = 0.018$) indicated that larger lesions tended to exhibit higher proliferative activity, echoing the size- and site-related gradients described by Wang et al. and others [4,13].

On multivariate analysis, tumor size >5 cm and Ki-67 >10% were associated with malignancy in this exploratory model (OR 3.5 and 2.9, respectively; both $p \leq 0.04$), whereas CD117 and DOG1 did not show significant associations after adjustment for proliferation and size. These findings parallel international data showing that Ki-67 thresholds around 10–15% stratify recurrence risk and survival in both GISTs and adenocarcinomas [10,11,13,22] and that elevated Ki-67 in small bowel adenocarcinomas is linked to nodal spread and poorer prognosis [11]. In NETs, our observations are concordant with the WHO 2019/2022 framework, in which Ki-67 remains the principal grading and prognostic parameter, with higher indices associated with nodal metastasis and early recurrence [3,16,18,27–30].

Cluster analysis further underscored the immunophenotypic heterogeneity of small bowel mesenchymal tumors, delineating three main profiles: classical GIST (CD117+/DOG1+/CD34+), a partial GIST/leiomyomatous pattern (CD117+/SMA+/CD34+), and a CD117−/DOG1− non-GIST group encompassing adenocarcinomas, NETs, and lymphomas. Together, these data support an integrated approach in which tumor size and Ki-67—interpreted alongside CD117, DOG1, and CD34, and complemented by molecular testing (KIT, PDGFRA, MMR status)—may contribute to diagnostic assessment and hypothesis generation for future risk stratification [2,16,31–33].

4.4. Strengths and Limitations

This study provides a comprehensive clinicopathological and immunohistochemical characterization of surgically treated small intestinal tumors, offering valuable insight into their histologic spectrum, biomarker expression, and clinicopathological correlations. Key strengths include the inclusion of multiple histologic subtypes (GIST, adenocarcinoma, neuroendocrine tumor, lymphoma, and others) within a single, well-defined surgical cohort; the use of standardized immunohistochemical markers (CD117, DOG1, CD34, SMA, and Ki-67) for precise tumor classification; and the application of multivariable and correlation analyses that identified exploratory associations between tumor size >5 cm, Ki-67 >10%, and malignancy. Nevertheless, the study has several limitations. Its retrospective and single-center design may introduce selection bias and limit the generalizability of the findings. The relatively small sample size (n = 61) restricts the statistical power for subgroup comparisons, and incomplete follow-up data precluded comprehensive survival analysis. Moreover, the absence of molecular profiling (e.g., KIT, PDGFRA, or MMR status) limits deeper biological interpretation. A key limitation is the absence of systematically recorded mitotic index in GISTs, preventing standard AFIP/NCCN risk stratification. The extreme imbalance between malignant and benign cases (59 vs. 2) limits the robustness of the logistic regression model, and therefore the multivariate results should be interpreted as exploratory. Given that only two benign cases were available, the number of events was insufficient for a stable multivariable logistic regression, and including multiple predictors introduces a high risk of overfitting. Consequently, the regression output should be regarded as exploratory and hypothesis-generating rather than confirmatory. The OR values <1 observed for CD117 and DOG1 in the multivariable model do not reflect a true protective effect; rather, they result from the strong collinearity between these markers and GIST histology, combined with the extremely small number of benign cases. These coefficients are therefore statistical artifacts and should not be interpreted biologically. Because the analytic cohort included biologically distinct tumor types (adenocarcinoma, GIST, NET, lymphoma), the multivariate model captures general predictors of malignancy rather than subtype-specific determinants. The inclusion of NET G1 within the malignant category may introduce heterogeneity, as G1 tumors show indolent biological behavior, although they remain classified as malignant neoplasms in current clinical staging frameworks. Therefore, the substantial heterogeneity across tumor types limits the generalizability of these predictors, which should be interpreted as exploratory. The MANOVA results should be interpreted with caution due to the small and unbalanced group sizes; the analysis was exploratory and primarily descriptive, and nonparametric tests (e.g., Kruskal–Wallis) provide more robust comparisons across tumor types. Future prospective, multicenter studies with integrated molecular analysis are warranted to validate and expand upon these findings. Incorporating molecular correlates such as KIT, PDGFRA, and MMR status in future cohorts will not only clarify the genetic landscape of small intestinal tumors but also strengthen the translational link between immunohistochemical features and targeted therapeutic strategies. Although the cohort is small and the multivariable analysis exploratory, single-center descriptive series remain relevant in the context of rare small bowel tumors. Site-specific data are scarce, as most studies combine gastric and intestinal cases. The present dataset provides detailed histopathological and immunohistochemical characterization and may support hypothesis generation and inform the design of future multicenter studies. Accordingly, the findings should be interpreted as complementary rather than confirmatory. Comprehensive survival analysis, including Kaplan–Meier curves and Cox regression, could not be conducted because of incomplete follow-up information and the retrospective nature of the study.

4.5. Future Directions

Future research on small intestinal tumors should prioritize multicentric validation and the incorporation of prospective survival analyses. Given the rarity and biological heterogeneity of these neoplasms, collaborative, large-scale studies are essential to achieve representative cohorts across all histologic subtypes and to enhance the external validity of current findings.

The establishment of prospective, multicenter registries with standardized diagnostic, histopathologic, and follow-up protocols will allow more accurate identification of prognostic determinants and refinement of existing risk stratification systems. Integrating molecular and genomic profiling, as recommended by recent NCCN and ENETS guidelines, is expected to further elucidate tumor biology and identify novel therapeutic targets.

In addition, future studies should combine clinical, morphological, and molecular parameters in survival-based models to enable personalized prognostic assessment and optimize multidisciplinary treatment strategies. Such integrated approaches will contribute to the development of precision medicine paradigms for small bowel malignancies and improve patient outcomes.

In summary, the present analysis integrates clinicopathological, immunohistochemical, and proliferative parameters to provide a unified view of small intestinal tumors. The consistent association between CD117/DOG1 expression and GIST histology, together with the exploratory associations of tumor size and Ki-67 with histologic malignancy, highlights the complementary role of morphological and immunohistochemical markers in diagnostic evaluation. These results bridge diagnostic accuracy with clinical relevance, offering a preliminary descriptive framework and paving the way for molecularly integrated, multicenter validation studies.

5. Conclusions

In this surgically treated cohort, adenocarcinomas represented the most frequent primary small bowel tumors, followed by GISTs and NETs, consistent with contemporary epidemiological data. CD117 and DOG1 reliably confirmed GIST diagnosis with high specificity, whereas CD34 expression supported stromal differentiation. In the exploratory multivariable analysis, tumor size >5 cm and Ki-67 >10% were associated with histological malignancy; however, these observations should be interpreted with caution due to sample imbalance and the absence of systematic outcome data. A positive correlation between tumor size and Ki-67 further suggests that larger lesions may exhibit higher proliferative activity.

Overall, combining immunohistochemical markers with Ki-67 and tumor size may support diagnostic evaluation and inform future risk stratification, but does not allow definitive prognostic or therapeutic conclusions. Prospective studies with standardized follow-up and adequate statistical power are required to validate these findings.

Author Contributions: Conceptualization L.A.B. and N.-D.M., writing—original draft L.A.B. and T.S.Ț.C., resources L.V., S.-S.M., T.S.Ț.C. and V.Ș., supervision S.-S.M. and L.C., investigation D.M., L.C., L.V., V.Ș. and L.V., writing—review L.A.B. and T.S.Ț.C., validation L.V., S.-S.M. and N.-D.M., software L.C., and D.M., visualization D.M. and L.C., data curation D.M., T.S.Ț.C. and N.-D.M., project administration L.A.B. and V.Ș., formal analysis S.-S.M. and N.-D.M., methodology D.M., L.V., and V.Ș. All authors have read and agreed to the published version of the manuscript.

Funding: The article processing charges were funded by the University of Medicine and Pharmacy of Craiova, Romania.

Institutional Review Board Statement: The study was conducted in accordance with the Declaration of Helsinki and was approved by the Ethics Committee of the Clinical Emergency County Hospital Craiova as a retrospective analysis of anonymized clinical data (Approval No. 55515, 18 November 2025). All surgical procedures and histopathological assessments took place during routine clinical care between 2020 and 2024, before the retrospective study protocol was submitted. Given the retrospective design and full anonymization of the dataset, the Ethics Committee waived the requirement for informed consent.

Informed Consent Statement: Given the retrospective design and full anonymization of the dataset, the Ethics Committee waived the requirement for individual informed consent.

Data Availability Statement: The data presented in this study are available on request from the corresponding author. The data are not publicly available due to patient confidentiality.

Conflicts of Interest: The authors declare that there are no conflicts of interest.

References

1. Benson, A.B.; Venook, A.P.; Al-Hawary, M.M.; Arain, M.A.; Chen, Y.J.; Ciombor, K.K.; Cohen, S.A.; Cooper, H.S.; Deming, D.A.; Garrido-Laguna, I.; et al. Small Bowel Adenocarcinoma, Version 1.2020, NCCN Clinical Practice Guidelines in Oncology. *J. Natl. Compr. Canc. Netw.* **2019**, *17*, 1109–1133. [CrossRef] [PubMed]
2. Khosla, D.; Dey, T.; Madan, R.; Gupta, R.; Goyal, S.; Kumar, N.; Kapoor, R. Small bowel adenocarcinoma: An overview. *World J. Gastrointest. Oncol.* **2022**, *14*, 413–422. [CrossRef] [PubMed]
3. Kupietzky, A.; Dover, R.; Mazeh, H. Surgical aspects of small intestinal neuroendocrine tumors. *World J. Gastrointest. Surg.* **2023**, *15*, 566–577. [CrossRef] [PubMed]
4. Wang, Q.; Li, M.; Bai, X.; Zhang, R.; Ruan, S.; Ou, C.; Li, J.; Li, J. Unraveling the site-specific features in small intestinal stromal tumors: A retrospective study. *BMC Gastroenterol.* **2025**, *25*, 337. [CrossRef]
5. Iwamuro, M.; Tanaka, T.; Okada, H. Review of lymphoma in the duodenum: An update of diagnosis and management. *World J. Gastroenterol.* **2023**, *29*, 1852–1862. [CrossRef]
6. Liu, F.Y.; Qi, J.P.; Xu, F.L.; Wu, A.P. Clinicopathological and immunohistochemical analysis of gastrointestinal stromal tumor. *World J. Gastroenterol.* **2006**, *12*, 4161–4165. [CrossRef]
7. Wongsiriamnuey, T.; Limsrivilai, J. Current perspectives on small bowel tumors: Overview of prevalence, clinical manifestations, and treatment approaches. *Siriraj Med. J.* **2024**, *76*, 225–233. [CrossRef]
8. Kim, S.H.; Kim, J.W. Small Bowel Malignancies in Patients Undergoing Capsule Endoscopy for Iron Deficiency Anemia. *Diagnostics* **2022**, *12*, 91. [CrossRef]
9. Cazacu, S.M.; Cârțu, D.; Popescu, M.; Streba, L.; Ungureanu, B.S.; Iovănescu, V.F.; Cimpoeru, M.; Mirea, C.S.; Surlin, V.M.; Mogoantă, S.; et al. Small Bowel Tumors: A 7-Year Study in a Tertiary Care Hospital. *Cancers* **2025**, *17*, 1465. [CrossRef]
10. Aparicio, T.; Pachev, A.; Laurent-Puig, P.; Svrcek, M. Epidemiology, Risk Factors and Diagnosis of Small Bowel Adenocarcinoma. *Cancers* **2022**, *14*, 2268. [CrossRef]
11. Turpin, A.; El Amrani, M.; Zaanan, A. Localized Small Bowel Adenocarcinoma Management: Evidence Summary. *Cancers* **2022**, *14*, 2892. [CrossRef]
12. Seo, H.S.; Hyeon, J.Y.; Shin, O.R.; Lee, H.H. C-Kit-Negative Gastrointestinal Stromal Tumor in the Stomach. *J. Gastric Cancer* **2015**, *15*, 290–294. [CrossRef]
13. Varshney, V.K.; Gupta, R.K.; Saluja, S.S.; Tyagi, I.; Mishra, P.K.; Batra, V.V. Analysis of clinicopathological and immunohistochemical parameters and correlation of outcomes in gastrointestinal stromal tumors. *Indian J. Cancer* **2019**, *56*, 135–143. [CrossRef]

14. Ríos-Moreno, M.J.; Jaramillo, S.; Pereira Gallardo, S.; Vallejo, A.; Mora, M.; García-Escudero, A.; Amérigo, J.; González-Cámpora, R. Gastrointestinal stromal tumors (GISTs): CD117, DOG-1 and PKCθ expression. Is there any advantage in using several markers? *Pathol. Res. Pract.* **2012**, *208*, 74–81. [CrossRef] [PubMed]
15. Şahin, S.; Ekinci, Ö.; Seçkin, S.; Dursun, A. The Diagnostic and Prognostic Utility of DOG1 Expression on Gastrointestinal Stromal Tumors. *Turk. Patoloji Derg.* **2017**, *33*, 1–8. [CrossRef] [PubMed]
16. Lim, J.Y.; Pommier, R.F. Clinical Features, Management, and Molecular Characteristics of Familial Small Bowel Neuroendocrine Tumors. *Front. Endocrinol.* **2021**, *12*, 622693. [CrossRef]
17. Dinu, A.; Aşchie, M.; Deacu, M.; Chisoi, A.; Enciu, M.; Cojocaru, O.; Vlad, S.E. Clinico-Morphological Correlations with Ki-67 and p53 Immunohistochemical Expression in High-Grade Gastrointestinal Neuroendocrine Neoplasms. *Gastrointest. Disord.* **2025**, *7*, 51. [CrossRef]
18. Kaçmaz, E.; Chen, J.W.; Tanis, P.J.; Nieveen van Dijkum, E.J.M.; Engelsman, A.F. Postoperative morbidity and mortality after surgical resection of small bowel neuroendocrine neoplasms: A systematic review and meta-analysis. *J. Neuroendocrinol.* **2021**, *33*, e13008. [CrossRef]
19. Pandya, K.; Overman, M.J.; Gulhati, P. Molecular Landscape of Small Bowel Adenocarcinoma. *Cancers* **2022**, *14*, 1287. [CrossRef] [PubMed]
20. Vanoli, A.; Grillo, F.; Furlan, D.; Arpa, G.; Grami, O.; Guerini, C.; Riboni, R.; Mastracci, L.; Di Sabatino, A. Small Bowel Epithelial Precursor Lesions: A Focus on Molecular Alterations. *Int. J. Mol. Sci.* **2021**, *22*, 4388. [CrossRef]
21. Gama, J.M.; Oliveira, R.C. Mesenchymal Tumors of the Gastrointestinal Tract—Beyond GIST—A Review. *Gastrointest. Disord.* **2024**, *6*, 257–291. [CrossRef]
22. Terada, T. Malignant tumors of the small intestine: A histopathologic study of 41 cases among 1,312 consecutive specimens of small intestine. *Int. J. Clin. Exp. Pathol.* **2012**, *5*, 203–209.
23. Usama, F.; Rasikh, R.; Hassam, K.; Rahman, M.; Khalil Ur Rehman, F.; Khan, I.W.; Lau, D.T. An update on gastrointestinal stromal tumors (GISTs) with a focus on extragastrointestinal stromal tumors (EGISTs). *Gastroenterol. Rep.* **2025**, *13*, goaf068. [CrossRef] [PubMed]
24. Ahmed, M. Recent advances in the management of gastrointestinal stromal tumor. *World J. Clin. Cases* **2020**, *8*, 3142–3155. [CrossRef] [PubMed]
25. Lim, K.T. Current surgical management of duodenal gastrointestinal stromal tumors. *World J. Gastrointest. Surg.* **2021**, *13*, 1166–1179. [CrossRef] [PubMed]
26. Sözütek, D.; Yanık, S.; Akkoca, A.N.; Sözütek, A.; Ozdemir, Z.T.; Avşar, C.U.; Günaldı, M.; Sahin, B.; Doron, F. Diagnostic and prognostic roles of DOG1 and Ki-67, in GIST patients with localized or advanced/metastatic disease. *Int. J. Clin. Exp. Med.* **2014**, *7*, 1914–1922.
27. Yano, T.; Yamamoto, H. Endoscopic Diagnosis of Small Bowel Tumor. *Cancers* **2024**, *16*, 1704. [CrossRef]
28. Tian, J.; Chen, W. Prediction of Ki-67 expression and malignant potential in gastrointestinal stromal tumors: Novel models based on CE-CT and serological indicators. *BMC Cancer* **2024**, *24*, 1412. [CrossRef]
29. Barbu, L.A.; Vasile, L.; Cercelaru, L.; Șurlin, V.; Mogoantă, S.-Ș.; Mogoș, G.F.R.; Țenea Cojan, T.S.; Mărgăritescu, N.-D.; Iordache, M.P.; Buliman, A. Aggressiveness in Well-Differentiated Small Intestinal Neuroendocrine Tumors: A Rare Case and Narrative Literature Review. *J. Clin. Med.* **2025**, *14*, 5821. [CrossRef]
30. Vasile, L.; Barbu, L.A.; Mogoş, G.F.R.; Şurlin, V.; Vîlcea, I.D.; Cercelaru, L.; Mogoantă, S.Ş.; Mărgăritescu, N.D.; Nimigean, V.; Nimigean, V.R.; et al. Neuroendocrine tumors of the appendix: A comprehensive review of the literature and case presentation. *Rom. J. Morphol. Embryol.* **2025**, *66*, 269–278. [CrossRef]
31. Țenea Cojan, T.S.; Șurlin, V.; Mogoantă, S.-S.; Mărgăritescu, N.-D.; Caragea, D.-C.; Țenea Cojan, I.-A.; Căluianu, V.; Marinaș, M.C.; Mogoș, G.F.R.; Vasile, L.; et al. Synchronous Ileal Metastasis from Pancreatic Ductal Adenocarcinoma: Case Report and Narrative Review with Practical Diagnostic and Management Points. *Life* **2025**, *15*, 1684. [CrossRef]
32. Barbu, L.A.; Cercelaru, L.; Vîlcea, I.-D.; Șurlin, V.; Mogoantă, S.-S.; Țenea Cojan, T.S.; Mărgăritescu, N.-D.; Țenea Cojan, A.-M.; Căluianu, V.; Popescu, M.; et al. Enteroenteric Fistula Following Multiple Magnet Ingestion in an Adult: Case Report, Literature Review and Management Algorithm. *Healthcare* **2025**, *13*, 2523. [CrossRef]
33. Wonglhow, J.; Sunpaweravong, P.; Sathitruangsak, C.; Dechaphunkul, A.; Wetwittayakhlang, P. A 20-Year Real-World Study of Small Bowel Cancers: Histologic Subtypes, Clinical Features, and Survival Implications. *J. Clin. Med.* **2025**, *14*, 6962. [CrossRef]

life

MDPI

Review

Synchronous Ileal Metastasis from Pancreatic Ductal Adenocarcinoma: Case Report and Narrative Review with Practical Diagnostic and Management Points

Tiberiu Stefăniță Țenea Cojan [1], Valeriu Șurlin [2], Stelian-Stefaniță Mogoantă [2], Nicolae-Dragoș Mărgăritescu [2], Daniel-Cosmin Caragea [3], Ioana-Alexia Țenea Cojan [4], Valentina Căluianu [1], Marius Cristian Marinaș [5], Gabriel Florin Răzvan Mogoș [1,*], Liviu Vasile [2] and Laurențiu Augustus Barbu [1]

[1] Department of Surgery, Railway Clinical Hospital Craiova, University of Medicine and Pharmacy of Craiova, 2 Petru Rares Street, 200349 Craiova, Romania; tiberiu.tenea@umfcv.ro (T.S.Ț.C.); valentina.andronache@yahoo.com (V.C.); laurentiu.barbu@umfcv.ro (L.A.B.)

[2] Department of Surgery, Emergency County Hospital, University of Medicine and Pharmacy of Craiova, 2 Petru Rares Street, 200349 Craiova, Romania; vsurlin@gmail.com (V.Ș.); ssmogo@yahoo.com (S.-S.M.); dmargaritescu@yahoo.com (N.-D.M.); vliviu777@yahoo.com (L.V.)

[3] Department of Internal Medicine, University of Medicine and Pharmacy of Craiova, 200349 Craiova, Romania; daniel.caragea@umfcv.ro

[4] Faculty of Medicine, University of Medicine and Pharmacy of Craiova, 200349 Craiova, Romania; teneaioana6@gmail.com

[5] Department of Obstetrics and Gynecology, Emergency County Hospital, University of Medicine and Pharmacy of Craiova, 2 Petru Rares Street, 200349 Craiova, Romania; cristian.marinas@umfcv.ro

* Correspondence: gabriel.mogos@umfcv.ro; Tel.: +40-722-669-232

Abstract: Background: Pancreatic ductal adenocarcinoma (PDAC) is an aggressive malignancy with poor prognosis, most frequently metastasizing to the liver, peritoneum, and lungs. Intestinal metastases are exceptionally rare and easily misinterpreted as primary small-bowel tumors, typically presenting with acute complications such as obstruction, perforation, or bleeding. **Methods**: We combined a detailed case description with a narrative literature review. PubMed/MEDLINE and Embase (2000–2025) were searched for case reports and case series describing intestinal metastases from PDAC with histopathological and immunohistochemical confirmation. **Case presentation**: We report a female patient presenting with acute intestinal obstruction caused by a synchronous ileal metastasis from PDAC. Imaging revealed an ileal stenosing lesion and a pancreatic body mass. An exploratory laparotomy identified a 3 cm transmural ileal tumor with additional serosal nodules. Histopathology confirmed a moderately differentiated adenocarcinoma. Immunohistochemistry supported pancreatic origin (CK7+, CA19-9+, faint CDX2), with mutant-type p53 positivity, ultra-low HER2/Neu expression, and a Ki-67 index of ~50%. The patient underwent segmental enterectomy with terminal ileostomy, followed by systemic therapy. **Conclusions**: This represents an exceptional and rare clinical finding rather than a presentation from which broad conclusions can be drawn. Histopathological and immunohistochemical analysis supported pancreatic origin and helped avoid misclassification as a primary intestinal neoplasm. It underscores the importance of careful clinicopathological correlation and multidisciplinary evaluation in atypical metastatic scenarios, while illustrating how surgery can provide symptom control and enable systemic therapy. Given its rarity, these observations should be interpreted with caution and regarded as descriptive rather than generalizable.

Keywords: pancreatic ductal adenocarcinoma; synchronous metastasis; ileal obstruction; intestinal metastasis; immunohistochemistry; p53; CK7; CA19-9; palliative surgery

 https://doi.org/10.3390/life15111684

1. Introduction

Pancreatic ductal adenocarcinoma (PDAC) is a highly aggressive gastrointestinal malignancy, typically diagnosed at an advanced stage, with limited therapeutic options and poor survival outcomes. The 5-year survival rate remains below 10% overall and under 3% in metastatic disease. The liver, peritoneum, and lungs represent the most common metastatic sites, and systemic therapy remains the standard of care according to current ESMO and ASCO guidelines [1–7].

In contrast, small bowel metastases from PDAC are exceptionally rare, with only isolated reports in the literature [8–11]. When present, they often manifest through acute complications such as obstruction or bleeding, and synchronous presentations are particularly uncommon. We present a case of synchronous ileal metastasis causing acute small bowel obstruction, underscoring the diagnostic challenges of atypical metastatic patterns and the critical role of timely surgical palliation to enable systemic therapy.

2. Case Presentation

2.1. Patient Information

A female patient, previously diagnosed by imaging with a pancreatic tumor, was admitted to the Department of Surgery, Railway Clinical Hospital Craiova. Her medical history was significant for arterial hypertension and dyslipidemia. She presented with diffuse abdominal pain, absence of intestinal transit for feces and gas, and fecaloid vomiting with onset 2 days prior to admission.

2.2. Clinical Findings

On examination, the abdomen was mobile with respiratory movements, diffusely tender on palpation, distended in volume, and showed diffuse muscular guarding. Abdominal resonance was absent.

2.3. Timeline

A structured timeline of the patient's clinical course, diagnostic workup, surgical intervention, and postoperative recovery is summarized below (Table 1).

Table 1. Clinical Timeline of Patient Presentation and Management.

Day	Clinical Event
Day 0	Onset of diffuse abdominal pain, fecaloid vomiting, and absence of intestinal transit.
Day 2	Admission to hospital; clinical and imaging workup performed.
Day 2 (evening)	Decision for surgical intervention; exploratory laparotomy performed.
Postoperative Days 1–3	Gradual clinical improvement; ileostomy functional; oral intake initiated.
Postoperative Days 4–9	Continued recovery without complications.
Postoperative Day 10	Discharged home in good general condition.

2.4. Diagnostic Assessment

Abdominal radiography: No pneumoperitoneum; hydro-aerial levels in the mesogastrium.

Ultrasonography: Dilated intestinal loops with liquid content and hypermotility; no abdominopelvic free fluid.

CT abdomen and pelvis: Focal, irregular parietal thickening with stenosing features located in the ileum, producing upstream intestinal distension with fluid content and hydro-aerial levels, without pneumoperitoneum (Figure 1). At the pancreatic body, a spontaneously isodense lesion with discrete iodophilia was identified, measuring 3.2 cm in axial diameter, without ductal dilatation (Figure 2). Given the acute obstructive presentation and the patient's overall clinical status, EUS-FNB of the pancreatic mass was not performed preoperatively. This decision was agreed upon in a multidisciplinary tumor board, with the plan to reassess the lesion at a later stage for histological confirmation.

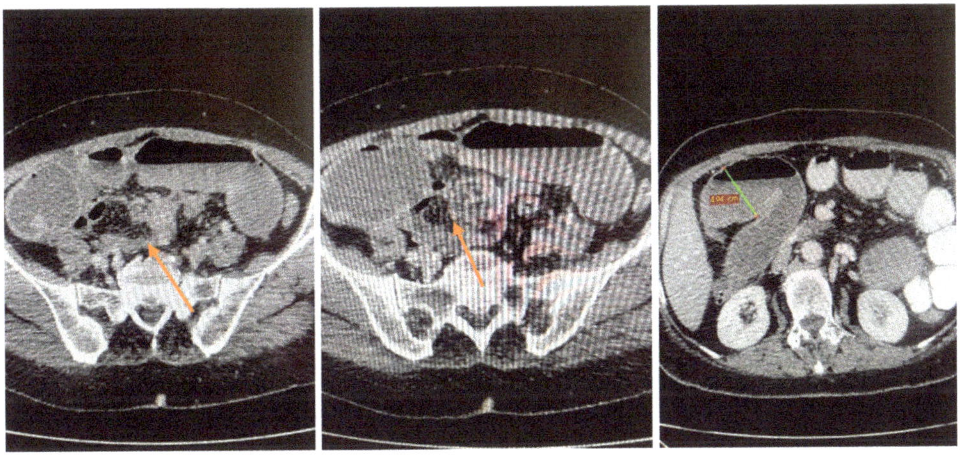

(a) (b) (c)

Figure 1. CT examination of the ileum. (**a**) Focal irregular parietal thickening (orange arrow). (**b**) Stenosing lesion (orange arrow). (**c**) Upstream intestinal dilatation (green measurement line).

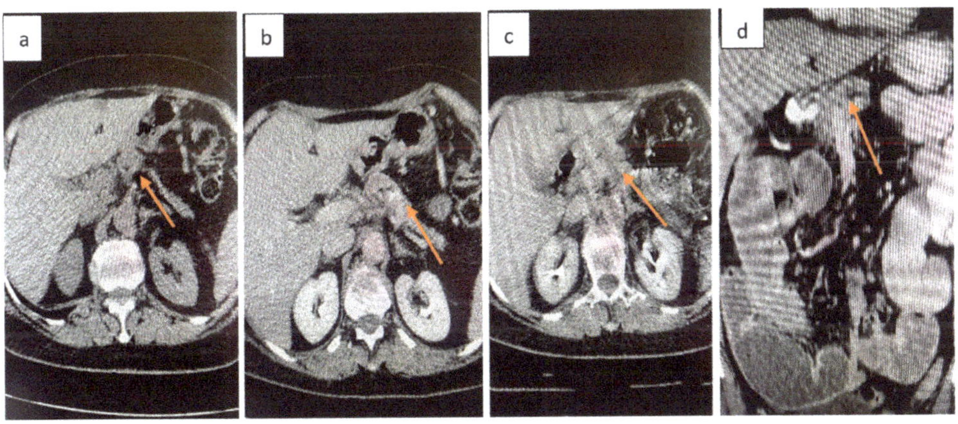

Figure 2. Contrast-enhanced abdominal CT. At the pancreatic body, a spontaneously isodense lesion with discrete iodophilia was identified, measuring 3.2 cm in axial diameter, without ductal dilatation (orange arrow). (**a**) Non-contrast phase. (**b**) Arterial phase. (**c**) Venous phase. (**d**) Delayed phase.

Laboratory investigations upon admission demonstrated leukocytosis with neutrophilia, indicating an acute inflammatory response. Coagulation studies were at the upper normal limit, while fibrinogen and ESR were markedly elevated, consistent with systemic inflammation. Renal function was preserved. Tumor markers showed a normal CEA but a mildly elevated CA 19-9, supporting possible pancreatic involvement (Table 2).

Table 2. Laboratory tests upon admission.

Parameter	Result	Normal Range
White blood cell count	$13.40 \times 10^3/\mu L$	$4–10 \times 10^3/\mu L$
Neutrophil proportion	77.9%	40–70%
Hemoglobin	13.4 g/dL	12–16 g/dL
Platelet count	$304 \times 10^3/\mu L$	$150–450 \times 10^3/\mu L$
Creatinine	0.7 mg/dL	0.6–1.3 mg/dL
Urea	28.37 mg/dL	15–45 mg/dL
INR	1.21	0.8–1.2
Prothrombin time	14.3 s	11–15 s
Fibrinogen	1115 mg/dL	200–400 mg/dL
C-reactive protein	—	<0.5 mg/dL
ESR	55 mm/h	<20 mm/h
CEA	1.23 ng/mL	<5 ng/mL
CA 19-9	53.11 U/mL	<37 U/mL

2.5. Therapeutic Intervention

Exploratory laparotomy revealed multiple dilated small bowel loops (8–10 cm in diameter, with thin walls). Approximately 50 cm proximal to the ileocecal valve, a 3 cm stenosing tumor extending beyond the serosa was identified. Two additional non-stenosing serosal nodules (1 cm and 1.5 cm, respectively) were also found upstream of the stenosis. In the corporeocaudal region of the pancreas, a firm, fixed mass measuring 5–5.5 cm was palpated, adherent posteriorly (Figure 3). The stomach and duodenum were markedly distended.

A segmental enterectomy was performed with terminal ileostomy in a "double-barrel" configuration.

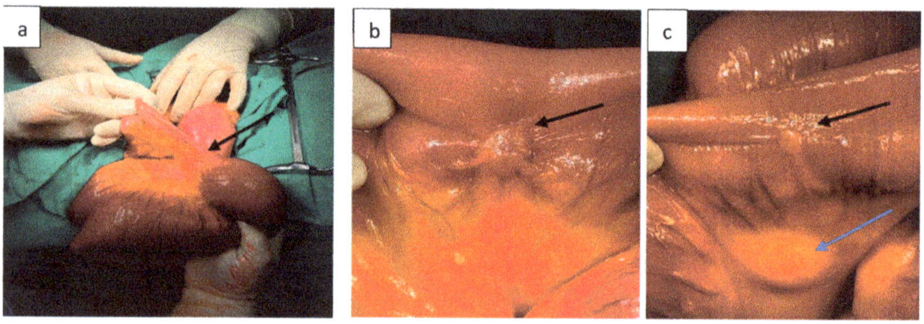

Figure 3. Intraoperative findings. (**a**) Stenosing ileal tumor (black arrow) with markedly dilated small bowel loops upstream and collapsed loops downstream. (**b**) Serosal tumor measuring 1.5 cm (black arrow). (**c**) Serosal tumor of 1 cm (black arrow) associated with intestinal lymphadenopathy (blue arrow).

2.6. Follow-Up and Outcomes

The postoperative course was favorable. The patient tolerated oral intake, had a functional ileostomy, and was discharged on postoperative day 10 in good general condition. She was subsequently referred to the oncology department and initiated systemic oncological treatment.

2.7. Histopathological Findings

Histopathological evaluation of the resected small bowel segment revealed a moderately differentiated adenocarcinoma, measuring 3 cm, with transmural infiltration and extension beyond the serosa (Figure 4). Immunohistochemical staining demonstrated CK7 (Figure 5) and CA19-9 positivity, with only faint CDX2 expression (Figure 6), consistent with a pancreatic origin. Tumor cells exhibited strong and diffuse mutant-type p53 positivity (Figure 7a), ultra-low HER2/Neu expression (Figure 7b,c), and a Ki-67 proliferation index of approximately 50% (Figure 8a). Scant mucinous secretion in tubular lumina and within some tumor cells was highlighted by PAS staining (Figure 8b). MMR protein expression was preserved, indicating a low probability of high microsatellite instability (MSI-H). Taken together, these findings supported the diagnosis of intestinal metastasis from a moderately differentiated pancreatic adenocarcinoma. We expanded the IHC panel to differentiate from a primary colonic or ileal tumor (CK20, SATB2, MUC1, SMAD4, CK19). The resulting profile (CK7+, CA19-9+, CK20−, SATB2−, MUC1+, SMAD4 loss, very faint CDX2) supports a pancreatic origin; however, in the absence of a pancreatic mass biopsy, the conclusion remains qualified as probable.

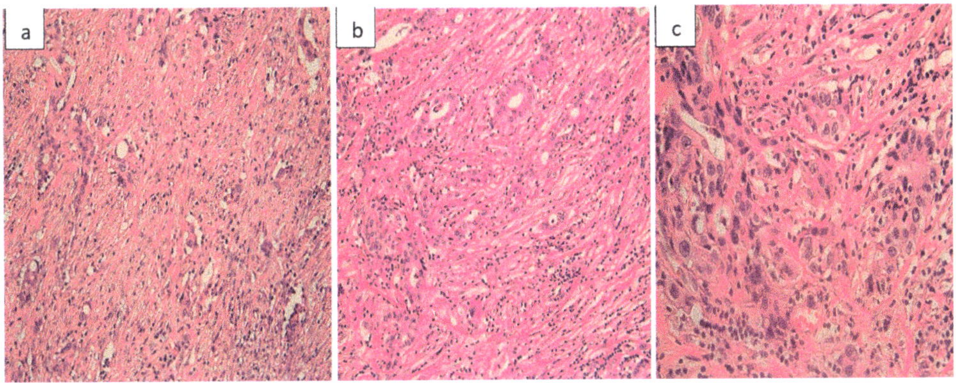

Figure 4. Moderately differentiated pancreatic adenocarcinoma. (**a**) Tumoral ducts with cuboidal cells, polymorphous nuclei, and frequent mitoses (H&E, 200×). (**b**) Cribriform structures and solid nests with desmoplastic stroma (H&E, 200×). (**c**) High-power view showing marked atypia and numerous mitotic figures (H&E, 400×).

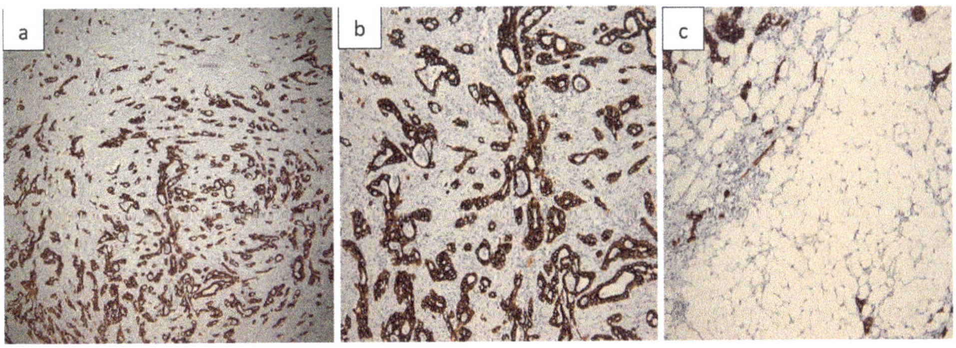

Figure 5. CK7 immunostaining. (**a**) Tubular pattern with complex architecture and isolated tumor cells at the invasion front (40×). (**b**) CK7 positivity highlighting the architectural complexity (100×). (**c**) Peripancreatic fat invasion on CK7 stain (100×).

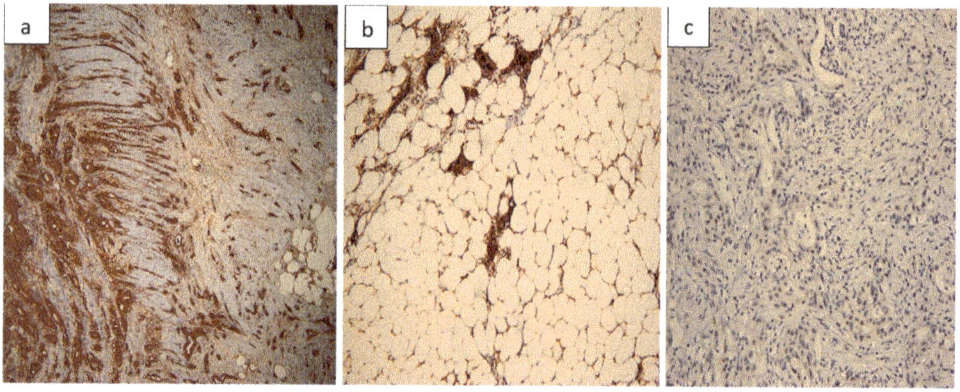

Figure 6. CA19-9/CDX2 immunoprofile. (**a**) CA19-9 positivity showing radial invasion in the muscularis propria of the duodenum (40×). (**b**) Peripancreatic fat invasion highlighted on CA19-9 stain (100×). (**c**) Very faint nuclear positivity for CDX2 in tumor cells (100×).

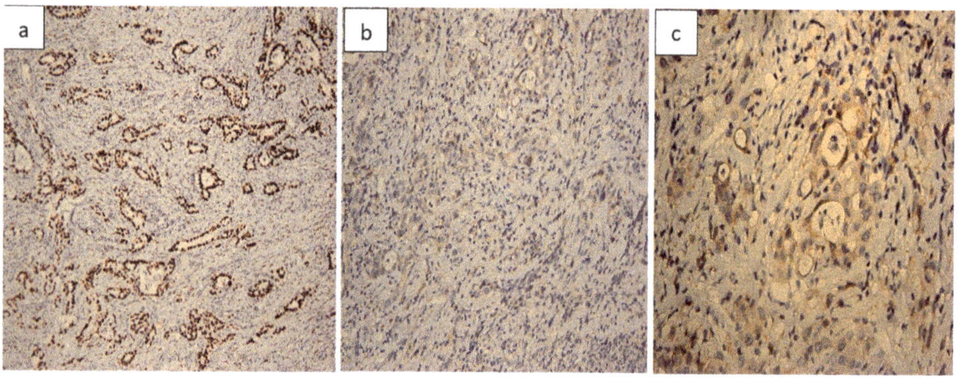

Figure 7. p53 and HER2/Neu immunoprofile. (**a**) Strong and diffuse mutant-type p53 positivity in tumor cells, with lighter wild-type staining in stromal cells (100×). (**b**) HER2/Neu ultra-low expression, with very faint membranous staining (20×). (**c**) Faint, discontinuous HER2/Neu immunostaining in scattered tumor cells ("hot spot") (40×).

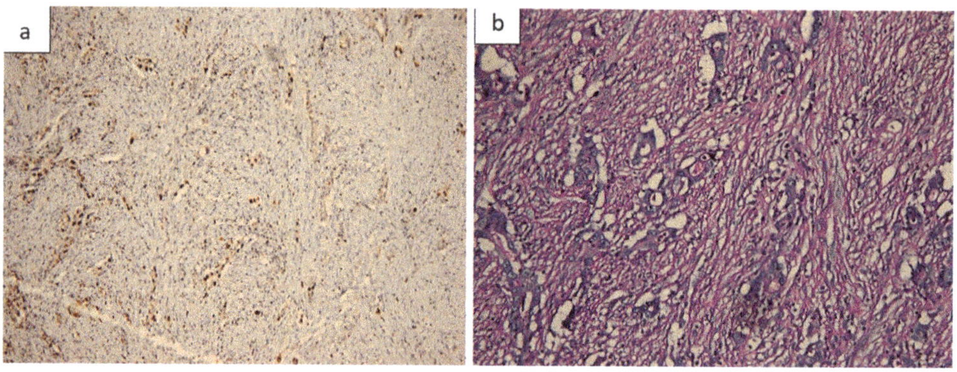

Figure 8. Ki-67 and PAS staining. (**a**) Ki-67 immunostaining showing a proliferation index of ~50% in tumor cells (100×). (**b**) Scant mucinous secretion in tubular lumina and within some tumor cells, highlighted by PAS staining (200×).

3. Materials and Methods

3.1. Literature Search and Selection

A narrative literature review was performed in PubMed/MEDLINE and Embase databases, covering the period 2000–2025. The following search terms were applied: *"pancreatic ductal adenocarcinoma" OR "PDAC" AND "intestinal metastasis" OR "small bowel metastasis" OR "colonic metastasis"*. In addition, the reference lists of relevant articles were screened manually to identify further eligible studies.

Inclusion criteria were case reports or case series reporting histologically confirmed intestinal metastases from PDAC. Studies were excluded if they described direct contiguous invasion without evidence of metastatic spread, lacked immunohistochemical confirmation, or were published in languages other than English.

3.2. Limitations

The evidence base is restricted to isolated case reports, which are inherently prone to publication bias. Further heterogeneity results from variability in immunohistochemical panels and occasional diagnostic uncertainty in differentiating true metastases from direct invasion. Consequently, quantitative synthesis was not feasible, and the results were analyzed qualitatively.

4. Discussion

More than half of patients with pancreatic ductal adenocarcinoma (PDAC) present with metastatic disease at diagnosis, most frequently involving the liver, peritoneum, and lungs [1,2]. Reports of small-bowel metastases are limited to isolated case descriptions, and no reliable incidence data are available [8–10].

4.1. Epidemiology and Mechanisms of Spread

Pancreatic ductal adenocarcinoma (PDAC) is one of the most lethal gastrointestinal malignancies and currently the seventh leading cause of cancer-related death worldwide, projected to rank second by 2030 [1,2]. Despite therapeutic progress, the 5-year survival remains 6–10%, and below 3% in metastatic disease [1]. Over half of patients present with advanced disease, with the liver (60–70%), peritoneum (20–40%), and lungs (10–20%) as the predominant metastatic sites [2,3]. Gastrointestinal involvement is exceptionally rare and reported almost exclusively as isolated case reports, with colonic and small-bowel metastases documented by immunohistochemical confirmation of pancreatic origin [8–10].

Three main mechanisms are proposed to explain these rare metastatic patterns. Hematogenous dissemination may account for distant intestinal lesions via tumor thrombi in the portal or systemic circulation, often without peritoneal involvement [1,3,11]. Lymphatic spread through mesenteric or retroperitoneal pathways can lead to skip metastases in the absence of dominant hepatic disease [3,9]. Finally, peritoneal seeding through transcoelomic spread allows exfoliated tumor cells to implant on the bowel surface and invade the wall, particularly in carcinomatosis or ascites, explaining some synchronous obstructive presentations [10,11].

4.2. Correlation with Reported Cases

Published cases illustrate these mechanisms (Figure 9). Metachronous jejunal and colonic metastases occurring after pancreaticoduodenectomy presented with obstruction and fever, requiring emergency resection; the patient died within seven months, consistent with aggressive disease and hematogenous or lymphatic spread [9]. A jejunal metastasis diagnosed five years after curative resection, confirmed by IHC (CK7+, CK20−), was resected with favorable recovery, and the absence of peritoneal disease suggested hematogenous or lymphatic dissemination [8]. A synchronous sigmoid metastasis with pancreatic-type IHC (CK7+, CK20−) was reported as an unusual metastatic pattern, with hematogenous, lymphatic, and transcoelomic routes considered plausible [11].

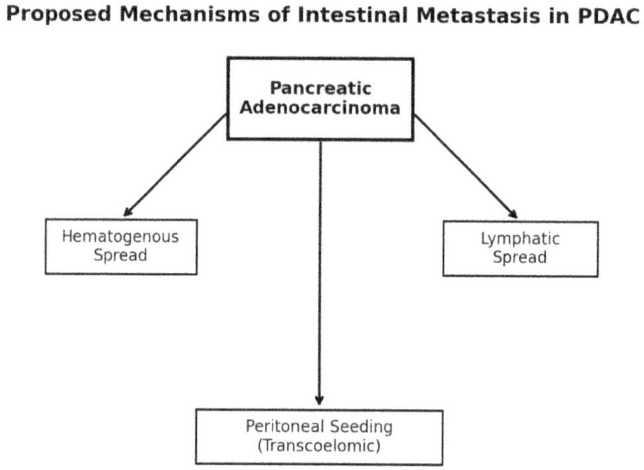

Figure 9. Proposed mechanisms of intestinal metastasis in PDAC. Legend: Three main routes have been proposed—(1) hematogenous dissemination to distant bowel, (2) lymphatic spread via mesenteric/retroperitoneal channels, and (3) peritoneal seeding with secondary bowel wall invasion [1,3,10].

4.3. Clinical Presentation and Diagnostic Work-Up

The clinical presentation of intestinal metastases from pancreatic ductal adenocarcinoma (PDAC) is nonspecific and often leads to delayed diagnosis. Typical symptoms include abdominal pain, nausea, vomiting, altered bowel habits, and signs of subocclusion or obstruction [9,10]. Occult gastrointestinal bleeding with anemia may be the initial manifestation [8], while hematemesis, melena, and iron-deficiency anemia can mimic other acute gastrointestinal conditions [12]. Obstructive symptoms may resemble mesenteric lymphatic cysts or appendiceal tumors [13,14]. Rarely, patients present with perforation and peritonitis requiring emergency surgery [10], and differential diagnoses should include colonic, rectal, or retroperitoneal pathologies [15]. Because of its rarity, intestinal involvement is often mistaken for a primary gastrointestinal tumor, underscoring the importance of histopathological confirmation.

The diagnosis is challenging and relies on appropriate imaging and histopathology. Contrast-enhanced CT is the first-line investigation to assess obstruction and metastatic spread [1], but sensitivity decreases for small or early lesions. Careful review of multiphasic CT is important in pancreatic tail primaries near the splenic hilum or flexure, where direct invasion may mimic metastasis. PET-CT can identify hypermetabolic bowel lesions when CT or endoscopy are inconclusive, as shown in a reported case of jejunal recurrence [8]. Endoscopy or capsule endoscopy may detect intraluminal lesions but have limited value for extramural disease. A definitive diagnosis requires histopathological and immunohistochemical confirmation of pancreatic origin [1].

4.4. Histopathological and Immunohistochemical Evidence

True small-bowel metastases from pancreatic ductal adenocarcinoma (PDAC) must be differentiated from direct invasion of adjacent loops and from primary intestinal adenocarcinoma. Immunohistochemistry (IHC) plays a key role in this distinction; a CK7+/CK20−/CDX2− profile supports pancreatic origin, while CK20+/CDX2+/SATB2+

suggests a colorectal primary [8,11]. Neuroendocrine tumors (NETs) of the small intestine, another important differential diagnosis, are typically chromogranin A and synaptophysin positive and may present with obstruction, anemia, or abdominal pain [16]. Primary intestinal lymphomas can also mimic these presentations, often debuting with obstruction or upper gastrointestinal symptoms [17].

Histologically, PDAC metastases usually involve the subserosa or submucosa with preservation of the mucosa. Deep biopsies are recommended because superficial samples can mimic a colorectal phenotype overlying a pancreatic metastasis. A practical diagnostic profile includes CK7+/CK20−/CDX2−, often MUC1+, with possible SMAD4 loss, whereas colorectal primaries are typically CK20+/CDX2+/SATB2+ and CK7−. Additional markers such as CK19 and CA19-9 may provide further support. Strong and diffuse p53 positivity, as in our case, is consistent with tumor progression and aids in distinguishing PDAC metastases [18].

Published reports describe identical IHC profiles in pancreatic primaries and intestinal lesions, most commonly diffuse CK7 positivity with CK20 negativity, supporting the diagnosis of metastatic spread rather than synchronous primaries [8,11]. This confirmation often guides therapy, favoring palliative surgery followed by systemic treatment. When feasible, pancreatic mass biopsy with IHC comparison (±KRAS/SMAD4) is recommended to exclude a synchronous luminal primary. If biopsy is not possible, extended IHC on the metastasis, correlated with morphology and imaging, helps reduce misclassification, though the conclusion remains probabilistic. Because aberrant marker expression may occur, final diagnosis should integrate clinical, radiologic, and pathological data, and when necessary, additional molecular testing.

4.5. Molecular and Therapeutic Considerations

Molecular profiling complements histopathology and immunohistochemistry in pancreatic ductal adenocarcinoma (PDAC) by identifying clinically relevant alterations. KRAS mutations are present in approximately 95% of cases, with the G12R variant—around 15%—showing distinct signaling that may confer relative sensitivity to MEK inhibition, though this remains investigational [19–21]. A subset of tumors harbor DNA damage repair alterations (BRCA1, BRCA2, PALB2), associated with platinum sensitivity and potential response to PARP inhibitors. Rare MSI-high tumors may benefit from immune checkpoint blockade [22,23]. For this reason, baseline next-generation sequencing is increasingly recommended in advanced PDAC to identify actionable targets, in line with ESMO, NCCN, and ASCO guidelines [6,24,25].

Accurate classification of intestinal lesions—distinguishing metastasis from a primary tumor or direct invasion—is crucial for therapeutic planning. Surgery or endoscopic procedures are typically reserved for complications such as obstruction or bleeding, or for carefully selected oligometastatic cases, while systemic therapy remains the standard of care [26]. Surgical intervention is most often used for acute complications, with reported procedures including segmental bowel resection, bypass, or stoma formation, resulting in short-term symptom relief [8–10]. Endoscopic palliation with self-expanding metal stents can decompress obstructive colonic lesions and serve as a bridge to systemic treatment. Chemotherapy regimens include FOLFIRINOX for fit patients and gemcitabine plus nab-paclitaxel for those with lower performance status, often initiated or resumed after palliation [2,27]. Given the aggressive course of PDAC, multidisciplinary decision-making is essential to balance surgical risks, expected benefits, and the feasibility of continuing systemic therapy.

4.6. Practical Management Algorithm for Intestinal Metastasis from PDAC

Step 1. Clinical suspicion

Patient with pancreatic adenocarcinoma presenting with abdominal pain, nausea, vomiting, subocclusion/obstruction, anemia, or GI bleeding [9,10].

Step 2. Diagnostic work-up

CT scan → first-line to assess site of obstruction and metastases [1].

PET-CT → for occult or equivocal lesions [8].

Histopathology + IHC (CK7+, CK19+, CA19-9+, CK20−, CDX2−) → confirm pancreatic origin [11].

Step 3. Emergency/urgent management

Endoscopic palliation (self-expanding metal stents) → in selected colonic obstruction.

Surgical resection (segmental bowel resection ± anastomosis or bypass) → for obstruction, perforation, bleeding [10,28].

Re-resection may be considered in oligometastatic disease with good performance status [8].

Step 4. Post-palliation systemic therapy

Resume or initiate systemic treatment:

FOLFIRINOX (fit patients).

Gemcitabine + nab-paclitaxel (more common in reported cases, tolerable) [2,27].

Step 5. Multidisciplinary follow-up

Regular monitoring with imaging + CA19-9.

Focus on symptom relief, nutritional support, and maintaining chemotherapy eligibility.

4.7. Prognosis and Clinical Lessons

The prognosis of pancreatic ductal adenocarcinoma (PDAC) remains poor, with a 5-year survival of 9–10% across all stages and less than 3% in metastatic disease [1,2]. Median survival in advanced or unresectable stages is short, underscoring the need for individualized multimodal strategies [1]. Outcomes of intestinal metastases are rarely documented; Miyasaka et al. reported death seven months after emergency resection for jejunal and colonic involvement [9], whereas Tseng et al. described favorable recovery and ongoing systemic therapy after re-resection of a metachronous jejunal metastasis nearly five years post-pancreatic surgery [8].

Prognosis is influenced by several factors. Tumor burden is critical—patients with oligometastatic disease may benefit from selective resection, while those with disseminated disease have a significantly worse outcome [8,9]. Performance status, reflected by ECOG score and suitability for systemic therapy (FOLFIRINOX or gemcitabine plus nab-paclitaxel), strongly impacts survival [1,8]. In selected patients, re-resection of intestinal metastases may offer symptom control and enable continuation of treatment [8].

Although long-term survival is uncommon, palliative surgery can provide rapid symptom relief, prevent life-threatening complications, and allow systemic therapy to continue. Miyasaka et al. reported good postoperative recovery with normalization of fever and inflammatory markers and hospital discharge [9]. Similarly, Meng et al. described initiation of gemcitabine plus nab-paclitaxel following IHC confirmation of pancreatic origin in a case of colonic metastasis [11].

4.8. Reported Cases in the Literature

A review of the literature (Table 3) highlights the extreme rarity of intestinal metastases from PDAC, with fewer than 15 well-documented cases over the last decade. Most cases were reported as **single case reports**, reflecting the anecdotal nature of the available evidence.

Table 3. Reported cases of intestinal metastases from pancreatic ductal adenocarcinoma (PDAC).

Author/Year	Patient (Age/Sex)	Interval from Primary PDAC	Site of Metastasis	Presentation	Management	Outcome
Fasano [10]	Long-term survivor (M)	Synchronous	Small bowel	Acute abdomen	Emergency small bowel resection	First described intestinal metastasis in long-term PDAC survivor with mesothelioma
Miyasaka [9]	63/M	3 months post-pancreaticoduodenectomy	Jejunum + colon	Abdominal pain, fever, diarrhea	Emergency resection (jejunum + colon)	Death at 7 months due to relapse
Nakaya [27]	72/M	Synchronous	Colon (within preexisting carcinoma)	Bowel obstruction	Colectomy	Rare phenomenon of PDAC metastasis colonizing colon carcinoma
Park [28]	73/F	Synchronous	Transverse colon	Large bowel obstruction	Segmental colectomy	Palliative survival, <1 year
Kahl [29]	91/F	Synchronous	Sigmoid colon	Large bowel obstruction	Sigmoid colectomy	Died shortly after surgery
Meng [11]	65/M	Concomitant	Sigmoid colon	Colon lesion detected on work-up	Diagnosis confirmed by IHC; chemotherapy	Extremely rare metastatic route
Ardalan [30]	66/F	Synchronous	Sigmoid colon	Acute obstruction	Emergency left hemicolectomy + IHC; FOLFIRINOX	Poor tolerance, palliative course
O'Sullivan [24]	Cases (2)	Synchronous	Rectum/colon	Obstruction, GI symptoms	Surgical resection/supportive	Reported as very rare synchronous cases
Tseng [8]	56/F	~5 years post-pancreaticoduodenectomy	Jejunum	Anemia (Hb 8–9 g/dL), occult bleeding	Segmental jejunal resection	Uneventful recovery; continued systemic therapy
Pacheco [31]	68/M	Metachronous (interval not specified)	Sigmoid colon	Symptomatic metastasis, bowel obstruction	Surgical resection	Reported as the third symptomatic colonic metastasis from PDAC
Present case (2025)	F	Concomitant	Ileum	Acute intestinal obstruction	Emergency ileal resection + anastomosis	Favorable recovery; referred to oncology.

Most patients with intestinal metastases from pancreatic ductal adenocarcinoma (PDAC) present with acute complications such as obstruction, abdominal pain, or perforation, while fewer are diagnosed incidentally during colonoscopy or imaging. Rare metachronous cases may occur years after pancreatic resection. The jejunum, ileum, and colon (sigmoid, transverse, rectum) are most often affected, with exceptional cases involving colonization of preexisting colorectal carcinoma, suggesting atypical spread [8–11].

Management is mainly palliative, typically involving emergency or symptom-driven segmental colectomy or enterectomy, with endoscopic stenting used selectively in colonic obstruction. Systemic chemotherapy (gemcitabine plus nab-paclitaxel or FOLFIRINOX) is often initiated or resumed after palliation. Prognosis remains poor, though re-resection may benefit carefully selected oligometastatic patients. In most cases, surgery provides symptom relief, improved quality of life, and enables continuation of systemic therapy [8–11].

4.9. Key Messages

Key practice points in diagnosing and managing intestinal metastases from PDAC are summarized in Table 4.

1. Intestinal metastases from PDAC are exceptional events, often presenting with acute surgical emergencies.
2. Surgical resection provides palliative benefit and may enable systemic therapy in selected patients.
3. The role of systemic chemotherapy is crucial, but evidence remains anecdotal.
4. Multidisciplinary evaluation is essential, as no standardized guidelines exist.

Table 4. Lessons learned/Practice points in diagnosing and managing intestinal metastases from PDAC.

Practice Point	Rationale
When technically feasible, target submucosa	Superficial mucosal biopsies may mimic a colorectal phenotype; submucosal sampling can improve diagnostic accuracy, but should not be considered mandatory
Always run CK7/CK20/CDX2/SATB2 ± MUC1/SMAD4	Distinguishes PDAC metastasis (CK7+/CDX2−/SATB2−) from primary intestinal adenocarcinoma.
Re-discuss at MDT before major surgery	Avoids inappropriate CRC-style resections and aligns care with systemic PDAC therapy. Avoiding inappropriate surgery in such rare scenarios is not based on a standardized algorithm, but rather on individualized, case-by-case multidisciplinary decision-making, aimed at aligning management with the underlying pancreatic primary.

Note: Adapted from published case reports and small series on intestinal metastases from PDAC [8–11,32–39].

4.10. Review Synthesis and Future Directions

Available evidence indicates that intestinal metastases from pancreatic ductal adenocarcinoma (PDAC) are exceptionally rare and usually present with obstruction, bleeding, or acute abdomen. Because clinical and imaging findings are nonspecific, histopathological and immunohistochemical confirmation is crucial. Although mainly palliative, surgery provides symptom relief and preserves eligibility for systemic therapy, the mainstay of treatment. Recognizing this entity helps avoid misdiagnosis and supports timely management.

Current knowledge relies on isolated case reports and small series, with no standardized guidelines. Future research should focus on registries to clarify incidence, risk factors, and outcomes, and on systematic reporting to refine diagnosis. Consensus recommendations are needed to standardize palliation, integrate systemic therapy, and optimize follow-up. This case adds to the limited literature by documenting a rare synchronous intestinal metastasis with acute obstruction and highlighting the value of such reports for future clinical practice.

5. Conclusions

Synchronous ileal metastasis from PDAC represents an exceptional and rare clinical finding, rather than a typical presentation from which general conclusions can be drawn. Histopathological and immunohistochemical analysis supported a pancreatic origin and helped avoid misclassification as a primary intestinal neoplasm. Surgical palliation provided symptom control and allowed systemic therapy to be initiated. As pancreatic mass biopsy was not performed in the acute setting, the diagnosis should be regarded as probable and interpreted cautiously, in conjunction with clinical, imaging, and IHC findings. This highlights the importance of multidisciplinary evaluation and careful, case-by-case decision-making in unusual metastatic scenarios, as well as the value of reporting rare cases to support future evidence-building rather than to establish clinical standards.

Author Contributions: Conceptualization L.A.B., D.-C.C. and N.-D.M.; writing—original draft L.A.B. and T.S.Ţ.C.; resources V.C., L.V., S.-S.M., G.F.R.M., T.S.Ţ.C. and V.Ş.; supervision M.C.M. and S.-S.M.; investigation M.C.M., V.C., L.V., G.F.R.M. and V.Ş.; writing—review M.C.M., L.A.B., T.S.Ţ.C. and G.F.R.M.; validation D.-C.C., L.V., S.-S.M. and N.-D.M.; software D.-C.C.,V.C. and I.-A.Ţ.C.; visualization V.C. and G.F.R.M.; data curation I.-A.Ţ.C., T.S.Ţ.C. and N.-D.M.; project administration L.A.B., D.-C.C. and V.Ş.; formal analysis M.C.M., I.-A.Ţ.C. and N.-D.M.; methodology I.-A.Ţ.C., L.V., S.-S.M. and V.Ş. All authors have read and agreed to the published version of the manuscript.

Funding: The article processing charges were funded by the University of Medicine and Pharmacy of Craiova, Romania.

Institutional Review Board Statement: The study was conducted in accordance with the Declaration of Helsinki and approved by the Ethics Committee of the Railway Clinical Hospital Craiova (approval no. 8457/24 September 2025).

Informed Consent Statement: Informed consent was obtained from the patient, whereby individual written informed consent was obtained, ensuring full compliance with ethical standards.

Data Availability Statement: The data presented in this study are available on request from the corresponding author. The data are not publicly available due to patient confidentiality.

Conflicts of Interest: The authors declare no conflicts of interest.

References

1. Pavlidis, E.T.; Galanis, I.N.; Pavlidis, T.E. Updates in the diagnosis and management of ductal adenocarcinoma of the pancreas. *World J. Clin. Oncol.* **2025**, *16*, 105601. [CrossRef]
2. Zhang, C.Y.; Liu, S.; Yang, M. Clinical diagnosis and management of pancreatic cancer: Markers, molecular mechanisms, and treatment options. *World J. Gastroenterol.* **2022**, *28*, 6827–6845. [CrossRef]
3. Cannistrà, M.; Ruggiero, M.; Zullo, A.; Serafini, S.; Grande, R.; Nardo, B. Metastases of pancreatic adenocarcinoma: A systematic review of literature and a new functional concept. *Int. J. Surg.* **2015**, *21* (Suppl. 1), S15–S21. [CrossRef] [PubMed]
4. Conroy, T.; Pfeiffer, P.; Vilgrain, V.; Lamarca, A.; Seufferlein, T.; O'Reilly, E.M.; Hackert, T.; Golan, T.; Prager, G.; Haustermans, K.; et al. Pancreatic cancer: ESMO Clinical Practice Guideline for diagnosis, treatment and follow-up. *Ann. Oncol.* **2023**, *34*, 987–1002. [CrossRef]
5. Springfeld, C.; Bailey, P.; Büchler, M.W.; Neoptolemos, J.P. ESMO 2023 pancreatic cancer guidelines signal stepwise progress. *Hepatobiliary Surg. Nutr.* **2024**, *13*, 362–365. [CrossRef]
6. Sohal, D.P.S.; Kennedy, E.B.; Cinar, P.; Conroy, T.; Copur, M.S.; Crane, C.H.; Garrido-Laguna, I.; Lau, M.W.; Johnson, T.; Krishnamurthi, S.; et al. Metastatic Pancreatic Cancer: ASCO Guideline Update. *J. Clin. Oncol.* **2020**, *38*, 3217–3230. [CrossRef]
7. Hayat, U.; Croce, P.S.; Saadeh, A.; Desai, K.; Appiah, J.; Khan, S.; Khan, Y.I.; Kumar, K.; Hanif, A. Current and Emerging Treatment Options for Pancreatic Cancer: A Comprehensive Review. *J. Clin. Med.* **2025**, *14*, 1129. [CrossRef] [PubMed]
8. Tseng, C.-W.; Tseng, I.-T.; Wu, C.-C. Rare Case of Metachronous Small-Bowel Metastasis from Pancreatic Cancer Presenting as Anemia Approximately 5 Years Postpancreatoduodenectomy. *J. Gastroenterol. Dig. Syst.* **2024**, *8*, 1–6. [CrossRef]
9. Miyasaka, M.; Noji, T.; Tanaka, K.; Nakanishi, Y.; Asano, T.; Ebihara, Y.; Kurashima, Y.; Nakamura, T.; Murakami, S.; Tsuchikawa, T.; et al. Oncological emergency surgery for metachronous large and small bowel metastases after pancreaticoduodenectomy for pancreatic cancer: A case report. *Surg. Case Rep.* **2018**, *4*, 99. [CrossRef]
10. Fasano, M.; Della Corte, C.M.; Vicidomini, G.; Scotti, V.; Rambaldi, P.F.; Fiorelli, A.; Accardo, M.; De Vita, F.; Santini, M.; Ciardiello, F.; et al. Small bowel metastasis from pancreatic cancer in a long-term survival patient with synchronous advanced malignant pleural mesothelioma: A case report and literature review. *Oncol. Lett.* **2016**, *12*, 4505–4509. [CrossRef]
11. Meng, N.; Han, P.; Liu, L.; Liu, J.; Liu, J. Colon Metastasis from Pancreatic Cancer: A Case Report. *OncoTargets Ther.* **2023**, *16*, 739–744. [CrossRef] [PubMed]
12. Barbu, L.A.; Vasile, L.; Cercelaru, L.; Şurlin, V.; Mogoantă, S.-S.; Mogoş, G.F.R.; Ţenea Cojan, T.S.; Mărgăritescu, N.-D.; Buliman, A. Non-Variceal Upper Gastrointestinal Bleeding: A Retrospective Cohort of 364 Cases, Historical Comparison, and Updated Management Algorithm. *Life* **2025**, *15*, 1320. [CrossRef]
13. Vasile, L.; Barbu, L.A.; Mogoş, G.F.R.; Şurlin, V.; Vîlcea, I.D.; Cercelaru, L.; Mogoantă, S.Ş.; Mărgăritescu, N.D.; Nimigean, V.; Nimigean, V.R.; et al. Neuroendocrine tumors of the appendix: A comprehensive review of the literature and case presentation. *Rom. J. Morphol. Embryol.* **2025**, *66*, 269–278. [CrossRef] [PubMed]

14. Barbu, L.A.; Cercelaru, L.; Vîlcea, I.-D.; Șurlin, V.; Mogoantă, S.-S.; Țenea Cojan, T.S.; Mărgăritescu, N.-D.; Popescu, M.; Mogoș, G.F.R.; Vasile, L. Coexistence of Acute Appendicitis and Mesenteric Cystic Lymphatic Malformation in an Adult: A Case Report and Narrative Review of Intraoperative Management Strategies. *Life* **2025**, *15*, 1390. [CrossRef]
15. Barbu, L.A.; Vasile, L.; Cercelaru, L.; Vîlcea, I.-D.; Șurlin, V.; Mogoantă, S.-S.; Mogoș, G.F.R.; Țenea Cojan, T.S.; Mărgăritescu, N.-D. Fused Ischiorectal Phlegmon with Pre- and Retroperitoneal Extension: Case Report and Narrative Literature Review. *J. Clin. Med.* **2025**, *14*, 4959. [CrossRef] [PubMed]
16. Calomino, N.; Fusario, D.; Cencini, E.; Lazzi, S. Two secondary localisation of non-Hodgkin's lymphomas in the upper gastrointestinal tract. *BMJ Case Rep.* **2022**, *15*, e247607. [CrossRef]
17. Waters, A.M.; Der, C.J. KRAS: The Critical Driver and Therapeutic Target for Pancreatic Cancer. *Cold Spring Harb. Perspect. Med.* **2018**, *8*, a031435. [CrossRef]
18. Ardalan, B.; Azqueta, J.; Sleeman, D. Cobimetinib Plus Gemcitabine: An Active Combination in KRAS G12R-Mutated Pancreatic Ductal Adenocarcinoma Patients in Previously Treated and Failed Multiple Chemotherapies. *J. Pancreat. Cancer* **2021**, *7*, 65–70. [CrossRef]
19. Mehdi, M.; Thalji, S.Z.; Shreenivas, A.; Chakrabarti, S.; Thomas, J.P.; Christians, K.K.; Evans, D.B.; Hall, W.A.; Erickson, B.; Thapa, B.; et al. MEK-Inhibitor (inh) and Hydroxychloroquine (HCQ) in KRAS-Mutated Advanced Pancreatic Ductal Adenocarcinoma (PDAC). *J. Clin. Oncol.* **2022**, *40*, e16260. [CrossRef]
20. Golan, T.; Hammel, P.; Reni, M.; Van Cutsem, E.; Macarulla, T.; Hall, M.J.; Park, J.O.; Hochhauser, D.; Arnold, D.; Oh, D.Y.; et al. Maintenance Olaparib for Germline *BRCA*-Mutated Metastatic Pancreatic Cancer. *N. Engl. J. Med.* **2019**, *381*, 317–327. [CrossRef]
21. Ghidini, M.; Lampis, A.; Mirchev, M.B.; Okuducu, A.F.; Ratti, M.; Valeri, N.; Hahne, J.C. Immune-Based Therapies and the Role of Microsatellite Instability in Pancreatic Cancer. *Genes* **2020**, *12*, 33. [CrossRef]
22. Mosele, F.; Remon, J.; Mateo, J.; Westphalen, C.B.; Barlesi, F.; Lolkema, M.P.; Normanno, N.; Scarpa, A.; Robson, M.; Meric-Bernstam, F.; et al. Recommendations for the use of next-generation sequencing (NGS) for patients with metastatic cancers: A report from the ESMO Precision Medicine Working Group. *Ann. Oncol.* **2020**, *31*, 1491–1505. [CrossRef]
23. Tempero, M.A.; Malafa, M.P.; Al-Hawary, M.; Behrman, S.W.; Benson, A.B.; Cardin, D.B.; Chiorean, E.G.; Chung, V.; Czito, B.; Del Chiaro, M.; et al. Pancreatic Adenocarcinoma, Version 2.2021, NCCN Clinical Practice Guidelines in Oncology. *J. Natl. Compr. Cancer Netw.* **2021**, *19*, 439–457. [CrossRef]
24. O'Sullivan, B.; Burton, T.; Van Dalen, R.; Welsh, F.; Pandita, A.; Fischer, J. Beware the pancreatic incidentaloma in colorectal tumours: Pancreatic adenocarcinoma with metastases to the colon and rectum. *J. Surg. Case Rep.* **2022**, *2022*, rjab629. [CrossRef]
25. Daamen, L.A.; Molenaar, I.Q.; Groot, V.P. Recent Advances and Future Challenges in Pancreatic Cancer Care: Early Detection, Liquid Biopsies, Precision Medicine and Artificial Intelligence. *J. Clin. Med.* **2023**, *12*, 7485. [CrossRef] [PubMed]
26. Bugazia, D.; Al-Najjar, E.; Esmail, A.; Abdelrahim, S.; Abboud, K.; Abdelrahim, A.; Umoru, G.; Rayyan, H.A.; Abudayyeh, A.; Al Moustafa, A.E.; et al. Pancreatic ductal adenocarcinoma: The latest on diagnosis, molecular profiling, and systemic treatments. *Front. Oncol.* **2024**, *14*, 1386699. [CrossRef] [PubMed]
27. Nakaya, T.; Oshiro, H.; Saito, T.; Sakuma, Y.; Horie, H.; Sata, N.; Tanaka, A. Metastasis of pancreatic cancer within primary colon cancer by overtaking the stromal microenvironment. *Int. J. Clin. Exp. Pathol.* **2018**, *11*, 3141–3146. [PubMed]
28. Park, D.Y.; Krishnamurthi, S.; Chahal, P.; Downs-Kelly, E.; Morris-Stiff, G. Pancreatic metastases to the colon: An unusual cause of colonic obstruction. *BMJ Case Rep.* **2019**, *12*, e228578. [CrossRef]
29. Kahl, R.; George, K.; Patel, K.; Stawick, L. Pancreatic Adenocarcinoma with Rare Sigmoid Colon Metastasis. *ACG Case Rep. J.* **2019**, *6*, e00132. [CrossRef]
30. Ardalan, B.; Azqueta, J.; England, J.; Hartmann, R. Pancreatic cancer presenting as bowel obstruction and role of next generation sequencing: A case report. *Int. J. Surg. Case Rep.* **2022**, *90*, 106654. [CrossRef]
31. Pacheco, F.; Luciano, E.; Hebert, D.; Marar, O. Metastatic pancreatic adenocarcinoma presenting as large bowel obstruction: A case report. *Int. J. Surg. Case Rep.* **2023**, *102*, 107801. [CrossRef]
32. Casolino, R.; Biankin, A.V. Treatment of pancreatic cancer in 2022. *Camb. Prism. Precis. Med.* **2023**, *1*, e14. [CrossRef]
33. Netto, D.; Frizziero, M.; Foy, V.; McNamara, M.G.; Backen, A.; Hubner, R.A. Systemic Therapy for Metastatic Pancreatic Cancer—Current Landscape and Future Directions. *Curr. Oncol.* **2024**, *31*, 5206–5223. [CrossRef]
34. Stoop, T.F.; Javed, A.A.; Oba, A.; Koerkamp, B.G.; Seufferlein, T.; Wilmink, J.W.; Besselink, M.G. Pancreatic cancer. *Lancet* **2025**, *405*, 1182–1202. [CrossRef] [PubMed]
35. Wainberg, Z.A.; Melisi, D.; Macarulla, T.; Pazo Cid, R.; Chandana, S.R.; De La Fouchardière, C.; Dean, A.; Kiss, I.; Lee, W.J.; Goetze, T.O.; et al. NALIRIFOX versus nab-paclitaxel and gemcitabine in treatment-naive patients with metastatic pancreatic ductal adenocarcinoma (NAPOLI 3): A randomised, open-label, phase 3 trial. *Lancet* **2023**, *402*, 1272–1281. [CrossRef]
36. Miyabayashi, K.; Nakagawa, H.; Koike, K. Molecular and Phenotypic Profiling for Precision Medicine in Pancreatic Cancer: Current Advances and Future Perspectives. *Front. Oncol.* **2021**, *11*, 682872. [CrossRef] [PubMed]
37. Ratner, E.S.; Sartorelli, A.C.; Lin, Z.P. Poly (ADP-ribose) polymerase inhibitors: On the horizon of tailored and personalized therapies for epithelial ovarian cancer. *Curr. Opin. Oncol.* **2012**, *24*, 564–571. [CrossRef]

38. Wang, H.; Li, Z.W.; Ou, Q.; Wu, X.; Nagasaka, M.; Shao, Y.; Ou, S.I.; Yang, Y. NTRK fusion positive colorectal cancer is a unique subset of CRC with high TMB and microsatellite instability. *Cancer Med.* **2022**, *11*, 2541–2549. [CrossRef] [PubMed]
39. Joshi, D.C.; Sharma, A.; Prasad, S.; Singh, K.; Kumar, M.; Sherawat, K.; Tuli, H.S.; Gupta, M. Novel therapeutic agents in clinical trials: Emerging approaches in cancer therapy. *Discov. Oncol.* **2024**, *15*, 342. [CrossRef]

life

MDPI

Article

Variceal Upper Gastrointestinal Bleeding: A Retrospective Cohort of 98 Cases, Historical Comparison, and Updated Management Algorithm

Laurențiu Augustus Barbu [1], Liliana Cercelaru [2], Ionică-Daniel Vîlcea [3], Valeriu Șurlin [3], Stelian-Stefaniță Mogoantă [3], Tiberiu Stefăniță Țenea Cojan [1], Nicolae-Dragoș Mărgăritescu [3,*], Ana-Maria Țenea Cojan [4], Valentina Căluianu [1], Daniela Marinescu [3], Gabriel Florin Răzvan Mogoș [1] and Liviu Vasile [3]

[1] Department of Surgery, Railway Clinical Hospital Craiova, University of Medicine and Pharmacy of Craiova, 2 Petru Rares Street, 200349 Craiova, Romania; laurentiu.barbu@umfcv.ro (L.A.B.); tiberiu.tenea@umfcv.ro (T.S.Ț.C.); valentina.andronache@yahoo.com (V.C.); gabriel.mogos@umfcv.ro (G.F.R.M.)

[2] Department of Embryology and Anatomy, University of Medicine and Pharmacy of Craiova, 200349 Craiova, Romania; liliana.cercelaru@umfcv.ro

[3] Department of Surgery, Emergency County Hospital, University of Medicine and Pharmacy of Craiova, 2 Petru Rares Street, 200349 Craiova, Romania; ionica.vilcea@umfcv.ro (I.-D.V.); vsurlin@gmail.com (V.Ș.); ssmogo@yahoo.com (S.-S.M.); dtmarinescu@yahoo.com (D.M.); vliviu777@yahoo.com (L.V.)

[4] Faculty of Medicine, University of Medicine and Pharmacy of Craiova, 200349 Craiova, Romania; anamariatenea0324@gmail.com

* Correspondence: dmargaritescu@yahoo.com; Tel.: +40-723-271-941

Abstract: Background: Variceal upper gastrointestinal bleeding (VUGIB) remains a major cause of short-term mortality in cirrhosis despite advances in endoscopic and pharmacological therapy. Prognostic factors and outcomes were evaluated in a historical cohort, and a guideline-aligned management algorithm is proposed. **Methods**: We conducted a retrospective study of 98 consecutive adults admitted with VUGIB to a tertiary surgical center in Romania (2009–2014). Demographics, etiology, admission hemoglobin (Hb), timing of presentation, endoscopic and surgical management, and outcomes were recorded. Survival was analyzed using Kaplan–Meier with log-rank tests; associations were tested with chi-square and *t*-tests; predictors of mortality were assessed with logistic regression. Receiver operating characteristic (ROC) curve analysis was used to evaluate the discriminatory ability of hemoglobin for in-hospital mortality. **Results**: Mean age was 57.8 ± 11.7 years; 60.2% were male. Cirrhosis etiology was alcoholic in 73%, viral in 18%, and metabolic in 9%. Endoscopy occurred within 48 h in 62% of patients, but only 4% underwent the procedure within 8 h. Overall mortality was 17.3%. Kaplan–Meier analysis showed no survival difference between alcoholic and viral cirrhosis (log-rank $p = 0.39$), but survival was markedly lower with Hb < 8 g/dL ($p < 0.001$). Admission delay was prognostic: >24 h was associated with worse survival ($p < 0.05$). On multivariable analysis (reference 1–2 days), admission at 3–4 days (OR 35.3, 95% CI 1.6–786, $p = 0.024$), >4 days (OR 71.0, 95% CI 2.16–2337, $p = 0.017$), and <6 h (OR 22.4, 95% CI 1.25–399.7, $p = 0.035$) independently predicted death. Admission Hb predicted mortality with an AUC of 0.79; the optimal cut-off was 4.3 g/dL (sensitivity 57%, specificity 95%). Limited use of pre-emptive TIPS likely contributed to outcomes. **Conclusions**: In this historical cohort, mortality from VUGIB was driven mainly by bleeding severity and admission delay, rather than by cirrhosis etiology. The study provides a historical benchmark for Eastern Europe, highlights gaps in adherence to contemporary standards, and supports restrictive transfusion, early vasoactive therapy, antibiotics, urgent endoscopy, and pre-emptive TIPS. The retrospective single-center design and limited therapies available during the study period remain important limitations.

https://doi.org/10.3390/life15101626

Keywords: variceal upper gastrointestinal bleeding; cirrhosis; admission delay; hemoglobin; Kaplan–Meier; restrictive transfusion; endoscopic band ligation; pre-emptive TIPS; portal hypertension; prognosis

1. Introduction

Upper gastrointestinal bleeding (UGIB) remains one of the most frequent and life-threatening emergencies encountered in gastroenterology and surgery. Despite significant advances in diagnosis and treatment, UGIB continues to be associated with considerable morbidity and mortality, with reported rates ranging from 7% to 10% in large international cohorts [1]. In Romania and many Eastern European countries, the burden of UGIB is particularly high due to the prevalence of alcohol-related liver disease and viral hepatitis, both of which are predisposed to variceal hemorrhage [2].

Variceal bleeding is the most severe form of UGIB, typically occurring in patients with advanced cirrhosis and portal hypertension. Approximately 50% of cirrhotic patients develop esophageal varices during the course of their disease, with a third of these experiencing at least one episode of variceal bleeding [3]. Mortality during the first episode remains high, ranging from 15% to 25%, largely due to hemodynamic instability, comorbidities, and the risk of early rebleeding [4]. Several prognostic factors have been identified, including advanced age, low hemoglobin at admission, hemodynamic shock, and delayed access to hospital care [5].

Current international guidelines emphasize that patients with suspected variceal upper gastrointestinal bleeding should receive vasoactive drugs at presentation, be managed with a restrictive transfusion policy, and undergo endoscopic treatment within 12 h after stabilization [6]. Nevertheless, observational studies continue to show delays in hospital referral and heterogeneity in treatment approaches, factors that may adversely influence prognosis [7].

The objective of this study was to identify prognostic factors for in-hospital mortality and to propose a management algorithm aligned with current international guidelines. The analysis focused on demographic and clinical characteristics to explore predictors of in-hospital mortality through multivariate modeling, the prognostic significance of admission hemoglobin using ROC curve analysis, and the interplay between anemia severity and admission delay. In addition, by contrasting our findings with previously published cohorts, we provide a management framework that reflects current international guideline recommendations [6,7].

2. Materials and Methods

2.1. Study Design and Setting

This retrospective observational cohort included 98 adult patients with variceal upper gastrointestinal bleeding admitted to the First Surgical Clinic of the Emergency County Clinical Hospital of Craiova, Romania, between 1 January 2009 and 31 December 2014.

2.2. Inclusion and Exclusion Criteria

Inclusion criteria were patients aged ≥18 years with a confirmed diagnosis of variceal UGIB, identified based on clinical presentation, laboratory data, and upper gastrointestinal endoscopy (UGIE). Exclusion criteria included non-variceal UGIB, lower gastrointestinal bleeding, incomplete medical records, and comorbidities significantly affecting the assessment of bleeding etiology (e.g., malignancies, hematological disorders).

2.3. Data Collection

For each patient, the following variables were recorded: demographics (age, sex, and place of residence—rural or urban); etiology of cirrhosis and relevant comorbidities (alcoholic, viral, or metabolic cirrhosis; chronic alcohol use; cardiovascular and gastrointestinal conditions, such as gastritis or peptic ulcer, as well as other significant medical disorders). Risk factors included chronic alcohol consumption, use of nonsteroidal anti-inflammatory drugs (NSAIDs), and anticoagulant therapy. Baseline laboratory parameters collected at admission comprised hemoglobin, hematocrit, platelet count, creatinine, urea, and other relevant values. Timing variables referred to the interval from the onset of bleeding to hospital admission, the time from admission to endoscopy, and the time from admission to surgery when applicable. Endoscopic findings were classified according to the lesions identified during upper gastrointestinal endoscopy. Therapeutic interventions were documented, including medical therapy (e.g., antisecretory drugs), endoscopic procedures (e.g., band ligation), and surgery where necessary. Finally, clinical outcomes were recorded, consisting of mortality, rebleeding episodes, and complications related to the administered therapies.

2.4. Endoscopic and Surgical Management

All patients underwent UGIE within 48 h of hospital admission according to ESGE guidelines. Endoscopic interventions included band ligation and sclerotherapy for variceal bleeding. Surgical interventions were performed in cases of failure of endoscopic treatment or recurrent bleeding, with trans-gastric ligation of esophageal varices being the most common surgical procedure.

Handling of Missing Data and Endoscopic Protocol

Cases with incomplete medical records were excluded from the analysis to avoid bias from missing data. No imputation methods were applied. All endoscopic procedures were performed according to the institutional protocol in place during 2009–2014, which was aligned with the then-current ESGE recommendations. Endoscopic evaluation and interventions (band ligation or sclerotherapy) were carried out by experienced endoscopists from the same surgical department, following a standardized approach.

2.5. Statistical Analysis

Descriptive statistics were used to report demographic and clinical characteristics as means $\pm$ standard deviation (SD) for continuous variables and frequencies (percentages) for categorical variables. Survival analysis was performed using Kaplan–Meier curves for categorical variables, and log-rank tests were used to compare survival distributions. Comparative analyses were performed with chi-square tests for categorical data and t-tests for continuous data. A p-value < 0.05 was considered statistically significant. Data were initially processed using Microsoft Excel 2016 (Microsoft Corp., Redmond, WA, USA) with XLSTAT 2022 (Addinsoft SARL, Paris, France). Statistical analyses were subsequently performed using SPSS version 25.0 (IBM Corp., Armonk, NY, USA).

2.6. Ethics Statement

This study was conducted in accordance with the Declaration of Helsinki and was approved by the Ethics Committee of the Emergency County Clinical Hospital (approval number 42408/9 September 2025). Informed consent for the use of medical data for research purposes was obtained in writing from all patients at the time of admission, in full compliance with ethical standards. For patients who subsequently died, informed consent had already been obtained at admission. All data were anonymized prior to analysis. Data analysis and manuscript submission were performed only after receiving this approval.

3. Results

The study cohort included 98 patients with variceal upper gastrointestinal bleeding. The majority were male (60.2%), with a mean age of 57.8 ± 11.7 years (Table 1). Most patients originated from rural areas (74.5%). Alcoholic cirrhosis was the leading etiology (73%), followed by viral (18%) and metabolic causes (9%). At admission, nearly half of the patients presented with Grade III bleeding severity (47%), while 16% were classified as Grade IV. Overall mortality was 17.3%.

Table 1. Baseline Characteristics of Patients with Variceal UGIB (n = 98).

Characteristic	Value
Total patients	98
Sex	Male 59 (60.2%), Female 39 (39.8%)
Mean age (years)	57.8 ± 11.7
Residence	Rural 73 (74.5%), Urban 25 (25.5%)
Etiology of cirrhosis	Alcoholic 72 (73%), Viral 18 (18%), Metabolic 8 (9%)
Severity grade (Hb)	Grade I: 10 (10%), Grade II: 26 (27%), Grade III: 46 (47%), Grade IV: 16 (16%)
Mortality	17 (17.3%)

In most patients, upper endoscopy was performed within 48 h of admission (61 cases, 62%). Only 4 patients (4%) underwent endoscopy within the first 8 h. A considerable proportion experienced delayed procedures: 24 patients (24%) between 3–4 days and 9 patients (9%) after more than 4 days (Table 2).

Table 2. Interval between hospital admission and endoscopy (EGD) in patients with variceal UGIB.

Interval	Cases (n)	Percentage (%)
<8 h	4	4%
≤48 h	61	62%
3–4 days	24	24%
>4 days	9	9%
Total	98	100%

Endoscopic evaluation confirmed that esophageal varices were the predominant source of upper gastrointestinal bleeding. A total of three patients required surgical intervention, all operated within the first 24 h. These cases underwent trans-gastric ligation of esogastric varices after failure of endoscopic and pharmacological therapy.

All patients received antisecretory medication during hospitalization. Combined therapy with both proton pump inhibitors (PPIs) and H2 receptor antagonists was the most frequently used regimen (51 cases, 52%). Monotherapy with PPIs was administered in 27 patients (28%), while 20 patients (20%) received only H2 receptor inhibitors (Table 3).

The majority of patients presented with a combination of hematemesis and melena (68 cases, 70%). Isolated hematemesis was reported in 18 patients (18%), while melena alone was observed in 12 patients (12%) (Table 4).

Table 3. Antisecretory therapy in patients with variceal UGIB (n = 98).

Therapy Type	Cases (n)	Percentage (%)
H2 receptor inhibitors	20	20%
Proton pump inhibitors	27	28%
Combined therapy	51	52%
Total	98	100%

Table 4. Clinical presentation in patients with variceal UGIB (n = 98).

Clinical Presentation	Cases (n)	Percentage (%)
Hematemesis	18	18%
Melena	12	12%
Hematemesis + Melena	68	70%
Total	98	100%

At admission, bleeding had already stopped in the majority of patients (60 cases, 61%). Continuous active bleeding was present in 20 patients (20%), while 18 patients (18%) presented with recurrent episodes (Table 5).

Table 5. Evolution of bleeding in patients with variceal UGIB (n = 98).

Form of Bleeding	Cases (n)	Percentage (%)
Stopped	60	61%
Continuous	20	20%
Recurrent	18	18%
Total	98	100%

Regarding past medical history, the most frequent associated condition was chronic alcohol use, reported in 57% of patients. Cardiovascular comorbidities were found in 19% of cases, while gastrointestinal conditions such as gastritis and peptic ulcer were reported in 9% each. Pulmonary disorders were noted in 5% of patients, and osteoarticular conditions were rare (1%) (Figure 1).

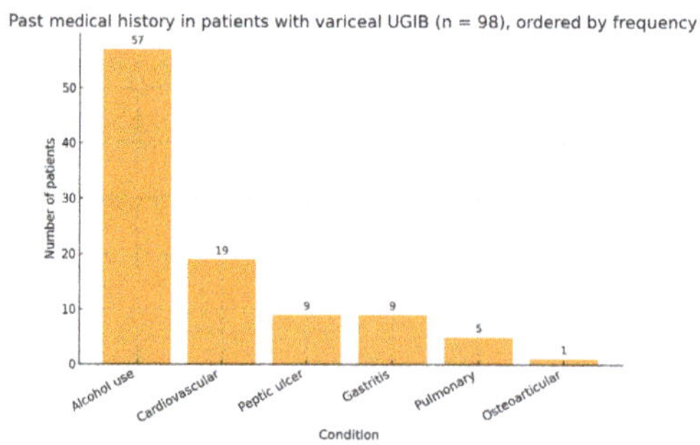

Figure 1. Past medical history in patients with variceal UGIB (n = 98).

Kaplan–Meier survival curves showed no significant survival difference between alcoholic and viral cirrhosis (Figure 2). In contrast, survival was significantly lower in patients admitted with Hb < 8 g/dL (Figure 3) and in those admitted more than 24 h after bleeding onset (Figure 4).

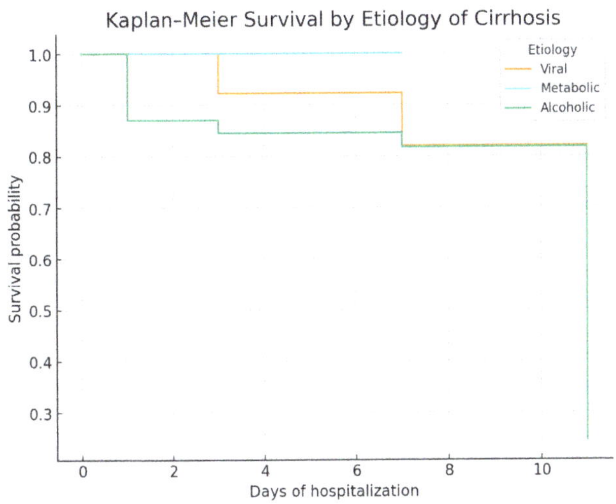

Figure 2. Kaplan–Meier survival curves stratified by the etiology of cirrhosis (alcoholic, viral, metabolic). Survival probability did not differ significantly between alcoholic and viral cirrhosis (log-rank $p = 0.39$). The metabolic subgroup was underrepresented and not suitable for meaningful comparison.

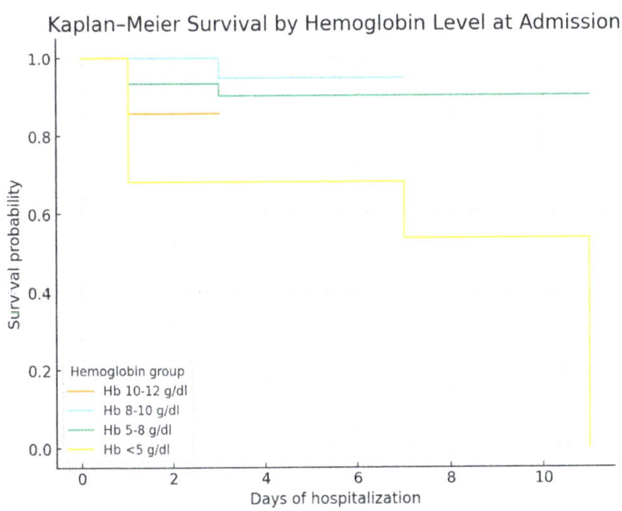

Figure 3. Kaplan–Meier survival by hemoglobin level at admission. Groups: <5 g/dL (n = 16), 5–8 g/dL (n = 46), 8–10 g/dL (n = 26), 10–12 g/dL (n = 10). Survival differed significantly across groups (log-rank $p < 0.001$). Total deaths: 17/98.

Kaplan–Meier survival analysis stratified by severity grade (Figure 5) showed a clear prognostic gradient: patients with Grade III (Hb 5–8 g/dL) and Grade IV (Hb < 5 g/dL) had markedly lower survival compared with Grade I–II (Hb $\geq$ 8 g/dL; log-rank $p < 0.001$). These findings were consistent with Chi-square analysis, which also demonstrated that variceal UGIB grade, admission delay, and length of hospital stay were significantly associated with mortality, while cirrhosis etiology was not.

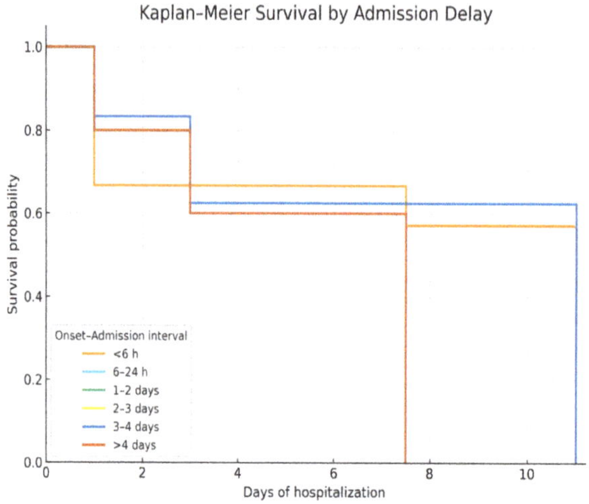

Figure 4. Kaplan–Meier survival curves stratified by admission delay (<6 h, 6–24 h, 1–2 days, 2–3 days, >3 days). Patients admitted more than 24 h after the onset of bleeding had significantly worse survival compared with those admitted earlier (log-rank $p < 0.05$).

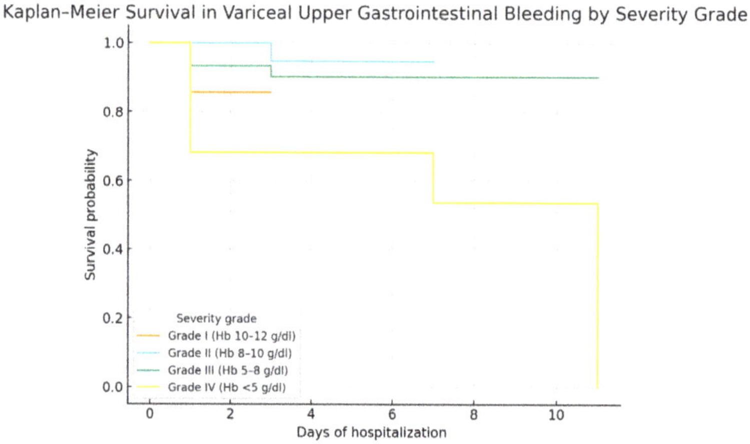

Figure 5. Kaplan–Meier survival curves stratified by severity grade of variceal upper gastrointestinal bleeding (Grade I–IV, defined by hemoglobin level at admission). Survival probability was significantly lower in patients with Grade III (Hb 5–8 g/dL) and Grade IV (Hb < 5 g/dL) compared with those in Grade I–II (Hb $\geq$ 8 g/dL; log-rank $p < 0.001$).

The final regression model showed a good fit (McFadden's $R^2 = 0.56$; AIC = 65.6; N = 98, deaths = 17). Multivariate logistic regression (Table 6) showed that interval admission delay was a significant predictor of mortality. Compared with patients admitted after 1–2 days, those admitted very early (<6 h) had higher odds of death (OR 22.4, 95% CI 1.25–399.7, $p = 0.035$). Similarly, delayed admission of 3–4 days (OR 35.3, 95% CI 1.59–786.1, $p = 0.024$) or more than 4 days (OR 71.0, 95% CI 2.16–2337.1, $p = 0.017$) was strongly associated with increased mortality. In contrast, etiology, age group, and variceal bleeding grade were not significantly associated with outcome.

Table 6. Multivariate logistic regression analysis of predictors of mortality in patients with variceal upper gastrointestinal bleeding (UGIB). Odds ratios (ORs) with 95% confidence intervals (CIs) and *p*-values are shown.

Variable (Reference)	Category	OR	95% CI	*p*-Value
Interval admission delay (ref: 1–2 days)	<6 h	22.4	1.25–399.7	**0.035**
	6–24 h	5.1	0.37–70.8	**0.220**
	3–4 days	35.3	1.59–786.1	**0.024**
	>4 days	71.0	2.16–2337.1	**0.017**
Etiology (ref: Other)	Alcoholic	1.4	0.35–5.4	**0.640**
Age group (ref: 31–40 year)	41–50 y	1.9	0.13–28.5	**0.620**
	51–60 y	0.8	0.05–13.5	**0.870**
	61–70 y	2.3	0.18–29.8	**0.520**
	>70 y	1.6	0.09–27.9	**0.740**
Variceal UGIB grade **(ref: 10–12)**	5–8	0.4	0.02–8.3	**0.550**
	8–10	0.3	0.01–6.7	**0.450**
	<5	2.8	0.15–51.8	**0.490**

In the univariate analysis, admission delay ≥3 days was likewise significantly associated with mortality (OR 6.82, 95% CI 1.87–24.9, $p = 0.004$), while admission delay >24 h alone was not (OR 0.88, $p = 0.805$) (Table 7).

Table 7. Univariate logistic regression analysis of mortality predictors.

Variable	OR	95% CI	*p*-Value
Admission delay >24 h vs. ≤24 h	0.88	0.30–2.53	**0.805**
Admission delay ≥3 days vs. ≤2 days	6.82	1.87–24.9	**0.004**

Mortality was highest in patients with Hb < 5 g/dL and in those admitted after >4 days or within 6 h of bleeding onset (Table 8).

Table 8. Cross-tabulation of mortality by VUGIB grade and admission delay.

Variable	Category	Survivors n (%)	Deaths n (%)	Total
VUGIB grade (Hb)	<5 g/dL	5 (31.3%)	11 (68.7%)	16
	5–8 g/dL	42 (91.3%)	4 (8.7%)	46
	8–10 g/dL	25 (96.2%)	1 (3.8%)	26
	10–12 g/dL	9 (90.0%)	1 (10.0%)	10
Admission delay	<6 h	6 (40.0%)	9 (60.0%)	15
	6–24 h	39 (97.5%)	1 (2.5%)	40
	1–2 days	30 (96.8%)	1 (3.2%)	31
	3–4 days	4 (57.1%)	3 (42.9%)	7
	>4 days	2 (40.0%)	3 (60.0%)	5
Total		81 (82.7%)	17 (17.3%)	98

The discriminative ability of hemoglobin levels at admission for predicting mortality was assessed using ROC curve analysis (Figure 6). Hemoglobin showed good predictive performance with an AUC of 0.79 (95% CI 0.68–0.89, $p < 0.01$). The optimal cut-off identified by the Youden index was 4.3 g/dL, providing a sensitivity of 57% and a specificity of 95% for mortality prediction.

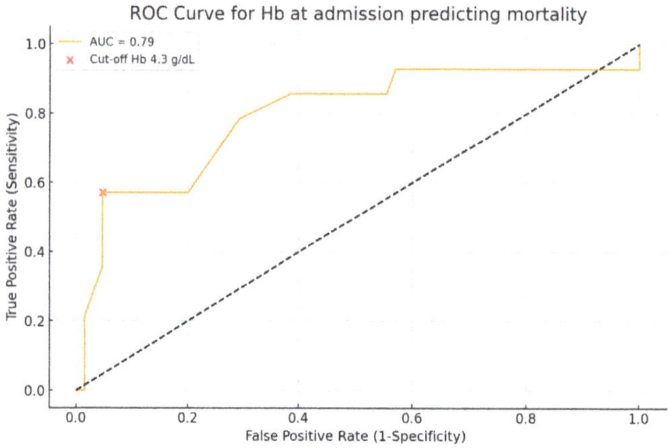

Figure 6. ROC curve of admission hemoglobin predicting in-hospital mortality (AUC = 0.79; optimal cut-off = 4.3 g/dL).

Patients admitted ≥3 days after bleeding onset had a significantly higher risk of mortality compared with those admitted within ≤2 days (50% vs. 12.8%). This corresponded to a relative risk of 3.9 and an odds ratio of 6.8 (95% CI 1.9–24.9, $p = 0.0056$) (Table 9).

Table 9. Risk estimates for admission delay ≥3 days vs. ≤2 days.

Comparison	Risk in Exposed	Risk in Unexposed	Relative Risk (RR)	Odds Ratio (OR)	95% CI (Approx.)	*p*-Value (Fisher)
Admission delay ≥3 days vs. ≤2 days	50% (6/12)	12.8% (11/86)	3.91	6.82	1.9–24.9	**0.0056**

Mortality was strongly influenced by both admission delay and hemoglobin level (Table 10). Patients admitted within ≤2 days and with Hb ≥ 8 g/dL had excellent survival (>95%), whereas those with delayed admission (≥3 days) and severe anemia (Hb < 8 g/dL) experienced the highest mortality (>70%). Early admission appeared to attenuate the adverse impact of low hemoglobin.

Table 10. Mortality stratified by admission delay and hemoglobin.

Group	Survivors n (%)	Deaths n (%)
≤2 days + Hb ≥ 8 g/dL	High survival (≈95%)	Very few deaths (≈5%)
≤2 days + Hb < 8 g/dL	Survival ~80%	Mortality ~20%
≥3 days + Hb ≥ 8 g/dL	Survival drops	Mortality ~40%
≥3 days + Hb < 8 g/dL	Very poor survival	Mortality > 70%

Mortality was stratified by cirrhosis etiology and hemoglobin level (Table 11). In alcoholic cirrhosis, patients with Hb < 8 g/dL had markedly higher mortality (~31%) compared with those with Hb ≥ 8 g/dL (~9%). In contrast, non-alcoholic patients showed overall lower mortality, with only ~13% deaths in the low hemoglobin group and none in the high hemoglobin group.

Table 11. Mortality stratified by etiology and hemoglobin.

Group	Survivors n (%)	Deaths n (%)	Total
Non-alcoholic + Hb ≥ 8 g/dL	100% survival	0% mortality	9
Non-alcoholic + Hb < 8 g/dL	~87% survival	~13% mortality	15
Alcoholic + Hb ≥ 8 g/dL	~91% survival	~9% mortality	23
Alcoholic + Hb < 8 g/dL	~69% survival	~31% mortality	32

4. Discussion

In this retrospective cohort of 98 patients admitted for variceal upper gastrointestinal bleeding between 2009 and 2014, we observed outcomes that are consistent with the historical burden of this condition. Despite advances in diagnosis and endoscopic therapy, VUGIB continues to carry substantial short-term mortality, in line with the reported 6-week mortality of 15–20% in international cohorts [1]. Our findings underscore the importance of early recognition, timely admission, and the adoption of evidence-based therapeutic strategies.

Our study confirms that mortality in VUGIB is driven primarily by the severity of hemorrhage at admission and by delays in hospital presentation, rather than by the underlying etiology of cirrhosis. In our cohort, alcoholic cirrhosis was predominant, in accordance with regional epidemiology and prior Eastern European studies, while viral and metabolic etiologies were less frequent. The predominance of alcoholic cirrhosis may reflect the regional patterns of alcohol consumption and the associated liver disease burden. These findings highlight the need for rapid intervention and appropriate risk stratification regardless of cirrhosis etiology.

4.1. Prognostic Factors and Comparison with Literature

Our study confirms that mortality in variceal upper gastrointestinal bleeding (UGIB) is determined mainly by hemorrhage severity at admission and delays in hospital presentation, rather than by cirrhosis etiology. Alcoholic cirrhosis predominated in our cohort (73%), consistent with Romanian and international data [8,9], while esophageal varices were the leading bleeding source [10]. The overall mortality of 17.3% aligns with European reports (15–22%) [11].

Hemoglobin on admission was a strong prognostic marker: patients with Hb < 5 g/dL had the poorest survival, consistent with the concept that profound anemia reflects uncontrolled bleeding and limited reserve. ROC curve analysis confirmed its discriminative value (AUC 0.79), though interpretation should consider other clinical factors [12,13]. Admission delay was also critical: both late presentation (>48–72 h) and very early admission (<6 h) were linked to higher mortality, reflecting the combined risks of uncontrolled bleeding and delayed intervention [14].

The underuse of pre-emptive TIPS in our historical cohort may have contributed to higher mortality. Prospective trials, notably García-Pagán et al., demonstrated survival benefit from early TIPS in Child–Pugh B/C patients [13], supporting current Baveno VII consensus, which emphasizes immediate vasoactive therapy, prophylactic antibiotics, and endoscopy within 12 h [15].

Taken together, our findings highlight hemoglobin levels and admission delay as key prognostic factors, reinforcing the importance of rapid referral, early endoscopy, and optimized transfusion strategies. These elements should be integrated into risk stratification and management algorithms to improve outcomes in variceal UGIB [13–19].

4.2. Etiology and Risk Stratification

In our cohort, patients admitted more than 24 h after bleeding onset had significantly worse outcomes, underscoring the importance of rapid referral and early specialized care. Previous studies consistently show that postponing admission or delaying therapeutic endoscopy increases mortality due to uncontrolled bleeding and early rebleeding [20–22]. Current guidelines, including ESGE and Baveno VII, recommend endoscopy within 12 h of stabilization, and our results support this timeframe [15,23].

Bleeding severity was another strong predictor: profound anemia (Hb < 8 g/dL, especially <5 g/dL) was closely linked to mortality, consistent with evidence that hemoglobin reflects both blood loss and prognosis [24–27]. Restrictive transfusion strategies (Hb 7–9 g/dL) have been shown to reduce rebleeding and death, with the pivotal trial by Villanueva et al. confirming improved survival and bleeding control [12,28,29].

Anemia severity and admission delay often coexisted, with late presenters showing greater hemodynamic instability, deeper anemia, and organ dysfunction, all contributing to poor outcomes [20,21,27]. These findings emphasize the need for efficient prehospital triage, early vasoactive therapy, restrictive but timely transfusion, and urgent endoscopic intervention.

In summary, our findings identify delayed presentation and severe anemia at admission as critical predictors of mortality in variceal bleeding, reinforcing the importance of rapid referral systems and adherence to guideline-based transfusion and endoscopic strategies [15,23,28].

4.3. Impact of Admission Delay and Initial Severity

Admission delay beyond 24 h was strongly associated with reduced survival, emphasizing the importance of timely referral and early intervention in variceal upper gastrointestinal bleeding (VUGIB). Prior studies have shown that postponing hospital admission or endoscopic therapy significantly increases mortality through uncontrolled hemorrhage and early rebleeding [20–22]. Current ESGE and Baveno VII recommendations advise endoscopy within 12 h of stabilization, and our findings support this threshold [15,23].

Bleeding severity was another major prognostic factor. Severe anemia (Hb < 8 g/dL), particularly <5 g/dL, was independently linked to mortality, consistent with evidence that low hemoglobin reflects both bleeding severity and poor prognosis [24,25,27]. Randomized trials and meta-analyses confirm that a restrictive transfusion strategy (Hb 7–9 g/dL) lowers rebleeding and mortality compared with liberal thresholds [28,29], as demonstrated in the pivotal trial by Villanueva et al. [12].

Notably, admission delay and anemia severity are interrelated, with late presenters more likely to exhibit hemodynamic instability, profound anemia, and multi-organ dysfunction, thereby amplifying risk [20,21,27]. This interplay underscores the need for coordinated prehospital triage, early vasoactive therapy, restrictive transfusion, and urgent endoscopy.

Overall, our findings confirm that delayed admission and severe anemia are key predictors of mortality in VUGIB, consistent with international guidelines [15,23,28], and highlight opportunities to improve survival through optimized referral systems and adherence to restrictive transfusion policies.

4.4. Therapeutic Strategies and Historical Context

During the study period (2009–2014), endoscopic therapy—mainly band ligation and, less frequently, sclerotherapy—was the cornerstone of treatment for variceal upper gastrointestinal bleeding in our center. Pharmacological therapy with vasoactive agents was inconsistently administered, and pre-emptive TIPS was rarely available. These limitations, reflecting both therapeutic standards of the time and resource constraints typical of many Eastern European centers, likely contributed to the suboptimal survival compared with contemporary series from Western Europe and North America [30,31].

Since then, therapeutic strategies have evolved substantially. Current consensus emphasizes a combined approach: immediate initiation of vasoactive therapy, routine administration of broad-spectrum antibiotics, and endoscopic band ligation within 12 h of admission [32]. Endoscopic sclerotherapy, once common, has been largely abandoned in favor of band ligation due to its superior safety profile [32].

A major advance has been the use of pre-emptive TIPS in selected high-risk patients (Child–Pugh C < 14 or Child–Pugh B > 7 with active bleeding). Randomized trials demonstrated that early TIPS reduces treatment failure and improves survival [33], although access remains limited in many low- and middle-income countries [34].

Our findings underscore the gap between available therapies during the study period and current evidence-based standards. Patients were treated mainly with conventional endoscopic procedures, while interventions now considered essential—such as early vasoactive therapy, prophylactic antibiotics, and pre-emptive TIPS—were not systematically applied. This therapeutic gap likely contributed to the higher mortality observed, reinforcing that adherence to guideline-based protocols can significantly improve prognosis in acute variceal bleeding [32,33]. It should be emphasized that our cohort reflects a historical period (2009–2014), when current standards of care such as early vasoactive therapy, routine prophylactic antibiotics, restrictive transfusion, and pre-emptive TIPS were not consistently applied. Therefore, the outcomes observed in our series should not be interpreted as representative of present-day management but rather as a benchmark of real-world practice in Eastern Europe at that time. This historical perspective also highlights the progress achieved over the last decade and underscores the survival gains expected with contemporary evidence-based strategies.

4.5. Strategies for the Primary Prevention of Variceal Bleeding

Primary prevention of variceal hemorrhage remains central to portal hypertension management. Current consensus recommends non-selective beta-blockers (NSBBs) as first-line therapy, with carvedilol increasingly favored due to its greater reduction in portal pressure compared with propranolol or nadolol [15]. Endoscopic variceal ligation (EVL) is an effective alternative when NSBBs are contraindicated or not tolerated [35]. Recent randomized data, including the CAVARLY trial, indicate that combining carvedilol with EVL may further reduce first bleeding events and one-year mortality [36]. For gastric varices, balloon-occluded retrograde transvenous obliteration (BRTO) shows promise, although current evidence is limited [37]. Overall, NSBBs remain the backbone of primary prophylaxis, with combination strategies considered in selected high-risk patients.

4.6. Secondary Prophylaxis of Variceal Hemorrhage

For secondary prevention of variceal hemorrhage, current consensus supports combining non-selective beta-blockers (NSBBs) with endoscopic variceal ligation (EVL), which is more effective than either therapy alone in reducing rebleeding [15,27,38,39]. EVL monotherapy is reserved for patients intolerant to NSBBs. Among beta-blockers, carvedilol is increasingly used due to its stronger effect on portal pressure, although propranolol and nadolol remain widely prescribed [15,35]. In gastric varices, emerging evidence suggests that adding NSBBs to endoscopic therapy may lower rebleeding risk, though survival benefit is less clear [37]. In high-risk patients or those with recurrent bleeding despite optimized prophylaxis, early trans-jugular intrahepatic portosystemic shunt (TIPS) offers an effective rescue option [27,35].

4.7. Endoscopic Therapy

Endoscopic variceal ligation has become the dominant endoscopic method for secondary prevention of variceal hemorrhage, progressively replacing endoscopic sclerotherapy (EIS). Evidence from meta-analyses demonstrates that EVL achieves superior variceal eradication and is associated with lower risks of rebleeding and adverse events compared with EIS [40]. Major consensus statements, including Baveno VII and the most recent AASLD guidance, recommend EVL in combination with nonselective beta-blockers (NSBBs) as the preferred strategy for secondary prophylaxis, as this dual approach lowers both rebleeding and mortality rates more effectively than either modality alone [15,41,42]. By contrast, combining EVL with sclerotherapy has not been shown to confer additional benefit and may increase complications, so it is not advised [25]. In the context of gastric varices, endoscopic cyanoacrylate injection remains the treatment of choice, with EVL considered only in selected situations [15]. Taken together, current data reinforce the role of EVL as the foundation of endoscopic management of variceal bleeding [43].

4.8. Efficacy and Limitations

Endoscopic variceal ligation (EVL) remains the primary endoscopic therapy for esophageal variceal hemorrhage, achieving initial hemostasis in 85–95% of cases [27,40]. Compared with sclerotherapy, EVL provides higher eradication rates, fewer recurrences, and fewer complications [40]. Because it does not address portal hypertension, recurrence is common unless combined with non-selective beta-blockers (NSBBs) [15]. Despite advances, rebleeding still occurs in 7–10% of patients within 6 weeks, and post-banding ulcer bleeding remains a relevant complication (2–10%) [44,45]. Current consensus supports EVL plus NSBBs as the most effective strategy for secondary prophylaxis, while combining EVL with sclerotherapy is discouraged due to excess adverse events [15,27,46]. For gastric varices, cyanoacrylate injection is preferred, with early trans-jugular intrahepatic portosystemic shunt (TIPS) considered in selected high-risk cases [1,27,47,48].

4.9. Coagulation Management and Adjunctive Therapies

Traditionally, cirrhosis was viewed as a hypo-coagulable state, with variceal hemorrhage attributed to impaired clotting factor synthesis and thrombocytopenia. More recent data support the concept of "rebalanced hemostasis," in which decreased procoagulant activity is offset by reduced anticoagulant function and endothelial dysfunction, placing patients at risk for both bleeding and thrombosis, particularly portal vein thrombosis [30,32,42].

These insights have reshaped transfusion strategies. Fresh frozen plasma and platelet concentrates were previously given prophylactically for elevated INR or low platelet counts, but evidence shows that INR is not a reliable predictor of bleeding and that indiscriminate transfusion may increase portal pressure and rebleeding risk [30]. Current guidelines therefore recommend restricting transfusion to cases of severe thrombocytopenia (<50,000/μL) or uncontrolled hemorrhage [33,49].

Viscoelastic assays such as thrombo-elastography (TEG) and rotational thromboelastometry (ROTEM) provide real-time assessment of clot dynamics, offering a more accurate measure of hemostasis than conventional assays. Their use can reduce unnecessary transfusions without increasing bleeding complications in cirrhotic patients undergoing invasive procedures [34].

Adjunctive pharmacologic measures remain crucial. Prophylactic antibiotics are essential given the adverse impact of bacterial infections on outcomes [50], while proton pump inhibitors are often used peri-endoscopically to minimize post-procedural ulcer risk. Antifibrinolytics have been explored but lack sufficient evidence for routine use.

In summary, coagulation management in cirrhosis should balance bleeding and thrombosis risk through restrictive transfusion policies, integration of viscoelastic testing, and targeted adjunctive therapies as part of evidence-based variceal bleeding care.

4.10. Clinical Implications and Proposal for an Updated Algorithm

The findings of our study have important clinical implications. Despite therapeutic advances, outcomes in variceal upper gastrointestinal bleeding (VUGIB) remain largely determined by admission delay and bleeding severity. This underscores the need for streamlined pathways that enable early recognition, rapid referral, and strict adherence to evidence-based protocols.

Recent consensus statements, including ESGE (2022), Baveno VII (2022), and AEEH (2025), provide standardized frameworks for acute variceal bleeding management. Integrating these recommendations with our observations, we propose a revised diagnostic and therapeutic algorithm that reflects contemporary standards while addressing gaps identified in routine practice [15,51]:

1. Early triage and resuscitation with restrictive transfusion—Patients should be rapidly identified at first contact and transferred to specialized centers whenever possible. Hemodynamic stabilization must be prioritized, with a restrictive transfusion strategy (target Hb 7–9 g/dL), as liberal transfusion has been associated with increased portal pressure and higher risk of rebleeding [15,23].
2. Prompt initiation of vasoactive drugs and antibiotics—Vasoactive agents (terlipressin, somatostatin, or octreotide) should be started immediately upon suspicion of variceal bleeding, before endoscopic confirmation, and continued for 2–5 days. In parallel, broad-spectrum antibiotics are mandatory to reduce the incidence of bacterial infections, which can precipitate rebleeding and worsen survival [42,51].
3. Early endoscopy within 12 h—Endoscopic band ligation is the first-line treatment for esophageal varices and should be performed within 12 h of admission, once the patient is stabilized. Sclerotherapy may be considered only if band ligation is not feasible. For gastric varices, cyanoacrylate injection is recommended [42,51–53].
4. Pre-emptive TIPS in high-risk patients—In patients with advanced liver disease (Child–Pugh C < 14 points or Child–Pugh B > 7 with active bleeding), early TIPS placement within 72 h has been shown to reduce treatment failure and improve survival [42,53]. The adoption of this strategy represents a paradigm shift compared to the period covered by our study, when TIPS was rarely available.
5. Secondary prophylaxis with non-selective beta-blockers (NSBBs) plus endoscopic surveillance—To prevent recurrent bleeding, combination therapy with NSBBs (e.g., propranolol or carvedilol) and repeated band ligation is recommended. This approach reduces both rebleeding rates and overall mortality [12,42].

The implementation of such an algorithm is expected to improve both short- and long-term outcomes, particularly in healthcare settings where gaps between guideline recommendations and real-world practice remain (Figure 7). The diagnostic and therapeutic algorithm proposed here does not aim to introduce novel concepts beyond established international guidelines. Its main value lies in contextualizing these recommendations for Eastern European healthcare systems, where resources may be limited and access to advanced interventions such as pre-emptive TIPS remains restricted. By integrating evidence-based strategies into a practical framework adapted to local realities, the algorithm provides clinicians with a structured approach to patient management in similar settings. Moreover, it illustrates the progress achieved since the 2009–2014 study period and highlights the contrast between historical practices and current standards of care.

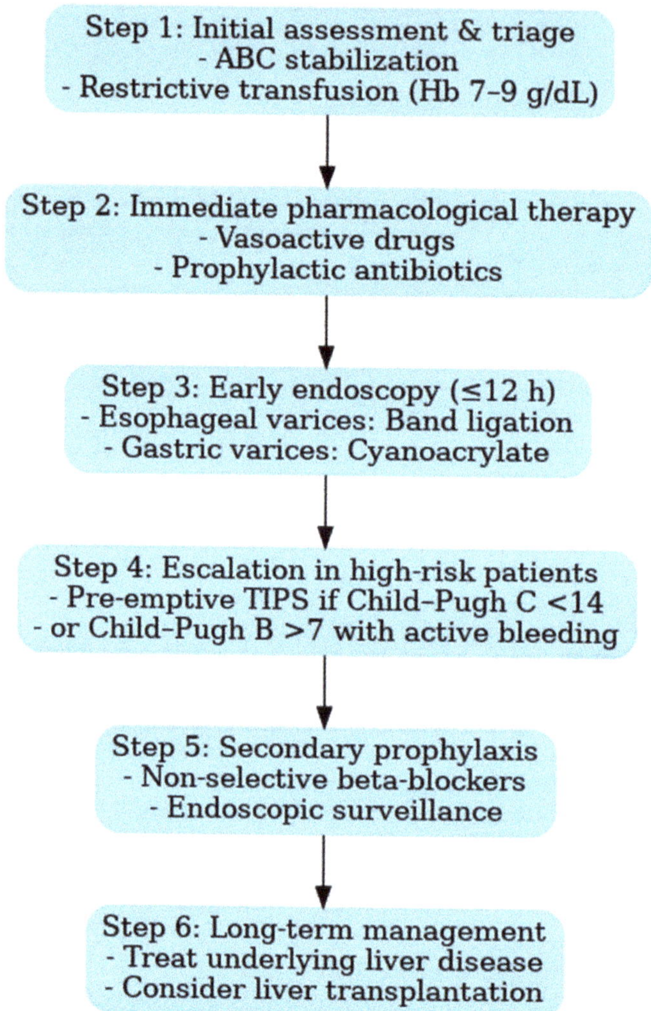

Figure 7. Proposed management algorithm for variceal upper gastrointestinal bleeding, integrating current guideline recommendations. Legend: ABC = Airway, Breathing, Circulation; TIPS = Transjugular Intrahepatic Portosystemic Shunt.

4.11. *Strengths and Limitations*

This study has notable strengths, including its status as one of the largest single-center retrospective cohorts of variceal upper gastrointestinal bleeding (VUGIB) from Eastern Europe, comprising 98 consecutive cases over a six-year period. The comprehensive collection of clinical, laboratory, and survival data enabled robust subgroup analyses, including risk stratification by etiology, hemoglobin levels at admission, and admission delay. Additionally, survival analysis using Kaplan–Meier curves provide valuable prognostic insights and establishes a historical benchmark for evaluating practice improvements. A further strength is the comparison of our findings with contemporary international guidelines, allowing for the development of an updated diagnostic and therapeutic algorithm applicable to both high-resource and resource-limited settings.

However, several limitations must be acknowledged. The retrospective design introduces potential biases related to data completeness and accuracy. As a retrospective study, it is susceptible to selection bias, reporting bias, and missing data, which can affect the reliability of the findings. Furthermore, the single-center nature of the study limits the generalizability of the findings to other healthcare systems, particularly in countries with different clinical settings and resources. As a tertiary surgical referral center, our hospital may also have received disproportionately severe cases, potentially inflating mortality rates compared with community hospitals. The single-center design, modest sample size, and retrospective methodology inherently constrain the external validity and generalizability of our findings. These limitations should be considered when interpreting the results.

Although relatively large for a single-center study in Eastern Europe, the sample size remains modest compared with multinational cohorts, limiting the statistical power of subgroup and regression analyses. The lack of standardized hemodynamic assessment (e.g., hepatic venous pressure gradient [HVPG]) precludes a precise characterization of portal hypertension severity, an increasingly important prognostic factor in cirrhosis. Additionally, systematic information on concomitant medications, including nonsteroidal anti-inflammatory drugs (NSAIDs), antiplatelet agents, beta-blockers, anticoagulants, and antiviral therapies, was not available, limiting our ability to assess their influence on bleeding risk and survival. Although comorbidities such as cardiovascular disease, diabetes, and renal dysfunction were documented, their independent prognostic impact was not evaluated. Moreover, data on alcohol abstinence and viral suppression were lacking, which limits the ability to contextualize outcomes based on etiology.

The incomplete information regarding the dose and duration of therapies, including vasoactive agents, antibiotics, and transfusions, reduces comparability with more contemporary cohorts. Importantly, during the study period (2009–2014), all patients were admitted and managed within the Surgical Department, in line with institutional protocols of that time. This organizational factor partly explains the limited use of vasoactive drugs, prophylactic antibiotics, and pre-emptive TIPS compared with current standards of care. An important limitation of our study is therefore the outdated timeframe (2009–2014). The cohort predates key advances in variceal bleeding management, including systematic use of vasoactive drugs at presentation, prophylactic antibiotics, restrictive transfusion strategies, and early pre-emptive TIPS in high-risk patients. Consequently, the direct clinical applicability of our findings to current practice is limited. However, this limitation also provides value: the data serve as a historical benchmark for Eastern Europe, allowing meaningful comparison with contemporary outcomes and illustrating the improvements achieved by guideline-based care.

Finally, the lack of long-term follow-up beyond hospitalization and six-week survival data prevented the evaluation of recurrent bleeding and long-term prognosis, which remains a critical aspect of VUGIB management. Taken together, the strengths and limitations of this study provide context for our findings and highlight the need for future multicenter prospective studies with standardized data collection, including detailed medication history, comorbidity assessment, and therapy protocols. Such studies should integrate validated risk scores (e.g., Child–Pugh, MELD), evaluate modern therapies such as early TIPS, and bridge the gap between guideline recommendations and real-world practice.

5. Conclusions

This study shows that variceal upper gastrointestinal bleeding (VUGIB) remains a major cause of morbidity and mortality, primarily influenced by bleeding severity at admission and delays in hospital presentation. Admission delay beyond 24 h and severe anemia are key prognostic factors. While alcoholic cirrhosis predominated in our cohort, etiology did not affect survival, highlighting the importance of timely intervention. Our findings support early vasoactive agents, restrictive transfusion, and urgent endoscopy. The underuse of pre-emptive TIPS indicates a gap in care. The proposed management algorithm aims to improve survival, and future studies are needed to refine prognostic models and optimize treatment strategies for VUGIB.

Author Contributions: Conceptualization, L.A.B. and N.-D.M.; writing—original draft, L.A.B. and T.S.Ț.C.; resources, V.C., L.C., L.V., S.-S.M., G.F.R.M., T.S.Ț.C. and V.Ș.; supervision, S.-S.M. and I.-D.V.; investigation, D.M., V.C., L.C., L.V., G.F.R.M., V.Ș. and I.-D.V.; writing—review, L.A.B., T.S.Ț.C. and G.F.R.M.; validation, L.V., S.-S.M. and N.-D.M.; software, V.C., A.-M.Ț.C., L.C. and I.-D.V.; visualization, D.M., V.C., G.F.R.M., L.C. and I.-D.V.; data curation, D.M., A.-M.Ț.C., T.S.Ț.C. and N.-D.M.; project administration, L.A.B. and V.Ș.; formal analysis, A.-M.Ț.C. and N.-D.M.; methodology, D.M., A.-M.Ț.C., L.V., S.-S.M. and V.Ș. All authors have read and agreed to the published version of the manuscript.

Funding: The article processing charges were funded by the University of Medicine and Pharmacy of Craiova, Romania.

Institutional Review Board Statement: The study was conducted in accordance with the Declaration of Helsinki and approved by the Ethical Committee of the Clinical Emergency County Hospital Craiova (no. 42408/9 September 2025).

Informed Consent Statement: Informed consent was obtained from the patient, whereby individual written informed consent was obtained, ensuring full compliance with ethical standards.

Data Availability Statement: The data presented in this study are available on request from the corresponding author. The data are not publicly available due to patient confidentiality.

Conflicts of Interest: The authors declare that there are no conflicts of interest.

Abbreviations

UGIB	Upper gastrointestinal bleeding
VUGIB	Variceal upper gastrointestinal bleeding
Hb	Hemoglobin
UGIE	Upper gastrointestinal endoscopy
ESGE	European Society of Gastrointestinal Endoscopy
TIPS	Trans-jugular intrahepatic portosystemic shunt
NSBB	Non-selective beta-blockers
EVL	Endoscopic variceal ligation
EIS	Endoscopic injection sclerotherapy
ROC	Receiver operating characteristic
AUC	Area under the curve
OR	Odds ratio
CI	Confidence interval

References

1. Almadi, M.A.; Almutairdi, A.; Alruzug, I.M.; Aldarsouny, T.A.; Semaan, T.; Aldaher, M.K.; AlMustafa, A.; Azzam, N.; Batwa, F.; Albawardy, B.; et al. Upper gastrointestinal bleeding: Causes and patient outcomes. *Saudi J. Gastroenterol.* **2021**, *27*, 20–27. [CrossRef]
2. Mertens, A.; Essing, T.; Kunstein, A.; Weigel, C.; Bode, J.; Roderburg, C.; Luedde, T.; Kandler, J.; Loosen, S.H. Acute Variceal Hemorrhage in Germany-A Nationwide Study of 65,357 Hospitalized Cases: Variceal Hemorrhage in Germany. *Can. J. Gastroenterol. Hepatol.* **2024**, *2024*, 5453294. [CrossRef]
3. Thörn, R.; Christensen, E.; Wixner, J.; Karling, P.; Werner, M. Survival after first diagnosis of oesophageal or gastric varices in a single centre in northern Sweden: A retrospective study. *Clin. Exp. Hepatol.* **2022**, *8*, 103–110. [CrossRef]

4. Tari, E.; Frim, L.; Stolcz, T.; Teutsch, B.; Veres, D.S.; Hegyi, P.; Erőss, B. At admission hemodynamic instability is associated with increased mortality and rebleeding rate in acute gastrointestinal bleeding: A systematic review and meta-analysis. *Ther. Adv. Gastroenterol.* **2023**, *16*, 17562848231190970. [CrossRef] [PubMed]
5. Lee, Y.R.; Park, S.Y.; Tak, W.Y. Treatment Outcomes and Prognostic Factors of Acute Variceal Bleeding in Patients with Hepatocellular Carcinoma. *Gut Liver* **2020**, *14*, 500–508. [CrossRef] [PubMed]
6. Orpen-Palmer, J.; Stanley, A.J. Update on the management of upper gastrointestinal bleeding. *BMJ Med.* **2022**, *1*, e000202. [CrossRef] [PubMed]
7. Nguyen, K.P.; Van Nguyen, X.; Doan, T.H. Impact of timing of endoscopy on clinical outcomes in cirrhotic patients with esophageal variceal bleeding: A monocentric retrospective study from Vietnam. *BMC Gastroenterol.* **2025**, *25*, 565. [CrossRef]
8. Matei, D.; Groza, I.; Furnea, B.; Puie, L.; Levi, C.; Chiru, A.; Cruciat, C.; Mester, G.; Vesa, S.C.; Tantau, M. Predictors of variceal or nonvariceal source of upper gastrointestinal bleeding. An etiology predictive score established and validated in a tertiary referral center. *J. Gastrointest. Liver Dis.* **2013**, *22*, 379–384.
9. Botianu, A.; Matei, D.; Tantau, M.; Acalovschi, M. Mortality and need of surgical treatment in acute upper gastrointestinal bleeding: A one year study in a tertiary center with a 24 hours/day-7 days/week endoscopy call. Has anything changed? *Chirurgia* **2013**, *108*, 312–318.
10. Holster, I.L.; Kuipers, E.J. Management of acute nonvariceal upper gastrointestinal bleeding: Current policies and future perspectives. *World J. Gastroenterol.* **2012**, *18*, 1202–1207. [CrossRef]
11. Alharbi, A.; Almadi, M.; Barkun, A.; Martel, M.; REASON Investigators. Predictors of a variceal source among patients presenting with upper gastrointestinal bleeding. *Can. J. Gastroenterol. Hepatol.* **2012**, *26*, 187–192. [CrossRef]
12. Villanueva, C.; Colomo, A.; Bosch, A.; Concepción, M.; Hernandez-Gea, V.; Aracil, C.; Graupera, I.; Poca, M.; Alvarez-Urturi, C.; Gordillo, J.; et al. Transfusion strategies for acute upper gastrointestinal bleeding. *N. Engl. J. Med.* **2013**, *368*, 11–21. [CrossRef]
13. García-Pagán, J.C.; Caca, K.; Bureau, C.; Laleman, W.; Appenrodt, B.; Luca, A.; Abraldes, J.G.; Nevens, F.; Vinel, J.P.; Mössner, J.; et al. Early TIPS (Transjugular Intrahepatic Portosystemic Shunt) Cooperative Study Group. Early use of TIPS in patients with cirrhosis and variceal bleeding. *N. Engl. J. Med.* **2010**, *362*, 2370–2379. [CrossRef]
14. Wong, Y.J.; Ho, W.L.D.; Abraldes, J.G. Pre-emptive TIPSS in Acute Variceal Bleeding: Current Status, Controversies, and Future Directions. *J. Clin. Transl. Hepatol.* **2022**, *10*, 1223–1228. [CrossRef] [PubMed]
15. de Franchis, R.; Bosch, J.; Garcia-Tsao, G.; Reiberger, T.; Ripoll, C.; on behalf of the Baveno VII Faculty. Baveno VII—Renewing consensus in portal hypertension. *J. Hepatol.* **2021**, *76*, 959–974. [CrossRef] [PubMed]
16. Zullo, A.; Soncini, M.; Bucci, C.; Marmo, R.; Gruppo Italiano per lo Studio dell'Emorragia Digestiva (GISED) (Appendix). Clinical outcomes in cirrhotics with variceal or nonvariceal gastrointestinal bleeding: A prospective, multicenter cohort study. *J. Gastroenterol. Hepatol.* **2021**, *36*, 3219–3223. [CrossRef] [PubMed]
17. Chalasani, N.; Kahi, C.; Francois, F.; Pinto, A.; Marathe, A.; Bini, E.J.; Pandya, P.; Sitaraman, S.; Shen, J. Improved patient survival after acute variceal bleeding: A multicenter, cohort study. *Am. J. Gastroenterol.* **2003**, *98*, 653–659. [CrossRef]
18. Reverter, E.; Tandon, P.; Augustin, S.; Turon, F.; Casu, S.; Bastiampillai, R.; Keough, A.; Llop, E.; González, A.; Seijo, S.; et al. A MELD-based model to determine risk of mortality among patients with acute variceal bleeding. *Gastroenterology* **2014**, *146*, 412–419.e3. [CrossRef]
19. Kulkarni, A.V.; Rabiee, A.; Mohanty, A. Management of Portal Hypertension. *J. Clin. Exp. Hepatol.* **2022**, *12*, 1184–1199. [CrossRef]
20. Lazăr, D.C.; Ursoniu, S.; Goldiş, A. Predictors of rebleeding and in-hospital mortality in patients with nonvariceal upper digestive bleeding. *World J. Clin. Cases* **2019**, *7*, 2687–2703. [CrossRef]
21. Xia, X.F.; Chiu, P.W.Y.; Tsoi, K.K.F.; Chan, F.K.L.; Sung, J.J.Y.; Lau, J.Y.W. The effect of off-hours hospital admission on mortality and clinical outcomes for patients with upper gastrointestinal hemorrhage: A systematic review and meta-analysis of 20 cohorts. *United Eur. Gastroenterol. J.* **2017**, *6*, 367–381. [CrossRef] [PubMed]
22. Barbu, L.A.; Vasile, L.; Cercelaru, L.; Şurlin, V.; Mogoantă, S.-S.; Mogoș, G.F.R.; Cojan, T.S.Ț.; Mărgăritescu, N.-D.; Buliman, A. Non-Variceal Upper Gastrointestinal Bleeding: A Retrospective Cohort of 364 Cases, Historical Comparison, and Updated Management Algorithm. *Life* **2025**, *15*, 1320. [CrossRef] [PubMed]
23. Gralnek, I.M.; Stanley, A.J.; Morris, A.J.; Camus, M.; Lau, J.; Lanas, A.; Laursen, S.B.; Radaelli, F.; Papanikolaou, I.S.; Gonçalves, T.C.; et al. Endoscopic diagnosis and management of nonvariceal upper gastrointestinal hemorrhage (NVUGIH): European Society of Gastrointestinal Endoscopy (ESGE) Guideline—Update 2021. *Endoscopy* **2021**, *53*, 300–332. [CrossRef]
24. Qamar, A.A.; Grace, N.D. Abnormal hematological indices in cirrhosis. *Can. J. Gastroenterol. Hepatol.* **2009**, *23*, 441–445. [CrossRef]
25. Marinescu, D.; Lazar, M.; Zaharie, S.; Comanescu, C.; Tudoran, C.; Bica, M.; Barbu, L. Upper Gastrointestinal Bleeding in Chronic Kidney Disease Patients. *Curr. Health Sci. J.* **2016**, *42*, 226–230.
26. Barbu, L.A.; Mărgăritescu, N.-D.; Cercelaru, L.; Caragea, D.-C.; Vîlcea, I.-D.; Şurlin, V.; Mogoantă, S.; Mogoș, G.F.R.; Vasile, L.; Cojan, T.Ș.Ț. Can Thrombosed Abdominal Aortic Dissecting Aneurysm Cause Mesenteric Artery Thrombosis and Ischemic Colitis?—A Case Report and a Review of Literature. *J. Clin. Med.* **2025**, *14*, 3092. [CrossRef]
27. Garcia-Tsao, G. Overview of Current Management of Portal Hypertension. *Gastroenterol. Hepatol.* **2021**, *17*, 40–42.

28. Teutsch, B.; Veres, D.S.; Pálinkás, D.; Simon, O.A.; Hegyi, P.; Erőss, B. Potential benefits of restrictive transfusion in upper gastrointestinal bleeding: A systematic review and meta-analysis of randomised controlled trials. *Sci. Rep.* **2023**, *13*, 17301. [CrossRef]
29. Wang, J.; Bao, Y.-X.; Bai, M.; Zhang, Y.-G.; Xu, W.-D.; Qi, X.-S. Restrictive *vs* liberal transfusion for upper gastrointestinal bleeding: A meta-analysis of randomized controlled trials. *World J. Gastroenterol.* **2013**, *19*, 6919–6927. [CrossRef]
30. Tripodi, A.; Mannucci, P.M. The coagulopathy of chronic liver disease. *N. Engl. J. Med.* **2011**, *365*, 147–156. [CrossRef]
31. Singh, A.D.; Mucha, S.R.; Lindenmeyer, C.C. Cirrhotic coagulopathy: A rebalanced hemostasis. *Clevel. Clin. J. Med.* **2022**, *89*, 523–533. [CrossRef] [PubMed]
32. Lisman, T.; Leebeek, F.W. Hemostatic alterations in liver disease: A review on pathophysiology, clinical consequences, and treatment. *Dig. Surg.* **2007**, *24*, 250–258. [CrossRef] [PubMed]
33. Northup, P.G.; Caldwell, S.H. Coagulation in liver disease: A guide for the clinician. *Clin. Gastroenterol. Hepatol.* **2013**, *11*, 1064–1074. [CrossRef] [PubMed]
34. De Pietri, L.; Bianchini, M.; Rompianesi, G.; Bertellini, E.; Begliomini, B. Thromboelastographic reference ranges for a cirrhotic patient population undergoing liver transplantation. *World J. Transplant.* **2016**, *6*, 583–593. [CrossRef]
35. Tripathi, D.; Handley, K.; Holden, L.; Abdali, Z.; Jowett, S.; Mathers, J.; Poyner, C.; Richardson, P.; Ferguson, J.; Rowe, I.; et al. Clinical Trial: A Multicentre Randomised Controlled Trial of Carvedilol Versus Variceal Band Ligation in Primary Prevention of Variceal Bleeding in Liver Cirrhosis (CALIBRE Trial). *Aliment. Pharmacol. Ther.* **2025**, *61*, 1740–1754. [CrossRef]
36. Kaplan, D.E.; Ripoll, C.; Thiele, M.; Fortune, B.E.; Simonetto, D.A.; Garcia-Tsao, G.; Bosch, J. AASLD Practice Guidance on risk stratification and management of portal hypertension and varices in cirrhosis. *Hepatology* **2023**, *79*, 1180–1211. [CrossRef]
37. Park, J.K.; Saab, S.; Kee, S.T.; Busuttil, R.W.; Kim, H.J.; Durazo, F.; Cho, S.-K.; Lee, E.W. Balloon-Occluded Retrograde Transvenous Obliteration (BRTO) for Treatment of Gastric Varices: Review and Meta-Analysis. *Dig. Dis. Sci.* **2014**, *60*, 1543–1553. [CrossRef]
38. Wu, L.; Huang, X.; Li, F.; Jiang, S.; Ni, L.; Ai, Y.; Schuppan, D.; Chen, S. Secondary Prophylaxis of Cirrhotic Gastric Variceal Bleeding: Addition of Non-Selective Beta-Blockers to Endoscopic Combined Treatment. *United Eur. Gastroenterol. J.* **2024**, *13*, 586–598. [CrossRef]
39. Cordon, J.P.; Torres, C.F.; García, A.B.; Rodriguez, F.G.; de Parga, J.M.S. Endoscopic management of esophageal varices. *World J. Gastrointest. Endosc.* **2012**, *4*, 312–322. [CrossRef]
40. Dai, C.; Liu, W.-X.; Jiang, M.; Sun, M.-J. Endoscopic variceal ligation compared with endoscopic injection sclerotherapy for treatment of esophageal variceal hemorrhage: A meta-analysis. *World J. Gastroenterol.* **2015**, *21*, 2534–2541. [CrossRef]
41. Singh, J.; Ebaid, M.; Saab, S. Advances in the management of complications from cirrhosis. *Gastroenterol. Rep.* **2023**, *12*, goae072. [CrossRef] [PubMed]
42. Villanueva, C.; Albillos, A.; Genescà, J.; Garcia-Pagan, J.C.; Calleja, J.L.; Aracil, C.; Bañares, R.; Morillas, R.M.; Poca, M.; Peñas, B.; et al. β blockers to prevent decompensation of cirrhosis in patients with clinically significant portal hypertension (PREDESCI): A randomised, double-blind, placebo-controlled, multicentre trial. *Lancet* **2019**, *393*, 1597–1608. [CrossRef] [PubMed]
43. Li, Y.; Du, L.; Zhang, S.; Liu, C.; Ma, C.; Liu, X.; Xu, H.; Fan, Z.; Hu, S.; Wang, J.; et al. Endoscopic variceal ligation combined with carvedilol versus endoscopic variceal ligation combined with propranolol for the treatment of oesophageal variceal bleeding in cirrhosis: Study protocol for a multicentre, randomised controlled trial. *BMJ Open* **2025**, *15*, e093866. [CrossRef] [PubMed]
44. Pallio, S.; Melita, G.; Shahini, E.; Vitello, A.; Sinagra, E.; Lattanzi, B.; Facciorusso, A.; Ramai, D.; Maida, M. Diagnosis and Management of Esophagogastric Varices. *Diagnostics* **2023**, *13*, 1031. [CrossRef]
45. Amin, N.; Ayoub, M.; Tomanguillo, J.; Chela, H.; Tahan, V.; Daglilar, E. Outcomes of Outpatient Elective Esophageal Varices Band Ligation in Cirrhosis Patients with Significant Thrombocytopenia. *Diseases* **2025**, *13*, 27. [CrossRef]
46. Pfisterer, N.; Unger, L.W.; Reiberger, T. Clinical algorithms for the prevention of variceal bleeding and rebleeding in patients with liver cirrhosis. *World J. Hepatol.* **2021**, *13*, 731–746. [CrossRef]
47. Shalaby, S.; Nicoară-Farcău, O.; Perez-Campuzano, V.; Olivas, P.; Torres, S.; García-Pagán, J.C.; Hernández-Gea, V. Transjugular Intrahepatic Portosystemic Shunt (TIPS) for Treatment of Bleeding from Cardiofundal and Ectopic Varices in Cirrhosis. *J. Clin. Med.* **2024**, *13*, 5681. [CrossRef]
48. Mohanty, A.; Garcia-Tsao, G. Management of acute variceal bleeding. *Clin. Liver Dis.* **2024**, *23*, e0176. [CrossRef]
49. Friedman, M.; Costa, V.; Rafiee, B.; Hilbert, T.; Jafri, M.; Wu, D.W. Platelet Transfusions: Current Practices and Emerging Alternatives in the United States. *Life* **2025**, *15*, 985. [CrossRef]
50. Lee, Y.Y.; Tee, H.-P.; Mahadeva, S. Role of prophylactic antibiotics in cirrhotic patients with variceal bleeding. *World J. Gastroenterol.* **2014**, *20*, 1790–1796. [CrossRef]
51. Albillos, A.; Bañares, R.; Hernández-Gea, V. Grupo Español de Consenso en Hipertensión Portal. Portal hypertension: Recommendations for diagnosis and treatment. Consensus document sponsored by the Spanish Association for the Study of the Liver (AEEH) and the Biomedical Research Network Center for Liver and Digestive Diseases (CIBERehd). *Rev. Esp. Enferm. Dig.* **2025**, *117*, 14–57. [CrossRef]

52. Barbu, L.A.; Mărgăritescu, N.D.; Ghiluşi, M.C.; Belivacă, D.; Georgescu, E.F.; Ghelase, Ş.M.; Marinescu, D. Severe upper gastrointestinal bleeding from gastrointestinal stromal tumor of the stomach. *Rom. J. Morphol. Embryol.* **2016**, *57*, 1397–1401. [PubMed]
53. Diaz-Soto, M.P.; Garcia-Tsao, G. Management of varices and variceal hemorrhage in liver cirrhosis: A recent update. *Ther. Adv. Gastroenterol.* **2022**, *15*, 17562848221101712. [CrossRef]

life

MDPI

Article

Metabolic Dysfunction-Associated Steatotic Liver Disease in a Patient with Phelan–McDermid Syndrome

Luigi Boccuto [1], Giuseppe Guido Maria Scarlata [2], Bridgette A. Moffitt [1], Sara M. Sarasua [1], Katy Phelan [3], Curtis Rogers [4] and Ludovico Abenavoli [2,*]

[1] Healthcare Genetics and Genomics Program, School of Nursing, College of Behavioral, Social and Health Sciences, Clemson University, Clemson, SC 29634, USA; lboccut@clemson.edu (L.B.); smsaras@clemson.edu (S.M.S.)

[2] Department of Health Sciences, University "Magna Græcia", 88100 Catanzaro, Italy; giuseppeguidomaria.scarlata@unicz.it

[3] Genetics Laboratory, Florida Cancer Specialists and Research Institute, Fort Myers, FL 33908, USA; kphelan@flcancer.com

[4] Greenwood Genetic Center, Greenville, SC 29605, USA; rcrgenetics@gmail.com

* Correspondence: l.abenavoli@unicz.it; Tel.: +39-0961-369-4387

Abstract: Background: Phelan–McDermid syndrome (PMS), caused by *SHANK3* variants or 22q13.3 deletions, often includes systemic features such as gastrointestinal and hepatic abnormalities. This study highlights the overlap between PMS and metabolic-associated steatotic liver disease (MASLD), focusing on *PNPLA3* variants and underscoring the need for structured metabolic monitoring. Methods: We describe a 25-year-old male with PMS due to a 22q13.33 microdeletion involving *SHANK3*. He exhibited developmental delay, seizures, and hypotonia. Genetic testing revealed homozygosity for the *PNPLA3* p.I148M variant. Clinical, anthropometric, biochemical, imaging, and metabolic investigations were performed, including liver ultrasound and metabolic profiling of lymphoblastoid cell lines. Results: Ultrasound revealed moderate hepatic steatosis consistent with MASLD. After ursodeoxycholic acid treatment and a Mediterranean-style diet, steatosis improved to mild. Metabolic profiling demonstrated increased nicotinamide adenine dinucleotide generation under metabolic stimuli, suggesting altered energy homeostasis. Conclusions: We highlight the contribution of *PNPLA3* to MASLD in PMS and support systematic hepatic monitoring. Genotype–phenotype associations in PMS may provide insights relevant to MASLD research and clinical management.

Keywords: guidelines; diagnosis; treatment; liver steatosis; genetic mutations; pathogenesis

1. Introduction

Phelan–McDermid syndrome (PMS), also known as 22q13 deletion syndrome, is a rare genetic disorder caused by deletions in chromosome 22q13.3 or mutations in the *SHANK3* gene located in the same region [1]. This syndrome is characterized by a wide spectrum of clinical manifestations (Table 1), including intellectual disability, delayed or absent speech, and various physical abnormalities. PMS is considered a significant medical condition due to its profound impact on the quality of life of affected individuals and their families [2]. Epidemiologically, PMS is estimated to occur in 1 in 8000 to 1 in 15,000 individuals, making it a relatively uncommon but noteworthy genetic disorder that necessitates further research and awareness [3]. The pathogenesis of PMS is primarily linked to the disruption of the *SHANK3* gene, which plays a crucial role in the development and function of synapses in the brain. This disruption leads to the neurological and developmental issues observed

https://doi.org/10.3390/life15101586

in PMS patients. The clinical presentation of PMS varies widely but often includes neurological traits such as developmental delay, language delay, motor impairment, hypotonia, seizures, sleep disturbances, and autism spectrum disorder [1–4]. Systemic features are also commonly reported and include gastrointestinal issues, renal disorders and lymphedema [1,5–8]. Currently, there is no cure for PMS, and treatment is primarily supportive, focusing on managing symptoms and improving the quality of life [7,9]. Interventions may include physical therapy, speech therapy, occupational therapy, and medications to control seizures and other associated conditions [9,10]. Among the non-neurological features of PMS, gastrointestinal issues are often overlooked and underdiagnosed due to the language impairment of the affected individuals and the difficulties in following a regular dietary regimen in the presence of complicating factors such as hypotonia and behavioral issues. Moreover, while digestive problems associated with gastroesophageal reflux or abnormal intestinal motility may be managed by parents or caregivers, signs and symptoms of liver disease often go unnoticed unless tests are performed, even though at least two major candidate genes for liver disease have been identified in the 22q13 region (*patatin-like phospholipase domain containing 3*, *PNPLA3*, and *cytochrome P450 2D6*, *CYP2D6*) and liver dysfunction might exert secondary effects on other PMS phenotypes [5,6,8,11]. A growing body of evidence supports the multisystemic impact of liver disease, with disruptive consequences on the cardiovascular system and lipid metabolism. Metabolic-associated steatotic liver disease (MASLD), previously known as non-alcoholic fatty liver disease (NAFLD), represents a spectrum of liver conditions ranging from simple steatosis to metabolic dysfunction-associated steatohepatitis (MASH), which can progress to fibrosis, cirrhosis, and hepatocellular carcinoma (HCC) [5]. The change in nomenclature from NAFLD to MASLD reflects a broader understanding of the disease's metabolic roots and its association with metabolic syndrome components, such as overweight or obesity, hypertension, type 2 diabetes mellitus (T2DM), and dyslipidemia [12]. MASLD is now recognized as the most common chronic liver disease worldwide, affecting approximately 25% of the global population [13–15]. Emerging research highlights a potential interplay between MASLD and PMS, particularly involving the *PNPLA3* gene and its product, adiponutrin, which is known to influence lipid metabolism and liver fat accumulation. *PNPLA3* is located on chromosome 22q13.31 and is sometimes co-deleted in PMS due to deletions of 22q13. In addition to the loss of a copy of *PNPLA3*, variants can be present in the gene. Variants in the *PNPLA3* gene, especially the I148M polymorphism, have been implicated in increased susceptibility to liver disease and MASLD in particular [5,16–19]. Moreover, the *PNPLA3* I148M variant is the primary driver of weight gain following hepatitis C virus cure [20]. At the same time, a recent observational study of 298 MASLD patients underscored the impact of genetic risk on disease progression, demonstrating that the *PNPLA3* variant is linked to elevated aspartate aminotransferase levels [21]. Given that individuals with PMS may have altered metabolic profiles and a higher prevalence of obesity and related metabolic conditions, understanding the interaction between PMS and MASLD at the genetic level is crucial for developing targeted therapeutic strategies [22–24]. There is an urgent need to apply the new MASLD definition in patients with PMS to enhance the understanding and management of liver-related complications in this population. At the same time, there is an international consensus regarding the management of patients with PMS and NAFLD, but not for MASLD [9]. Recognizing MASLD in the context of PMS is pivotal for early diagnosis, appropriate management, and the prevention of advanced liver disease. In consideration of the pivotal role of *PNPLA3* variants in the pathogenesis of MASLD, PMS may indeed be considered a model disease that will allow researchers and physicians to explore dysmetabolic dynamics and identify molecular targets for potential treatment development. This study aims to contribute to this growing body of knowledge by presenting a case of a 25-year-old male with PMS and MASLD, highlighting the clinical, genetic, and metabolic intersections of these two conditions.

Table 1. Summary of the clinical manifestations in patients with PMS.

Domain	Clinical Manifestations
Neurological/Developmental	Intellectual disability Developmental delay Language delay or absent speech Motor impairment Hypotonia Seizures Sleep disturbances Autism spectrum disorder/autistic traits
Systemic	Gastrointestinal diseases Kidney diseases Lymphedema
Hepatic/Metabolic	MASLD Metabolic syndrome
Other features	Minor dysmorphic traits

Abbreviations: MASLD, metabolic-associated steatotic liver disease.

2. Patients and Methods

2.1. Clinical Presentation

At the latest evaluation, the patient, a Caucasian 25-year-old male, presented with developmental delay, minor hypotonia, seizures, and minor facial dysmorphic traits, including facial asymmetry, bulbous nose, broad nasal root, large fleshy ears, cupid-bow sign in the upper lip, and large lower lip (Figure 1). When compared to the previous clinical report, when the subject was 20 years old, his cognitive and behavioral condition improved, and he developed a better sleep regimen [5]. However, more severe and frequent episodes of seizures—up to 2–3 events per day—have been noted until a month before the evaluation, when they seem to have responded positively to the introduction of cenobamate. Regression has been reported, mainly affecting motor and communication skills. For this reason, a sedentary lifestyle was highlighted. A negative response to gastroprotective drugs (i.e., pantoprazole) has been noted, with main consequences on behavior (agitation, irritability), hypotonia, and sleep (insomnia); the symptoms resolved drastically after the suspension of the drugs.

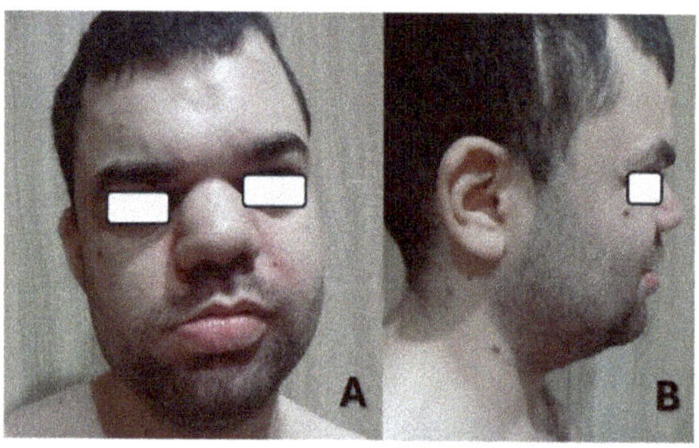

Figure 1. Frontal (**A**) and lateral (**B**) pictures of the index case at age 25 showing minor dysmorphic traits.

2.2. Genetic Tests

As previously reported, genetic tests identified an approximately 100-Kb 22q13.33 deletion (chr22:51,123,491-51,224,252/hg19; chr22:51,199,330-51,299,321/hg38, Figure 2) within the *SHANK3* gene and the homozygous c. 444C > G variant (p.I148M, SNP rs738409, CADD score 13.7) in the *PNPLA3* gene [5]. Although this variant is relatively common in the general population (G: 23.25%, gnomAD v. 4.1.0), it has been thoroughly associated with various degrees of liver disease due to its predisposing effect to lipid accumulation in hepatocytes [17].

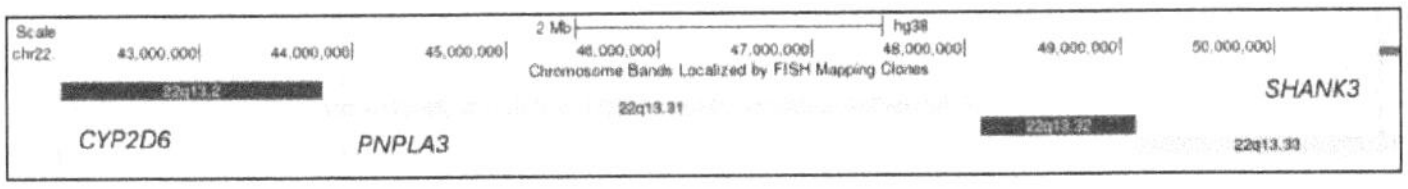

Figure 2. Graphic representation of the location of the main genes of interest (*CYP2D6*, *PNPLA3*, and *SHANK3*) on chromosome 22q13. The gene loci are highlighted in light blue, the deletion detected in the subject is indicated by the red bar (generated using UCSC Genome Browser, GRCh38/hg38, https://genome.ucsc.edu/index.html) (accessed on 12 May 2025).

2.3. Lymphoblastoid Cell Lines

Lymphoblastoid cell lines (LCLs) were established from peripheral blood samples collected by venipuncture from 43 individuals, using lymphocyte immortalization Via Epstein–Barr virus for the purpose of obtaining a metabolic profile. LCLs were harvested in Sigma RPMI-1640 with 15% fetal bovine serum from Atlanta Biological (Flowery Branch, GA, USA), 2 mM L-Glutamine, 100 U/mL Penicillin, and 100 µg/mL Streptomycin from Sigma-Aldrich (St. Louis, MO, USA).

2.4. Metabolic Profiling via Biolog Phenotype Mammalian Microarrays

We assessed the metabolic signature of the proband's LCLs using the Phenotype Mammalian MicroArray (PM-M) technology developed by Biolog (Hayward, CA, USA). The PM-M plates are designed to assess metabolic activity by measuring the cellular production of nicotinamide adenine dinucleotide (NADH) in the presence of different compounds. The methodology employed microplates with different molecules, which acted either as energy sources (plates PM–M1 to M4) or as metabolic effectors (plates PM–M5 to M8). Each well contained a single chemical, and the production of NADH per well was monitored using a colorimetric redox dye chemistry. In this way, NADH production was used as an indicator of metabolic dysregulation. The energy sources included carbohydrates, nucleotides, carboxylic acids, and ketone bodies in plate PM–M1, and amino acids, both alone and as dipeptides in plates PM–M2 to M4. The metabolic effectors included ions (PM–M5), hormones, growth factors, and cytokines (PM–M6 to M8). The relative absorbance ($A_{590-750}$) was calculated per well, and these absorbance endpoint readings were used as a measure of metabolite usage. Readings were normalized using triplicate absorbance readings from the corresponding empty plate (plates run with just media and dye, without cells). Data were analyzed using a custom R package (version 4.1.2) and the opm R package (version 4.1.2). These values were then transformed to a logarithmic scale for analysis and compared with the average values generated by the 50 LCLs from typically developing controls. The main goal was to identify significant abnormalities in metabolic pathways and responses to effectors, specifically compounds differentially metabolized by participants and controls.

2.5. Statistical Analysis

Comparisons of means were performed using two-sided *t*-tests. Chi-square tests to measure associations between categorical values used the Mid-P exact two-tailed test as provided by OpenEpi [25]. The metabolic profile data were analyzed by the non-parametric Mann–Whitney two-sided test, with a cut-off of p-value ≤ 0.05 after applying the Benjamini–Hochberg correction (R method: p.adjust) for multiple testing (FDR).

3. Results

The subject is currently following a clinical follow-up protocol for his gastrointestinal symptoms, including dyspepsia and constipation. As part of such protocol and in consideration of the evidence reported regarding the *PNPLA3* p.I148M variant, the subject underwent an abdominal ultrasound, which revealed the presence of moderate liver steatosis, as shown in Figure 3, indicating a slight improvement from the previous report, most likely due to the therapeutic dietary regimen.

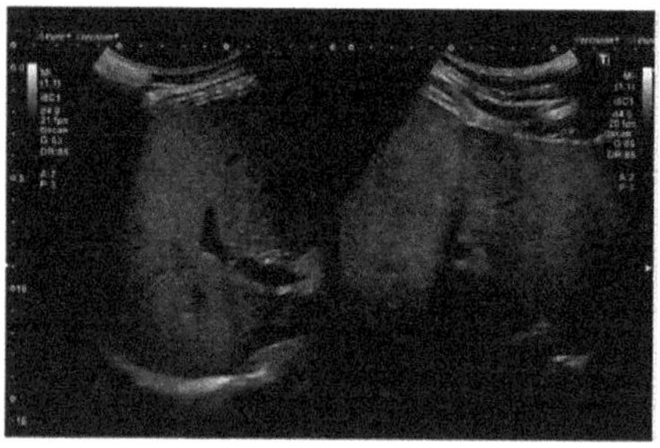

Figure 3. Abdominal ultrasound performed at baseline showed a diffuse increase in liver echogenicity and slight inhomogeneity, with a liver size of 16 cm, suggesting the presence of moderate liver steatosis. No additional focal liver lesions or signs of advanced liver disease are identified.

Due to this finding, certain anthropometric and laboratory indices associated with the diagnosis of MASLD were evaluated according to international guidelines. Specifically, steatotic liver disease (SLD) with at least one of five cardiometabolic risk factors such as (i) body mass index (BMI) $\geq$ 25 kg/m^2 or waist circumference > 94 cm; (ii) fasting serum glucose $\geq$ 100 mg/dL or diagnosis of T2DM or receiving treatment for T2DM; (iii) blood pressure $\geq$ 135/85 mmHg or taking specific antihypertensive medication; (iv) plasma triglycerides $\geq$ 150 mg/dL or undergoing lipid-lowering therapy; (v) plasma high-density lipoproteins (HDL) $\leq$ 40 mg/dL or undergoing lipid-lowering therapy [26]. The patient met the criteria outlined in Table 2 and was therefore diagnosed with MASLD.

Table 2. MASLD criteria—SLD plus at least one of five cardiometabolic risk factors.

MASLD Criterium	Value	Satisfied
SLD	Moderate SLD	Yes
BMI $\geq$ 25 kg/m^2 or waist circumference > 94 cm	BMI 26.57 kg/m^2 Waist circumference 101 cm	Yes
Fasting serum glucose $\geq$ 100 mg/dL or diagnosis of T2DM	93 mg/dL	No
Blood pressure $\geq$ 135/85 mmHg	120/80 mmHg	No
Triglycerides $\geq$ 150 mg/dL	111 mg/dL	No
HDL $\leq$ 40 mg/dL	62 mg/dL	No

Abbreviations: SLD: steatotic liver disease; BMI: body mass index; T2DM: type 2 diabetes mellitus; HDL: high-density lipoproteins.

The subject was treated with ursodeoxycholic acid 450 mg 1/daily and a low-fat, high-fiber diet following the Mediterranean dietary regimen for 6 months, in accordance with international guidelines for MASLD treatment [26–30]. This therapeutic approach resulted in a reduction in liver steatosis from moderate (Figure 3) to mild after 6 months, which was confirmed with ultrasound (no ultrasound image available). Currently, the patient is stable from a hepatic and metabolic standpoint and is continuing follow-up at our Centers.

Metabolic profiling of LCLs from the patient measured the production of energy in the form of NADH in the presence of various compounds, assessing the capacity of the cells to generate energy in response to different metabolic conditions. When compared to the profile of 50 controls, the patient cells showed increased energy production when exposed to several compounds (Figure 4). Even if no difference reached statistical significance (p-value < 0.05) due to the comparison of a single case sample versus a control cohort, the results indicated insightful trends with unadjusted p-values < 0.1 and suggested possible alterations of multiple metabolic pathways, ranging from hormones (thyroxine or T4, beta-estradiol, insulin) to growth factors (insulin-like growth factor-1, IGF-1, platelet-derived growth factor-AB, PDGF-AB).

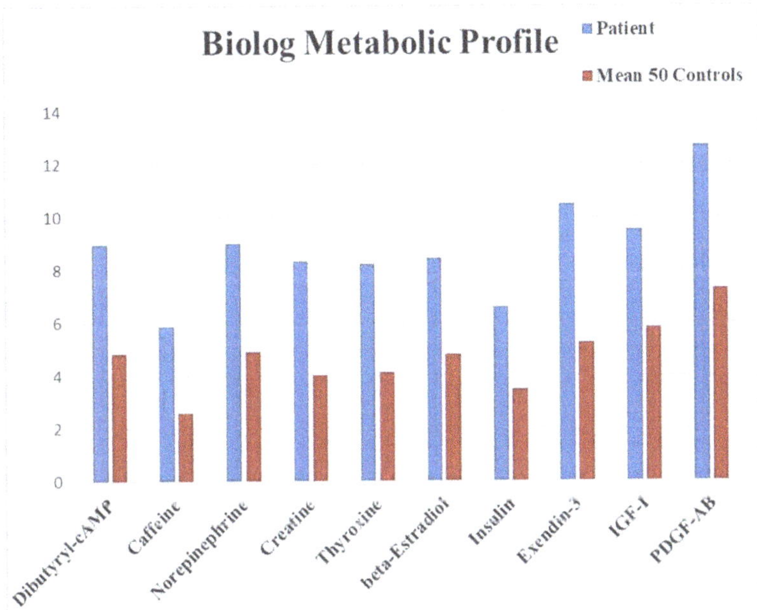

Figure 4. Metabolic profile obtained from LCLs tested on Biolog PM-Ms. The graphic shows endpoint absorbance values (y axis) indicating the levels of NADH produced from glucose in the presence of the listed compounds (x axis). All differences had an unadjusted p-value < 0.1. Abbreviations: IGF-1, insulin-like growth factor-1; PDGF-AB, platelet-derived growth factor-AB.

The data emerging from the metabolic profile indicate an increased responsivity of the patient's cells to hormones and growth factors like thyroxine (T4), insulin, IGF-1, and PDGF-AB that promote cellular growth, proliferation, protein synthesis, and storage of energy sources. These metabolic findings indicate that LCLs from the proband tend to increase their production of NADH more than control cells when exposed to hormones or growth factors promoting tissue building and fat accumulation. This trend suggests a predisposition towards an anabolic profile and is in line with the observed clinical presentation, characterized by obesity and liver steatosis. Recognizing a genetic predisposition to an anabolic profile bears relevant translational implications for the clinical and dietary management of the patient.

Another relevant trend is characterized by the increased response to stimulatory compounds, such as dibutyril-cAMP, caffeine, norepinephrine, and creatine. The elevated energy production in LCLs in the presence of such compounds may be compatible with an impaired metabolic activity, which would require a disproportionate amount of energy sources.

4. Discussion

4.1. PMS and MASLD Interplay

The reported case with a diagnosis of PMS due to a small deletion on chromosome 22q13.33 and MASLD is likely associated with a homozygous p.I148M variant in *PNPLA3*. Although the two conditions are etiologically independent, the *PNPLA3* gene maps on chromosome 22q13.31 and is often deleted in cases of PMS caused by large chromosomal deletions (>5 Mb, see Figure 2) [11]. Despite its deleterious effects on liver function and lipid metabolism, this variant is relatively common in the general population, making it the main genetic factor predisposing to various liver diseases, including MASLD. In cases of PMS, due to larger deletions, one copy of *PNPLA3* may be deleted. The combination of the p.I148M variant on one allele of *PNPLA3* with the deletion of the other allele would amplify the deleterious effects of the variant. It has been shown that the liver phenotype associated with a combination of a 22q13.3 deletion including *PNPLA3* and a p.I148M variant is virtually indistinguishable from the one caused by a homozygous p.I148M variant [5]. The study presents clinical, imaging, and laboratory data on an individual previously described for his liver phenotype, highlighting the multisystemic evolution of his condition, now satisfying the clinical criteria for MASLD [5]. Functional in vitro studies on cells from the reported case subject revealed abnormal metabolic trends with altered energetic responses to hormones either produced by the liver (like IGF-1) or targeting it (thyroxine). Even if the results failed to reach statistical significance because only one case sample was available, it is plausible to postulate that further studies may validate a potential metabolomic profile characterizing individuals with PMS and homozygous *PNPLA3* variants. The results emerging from this longitudinal assessment underline the complexity of the phenotype associated with *PNPLA3* variants and suggest a pivotal role for this gene in the gastrointestinal phenotype of PMS as well as in the genetic predisposition to liver disease in general and MASLD in particular. The data emerging here reported are in line with the current literature and validate the pivotal role of *PNPLA3* variants in MASLD, highlighting the multisystemic implications of the metabolic disruption caused by the abnormal *PNPLA3* function in hepatocytes [5,16–19]. In fact, our longitudinal investigation allowed us to describe how the evolution of the *PNPLA3*-associated phenotype incorporates the involvement of signs and symptoms beyond the liver, such as obesity, while other parameters might be within normal ranges thanks to the therapeutic regimen. These findings indicate that individuals with PMS caused by large (>5 Mb) 22q13.3 deletions may be at risk for liver disease and, in the long term, MASLD. The same predisposition may affect individuals with homozygous *PNPLA3* variants only. The dynamic phenotype associated with variants in this gene also emphasizes the need for a multidisciplinary approach to MASLD, with guidelines focusing on monitoring lipid and glucose metabolism and the cardiovascular system. Moreover, in cases of large 22q13.3 deletions where *PNPLA3* may be deleted, clinicians should investigate whether the deletion also encompasses the *CYP2D6* gene, one of the most critical pharmacogenes, mapping on chromosome 22q13.2 (Figure 2) [8,11,31]. Loss of one active copy of *CYP2D6*, in the presence of impaired liver function, may increase the risk for adverse reactions to medications, complicating the overall phenotype [32,33].

4.2. Strengths and Limitations

Our report presents several notable strengths. First, it integrates detailed clinical, genetic, imaging, and metabolomic data from a single patient with PMS carrying a homozygous *PNPLA3* p.I148M variant, thereby providing a unique longitudinal perspective. The availability of repeated clinical assessments over time, including neurodevelopmental, metabolic, and hepatological parameters, allows for a dynamic evaluation of the patient's phenotype. Such a longitudinal approach is rarely available in rare genetic syndromes, and it offers valuable insights into the natural history of disease progression and therapeutic response. Second, the use of LCLs and PM-Ms technology enabled functional testing beyond descriptive clinical observation. This methodological strength provided preliminary evidence of altered metabolic responses to hormones and growth factors, which may represent a candidate biomarker signature for patients with PMS and *PNPLA3* variants. Although the presented results are promising, they were generated on a single patient and require validation on a much larger cohort. Third, the incorporation of imaging data and compliance with internationally accepted MASLD diagnostic criteria strengthen the reliability of the liver disease diagnosis and its correlation with genetic findings. Finally, the present report contributes to a growing body of literature emphasizing the multisystemic impact of *PNPLA3* variants, underlining the importance of considering liver disease surveillance in syndromic patients. Nevertheless, important limitations must be acknowledged. Foremost, this is a single-case study, which inherently limits generalizability: we aimed to perform an exploratory longitudinal study to monitor the possible evolution of the gastrointestinal and metabolic phenotype in an individual with PMS. Although the genetic predisposition to abnormal liver function reported in this condition makes it a good model disorder for MASLD and other liver diseases, the rarity and phenotypical variability of PMS suggest that further validation is necessary before translating these results to clinical protocols. Indeed, observed associations between PMS, *PNPLA3* homozygosity, and MASLD must therefore be interpreted with caution until confirmed in larger cohorts. The absence of a family-based genetic analysis also prevents a more complete understanding of inheritance patterns and penetrance in this case. Furthermore, the metabolic profiling findings, while suggestive, did not achieve statistical significance after correction for multiple testing. This limitation reflects both the low statistical power of a single sample and the technical variability intrinsic to in vitro assays. Another limitation is the role of ultrasound imaging as the primary tool in the follow-up of liver steatosis. Although widely available and noninvasive, ultrasound lacks the sensitivity of advanced imaging modalities such as transient elastography, which could have provided more accurate quantification of hepatic fat and fibrosis. Finally, environmental and lifestyle factors, including adherence to the Mediterranean diet, may have influenced the clinical course but could not be rigorously quantified in our investigation.

5. Conclusions and Future Perspectives

Although PMS is a relatively rare genetic disorder, the clinical and functional investigation of the phenotypes associated with mutations of the genes in the 22q13.3 region may bring to light valuable genotype–phenotype correlations that may apply to non-syndromic cases as well. In our experience, we provided further evidence supporting the pathogenic role of *PNPLA3* variants in the pathogenesis of MASLD in a subject with PMS, suggesting that the phenotype would evolve with time and highlighting the importance of a thorough multidisciplinary surveillance protocol in individuals with large 22q13.3 deletions. Building on our findings, several valuable avenues for future research emerge. First, expanding the study to larger cohorts of individuals with PMS, especially those harboring *PNPLA3* variants, would help establish genotype–phenotype correlations and assess the generalizability of our observations in MASLD evolution. Indeed, large-scale epidemiological and sequencing studies have demonstrated that the *PNPLA3* I148M variant is the most impactful genetic determinant of MASLD worldwide, responsible for significant variation in disease severity and outcomes across populations [34]. Second, exploring the mechanistic underpinnings of *PNPLA3*-driven hepatic pathology in PMS is critical. A recent study has revealed an association between the *PNPLA3* I148M variant and increased immune cell infiltration and activation in MASLD onset, highlighting a possible inflammatory axis to disease progression [19]. Delineating these immune-mediated pathways could unveil novel therapeutic targets. Third, the advent of precision-medicine approaches, such as RNA silencing therapies targeting *PNPLA3*, offers promising translational potential. Preclinical models and early-phase trials have already demonstrated a reduction in liver fat content in carriers of the risk allele, supporting the feasibility of this intervention [35]. At the same time, ARO-PNPLA3, an RNA interference–based therapy, was recently designed to reduce hepatic *PNPLA3* expression in patients with MASH. Specifically, in a Phase 1 clinical trial (NCT04844450), a single-dose treatment produced encouraging results, achieving dose-dependent reductions of nearly 40% in liver fat content among individuals homozygous for the I148M mutation [36]. Finally, integrating polygenic risk scores that include *PNPLA3* alongside clinical scores (e.g., Fibrosis-4 index) could refine risk stratification for liver-related events in MASLD. In longitudinal cohorts, combined genetic-clinical models have shown markedly improved prediction of adverse outcomes [37]. In addition, future research should also investigate environmental and lifestyle modifiers that could interact with *PNPLA3*-driven susceptibility in PMS. Diet, physical activity, and alcohol consumption are well-established contributors to MASLD severity, and their potential synergistic or mitigating effects in genetically predisposed individuals remain incompletely understood. For example, adherence to a Mediterranean diet has been linked to improved hepatic outcomes in *PNPLA3* carriers, suggesting that nutritional interventions may be particularly beneficial in this subgroup of patients [38]. Similarly, studies of gut microbiota composition in PMS patients could provide insight into whether alterations in the gut-liver axis further exacerbate *PNPLA3*-related hepatic vulnerability [39]. Another important direction lies in longitudinal natural-history studies of PMS individuals carrying *PNPLA3* variants. Such efforts would clarify whether the onset of MASLD-related complications, such as fibrosis progression or HCC, follows a predictable trajectory, and whether early lifestyle or pharmacological interventions can alter this course [40]. Importantly, incorporating advanced imaging modalities (e.g., transient elastography, contrast-enhanced ultrasound, or magnetic resonance imaging-based biomarkers) could improve noninvasive monitoring and reduce reliance on liver biopsy [41]. Ultimately, these integrated approaches underscore the importance of multidisciplinary care in PMS patients, encompassing genetics, hepatology, neurology, and nutrition. By characterizing the complex interplay between genetic and environmental factors, and by translating mechanistic insights into therapeutic strategies, future studies may substantially improve both the quality of life and long-term outcomes of individuals with PMS who are at risk for MASLD [42]. Moreover, the clinical significance of integrating genetic counseling into the management of PMS cannot be overlooked. Families affected by large 22q13.3 deletions would greatly benefit from structured counseling programs that include information on MASLD risk, lifestyle modifications, and potential participation in clinical trials targeting *PNPLA3*. Educational initiatives could also empower caregivers to recognize early metabolic or hepatic warning signs, prompting timely specialist referral [43]. From a healthcare perspective, these measures would not only enhance personalized care but also generate valuable real-world evidence to guide broader recommendations for rare genetic syndromes intersecting with common metabolic diseases. Overall, the results emerging from this study describe the longitudinal evolution of the liver phenotype from steatosis to MASLD in a subject with PMS and provide functional evidence of pathogenic mechanisms based on a predisposing genetic background. Although these findings were reported in a patient with a rare genetic disorder, it is plausible that similar mechanisms and clinical patterns apply to sporadic cases as well, providing relevant information about the risk of MASLD and the possible evolution of the liver phenotype in predisposed subjects.

Author Contributions: Conceptualization, L.B., G.G.M.S. and L.A.; methodology, G.G.M.S., B.A.M. and L.A.; software, B.A.M.; validation, S.M.S., K.P. and C.R.; formal analysis, G.G.M.S. and B.A.M.; investigation, L.B., G.G.M.S., B.A.M., S.M.S. and L.A.; resources, L.A.; data curation, L.B., G.G.M.S. and L.A.; writing—original draft preparation, L.B., G.G.M.S. and B.A.M.; writing—review and editing, S.M.S., K.P., C.R. and L.A.; visualization, S.M.S., K.P. and C.R.; supervision, L.B. and L.A. All authors have read and agreed to the published version of the manuscript.

Funding: This research received no external funding.

Institutional Review Board Statement: The research was approved by the Self Regional Health System Institutional Review Board (Pro0057738) on 2017-08-01.

Informed Consent Statement: Informed consent was obtained from all subjects involved in the study. Informed consent for publication was obtained from all identifiable human participants.

Data Availability Statement: All data are available in the manuscript.

Acknowledgments: We would like to thank the Italian Phelan–McDermid Syndrome Association for supporting our research.

Conflicts of Interest: The authors declare no conflicts of interest.

Abbreviations

The following abbreviations are used in this manuscript:

BMI	Body mass index
CYP2D6	Cytochrome P450 2D6
HCC	Hepatocellular carcinoma
HDL	High-density lipoproteins
IGF-1	Insulin-like growth factor 1
LCLs	Lymphoblastoid cell lines
MASH	Metabolic dysfunction-associated steatohepatitis
MASLD	Metabolic-associated steatotic liver disease
NAFLD	Non-alcoholic fatty liver disease
NADH	Nicotinamide adenine dinucleotide
PDGF-AB	Platelet-derived growth factor-AB
PMS	Phelan–McDermid Syndrome
PNPLA3	Patatin-like phospholipase domain containing 3
PM-Ms	Phenotype Mammalian Microarrays
SLD	Steatotic liver disease
SNP	Single nucleotide polymorphism
T2DM	Type 2 diabetes mellitus

References

1. Schön, M.; Lapunzina, P.; Nevado, J.; Mattina, T.; Gunnarsson, C.; Hadzsiev, K.; Verpelli, C.; Bourgeron, T.; Jesse, S.; van Ravenswaaij-Arts, C.M.A.; et al. Definition and clinical variability of *SHANK3*-related Phelan-McDermid syndrome. *Eur. J. Med. Genet.* **2023**, *66*, 104754. [CrossRef] [PubMed]
2. Frank, Y.; Levy, T.; Lozano, R.; Friedman, K.; Underwood, S.; Kostic, A.; Walker, H.; Kolevzon, A. Gait Abnormalities in Children with Phelan-McDermid Syndrome. *J. Child Neurol.* **2023**, *38*, 665–671. [CrossRef] [PubMed]

3. Cammarata-Scalisi, F.; Callea, M.; Martinelli, D.; Willoughby, C.E.; Tadich, A.C.; Araya Castillo, M.; Lacruz-Rengel, M.A.; Medina, M.; Grimaldi, P.; Bertini, E.; et al. Clinical and Genetic Aspects of Phelan-McDermid Syndrome: An Interdisciplinary Approach to Management. *Genes* **2022**, *13*, 504. [CrossRef]
4. Delling, J.P.; Boeckers, T.M. Comparison of SHANK3 deficiency in animal models: Phenotypes, treatment strategies, and translational implications. *J. Neurodev. Disord.* **2021**, *13*, 55. [CrossRef]
5. Boccuto, L.; Abenavoli, L.; Cascio, L.; Srikanth, S.; DuPont, B.; Mitz, A.R.; Rogers, R.C.; Phelan, K. Variability in Phelan-McDermid syndrome: The impact of the PNPLA3 p.I148M polymorphism. *Clin. Genet.* **2018**, *94*, 590–591. [CrossRef]
6. Matuleviciene, A.; Siauryte, K.; Kuiper, E.; Grabrucker, A.M.; European Phelan-McDermid Syndrome Guideline Consortium. Consensus recommendations on chewing, swallowing and gastrointestinal problems in Phelan-McDermid syndrome. *Eur. J. Med. Genet.* **2023**, *66*, 104763. [CrossRef]
7. Levy, T.; Farmer, C.; Srivastava, S.; Johnson, K.; Trayvick, J.; Brune, C.; Massa, A.; Silver, H.; Siper, P.M.; Zweifach, J.; et al. Genetic Subtypes of Phelan-McDermid Syndrome Exhibit Similar Rates of Change Despite Differences in Level of Impairment in Developmental Constructs. *Am. J. Intellect. Dev. Disabil.* **2025**, *130*, 395–413. [CrossRef] [PubMed]
8. Nevado, J.; Escalada, B.; Muñoz-GªPorrero, Y.; Adan, C.; Tenorio-Castaño, J.; Lapunzina, P.D. Genotype-Phenotype Associations in Phelan-McDermid Syndrome: Insights into Novel Genes Beyond *SHANK3*. *Int. J. Mol. Sci.* **2025**, *26*, 4653. [CrossRef]
9. Srivastava, S.; Sahin, M.; Buxbaum, J.D.; Berry-Kravis, E.; Soorya, L.V.; Thurm, A.; Bernstein, J.A.; Asante-Otoo, A.; Bennett, W.E.; Betancur, C., Jr.; et al. Updated consensus guidelines on the management of Phelan-McDermid syndrome. *Am. J. Med. Genet. A* **2023**, *191*, 2015–2044. [CrossRef]
10. Kolevzon, A.; Angarita, B.; Bush, L.; Wang, A.T.; Frank, Y.; Yang, A.; Rapaport, R.; Saland, J.; Srivastava, S.; Farrell, C.; et al. Phelan-McDermid syndrome: A review of the literature and practice parameters for medical assessment and monitoring. *J. Neurodev. Disord.* **2014**, *6*, 39. [CrossRef]
11. Boccuto, L.; Mitz, A.; Abenavoli, L.; Sarasua, S.M.; Bennett, W.; Rogers, C.; DuPont, B.; Phelan, K. Phenotypic Variability in Phelan-McDermid Syndrome and Its Putative Link to Environmental Factors. *Genes* **2022**, *13*, 528. [CrossRef]
12. Colaci, C.; Gambardella, M.L.; Scarlata, G.G.M.; Boccuto, L.; Colica, C.; Luzza, F.; Scarpellini, E.; Mendez-Sanchez, N.; Abenavoli, L. Dysmetabolic comorbidities and non-alcoholic fatty liver disease: A stairway to metabolic dysfunction-associated steatotic liver disease. *Hepatoma Res.* **2024**, *10*, 16. [CrossRef]
13. Chan, W.K.; Chuah, K.H.; Rajaram, R.B.; Lim, L.L.; Ratnasingam, J.; Vethakkan, S.R. Metabolic Dysfunction-Associated Steatotic Liver Disease (MASLD): A State-of-the-Art Review. *J. Obes. Metab. Syndr.* **2023**, *32*, 197–213. [CrossRef]
14. Younossi, Z.M.; Golabi, P.; Paik, J.M.; Henry, A.; Van Dongen, C.; Henry, L. The global epidemiology of nonalcoholic fatty liver disease (NAFLD) and nonalcoholic steatohepatitis (NASH): A systematic review. *Hepatology* **2023**, *77*, 1335–1347. [CrossRef]
15. Le, M.H.; Yeo, Y.H.; Li, X.; Li, J.; Zou, B.; Wu, Y.; Ye, Q.; Huang, D.Q.; Zhao, C.; Zhang, J.; et al. 2019 Global NAFLD Prevalence: A Systematic Review and Meta-analysis. *Clin. Gastroenterol. Hepatol.* **2022**, *20*, 2809–2817.e28. [CrossRef] [PubMed]
16. Tsedendorj, Y.; Daramjav, D.; Enkhbat, Y.; Dondov, G.; Dashjamts, G.; Khayankhyarvaa, E.; Ganzorig, A.E.; Ulziitsogt, B.; Badamjav, T.; Batsaikhan, B.; et al. Genetic Risk of MASLD in Mongolians: Role of *PNPLA3* and *FTO SNPs*. *Curr. Issues Mol. Biol.* **2025**, *47*, 605. [CrossRef] [PubMed]
17. Gawrieh, S.; Yao, J.; Guo, X.; Diehl, A.M.; Rotter, J.I.; Chalasani, N.P. Biological age, PNPLA3 and risk of metabolic dysfunction-associated steatotic liver disease. *Clin. Gastroenterol. Hepatol.* **2025**, *ahead of print*. [CrossRef]
18. Romeo, S.; Valenti, L. Fifteen Years of PNPLA3: Transforming Hepatology Through Human Genetics. *Liver Int.* **2025**, *45*, e70240. [CrossRef]
19. Lee, J.; Cha, J.H.; Cho, H.S.; Yang, K.; Yang, H.; Nam, H.; Byun, M.Y.; Cho, S.K.; Park, J.; Ko, H.W.; et al. The PNPLA3 I148M variant is associated with immune cell infiltration and advanced fibrosis in MASLD: A prospective genotype-phenotype study. *J. Gastroenterol.* **2025**, *60*, 1284–1295. [CrossRef] [PubMed]
20. Pitova, V.; Frankova, S.; Holinka, M.; Merta, D.; Vesela, S.; Hubacek, J.A.; Jirsa, M.; Sperl, J. *PNPLA3* I148M variant is the main driver of weight gain after hepatitis C cure. *Sci. Rep.* **2025**, *15*, 25543. [CrossRef]
21. Torre, P.; Motta, B.M.; Sarcina, T.; Festa, M.; Masarone, M.; Persico, M. Early Insights from Metabolic Dysfunction-Associated Steatotic Liver Disease (MASLD) Patients: An Observational Study on Polygenic Risk and Liver Biomarkers. *Int. J. Mol. Sci.* **2025**, *26*, 8426. [CrossRef] [PubMed]
22. Eskridge, W.; Cryer, D.R.; Schattenberg, J.M.; Gastaldelli, A.; Malhi, H.; Allen, A.M.; Noureddin, M.; Sanyal, A.J. Metabolic Dysfunction-Associated Steatotic Liver Disease and Metabolic Dysfunction-Associated Steatohepatitis: The Patient and Physician Perspective. *J. Clin. Med.* **2023**, *12*, 6216. [CrossRef]
23. Hashim, M.M.A.; Khan, M.A.M.; Ashraf, M.U.; Mohsin, S.; Zahoor, K.; Niazi, J.; Khan, A.; Muzaffar, S.; Makhdumi, M.; Ibad, O.A.; et al. Pathological Evolution and Internal Medicine Management of Nonalcoholic Fatty Liver Disease (NAFLD) in the Era of Metabolic Dysfunction-Associated Steatotic Liver Disease (MASLD). *Cureus* **2025**, *17*, e86963. [CrossRef] [PubMed]

24. Sherman, D.J.; Liu, L.; Mamrosh, J.L.; Xie, J.; Ferbas, J.; Lomenick, B.; Ladinsky, M.S.; Verma, R.; Rulifson, I.C.; Deshaies, R.J. The fatty liver disease-causing protein PNPLA3-I148M alters lipid droplet-Golgi dynamics. *Proc. Natl. Acad. Sci. USA* **2024**, *121*, e2318619121. [CrossRef]
25. Sullivan, K.M.; Dean, A.; Soe, M.M. On Academics: OpenEpi: A web-based epidemiologic and statistical calculator for public health. *Public Health Rep.* **2009**, *124*, 471–474. [CrossRef]
26. Rinella, M.E.; Lazarus, J.V.; Ratziu, V.; Francque, S.M.; Sanyal, A.J.; Kanwal, F.; Romero, D.; Abdelmalek, M.F.; Anstee, Q.M.; Arab, J.P.; et al. A multisociety Delphi consensus statement on new fatty liver disease nomenclature. *J. Hepatol.* **2023**, *78*, 1966–1986. [CrossRef] [PubMed]
27. European Association for the Study of the Liver (EASL); European Association for the Study of Diabetes (EASD); European Association for the Study of Obesity (EASO). EASL-EASD-EASO Clinical Practice Guidelines on the management of metabolic dysfunction-associated steatotic liver disease (MASLD). *J. Hepatol.* **2024**, *81*, 492–542. [CrossRef]
28. Menotti, A.; Puddu, P.E. Ancel Keys, the Mediterranean Diet, and the Seven Countries Study: A Review. *J. Cardiovasc. Dev. Dis.* **2025**, *12*, 141. [CrossRef]
29. Zhang, W.; Tang, Y.; Huang, J.; Hu, H. Efficacy of ursodeoxycholic acid in nonalcoholic fatty liver disease: An updated meta-analysis of randomized controlled trials. *Asia Pac. J. Clin. Nutr.* **2020**, *29*, 696–705.
30. Perva, I.T.; Simina, I.E.; Bende, R.; Motofelea, A.C.; Chirita Emandi, A.; Andreescu, N.; Sima, A.; Vlad, A.; Sporea, I.; Zimbru, C.; et al. Use of a Micronutrient Cocktail to Improve Metabolic Dysfunction-Associated Steatotic Liver Disease (MASLD) in Adults with Obesity: A Randomized, Double-Blinded Pilot Clinical Trial. *Medicina* **2024**, *60*, 1366. [CrossRef]
31. Dyar, B.; Meaddough, E.; Sarasua, S.M.; Rogers, C.; Phelan, K.; Boccuto, L. Genetic Findings as the Potential Basis of Personalized Pharmacotherapy in Phelan-McDermid Syndrome. *Genes* **2021**, *12*, 1192. [CrossRef]
32. Kane, M. CYP2D6 Overview: Allele and Phenotype Frequencies. In *Medical Genetics Summaries [Internet]*; Pratt, V.M., Scott, S.A., Pirmohamed, M., Esquivel, B., Kattman, B.L., Malheiro, A.J., Eds.; 15 October 2021 [Updated 17 January 2025]; National Center for Biotechnology Information: Bethesda, MD, USA, 2012. Available online: https://www.ncbi.nlm.nih.gov/books/NBK574601/ (accessed on 28 September 2025).
33. Nahid, N.A.; Johnson, J.A. CYP2D6 pharmacogenetics and phenoconversion in personalized medicine. *Expert Opin. Drug Metab. Toxicol.* **2022**, *18*, 769–785. [CrossRef]
34. Kozlitina, J.; Sookoian, S. Global Epidemiological Impact of PNPLA3 I148M on Liver Disease. *Liver Int.* **2025**, *45*, e16123. [CrossRef]
35. Lindén, D.; Tesz, G.; Loomba, R. Targeting PNPLA3 to Treat MASH and MASH Related Fibrosis and Cirrhosis. *Liver Int.* **2025**, *45*, e16186. [CrossRef]
36. Josephine, B. *Arrowhead Pharmaceuticals Gains Full Rights to NASH Candidate ARO-PNPLA3 with Promising Phase 1 Results*; Arrowhead Pharmaceuticals Inc.: Pasadena, CA, USA, 2024. Available online: https://ir.arrowheadpharma.com/news-releases/news-release-details/arrowhead-pharmaceuticals-gains-full-rights-nash-candidate-aro (accessed on 28 September 2025).
37. Seko, Y.; Yamaguchi, K.; Shima, T.; Iwaki, M.; Takahashi, H.; Kawanaka, M.; Tanaka, S.; Mitsumoto, Y.; Yoneda, M.; Nakajima, A.; et al. Clinical Utility of Genetic Variants in *PNPLA3* and *TM6SF2* to Predict Liver-Related Events in Metabolic Dysfunction-Associated Steatotic Liver Disease. *Liver Int.* **2025**, *45*, e16124. [CrossRef] [PubMed]
38. Speliotes, E.K.; Schneider, C.V. PNPLA3 I148M Interacts With Environmental Triggers to Cause Human Disease. *Liver Int.* **2025**, *45*, e16106. [CrossRef] [PubMed]
39. Sato, S.; Iino, C.; Sasada, T.; Soma, G.; Furusawa, K.; Yoshida, K.; Sawada, K.; Mikami, T.; Nakaji, S.; Sakuraba, H.; et al. Epidemiological Study on the Interaction between the *PNPLA3* (rs738409) and Gut Microbiota in Metabolic Dysfunction-Associated Steatotic Liver Disease. *Genes* **2024**, *15*, 1172. [CrossRef] [PubMed]
40. Armandi, A.; Bugianesi, E. Dietary and pharmacological treatment in patients with metabolic-dysfunction associated steatotic liver disease. *Eur. J. Intern. Med.* **2024**, *122*, 20–27. [CrossRef]
41. Kokkorakis, M.; Muzurović, E.; Volčanšek, Š.; Chakhtoura, M.; Hill, M.A.; Mikhailidis, D.P.; Mantzoros, C.S. Steatotic Liver Disease: Pathophysiology and Emerging Pharmacotherapies. *Pharmacol. Rev.* **2024**, *76*, 454–499. [CrossRef]
42. Bolbocean, C.; Andújar, F.N.; McCormack, M.; Suter, B.; Holder, J.L., Jr. Health-Related Quality of Life in Pediatric Patients with Syndromic Autism and their Caregivers. *J. Autism Dev. Disord.* **2022**, *52*, 1334–1345. [CrossRef]
43. Landlust, A.M.; Koza, S.A.; Carbin, M.; Walinga, M.; Robert, S.; Cooke, J.; Vyshka, K.; European Phelan-McDermid syndrome consortium; van Balkom, I.D.C. van Ravenswaaij-Arts, C. Parental perspectives on Phelan-McDermid syndrome: Results of a worldwide survey. *Eur. J. Med. Genet.* **2023**, *66*, 104771. [CrossRef] [PubMed]

life

MDPI

Article

Non-Variceal Upper Gastrointestinal Bleeding: A Retrospective Cohort of 364 Cases, Historical Comparison, and Updated Management Algorithm

Laurențiu Augustus Barbu [1], Liviu Vasile [2], Liliana Cercelaru [3], Valeriu Șurlin [2], Stelian-Stefaniță Mogoantă [2], Gabriel Florin Răzvan Mogoș [1], Tiberiu Stefăniță Țenea Cojan [1], Nicolae-Dragoș Mărgăritescu [2,*] and Anca Buliman [4]

[1] Department of Surgery, Railway Clinical Hospital Craiova, University of Medicine and Pharmacy of Craiova, 2 Petru Rares Street, 200349 Craiova, Romania; laurentiu.barbu@umfcv.ro (L.A.B.); gabriel.mogos@umfcv.ro (G.F.R.M.); tiberiu.tenea@umfcv.ro (T.S.Ț.C.)

[2] Department of Surgery, Emergency County Hospital, University of Medicine and Pharmacy of Craiova, 2 Petru Rares Street, 200349 Craiova, Romania; vliviu777@yahoo.com (L.V.); vsurlin@gmail.com (V.Ș.); ssmogo@yahoo.com (S.-S.M.)

[3] Department of Embryology and Anatomy, University of Medicine and Pharmacy of Craiova, 200349 Craiova, Romania; liliana.cercelaru@umfcv.ro

[4] Department of Radiology, Faculty of Medicine, Titu Maiorescu University, 67A Gheorghe Petrașcu Street, 031593 Bucharest, Romania; buliman_anca@yahoo.com

* Correspondence: dmargaritescu@yahoo.com; Tel.: +40-723-271-941

Abstract: Background: Non-variceal upper gastrointestinal bleeding (NVUGIB) remains a critical medical–surgical emergency associated with significant morbidity, mortality, and healthcare burden worldwide. Despite advances in diagnostic and therapeutic modalities, NVUGIB continues to pose complex clinical challenges, particularly in resource-limited settings. **Methods**: This retrospective observational study analyzed 364 consecutive adult patients diagnosed with NVUGIB and hospitalized at the First Surgical Clinic of the County Emergency Clinical Hospital Craiova between January 2009 and December 2014. Inclusion criteria required a confirmed diagnosis based on clinical presentation, laboratory findings, and upper gastrointestinal endoscopy (UGIE). Demographic variables, etiology, comorbidities, drug-induced triggers, laboratory parameters, onset-to-admission and onset-to-surgery intervals, endoscopic findings, therapeutic interventions (medical, endoscopic, surgical), rebleeding rates, and mortality were recorded and analyzed. Results were descriptively compared with historical data from the national and international literature. Due to the retrospective and aggregate nature of the data, survival analysis (Kaplan–Meier) was not applicable. **Results**: Peptic ulcers, erosive gastritis, Mallory–Weiss syndrome, and gastric neoplasms were the predominant etiologies. NSAID use, oral anticoagulation, and alcohol consumption emerged as major risk factors. Endoscopic hemostasis was achieved in the majority of cases; surgical intervention was required in 11.5% of patients, mainly for refractory or recurrent bleeding. The overall mortality rate was 10.9%, consistent with historical benchmarks. Comparative analysis revealed trends in etiology and management reflecting evolving clinical practice standards. **Conclusions**: NVUGIB remains a significant clinical challenge with persistent mortality and rebleeding risks. This cohort highlights the need for timely diagnosis, risk stratification, and an evidence-based therapeutic strategy integrating modern endoscopic and surgical options. An updated diagnostic and management algorithm is proposed to guide practical decision-making and optimize outcomes in similar tertiary care settings.

 https://doi.org/10.3390/life15081320

Keywords: non-variceal upper gastrointestinal bleeding; peptic ulcer; retrospective cohort; endoscopic therapy; surgical intervention; risk factors; historical comparison; management algorithm

1. Introduction

Upper gastrointestinal bleeding (UGIB), defined as hemorrhage originating proximal to the ligament of Treitz, typically presents with hematemesis, coffee-ground emesis, or melena and remains a common medical emergency [1]. It accounts for over 300,000 hospital admissions annually in the United States, with mortality ranging from 3.5% to 10%, particularly affecting older adults and males [2]. While the incidence has declined due to a reduction in peptic ulcer disease (PUD), rebleeding remains a concern and is closely associated with increased mortality [3].

The most frequent causes of non-variceal UGIB are PUD (20–50%), gastroduodenal erosions (8–15%), esophagitis (5–15%), Mallory–Weiss tears (8–15%), vascular malformations, and neoplastic lesions [4,5]. Major risk factors include *Helicobacter pylori* infection, NSAID use, stress-related mucosal injury, and acid hypersecretion. Notably, *H. pylori*-positive ulcers are associated with better outcomes, while idiopathic ulcers (negative for NSAIDs and *H. pylori*) correlate with increased severity and systemic disease burden [5,6].

Endoscopic therapy remains the standard of care, with injection (e.g., epinephrine), thermal (e.g., argon plasma coagulation), and mechanical methods (e.g., hemoclips) applied based on lesion characteristics [7–10]. Novel agents such as TC-325 (Hemospray) provide non-contact hemostasis but are primarily used as adjuncts due to their transient mucosal effect [11–15].

Despite advances in diagnostic and therapeutic techniques, variability in outcomes persists across populations, and regional data from Eastern Europe—particularly Romania—remain limited and dispersed. National studies conducted more than a decade ago nonetheless provide a valuable basis for examining practice patterns and factors associated with outcomes in real-world settings.

The objective of this study was to analyze the clinical features, management strategies, and outcomes of patients with non-variceal upper gastrointestinal bleeding (NVUGIB) admitted to our center. A comparative assessment with data from the Romanian and international literature was conducted to identify relevant differences in epidemiology, treatment approaches, and prognostic factors. This analysis aimed to enhance the understanding of NVUGIB patterns in our setting and support evidence-based improvements in patient care.

2. Materials and Methods

2.1. Study Design and Setting

This retrospective observational study included 364 adult patients diagnosed with non-variceal upper gastrointestinal bleeding (NVUGIB), admitted to the First Surgical Clinic of the Emergency County Clinical Hospital of Craiova between 1 January 2009 and 31 December 2014.

2.2. Inclusion and Exclusion Criteria

Inclusion criteria comprised patients aged ≥18 years with a confirmed diagnosis of NVUGIB based on clinical presentation, laboratory data, and upper gastrointestinal endoscopy (UGIE). Exclusion criteria included variceal upper gastrointestinal bleeding, lower gastrointestinal bleeding, incomplete medical records, or comorbidities that could significantly confound bleeding etiology assessment.

2.3. Data Collection

The following variables were recorded for each patient:

- **demographics**: age, sex;
- **bleeding etiology** and **comorbidities**: cardiovascular, pulmonary, renal, and hepatic diseases;
- **risk factors**: prior peptic ulcer, gastritis, Mallory–Weiss syndrome, liver cirrhosis, chronic alcohol use, NSAIDs, acetylsalicylic acid, paracetamol, oral anticoagulants.

Pre-admission medications were abstracted verbatim from clinical charts and emergency department notes. Records did not consistently capture dose, duration, or concomitant use; therefore, each agent was categorized individually, and simultaneous NSAID co-use could not be confirmed.

- **Baseline laboratory parameters**: hemoglobin, hematocrit, platelet count, creatinine, urea;
- **timing variables**: onset-to-admission, admission-to-endoscopy, and onset-to-surgery intervals;
- **endoscopic findings**, lesion types and classification;
- **therapeutic interventions**: medical, endoscopic, and surgical;
- **clinical outcomes**: mortality, rebleeding, and drug-related bleeding.

2.4. Endoscopic and Surgical Management

All patients underwent UGIE within 24 h of admission, following ESGE guidelines. Therapeutic procedures included adrenaline injection and hemoclip placement. Surgery was reserved for patients with failed conservative management or recurrent bleeding.

Patients on oral anticoagulants (vitamin K antagonists or direct oral anticoagulants) were managed according to international guidelines. This included temporary cessation of anticoagulation, intravenous PPI therapy, and, when necessary, administration of prothrombin complex concentrate (PCC) or fresh frozen plasma (FFP), alongside tailored fluid and transfusion therapy.

2.5. Statistical Analysis

Descriptive statistics were reported as mean $\pm$ standard deviation (SD) for continuous variables. Due to the absence of time-to-event data, survival analyses were not performed. Comparative analyses with national and international data (e.g., Alharabi, Romcea, Matei, Botianu, Groza) were descriptively conducted. Inferential statistical tests included Student's t-test and Chi-square tests. A p-value < 0.05 was considered statistically significant. Data were processed using Microsoft Excel 2019 (Microsoft Corp., Redmond, WA, USA) with XLSTAT (Addinsoft SARL, Paris, France).

2.6. Ethics Statement

This study was conducted in accordance with the Declaration of Helsinki and was approved by the Ethics Committee of the Emergency County Clinical Hospital of Craiova (approval number 32909/14 July 2025). Informed consent for the use of medical data in research was obtained from all patients at admission, as part of the standard hospital documentation. This included patients who later died. All data were anonymized prior to analysis.

3. Results

The results section presents a detailed comparative analysis of our study population and the findings reported in the relevant literature. The data include demographic characteristics, clinical and endoscopic findings, baseline laboratory parameters, triggering factors, therapeutic approaches (medical, endoscopic, and surgical), as well as outcome measures such as mortality and rebleeding rates.

In our cohort, 364 patients were diagnosed with non-variceal upper gastrointestinal bleeding (NVUGIB). Of these, 256 were male (approximately 70%) and 108 were female (approximately 30%—Figure 1).

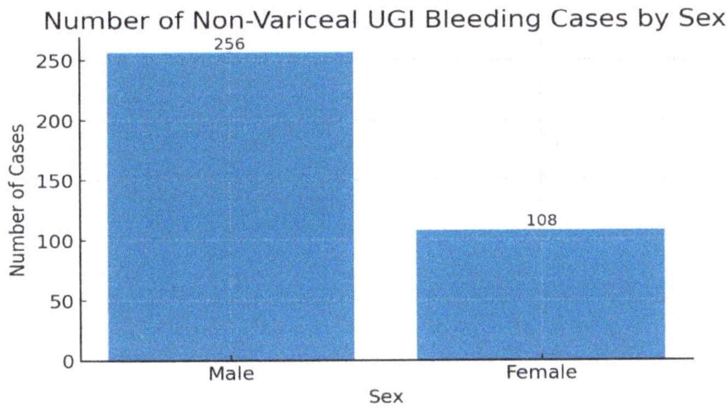

Figure 1. Sex distribution of patients with non-variceal upper gastrointestinal bleeding reported in our study.

The mean age and standard deviation of patients with upper gastrointestinal bleeding in our study are shown in Figure 2.

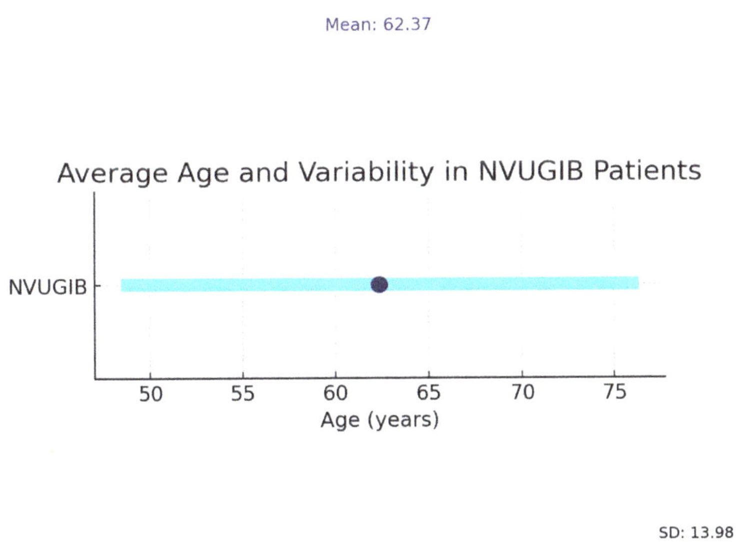

Figure 2. Mean age and standard deviation (SD) of patients with NVUGIB.

Analysis of the patients' personal medical history showed that the most frequent underlying condition was peptic ulcer disease, diagnosed in **192** patients (**52.7%**). Gastritis was reported in **132** cases, while liver cirrhosis was documented in **98** patients (**26.9%**).

Alcohol consumption was recorded in **206** individuals (**56.6%**). Additional comorbidities included cardiovascular disease (**145** cases), pulmonary disease (**41** cases) and osteoarticular conditions (**28** cases). These findings are summarized in Figure 3.

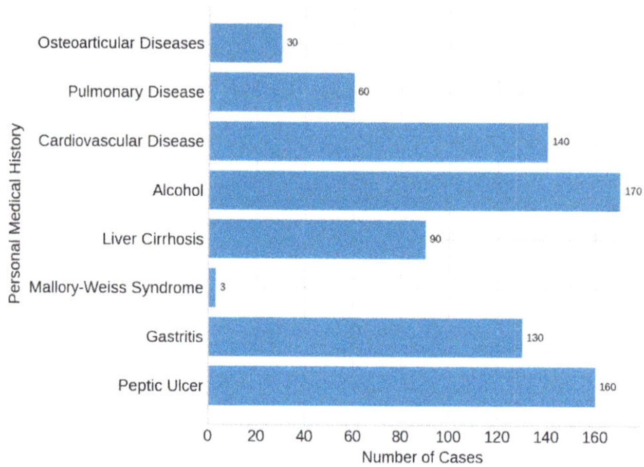

Figure 3. Patients' personal medical history in UGIB.

Endoscopic evaluation in our cohort revealed that gastroduodenal ulcers were the predominant finding among patients with non-variceal upper gastrointestinal bleeding (Figure 4).

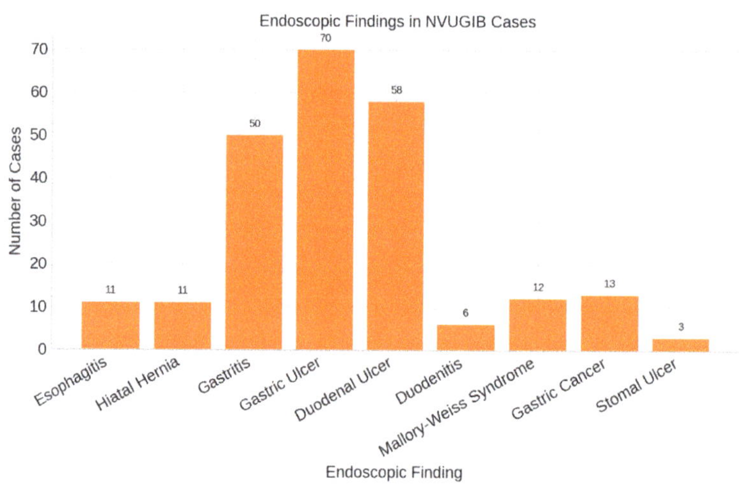

Figure 4. Endoscopic findings in NVUGIB.

In our cohort, drug-related triggers for upper gastrointestinal bleeding included non-steroidal anti-inflammatory drugs (NSAIDs) in 36.2% of patients, acetylsalicylic acid in 7.1%, paracetamol in 1.9%, anticoagulants in 9.3%, and corticosteroids in 2.5%. Alcohol consumption was recorded in 56.6% of patients. These data are summarized in Figure 5. Information on concomitant NSAID use (e.g., acetylsalicylic acid with another NSAID) was unavailable.

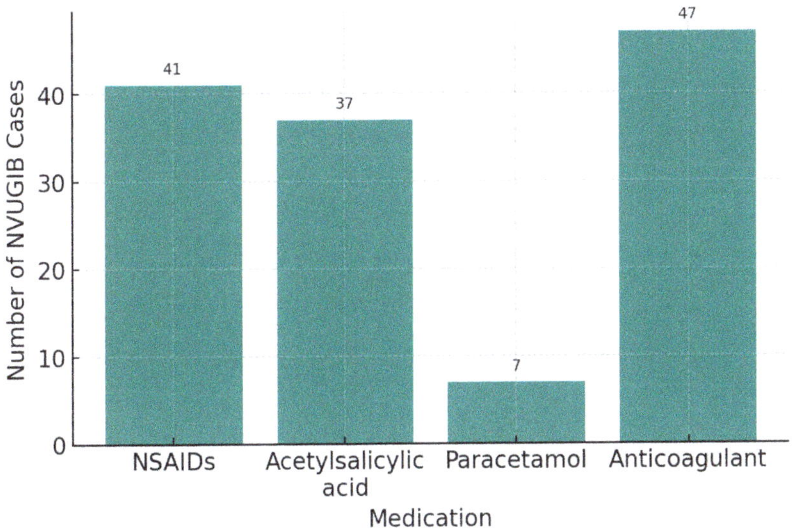

Figure 5. Medication use in NVUGIB cases. Legend: NSAIDs = non-steroidal anti-inflammatory drugs.

Among the 364 patients with non-variceal upper gastrointestinal bleeding, 49 (13.5%) were classified as Grade I (Hb 10–12 g/dL), 130 (35.7%) as Grade II (Hb 8–10 g/dL), 140 (38.5%) as Grade III (Hb 5–8 g/dL), and 45 (12.4%) as Grade IV (Hb < 5 g/dL). Grade III was the most frequent severity category observed (Figure 6).

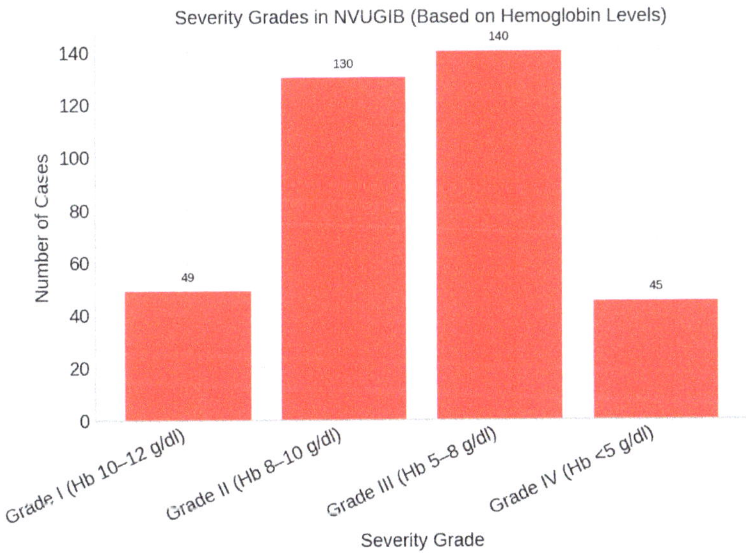

Figure 6. Severity grades in non-variceal upper gastrointestinal bleeding (based on hemoglobin levels).

The type of antisecretory therapy administered in non-variceal upper gastrointestinal bleeding was analyzed, with the distribution of patients receiving H2-receptor antagonists, proton pump inhibitors, or combination therapy (Figure 7).

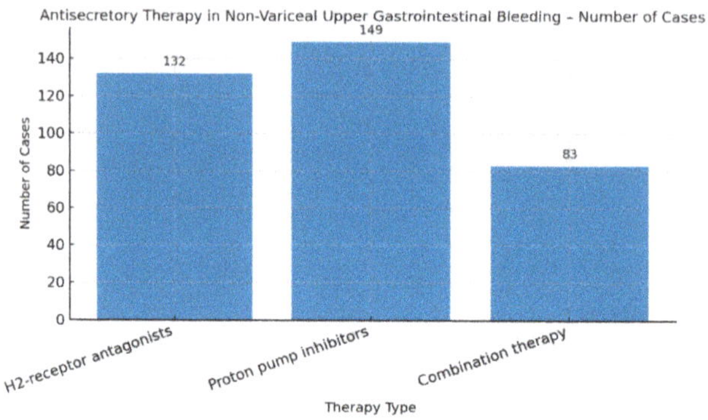

Figure 7. Distribution of antisecretory therapy types administered in non-variceal upper gastrointestinal bleeding. Legend: H2-receptor antagonists = histamine type 2 receptor antagonists.

In our study, bipolar electrocoagulation was the most frequently used endoscopic therapy for non-variceal upper gastrointestinal bleeding (Figure 8).

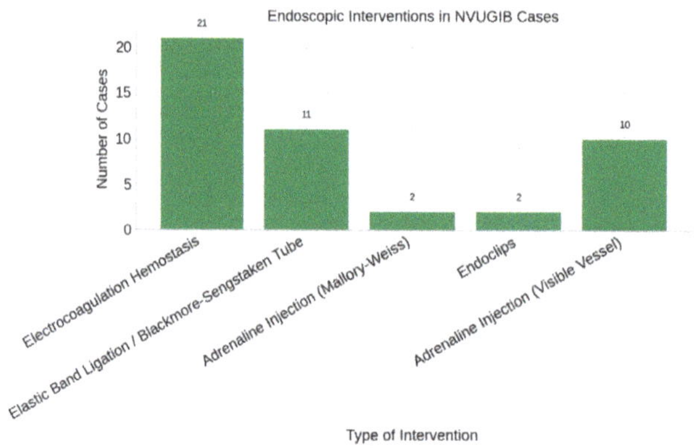

Figure 8. Endoscopic interventions performed in non-variceal upper gastrointestinal bleeding cases.

In our cohort, the mortality rate for non-variceal upper gastrointestinal bleeding was 10.9%, as shown in Figure 9.

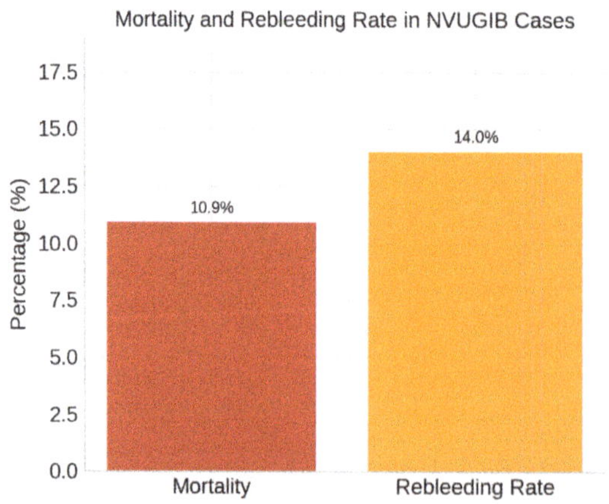

Figure 9. Mortality and rebleeding rate.

An important factor influencing patient outcomes in non-variceal upper gastrointestinal bleeding is the timing of surgical intervention (Figure 10).

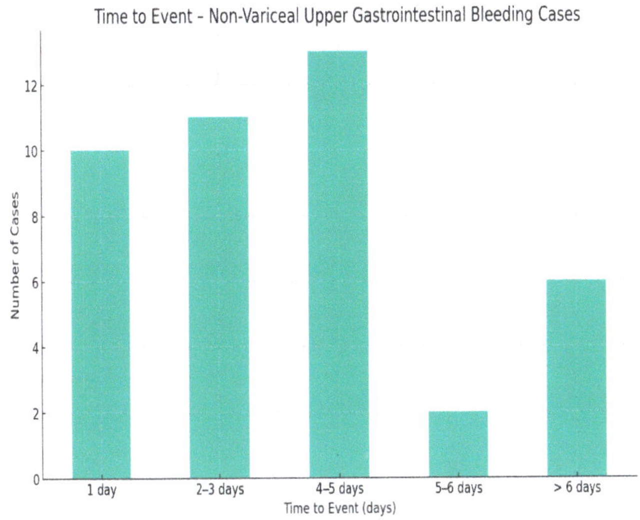

Figure 10. Distribution of cases by onset-to-surgery interval.

Rebleeding occurred more frequently in patients who underwent surgical treatment; however, this difference was not statistically significant in univariate analysis ($p > 0.05$) (Figure 11).

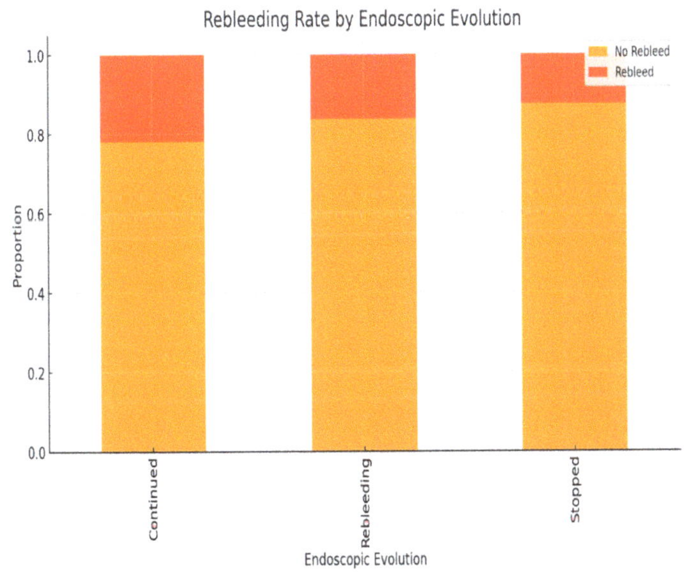

Figure 11. Proportion of patients with and without rebleeding, stratified by type of treatment (conservative vs. surgical).

NSAID use was associated with a higher proportion of rebleeding episodes. This difference reached statistical significance (χ^2 test, $p < 0.05$), suggesting that NSAIDs may be an independent risk factor for rebleeding (Figure 12).

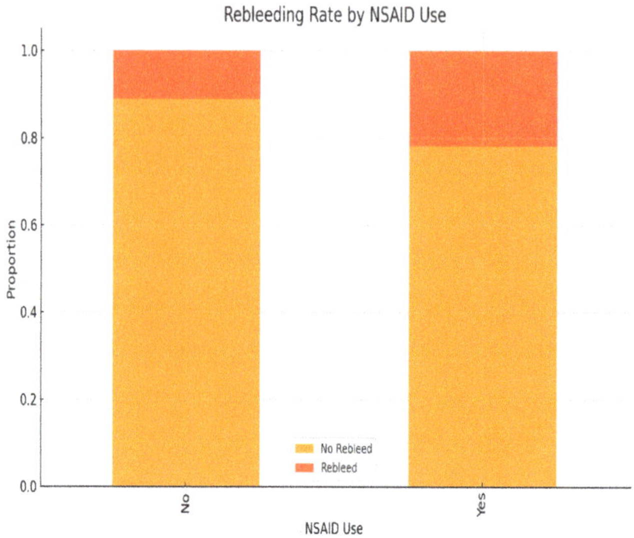

Figure 12. Comparison of rebleeding rates in patients with and without NSAID use.

As expected, rebleeding was more frequently observed in patients whose bleeding had initially continued or recurred after endoscopic management. The association was statistically significant ($p < 0.01$) (Figure 13).

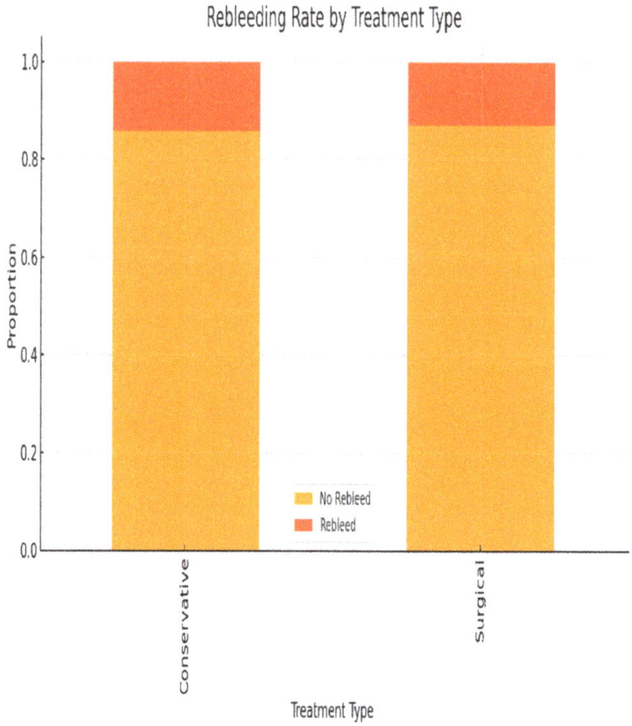

Figure 13. Rebleeding distribution based on the initial endoscopic evolution (bleeding stopped, continued, or recurred).

Multivariate logistic regression identified low hemoglobin at admission and alcohol use as independent predictors of rebleeding ($p < 0.05$). Endoscopic therapy was significantly associated with a reduced risk of rebleeding ($p < 0.01$). Age and NSAID use were not statistically significant in the multivariate model (Table 1).

Table 1. Multivariate logistic regression analysis of factors associated with rebleeding in NVUGIB (n = 364).

Variable	Odds Ratio (OR)	95% Confidence Interval	*p*-Value
Age (years)	1.04	1.01–1.07	0.011
Hemoglobin (g/dL)	0.82	0.69–0.97	0.017
Alcohol use (Yes vs. No)	2.15	1.18–3.91	0.013
Anticoagulant use (Yes vs. No)	2.45	1.21–4.98	0.012
Surgical intervention (Yes)	2.92	1.32–6.48	0.008

Legend: *p*-value = probability value.

The rate of surgical intervention for upper gastrointestinal bleeding was 11.5%. A comprehensive summary of the surgical techniques employed for non-variceal upper gastrointestinal bleeding, including the types of procedures and their respective case counts, is presented in Figure 14.

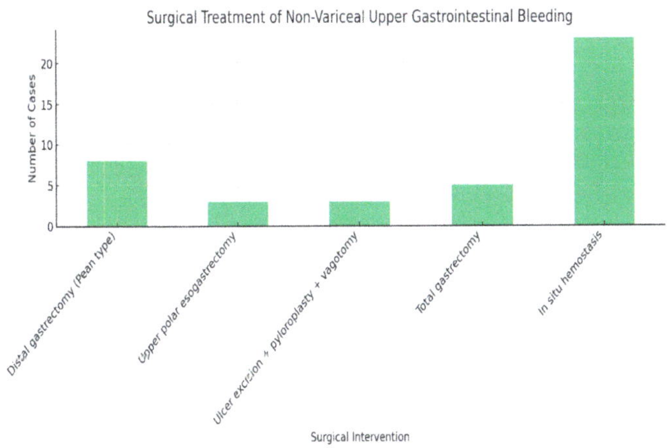

Figure 14. Surgical treatment of NVGIB.

Multivariate analysis showed that rebleeding, low hemoglobin levels, and ulcerative lesions were significantly associated with the need for surgical intervention, while age and alcohol use were not (Table 2).

Table 2. Multivariate logistic regression analysis of factors associated with surgical intervention in NVUGIB (n = 364).

Variable	Odds Ratio (OR)	95% Confidence Interval	*p*-Value
Age (years)	1.01	0.97–1.05	0.510
Hemoglobin (g/dL)	0.75	0.61–0.93	0.008
Rebleeding (Yes vs. No)	3.90	2.00–7.60	<0.001
Ulcerative lesion (Yes/No)	2.15	1.10–4.20	0.024
Alcohol use (Yes vs. No)	1.42	0.76–2.65	0.270

Legend: *p*-value = probability value.

Multivariate analysis identified older age, low hemoglobin levels, alcohol use, anticoagulant therapy, and surgical intervention as independent predictors of in-hospital mortality (Table 3).

Table 3. Multivariate logistic regression analysis of factors associated with in-hospital mortality in NVUGIB (n = 364).

Variable	Odds Ratio (OR)	95% Confidence Interval	*p*-Value
Age (years)	1.04	1.01–1.07	0.011
Hemoglobin (g/dL)	0.82	0.69–0.97	0.017
Alcohol use (Yes vs. No)	2.15	1.18–3.91	0.013
Anticoagulant use (Yes vs. No)	2.45	1.21–4.98	0.012
Surgical intervention (Yes)	2.92	1.32–6.48	0.008

Legend: *p*-value = probability value.

Student's *t*-test and Chi-square tests were used for statistical comparisons. Patients who died were significantly older than survivors (68.4 ± 11.2 vs. 61.6 ± 14.1 years; $p = 0.0005$). Alcohol consumption was not significantly associated with mortality ($p = 0.1001$). Type of antisecretory therapy showed significant distribution differences ($p = 0.0001$), while trends in endoscopic therapy ($p = 0.0911$) and timing of surgery ($p = 0.0565$) did not reach statistical significance. Surgical procedure types differed significantly across categories ($p < 0.0001$) (Table 4).

Table 4. Statistical comparison of clinical and therapeutic variables in relation to patient outcomes in non-variceal upper gastrointestinal bleeding.

Comparison	Test Type	Value	*p*-Value	Statistical Significance
Mean age: deceased vs. survivors	Student's *t*-test	t = 3.51	0.0005	significant
Mortality: alcohol users vs. non-users	Chi-square	$\chi^2 = 2.70$	0.1001	not significant
Type of antisecretory therapy	Chi-square	$\chi^2 = 19.36$	0.0001	significant
Type of endoscopic treatment	Chi-square	$\chi^2 = 4.79$	0.0911	borderline
Surgery timing intervals	Chi-square	$\chi^2 = 9.19$	0.0565	borderline
Types of surgical interventions	Chi-square	$\chi^2 = 33.71$	<0.0001	significant

Legend: *p*-value = probability value, Student's *t*-test = a statistical test used to compare the means of two groups, Chi-square = a statistical test used to determine whether there is a significant association between categorical variables, χ^2—Chi-square statistic, a measure used to evaluate the association between categorical variables. Statistical significance—interpretation of *p*-value results: significant ($p < 0.05$), not significant ($p \geq 0.05$), borderline (*p* close to 0.05).

4. Discussion

Upper gastrointestinal bleeding (UGIB) remains a critical medical–surgical emergency associated with significant morbidity, mortality, and healthcare burden, including in Eastern Europe [16–18]. Recent guidelines from the American College of Gastroenterology (ACG) have introduced key updates in the management of ulcer-related UGIB. These include a more selective approach to hospitalization, with outpatient management recommended for patients with a Glasgow-Blatchford Score (GBS) of 0–1, given their low risk of intervention or death. A restrictive transfusion strategy is also advised, with a hemoglobin threshold of 7 g/dL in stable patients, supported by evidence indicating lower rebleeding and mortality rates [18].

The ACG further recommends intravenous erythromycin prior to endoscopy to improve mucosal visualization and reduce the duration of hospitalization. Post-endoscopic care should involve high-dose proton pump inhibitor (PPI) therapy, either by continuous infusion or intermittent dosing, maintained for a minimum of 72 h. Additionally, advanced endoscopic techniques such as hemostatic powder spray (TC-325) and over-the-scope clips (OTSCs) are recognized as effective rescue tools for controlling active or recurrent bleeding [18].

In the present study, non-variceal UGIB was diagnosed in 364 patients, reflecting a high incidence consistent with the previous literature. Although data collection occurred before the widespread adoption of newer hemostatic methods and guideline updates, this study offers valuable real-world insight into clinical management within a tertiary care setting in Eastern Europe. Notably, male patients were nearly twice as frequently affected as females, likely due to increased exposure to modifiable risk factors including NSAID use, alcohol consumption, and smoking (Figure 1). This distribution aligns with prior European and global findings.

Incidence increased with age in our cohort, differing from findings by Pongprasobchai et al. [19], who observed stable rates across age groups, and Matei et al. [20], who reported overall lower incidence (Figure 2).

From patients' medical history, the main causes of non-variceal UGIB were gastroduodenal ulcers, gastritis, Mallory–Weiss syndrome, and liver cirrhosis. Key risk factors included alcohol use and comorbidities such as cardiovascular, pulmonary, and osteoarticular diseases. These findings align with Alharbi et al. [16], who also identified ulcers and cirrhosis as leading etiologies (Figure 3).

The predominance of gastroduodenal ulcers in our cohort is consistent with both Romanian and international data, where duodenal ulcer is the leading cause of non-variceal UGIB (Figure 4). Erosive gastritis is also common, though its prevalence varies due to differences in diagnostic methods and populations. Rare lesions, such as Dieulafoy's lesion and angiodysplasia, were infrequently observed. Overall, major etiologies appear consistent across studies, with variations shaped by local epidemiology and healthcare practices.

Although not statistically significant, the slightly higher rebleeding rate observed among surgically treated patients may reflect more advanced disease at presentation or suboptimal response to initial endoscopic management (Figure 11).

Our findings support the well-established role of NSAIDs as a risk factor for upper gastrointestinal mucosal damage and recurrence of bleeding, underlining the need for careful risk stratification and gastroprotective strategies in high-risk patients (Figure 12).

These findings reinforce the prognostic value of persistent or recurrent bleeding following endoscopic intervention and highlight the importance of close monitoring and timely escalation of care (Figure 13).

Our findings confirm that low hemoglobin levels and alcohol consumption significantly increase the risk of rebleeding, in line with previous reports. The protective effect of endoscopic therapy was also consistent with established data (Table 1).

The increased likelihood of surgical intervention in patients with rebleeding, low hemoglobin levels, or ulcerative lesions emphasizes the role of early risk stratification. Age and alcohol use did not reach statistical significance, suggesting a lesser impact on surgical decision-making in our cohort (Table 2).

These findings suggest that advanced age, anemia, alcohol use, and anticoagulant therapy contribute significantly to mortality risk in upper gastrointestinal bleeding. The association with surgical intervention may reflect the severity of cases requiring operative management. Early recognition of these high-risk factors is essential for optimizing patient outcomes (Table 3).

Older age was significantly associated with in-hospital mortality, confirming its role as a key risk factor in UGIB. Although alcohol use did not reach statistical significance, the observed trend suggests a potential contribution. The significant variation in antisecretory therapy and surgical procedures underscores the impact of individualized treatment strategies on clinical outcomes (Table 4).

4.1. Anticoagulation and Endoscopic Timing

Upper gastrointestinal bleeding (UGIB) in patients on chronic oral anticoagulants poses a therapeutic dilemma, requiring careful risk–benefit assessment between bleeding and thromboembolism. UGIB occurs in up to 20% of anticoagulated patients, with endoscopy essential for diagnosis and management, despite the absence of a consistent bleeding site.

Direct oral anticoagulants (DOACs), widely used for atrial fibrillation and venous thromboembolism, carry a bleeding risk comparable to or higher than warfarin. Although DOACs offer predictable pharmacokinetics and rapid clearance, they lack routine monitoring tools and universally available reversal agents. In acute UGIB, therapy should be promptly discontinued, with time serving as a key mitigating factor due to short half-lives. PCCs or activated PCCs may be used in severe cases; hemodialysis is effective only for dabigatran. Current guidance is largely expert-based, highlighting the need for robust clinical data [21–24].

In major bleeding, the American College of Clinical Pharmacology recommends prompt anticoagulant cessation and reversal with prothrombin complex concentrate (PCC) over fresh frozen plasma (FFP), along with 5–10 mg IV vitamin K [25]. PCCs, containing factors II, VII, IX, and X, offer rapid correction and are available in inactive or activated forms.

Conversely, the American College of Cardiology advises using FFP—without vitamin K—in patients with mechanical valves due to thrombosis risk [26].

Gastrointestinal bleeding under vitamin K antagonist (VKA) therapy requires urgent reversal, especially in unstable patients or those with high INR. ESGE guidelines favor PCC over FFP due to faster INR normalization, lower volume, and better bleeding control during endoscopy [26–28].

In anticoagulated patients, vitamin K antagonists (VKAs) should be withheld and reversed under specialist supervision. Recent guidelines recommend that direct oral anticoagulants (DOACs) should also be temporarily discontinued in the setting of acute non-variceal upper gastrointestinal bleeding (NVUGIB); however, endoscopy should not be delayed due to ongoing anticoagulation [1]. In cases of severe or life-threatening bleeding, reversal agents such as idarucizumab (for dabigatran) or andexanet alfa (for factor Xa inhibitors), or prothrombin complex concentrate (PCC), may be considered—although the evidence supporting their use is limited [2].

Resumption Strategies After Hemostasis

The 2022 International Consensus recommends resuming DOACs within 48–72 h after successful endoscopic hemostasis, in line with observational data showing no increased rebleeding risk. Acetylsalicylic acid for secondary prevention should be resumed within 3 days, provided bleeding is controlled [29].

Our data confirm NSAIDs and alcohol as leading triggers of NVUGIB, consistent with other Romanian and international studies. Compared to Alharbi et al. [16], who reported higher rates for paracetamol and anticoagulants, our lower values may reflect local prescribing patterns. Minor differences in acetylsalicylic acid and corticosteroid use across studies likely result from population risk profiles and access to gastroprotective strategies (Figure 5). These laboratory findings are comparable to those reported by Matei [20], indicating similar clinical profiles among patients with NVUGIB.

The ESGE guidelines recommend early assessment of hemodynamic status and prompt resuscitation with crystalloids in unstable patients. A restrictive transfusion strategy is advised, targeting hemoglobin 7–9 g/dL, with higher thresholds for those with cardiac comorbidities. Risk stratification, especially via the Glasgow-Blatchford Score (GBS), is essential to guide early discharge or urgent intervention [28].

4.2. Pharmacological Therapy

Proton pump inhibitors (PPIs) were the primary antisecretory therapy, used in 41% of non-variceal UGIB cases (Figure 7), while 36% received H2-receptor antagonists (H2RAs), and 23% a combination of both. These data reflect the preference for PPIs as first-line treatment.

H2RAs, though historically used, show limited efficacy in acute peptic ulcer bleeding due to rapid tolerance development and reduced acid suppression over time [30]. Comparative studies have shown PPIs maintain gastric pH more effectively than H2RAs. In our cohort, outcomes were similar between treatment groups, limiting definitive conclusions on superiority.

High-dose intravenous PPI therapy (80 mg bolus followed by 8 mg/h infusion for 72 h) has proven effective post-endoscopic treatment in patients with high-risk bleeding stigmata. Lau et al. reported a significant rebleeding reduction—from 22.5% to 6.7%—with PPI therapy [31].

In contrast, a large study (n = 1256) found no significant outcome difference between high-dose pantoprazole and ranitidine, though pantoprazole showed better overall efficacy. The unusually low rebleeding rate in the ranitidine group (3.2%) may explain this discrepancy [32].

A meta-analysis by Leontiadis et al. (24 RCTs, n = 4373) confirmed that PPIs significantly reduce rebleeding, surgery, repeat endoscopy, and mortality in non-variceal UGIB [33]. Similar benefits were reported by Laine et al., particularly with high-dose IV PPI therapy versus placebo [10].

Current guidelines support an 80 mg IV bolus followed by 8 mg/h infusion for 72 h, even without prior endoscopy, especially in patients with adherent clots [10,34]. Although Andriulli et al. found no dose-dependent differences, their results are limited by study design [34]. A meta-analysis by Wang et al. (7 RCTs, n = 1157) also found no clear advantage of high-dose over standard-dose PPI post-endoscopy [35].

Despite mixed findings, international consensus continues to recommend high dose PPI infusion post-endoscopic hemostasis, which aligns with our clinical practice [31].

Pre-endoscopic PPI therapy reduces high-risk stigmata and the need for intervention but has no clear effect on rebleeding, surgery, or mortality. Tranexamic acid may reduce mortality, though evidence is outdated and inconsistent. Somatostatin and octreotide offer limited benefit and are not routinely recommended. IV erythromycin improves gastric visualization and reduces transfusions, repeat endoscopy, and hospital stay. Metoclopramide is less studied and poses neurological risks, warranting cautious use [36,37].

In the 1980s, investigators such as Graham [38] and Peterson [39] questioned the routine use of endoscopy in upper gastrointestinal bleeding (UGIB) due to the limited availability of effective therapeutic interventions at the time. This perspective shifted following a landmark 1990 meta-analysis by Sacks et al. [40], which demonstrated that endoscopic hemostasis significantly reduced rebleeding, the need for surgery, and mortality. This established endoscopy as a cornerstone in UGIB management. However, concerns about the safety of early endoscopy emerged in the mid-1990s, as studies by Yen [41] and Hill [42] reported higher rates of oxygen desaturation during urgent procedures in high-risk, unsedated patients without oxygen supplementation—conditions that differ substantially from current clinical practice.

Beyond safety, routine early endoscopy poses logistical and financial challenges. Maintaining 24/7 endoscopy services requires substantial staffing and infrastructure, especially in non-tertiary centers. Additionally, early procedures may detect transient stigmata, leading to potentially unnecessary interventions and increased costs.

Despite initial concerns, subsequent evidence supports the benefit of early endoscopy (within 24 h) in most patients with UGIB. Meta-analyses and cohort studies show that early intervention is associated with reduced hospital stay, lower transfusion needs, and fewer complications, particularly in high-risk patients [43–46].

According to the updated ESGE 2024 guideline, very early endoscopy (<6 h) is recommended only in unstable patients, while routine early endoscopy (<24 h) remains the standard of care. Additionally, topical hemostatic agents such as Hemospray are now recognized as temporary rescue options when conventional endoscopic methods fail [30].

Massive UGIB requires emergency endoscopy after hemodynamic stabilization; in active bleeding, it may proceed during resuscitation. Caution is warranted in elderly and comorbid patients due to reduced tolerance to hypovolemia and increased risk of organ dysfunction.

Standard management includes endoscopic hemostasis followed by acid suppression, which lowers rebleeding risk and improves outcomes [43]. Gastric acidity impairs clot stability by inhibiting platelet function and promoting fibrinolysis. A gastric pH > 4–6 supports hemostasis, while pH < 2 activates pepsin, leading to clot lysis [44,45].

The rationale for acid suppression in UGIB lies in the negative impact of gastric acid on clot stability, including:

- inhibition of platelet aggregation;
- clot lysis via pepsin activation at low pH;
- enhanced fibrinolysis in acidic environments;
- optimal clot stability at pH 6–6.5, as shown in experimental models [46].

4.3. Endoscopic Therapy

Endoscopic therapy is the first-line treatment for bleeding gastroduodenal ulcers, including massive hemorrhage. It enables source identification, excludes variceal bleeding, and guides risk stratification via endoscopic stigmata. Early endoscopy improves outcomes, especially in cases with active bleeding or visible vessels.

ESGE recommends endoscopy within 24 h, or <12 h for high-risk patients. The Forrest classification is used to guide therapy: Forrest Ia, Ib, IIa, and IIb (after clot removal) require hemostasis, while IIc and III do not. Epinephrine should be combined with mechanical or thermal methods, not used alone [30].

For non-ulcer lesions (e.g., Mallory–Weiss, Dieulafoy, angioectasias, tumors), endoscopic therapy is recommended despite limited long-term data. If endoscopy fails or is not feasible, transcatheter angiographic embolization (TAE) or surgery should be considered [47].

Risk stratification in acute UGIH is critical for guiding intervention and determining inpatient vs. outpatient care. The Glasgow-Blatchford Score (GBS) and Rockall score are widely validated, predicting the need for intervention and mortality, respectively.

Recent APAGE recommendations support incorporating serum lactate levels alongside clinical scoring systems such as the Glasgow-Blatchford Score to better stratify high-risk patients with UGIB [48].

In our cohort, interventional endoscopy was performed in 19.8% of cases—lower than rates reported by Botianu et al. [49] (Figure 9). Techniques included epinephrine injection, hemoclips, and bipolar electrocoagulation in select cases, underscoring its role when pharmacologic therapy is insufficient.

A meta-analysis by Cook et al. (30 trials) confirmed that endoscopic therapy significantly reduces rebleeding, surgery, and mortality, particularly in patients with active bleeding or visible vessels [50]. Kahi et al. later showed that endoscopic treatment of ulcers with adherent clots reduced rebleeding (8.2%) compared to medical therapy alone (24.7%) [51].

Adding a second endoscopic modality during the same session reduces rebleeding (18.8% to 10.4%), need for surgery (10.8% to 7.1%), and mortality (5% to 2.5%), regardless of technique. Hemoclips and thermal coagulation are both effective, with hemoclips mimicking surgical ligation.

However, hemoclips may be technically limited in fibrotic ulcers, difficult angles, or multiple bleeding sites. In one RCT, deployment failure occurred in 10% of cases due to device-related issues [52].

4.4. Limitations of Endoscopic Therapy in Severe Gastrointestinal Bleeding

A key limitation of endoscopic hemostasis is bleeding from erosion into large-caliber arteries, where control is difficult. As per Poiseuille's law, small increases in vessel diameter lead to exponential rises in flow, complicating endoscopic efficacy.

In a pre-endoscopy era study, Swain et al. analyzed 27 emergency gastrectomies for bleeding ulcers and found average arterial diameters of 0.7 mm (range: 0.1–1.8 mm). Nearly half were subserosal vessels, with some showing aneurysmal dilation, especially in large, penetrating ulcers. These anatomical factors present major challenges for endoscopic treatment [53].

In a follow-up study, Swain reported a mean arterial diameter of 3.75 mm at bleeding sites in fatal gastric ulcer cases, highlighting the limitations of endoscopic therapy in large-vessel erosion [53].

For high-risk NVUGIB (Forrest Ia, Ib, IIa), endoscopic hemostasis—via injection, thermal, or mechanical methods—is superior to pharmacotherapy alone. Meta-analyses support combination therapy (e.g., epinephrine plus clips or thermal coagulation) as the most effective strategy to reduce rebleeding and surgical need [30,54].

Topical agents such as Hemospray are now endorsed in the ESGE 2024 guideline as temporary rescue options when standard endoscopic modalities fail [55,56].

While erosive esophagitis, gastritis, and duodenitis often respond to high-dose PPI therapy without endoscopy, early endoscopy remains critical for risk stratification and treatment of Mallory–Weiss tears, Dieulafoy lesions, angioectasias, and tumors. In these cases, combined endoscopic modalities offer improved hemostasis, though mortality benefits remain uncertain and require further evidence.

4.5. Post-Endoscopic Management

In post-endoscopic management of non-variceal upper gastrointestinal hemorrhage (NVUGIH), ESGE recommends high-dose PPI therapy (intravenous bolus followed by 72-h infusion) after successful hemostasis or in cases with adherent clots. Intermittent IV boluses or high-dose oral PPIs may be used in patients able to take oral medication.

The ACG guidelines emphasize that high-dose intravenous PPIs should be reserved for patients with high-risk endoscopic stigmata, while patients with clean-based ulcers may be managed with oral PPI therapy and do not require second-look endoscopy [18].

In cases of clinical rebleeding, repeat endoscopy is advised, with angiographic embolization or surgery if re-hemostasis fails.

Testing for *Helicobacter pylori* should be performed during the acute phase, with eradication therapy if positive and later confirmation of clearance.

Anticoagulation should be resumed based on individual thromboembolic risk, typically within 7–15 days, or earlier in high-risk patients. Recent international guidelines (e.g., ESGE, BSG, and ACG) recommend that acetylsalicylic acid used for secondary cardiovascular prevention should not be discontinued during episodes of non-variceal upper gastrointestinal bleeding (NVUGIB). If temporarily interrupted, acetylsalicylic acid therapy should be resumed as soon as hemostasis is confirmed endoscopically—ideally within 3 to 5 days. In contrast, in cases where acetylsalicylic acid is prescribed for primary prevention, discontinuation may be considered, and resumption should be carefully re-evaluated based on individual risk–benefit balance. For patients on dual antiplatelet therapy (DAPT), acetylsalicylic acid should be maintained and the P2Y12 inhibitor restarted after endoscopic hemostasis in consultation with cardiology. PPI co-therapy is strongly recommended to minimize gastrointestinal risk [18,57,58].

Evidence-based guidelines for NVUGIH recommend high-dose PPI therapy (80 mg IV bolus followed by 8 mg/h infusion for 72 h) after endoscopic hemostasis, based on data showing reduced rebleeding, surgery, and mortality. However, recent meta-analyses, including that by Sachar et al., suggest that intermittent PPI dosing—oral or IV—may be non-inferior, though slightly higher rebleeding rates may require retreatment [32].

High-dose oral PPI regimens appear to achieve similar intragastric pH levels, but larger trials are needed to confirm their efficacy across populations with varying metabolism profiles [30,58].

Hemostatic powders and over-the-scope clips (OTSCs) are promising salvage options for refractory bleeding. Routine second-look endoscopy remains controversial due to limited benefit and cost-effectiveness, except in high-risk patients.

Peptic ulcer disease, primarily linked to *Helicobacter pylori*, remains the most frequent NVUGIH cause. Delayed testing improves accuracy, and eradication confirmation is essential to prevent recurrence.

Observational data support resuming anticoagulation around 7 days post-bleed to reduce thromboembolic risk and improve survival. Individualized decisions, including bridging strategies, may be necessary in high-risk patients [30,59].

In NVUGIH, acetylsalicylic acid can be safely resumed by day 3 in patients with high-risk endoscopic stigmata, balancing rebleeding risk with thrombotic prevention. In patients without high-risk stigmata, immediate resumption is appropriate, as PPIs support ulcer healing irrespective of antiplatelet use.

Although initial concerns existed about a potential interaction between clopidogrel and PPIs, recent randomized trials and propensity-matched studies show no significant increase in cardiovascular events. Meanwhile, PPI co-therapy effectively reduces GI bleeding, supporting its continued use in patients on dual antiplatelet therapy [30,47].

4.6. Predictive Factors for Endoscopic Therapy Failure in Upper Gastrointestinal Bleeding

Elmunzer et al. reviewed ten prospective studies on predictors of endoscopic therapy failure in upper gastrointestinal bleeding, identifying hemodynamic instability and significant comorbidities as key pre-endoscopic risk factors [60]. Intra-procedural predictors included active bleeding, large ulcer size, and ulcer location on the lesser curvature of the stomach or posterior wall of the duodenal bulb.

These locations are prone to erosion into major arteries such as the gastroduodenal or left gastric artery, often resulting in bleeding that exceeds the hemostatic capacity of current endoscopic methods. Therefore, hemodynamic instability, ongoing hemorrhage, large ulcer size, and posterior duodenal location are strong predictors of rebleeding and treatment failure, underscoring the anatomical and technical limitations of endoscopic intervention.

Non-variceal upper gastrointestinal bleeding should be assessed within a broader vascular context, as thrombotic vascular conditions such as ischemic colitis secondary to a thrombosed aortic aneurysm may indicate an underlying prothrombotic state with implications for both prognosis and therapeutic strategy [61].

4.7. The Role and Timing of Surgical Intervention in Upper Gastrointestinal Bleeding

Surgical intervention remains the definitive treatment for patients in whom endoscopic hemostasis fails or is not feasible. While often considered a clinical endpoint in studies on endoscopic efficacy, the need for surgery has markedly decreased with advances in endoscopic techniques and is now typically reserved for cases of life-threatening hemorrhage.

In our cohort, endoscopy was used for both diagnosis and treatment in 50.2% of gastroduodenal ulcer cases. Combined medical and endoscopic therapy was successful in 89.7% of patients, while 10.3% required surgery. Predictors of endoscopic failure included gastric ulcer location, large ulcer size, and hemodynamic instability—present in 41.6% of surgically managed cases.

Mortality after failed endoscopic therapy ranges between 15% and 25% [62]. Risk factors for failure include massive hemorrhage with hypotension, recurrent bleeding, advanced age, and unfavorable ulcer characteristics such as large size and difficult location. The optimal timing of surgical intervention remains debated, particularly since the 1980s.

Reported mortality rates for non-variceal upper gastrointestinal bleeding (NVUGIB) vary widely, from 2.6% [63] to 14% [64], depending on factors such as timeliness of endoscopy, use of standardized protocols, patient comorbidity, and access to specialized care.

In our study, the mortality rate was 10.9%, consistent with international reports ranging from 2.6% to 14% and reflecting comparable outcomes across diverse clinical settings. This closely aligns with the 10.43% mortality rate reported by Botianu [49], suggesting similar patient management strategies and risk profiles in Romania. Conversely, the higher mortality rate of 18.7% reported by Dicu [65] may be attributed to delayed interventions or differences in patient comorbidities.

Multivariate analysis revealed that increased age, low hemoglobin levels at admission, alcohol use, anticoagulant therapy, and surgical intervention were independently associated with in-hospital mortality. These findings emphasize the need for early recognition and aggressive management of high-risk patients.

Statistical analysis using *t*-tests and Chi-square tests confirmed that mortality was significantly associated with older age and type of antisecretory therapy. Timing of surgery approached statistical significance, while alcohol use did not show a statistically significant association with mortality. Tailored surgical approaches were significantly associated with patient outcome (Table 4).

Rebleeding rates showed notable variation, with our study (14%) closely aligning with the 12.02% reported by Botianu et al [49]. In contrast, Dicu [65] observed a significantly higher rate of 40.2%, likely reflecting differences in endoscopic technique, hemostasis protocols, and post-procedural care.

These findings underscore the persistent burden of mortality and rebleeding in non-variceal upper gastrointestinal bleeding and reinforce the need for improved diagnostic accuracy and standardized therapeutic strategies.

The Birmingham study evaluated 104 patients with bleeding peptic ulcers, comparing early versus delayed surgical intervention [66]. Early surgery was indicated by transfusion of ≥4 units in 24 h, rebleeding, high-risk endoscopic stigmata, or recent upper GI bleeding history. Delayed surgery was reserved for more extensive transfusion needs or repeated rebleeding.

In patients under 60, early surgery was performed in 52% compared to 5% in the delayed group. For those over 60, early surgery occurred in 62% versus 27%, indicating that both age and timing significantly influence the need for surgical intervention.

Applying similar criteria in our study, immediate surgery within 24 h was performed in 29.1% of cases, delayed emergency surgery (within 72 h) in 25%, and late interventions (beyond 72 h) in 45.9%. Among patients under 60 years, early surgery was required in 35% of cases, compared to 25% among those undergoing late intervention.

Saperas et al. evaluated 69 patients over 50 years old with non-arterial bleeding or stigmata of recent hemorrhage without a visible vessel, showing that neither early nor delayed surgery was required, supporting conservative management in the absence of high-risk endoscopic features [67].

These findings, along with prior data, suggest that early surgery should generally be avoided unless high-risk endoscopic stigmata are present. Endoscopic therapy remains the first-line treatment for peptic ulcer bleeding, with surgery reserved for refractory cases.

In rebleeding scenarios, the decision between repeat endoscopy and surgery remains debated. While some elderly, high-risk patients may benefit from a second-look endoscopy, persistent hypotension or multiple failed endoscopic attempts may delay definitive treatment. In such cases, timely surgical intervention may improve outcomes [66].

Cheung et al. treated 1169 patients with peptic ulcer bleeding using epinephrine injection followed by thermal coagulation over a 40-month period [66]. Endoscopic hemostasis failed in 17 patients who required surgery. The rebleeding rate after successful endoscopic therapy was 8.7%. No significant differences were observed in 30-day mortality, hospital stay, or transfusion requirements. However, surgical patients had a higher rate of post-operative complications. Repeat endoscopy controlled rebleeding in 75% of cases, indicating it may be a viable alternative to surgery in selected patients.

Ulcer size > 2 cm and hypotension at rebleeding were independent predictors of endoscopic failure. In our cohort, these factors were present in 11 cases (9.73% of ulcer patients), accounting for 32.3% of surgeries for peptic ulcer bleeding.

Imhof et al. compared endoscopic fibrin glue injection to early surgery in patients with arterial bleeding or visible vessels ≥ 2 mm in peptic ulcers [68]. Rebleeding occurred in 50% of the endoscopy group versus 4% in the surgery group, with no significant difference in mortality. Early surgery offered more effective and definitive hemostasis in high-risk cases.

Bender et al. advocated for surgery in patients presenting with hemorrhagic shock, especially those over 65 years, with ulcers > 2 cm, high-risk stigmata, or prior ulcer complications [69]. Among 66 surgically treated patients followed over five years, no mortality was reported.

In our cohort, 211 patients were over 65 years; 38 had hemorrhagic shock and underwent surgery for bleeding peptic ulcers, including 4 with ulcers > 2 cm. Only one post-operative complication (anastomotic fistula) occurred, managed conservatively.

Mueller et al. operated on 157 patients with spurting hemorrhage, visible vessels in posterior duodenal ulcers, or transfusion needs >6 units in 24 h, or rebleeding within 48 h. The reported 30-day post-operative mortality was 7% [70].

4.8. Type of Surgical Intervention in Peptic Ulcer Bleeding

In the current era of proton pump inhibitors and *Helicobacter pylori* eradication, surgery in peptic ulcer bleeding aims primarily at achieving hemostasis rather than a definitive cure.

Poxon et al. [71] studied 137 patients treated surgically for bleeding ulcers. Rebleeding occurred in 6 of 62 patients undergoing oversewing, but none following conventional procedures (e.g., ulcer excision with vagotomy or gastrectomy). The trial was halted due to high fatal rebleeding rates in conservative surgery groups, with mortality reaching 26% for oversewing and 19% for conventional surgery.

In our cohort, no rebleeding was observed after in situ hemostasis. Post-operative complications were mostly infectious, such as wound infections and fistulas.

Most surgeries occurred within 1–5 days of symptom onset, supporting a stepwise approach favoring initial medical and endoscopic therapy. Delayed surgeries (beyond six days) likely reflect initially successful conservative management or late-onset complications requiring surgical resolution (Figure 10).

In our cohort, 11.5% of patients with non-variceal upper gastrointestinal bleeding required surgery, slightly exceeding the 7.66% reported by Botianu et al. [49]. This difference may reflect variations in case severity, patient selection, or differences in the availability and effectiveness of endoscopic hemostasis prior to surgical intervention. Given the retrospective nature of our study and the study period (2009–2014), these findings also likely reflect the healthcare context in Eastern Europe at that time, when financial and infrastructural constraints limited uniform 24/7 access to functional endoscopic services, potentially leading to a higher proportion of surgical cases.

Among the 42 surgically treated patients in our series, in situ hemostasis was the most common approach (54.8%), reflecting a preference for limited, targeted bleeding control (Figure 14). Distal gastrectomy (19%) and ulcer excision with pyloroplasty and vagotomy (7%) were selectively performed, while extensive procedures such as total gastrectomy or upper polar esogastrectomy were reserved for complex cases. These data support a tailored surgical strategy focused on hemostasis and organ preservation.

Angiographic therapy was introduced in the 1970s as a surgical alternative for massive peptic ulcer bleeding [71], predating endoscopic hemostasis. Technological advances—such as microcatheters and improved embolic agents—have enhanced safety and durability, reducing ischemic complications.

Refractory ulcers often erode into major arteries: gastric ulcers along the lesser curvature may affect branches of the left gastric artery, while posterior duodenal ulcers typically involve the gastroduodenal or pancreaticoduodenal arteries [72].

Eriksson et al. introduced a technique using endoscopic clip placement to guide angiographic localization of bleeding sites [73]. Various embolic agents—such as cyanoacrylate, microspheres, and gelatin particles—can be used alone or in combination for vessel occlusion. Complications include gastric or duodenal infarction, hepatic ischemia, and delayed duodenal strictures [74], with adhesive agents requiring caution due to potential reflux into non-target vessels.

Angiographic embolization is effective in high-risk surgical candidates, after failed endoscopy, or in post-operative rebleeding. Technical success ranges from 90 to 100%, with clinical success between 50 and 83%.

Ripoll et al. compared surgery versus embolization, noting similar rebleeding (29% vs. 23%) and mortality rates (26% vs. 21%) despite older age and more comorbidities in the embolization group [75]. Eriksson et al. also reported lower 30-day mortality in embolized patients compared to those undergoing surgery after failed endoscopy, supporting embolization as a safer option in selected high-risk cases [73].

Effective management of upper gastrointestinal bleeding (UGIB) requires timely, structured clinical decisions to reduce morbidity and mortality. We propose a practical stepwise algorithm to guide clinicians from emergency evaluation to post-endoscopic care (Figure 15). This approach integrates current evidence and best practices, emphasizing early risk stratification, optimal resource use, and individualized therapy.

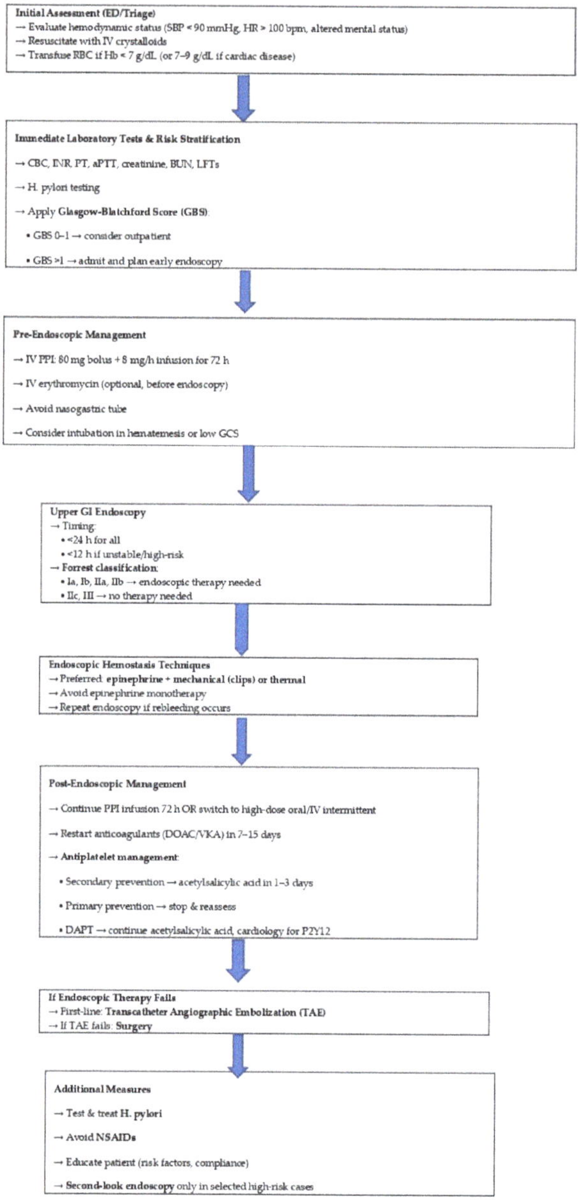

Figure 15. Stepwise approach to acute upper gastrointestinal bleeding.

4.9. Limitations

This study has several limitations. First, its retrospective design depends on the completeness and accuracy of medical records. Data on concurrent NSAID therapy—such as acetylsalicylic acid in combination with other non-steroidal anti-inflammatory drugs—were not systematically recorded, including dose and duration. Although comorbidities were documented, their influence on bleeding risk and patient outcomes was not explored in depth. These factors may affect the results and should be addressed in prospective studies with standardized data collection.

5. Conclusions

This retrospective study highlights that non-variceal upper gastrointestinal bleeding (NVUGIB) remains a significant clinical challenge, with peptic ulcer as the main cause. Independent risk factors for rebleeding and mortality were identified, including low hemoglobin at admission, alcohol use, advanced age, anticoagulant therapy, and the need for surgery. Endoscopic hemostasis significantly reduced the risk of rebleeding. Based on these findings, we propose an updated algorithm to optimize NVUGIB management, emphasizing early risk stratification, timely endoscopy, and individualized decisions regarding antithrombotic therapy.

Author Contributions: Conceptualization L.A.B. and N.-D.M.; writing—original draft L.A.B., A.B. and T.S.Ț.C.; resources L.C., L.V., S.-S.M., G.F.R.M., T.S.Ț.C. and V.Ș.; supervision S.-S.M.; investigation L.C., L.V., G.F.R.M. and V.Ș.; writing—review L.A.B., T.S.Ț.C. and G.F.R.M.; validation L.V., S.-S.M., V.Ș. and N.-D.M.; software L.C. and A.B.; visualization G.F.R.M. and L.C.; data curation T.S.Ț.C. and N.-D.M.; project administration L.A.B. and A.B.; formal analysis N.-D.M. and A.B.; methodology L.V., S.-S.M. and V.Ș. All authors have read and agreed to the published version of the manuscript.

Funding: The article processing charges were funded by the University of Medicine and Pharmacy of Craiova, Romania.

Institutional Review Board Statement: The study was conducted in accordance with the Declaration of Helsinki and approved by the Ethical Committee of the Clinical Emergency County Hospital Craiova (no. 32909/14 July 2025).

Informed Consent Statement: Informed consent was obtained from all subjects involved in the study.

Data Availability Statement: The data presented in this study are available on request from the corresponding author.

Conflicts of Interest: The authors declare no conflicts of interest.

References

1. Laine, L.; Shah, A. Randomized trial of urgent vs. elective colonoscopy in patients hospitalized with lower GI bleeding. *Am. J. Gastroenterol.* **2010**, *105*, 2636–2641; quiz 2642. [CrossRef]
2. Targownik, L.E.; Nabalamba, A. Trends in management and outcomes of acute nonvariceal upper gastrointestinal bleeding: 1993–2003. *Clin. Gastroenterol. Hepatol.* **2006**, *4*, 1459–1466. [CrossRef]
3. Lanas, A.; García-Rodríguez, L.A.; Polo-Tomás, M.; Ponce, M.; Alonso-Abreu, I.; Perez-Aisa, M.A.; Perez-Gisbert, J.; Bujanda, L.; Castro, M.; Muñoz, M.; et al. Time trends and impact of upper and lower gastrointestinal bleeding and perforation in clinical practice. *Am. J. Gastroenterol.* **2009**, *104*, 1633–1641. [CrossRef]
4. Wuerth, B.A.; Rockey, D.C. Changing Epidemiology of Upper Gastrointestinal Hemorrhage in the Last Decade: A Nationwide Analysis. *Dig. Dis. Sci.* **2018**, *63*, 1286–1293. [CrossRef]
5. Wollenman, C.S.; Chason, R.; Reisch, J.S.; Rockey, D.C. Impact of ethnicity in upper gastrointestinal hemorrhage. *J. Clin. Gastroenterol.* **2014**, *48*, 343–350. [CrossRef]
6. Sung, J.J.; Tsoi, K.K.; Ma, T.K.; Yung, M.Y.; Lau, J.Y.; Chiu, P.W. Causes of mortality in patients with peptic ulcer bleeding: A prospective cohort study of 10,428 cases. *Am. J. Gastroenterol.* **2010**, *105*, 84–89. [CrossRef] [PubMed]
7. Barbu, L.A.; Mărgăritescu, N.D.; Șurlin, M.V. Diagnosis and Treatment Algorithms of Acute Variceal Bleeding. *Curr. Health Sci. J.* **2017**, *43*, 191–200. [CrossRef] [PubMed]
8. Marinescu, D.; Lazar, M.; Zaharie, S.; Comanescu, C.; Tudoran, C.; Bica, M.; Barbu, L. Upper Gastrointestinal Bleeding in Chronic Kidney Disease Patients. *Curr. Health Sci. J.* **2016**, *42*, 226–230. [CrossRef]
9. Mărgăritescu, N.D.; Ciobanu, M.O.; Nemeş, R.N.; Ghelase, Ş.M.; Pleşea, R.M.; Georgescu, I.; Voinea, B.; Pleşea, I.E.; ChiuŢu, L.C. The morphological profile of small bowel tumors—Our experience. *Rom. J. Morphol. Embryol.* **2016**, *57*, 1241–1252. [PubMed]
10. Laine, L.; McQuaid, K.R. Endoscopic therapy for bleeding ulcers: An evidence-based approach based on meta-analyses of randomized controlled trials. *Clin. Gastroenterol. Hepatol.* **2009**, *7*, 33–47; quiz 1–2. [CrossRef]
11. Mujtaba, S.; Chawla, S.; Massaad, J.F. Diagnosis and Management of Non-Variceal Gastrointestinal Hemorrhage: A Review of Current Guidelines and Future Perspectives. *J. Clin. Med.* **2020**, *9*, 402. [CrossRef] [PubMed]

12. Holster, I.L.; van Beusekom, H.M.; Kuipers, E.J.; Leebeek, F.W.; de Maat, M.P.; Tjwa, E.T. Effects of a hemostatic powder hemospray on coagulation and clot formation. *Endoscopy* **2015**, *47*, 638–645. [CrossRef]
13. Changela, K.; Papafragkakis, H.; Ofori, E.; Ona, M.A.; Krishnaiah, M.; Duddempudi, S.; Anand, S. Hemostatic powder spray: A new method for managing gastrointestinal bleeding. *Therap. Adv. Gastroenterol.* **2015**, *8*, 125–135. [CrossRef]
14. Chen, Y.I.; Barkun, A.; Nolan, S. Hemostatic powder TC-325 in the management of upper and lower gastrointestinal bleeding: A two-year experience at a single institution. *Endoscopy* **2015**, *47*, 167–171. [CrossRef]
15. Pittayanon, R.; Rerknimitr, R.; Barkun, A. Prognostic factors affecting outcomes in patients with malignant GI bleeding treated with a novel endoscopically delivered hemostatic powder. *Gastrointest. Endosc.* **2018**, *87*, 994–1002. [CrossRef] [PubMed]
16. Alharbi, A.; Almadi, M.; Barkun, A.; Martel, M. REASON Investigators. Predictors of a variceal source among patients presenting with upper gastrointestinal bleeding. *Can. J. Gastroenterol.* **2012**, *26*, 187–192. [CrossRef]
17. Romcea, A.A.; Tanţău, M.; Seicean, A.; Pascu, O. The etiology of upper gastrointestinal bleeding in cirrhotic patients. *Clujul Med.* **2013**, *86*, 21–23. [PubMed]
18. Laine, L.; Barkun, A.N.; Saltzman, J.R.; Martel, M.; Leontiadis, G.I. ACG Clinical Guideline: Upper Gastrointestinal and Ulcer Bleeding. *Am. J. Gastroenterol.* **2021**, *116*, 899–917. [CrossRef]
19. Pongprasobchai, S.; Nimitvilai, S.; Chasawat, J.; Manatsathit, S. Upper gastrointestinal bleeding etiology score for predicting variceal and non-variceal bleeding. *World J. Gastroenterol.* **2009**, *15*, 1099–1104. [CrossRef]
20. Matei, D.; Groza, I.; Furnea, B.; Puie, L.; Levi, C.; Chiru, A.; Cruciat, C.; Mester, G.; Vesa, S.C.; Tantau, M. Predictors of variceal or nonvariceal source of upper gastrointestinal bleeding. An etiology predictive score established and validated in a tertiary referral center. *J. Gastrointest. Liver Dis.* **2013**, *22*, 379–384.
21. Chai-Adisaksopha, C.; Crowther, M.; Isayama, T.; Lim, W. The impact of bleeding complications in patients receiving target-specific oral anticoagulants: A systematic review and meta-analysis. *Blood* **2014**, *124*, 2450–2458. [CrossRef]
22. Ruff, C.T.; Giugliano, R.P.; Braunwald, E.; Hoffman, E.B.; Deenadayalu, N.; Ezekowitz, M.D.; Camm, A.J.; Weitz, J.I.; Lewis, B.S.; Parkhomenko, A.; et al. Comparison of the efficacy and safety of new oral anticoagulants with warfarin in patients with atrial fibrillation: A meta-analysis of randomised trials. *Lancet* **2014**, *383*, 955–962. [CrossRef]
23. Ansell, J.E.; Bakhru, S.H.; Laulicht, B.E.; Steiner, S.S.; Grosso, M.; Brown, K.; Dishy, V.; Noveck, R.J.; Costin, J.C. Use of PER977 to reverse the anticoagulant effect of edoxaban. *N. Engl. J. Med.* **2014**, *371*, 2141–2142. [CrossRef]
24. Abraham, N.S.; Castillo, D.L. Novel anticoagulants: Bleeding risk and management strategies. *Curr. Opin. Gastroenterol.* **2013**, *29*, 676–683. [CrossRef]
25. Holbrook, A.; Schulman, S.; Witt, D.M.; Vandvik, P.O.; Fish, J.; Kovacs, M.J.; Svensson, P.J.; Veenstra, D.L.; Crowther, M.; Guyatt, G.H. Evidence-based management of anticoagulant therapy: Antithrombotic Therapy and Prevention of Thrombosis, 9th ed: American College of Chest Physicians Evidence-Based Clinical Practice Guidelines. *Chest* **2012**, *141* (Suppl. S2), e152S–e184S. [CrossRef]
26. Baron, T.H.; Kamath, P.S.; McBane, R.D. New anticoagulant and antiplatelet agents: A primer for the gastroenterologist. *Clin. Gastroenterol. Hepatol.* **2014**, *12*, 187–195. [CrossRef]
27. Karaca, M.A.; Erbil, B.; Ozmen, M.M. Use and effectiveness of prothrombin complex concentrates vs fresh frozen plasma in gastrointestinal hemorrhage due to warfarin usage in the ED. *Am. J. Emerg. Med.* **2014**, *32*, 660–664. [CrossRef]
28. Barkun, A.N.; Almadi, M.; Kuipers, E.J.; Laine, L.; Sung, J.; Tse, F.; Leontiadis, G.I.; Abraham, N.S.; Calvet, X.; Chan, F.K.L.; et al. Management of Nonvariceal Upper Gastrointestinal Bleeding: Guideline Recommendations From the International Consensus Group. *Ann. Intern. Med.* **2019**, *171*, 805–822. [CrossRef]
29. Kang, S.J.; Tae, C.H.; Bang, C.S.; Shin, C.M.; Jeong, Y.H.; Choi, M.; Hwang, J.H.; Saito, Y.; Chiu, P.W.Y.; Rerknimitr, R.; et al. International Digestive Endoscopy Network Consensus on the Management of Antithrombotic Agents in Patients Undergoing Gastrointestinal Endoscopy. *Gut Liver* **2024**, *18*, 764–780. [CrossRef]
30. Gralnek, I.M.; Dumonceau, J.M.; Kuipers, E.J.; Lanas, A.; Sanders, D.S.; Kurien, M.; Rotondano, G.; Hucl, T.; Dinis-Ribeiro, M.; Marmo, R.; et al. Diagnosis and management of nonvariceal upper gastrointestinal hemorrhage: European Society of Gastrointestinal Endoscopy (ESGE) Guideline. *Endoscopy* **2015**, *47*, a1–a46. [CrossRef]
31. Lau, J.Y.; Sung, J.J.; Lee, K.K.; Yung, M.Y.; Wong, S.K.; Wu, J.C.; Chan, F.K.; Ng, E.K.; You, J.H.; Lee, C.W.; et al. Effect of intravenous omeprazole on recurrent bleeding after endoscopic treatment of bleeding peptic ulcers. *N. Engl. J. Med.* **2000**, *343*, 310–316. [CrossRef]
32. Sachar, H.; Vaidya, K.; Laine, L. Intermittent vs continuous proton pump inhibitor therapy for high-risk bleeding ulcers: A systematic review and meta-analysis. *JAMA Intern. Med.* **2014**, *174*, 1755–1762. [CrossRef] [PubMed]
33. Leontiadis, G.I.; Sharma, V.K.; Howden, C.W. Proton pump inhibitor therapy for peptic ulcer bleeding: Cochrane collaboration meta-analysis of randomized controlled trials. *Mayo Clin. Proc.* **2007**, *82*, 286–296. [CrossRef]
34. Andriulli, A.; Loperfido, S.; Focareta, R.; Leo, P.; Fornari, F.; Garripoli, A.; Tonti, P.; Peyre, S.; Spadaccini, A.; Marmo, R.; et al. High- versus low-dose proton pump inhibitors after endoscopic hemostasis in patients with peptic ulcer bleeding: A multicentre, randomized study. *Am. J. Gastroenterol.* **2008**, *103*, 3011–3018. [CrossRef]

35. Wang, C.H.; Ma, M.H.; Chou, H.C.; Yen, Z.S.; Yang, C.W.; Fang, C.C.; Chen, S.C. High-dose vs non-high-dose proton pump inhibitors after endoscopic treatment in patients with bleeding peptic ulcer: A systematic review and meta-analysis of randomized controlled trials. *Arch. Intern. Med.* **2010**, *170*, 751–758. [CrossRef]
36. Gluud, L.L.; Klingenberg, S.L.; Langholz, E. Tranexamic acid for upper gastrointestinal bleeding. *Cochrane Database Syst. Rev.* **2012**, *1*, CD006640. [CrossRef]
37. Theivanayagam, S.; Lim, R.G.; Cobell, W.J.; Gowda, J.T.; Matteson, M.L.; Choudhary, A.; Bechtold, M.L. Administration of erythromycin before endoscopy in upper gastrointestinal bleeding: A meta-analysis of randomized controlled trials. *Saudi J. Gastroenterol.* **2013**, *19*, 205–210. [CrossRef]
38. Graham, D.Y. Limited value of early endoscopy in the management of acute upper gastrointestinal bleeding. Prospective controlled trial. *Am. J. Surg.* **1980**, *140*, 284–290. [CrossRef]
39. Peterson, W.L.; Barnett, C.C.; Smith, H.J.; Allen, M.H.; Corbett, D.B. Routine early endoscopy in upper-gastrointestinal-tract bleeding: A randomized, controlled trial. *N. Engl. J. Med.* **1981**, *304*, 925–929. [CrossRef]
40. Sacks, H.S.; Chalmers, T.C.; Blum, A.L.; Berrier, J.; Pagano, D. Endoscopic hemostasis. An effective therapy for bleeding peptic ulcers. *JAMA* **1990**, *264*, 494–499. [CrossRef]
41. Yen, D.; Hu, S.C.; Chen, L.S.; Liu, K.; Kao, W.F.; Tsai, J.; Chern, C.H.; Lee, C.H. Arterial oxygen desaturation during emergent nonsedated upper gastrointestinal endoscopy in the emergency department. *Am. J. Emerg. Med.* **1997**, *15*, 644–647. [CrossRef]
42. Hill, D.B.; Stokes, B.; Gilinsky, N.H. Arterial oxygen saturation during emergency esophagogastroduodenoscopy. The effects of nasal oxygen. *J. Clin. Gastroenterol.* **1994**, *18*, 284–286. [CrossRef] [PubMed]
43. Chiu, P.W. Endoscopic Management of Peptic Ulcer Bleeding: Recent Advances. *Clin. Endosc.* **2019**, *52*, 416–418. [CrossRef] [PubMed]
44. Cipolletta, L.; Bianco, M.A.; Rotondano, G.; Marmo, R.; Piscopo, R. Outpatient management for low-risk nonvariceal upper GI bleeding: A randomized controlled trial. *Gastrointest. Endosc.* **2002**, *55*, 1–5. [CrossRef]
45. Vreeburg, E.M.; Levi, M.; Rauws, E.A.; Deventer, S.J.; Snel, P.; Bartelsman, J.W.; Ten Cate, J.W.; Tytgat, G.N. Enhanced mucosal fibrinolytic activity in gastroduodenal ulcer haemorrhage and the beneficial effect of acid suppression. *Aliment. Pharmacol. Ther.* **2001**, *15*, 639–646. [CrossRef] [PubMed]
46. Lin, K.J.; Hernández-Díaz, S.; García Rodríguez, L.A. Acid suppressants reduce risk of gastrointestinal bleeding in patients on antithrombotic or anti-inflammatory therapy. *Gastroenterology* **2011**, *141*, 71–79. [CrossRef]
47. Cardoso, R.N.; Benjo, A.M.; DiNicolantonio, J.J.; Garcia, D.C.; Macedo, F.Y.; El-Hayek, G.; Nadkarni, G.N.; Gili, S.; Iannaccone, M.; Konstantinidis, I.; et al. Incidence of cardiovascular events and gastrointestinal bleeding in patients receiving clopidogrel with and without proton pump inhibitors: An updated meta-analysis. *Open Heart* **2015**, *2*, e000248. [CrossRef]
48. Sung, J.J.; Chiu, P.W.; Chan, F.K.L.; Lau, J.Y.; Goh, K.L.; Ho, L.H.; Jung, H.Y.; Sollano, J.D.; Gotoda, T.; Reddy, N.; et al. Asia-Pacific working group consensus on non-variceal upper gastrointestinal bleeding: An update 2018. *Gut* **2018**, *67*, 1757–1768. [CrossRef]
49. Botianu, A.; Matei, D.; Tantau, M.; Acalovschi, M. Mortality and need of surgical treatment in acute upper gastrointestinal bleeding: A one year study in a tertiary center with a 24 hours/day-7 days/week endoscopy call. Has anything changed? *Chirurgia* **2013**, *108*, 312–318.
50. Cook, D.J.; Guyatt, G.H.; Salena, B.J.; Laine, L.A. Endoscopic therapy for acute nonvariceal upper gastrointestinal hemorrhage: A meta-analysis. *Gastroenterology* **1992**, *102*, 139–148. [CrossRef]
51. Kahi, C.J.; Jensen, D.M.; Sung, J.J.; Bleau, B.L.; Jung, H.K.; Eckert, G.; Imperiale, T.F. Endoscopic therapy versus medical therapy for bleeding peptic ulcer with adherent clot: A meta-analysis. *Gastroenterology* **2005**, *129*, 855–862. [CrossRef]
52. Lin, H.J.; Perng, C.L.; Sun, I.C.; Tseng, G.Y. Endoscopic haemoclip versus heater probe thermocoagulation plus hypertonic saline-epinephrine injection for peptic ulcer bleeding. *Dig. Liver Dis.* **2003**, *35*, 898–902. [CrossRef] [PubMed]
53. Swain, C.P.; Storey, D.W.; Bown, S.G.; Heath, J.; Mills, T.N.; Salmon, P.R.; Northfield, T.C.; Kirkham, J.S.; O'Sullivan, J.P. Nature of the bleeding vessel in recurrently bleeding gastric ulcers. *Gastroenterology* **1986**, *90*, 595–608. [CrossRef]
54. Raju, G.S.; Gajula, L. Endoclips for GI endoscopy. *Gastrointest. Endosc.* **2004**, *59*, 267–279. [CrossRef]
55. Alali, A.A.; Moosavi, S.; Martel, M.; Almadi, M.; Barkun, A.N. Topical hemostatic agents in the management of upper gastrointestinal bleeding: A meta-analysis. *Endosc. Int. Open* **2023**, *11*, E368–E385. [CrossRef] [PubMed]
56. Gralnek, I.M.; Stanley, A.J.; Morris, A.J.; Camus, M.; Lau, J.; Lanas, A.; Laursen, S.B.; Radaelli, F.; Papanikolaou, I.S.; Cúrdia Gonçalves, T.; et al. Endoscopic diagnosis and management of nonvariceal upper gastrointestinal hemorrhage (NVUGIH): European Society of Gastrointestinal Endoscopy (ESGE) Guideline—Update 2021. *Endoscopy* **2021**, *53*, 300–332. [CrossRef] [PubMed]
57. Grottke, O.; Afshari, A.; Ahmed, A.; Arnaoutoglou, E.; Bolliger, D.; Fenger-Eriksen, C.; von Heymann, C. Clinical guideline on reversal of direct oral anticoagulants in patients with life threatening bleeding. *Eur. J. Anaesthesiol.* **2024**, *41*, 327–350. [CrossRef]
58. Javid, G.; Zargar, S.A.; U-Saif, R.; Khan, B.A.; Yatoo, G.N.; Shah, A.H.; Gulzar, G.M.; Sodhi, J.S.; Khan, M.A. Comparison of p.o. or i.v. proton pump inhibitors on 72-h intragastric pH in bleeding peptic ulcer. *J. Gastroenterol. Hepatol.* **2009**, *24*, 1236–1243. [CrossRef]

59. Douketis, J.D.; Spyropoulos, A.C.; Spencer, F.A.; Mayr, M.; Jaffer, A.K.; Eckman, M.H.; Dunn, A.S.; Kunz, R. Perioperative management of antithrombotic therapy: Antithrombotic Therapy and Prevention of Thrombosis, 9th ed: American College of Chest Physicians Evidence-Based Clinical Practice Guidelines. *Chest* **2012**, *141* (Suppl. S2), e326S–e350S. [CrossRef]
60. Elmunzer, B.J.; Young, S.D.; Inadomi, J.M.; Schoenfeld, P.; Laine, L. Systematic review of the predictors of recurrent hemorrhage after endoscopic hemostatic therapy for bleeding peptic ulcers. *Am. J. Gastroenterol.* **2008**, *103*, 2625–2632; quiz 2633. [CrossRef]
61. Barbu, L.A.; Mărgăritescu, N.-D.; Cercelaru, L.; Caragea, D.-C.; Vîlcea, I.-D.; Șurlin, V.; Mogoantă, S.-Ș.; Mogoș, G.F.R.; Vasile, L.; Țenea Cojan, T.Ș. Can Thrombosed Abdominal Aortic Dissecting Aneurysm Cause Mesenteric Artery Thrombosis and Ischemic Colitis?—A Case Report and a Review of Literature. *J. Clin. Med.* **2025**, *14*, 3092. [CrossRef] [PubMed]
62. Robson, A.J.; Richards, J.M.; Ohly, N.; Nixon, S.J.; Paterson-Brown, S. The effect of surgical subspecialization on outcomes in peptic ulcer disease complicated by perforation and bleeding. *World J. Surg.* **2008**, *32*, 1456–1461. [CrossRef]
63. Paspatis, G.A.; Matrella, E.; Kapsoritakis, A.; Leontithis, C.; Papanikolaou, N.; Chlouverakis, G.J.; Kouroumalis, E. An epidemiological study of acute upper gastrointestinal bleeding in Crete, Greece. *Eur. J. Gastroenterol. Hepatol.* **2000**, *12*, 1215–1220. [CrossRef]
64. van Leerdam, M.E.; Vreeburg, E.M.; Rauws, E.A.; Geraedts, A.A.; Tijssen, J.G.; Reitsma, J.B.; Tytgat, G.N. Acute upper GI bleeding: Did anything change? Time trend analysis of incidence and outcome of acute upper GI bleeding between 1993/1994 and 2000. *Am. J. Gastroenterol.* **2003**, *98*, 1494–1499. [CrossRef]
65. Dicu, D.; Pop, F.; Ionescu, D.; Dicu, T. Comparison of risk scoring systems in predicting clinical outcome at upper gastrointestinal bleeding patients in an emergency unit. *Am. J. Emerg. Med.* **2013**, *31*, 94–99. [CrossRef]
66. Cheung, F.K.; Lau, J.Y. Management of massive peptic ulcer bleeding. *Gastroenterol. Clin. N. Am.* **2009**, *38*, 231–243. [CrossRef]
67. Saperas, E.; Piqué, J.M.; Pérez Ayuso, R.; Bordas, J.M.; Terés, J.; Pera, C. Conservative management of bleeding duodenal ulcer without a visible vessel: Prospective randomized trial. *Br. J. Surg.* **1987**, *74*, 784–786. [CrossRef]
68. Imhof, M.; Ohmann, C.; Röher, H.D.; Glutig, H.; DUESUC Study Group. Endoscopic versus operative treatment in high-risk ulcer bleeding patients—Results of a randomised study. *Langenbecks Arch. Surg.* **2003**, *387*, 327–336. [CrossRef]
69. Bender, J.S.; Bouwman, D.L.; Weaver, D.W. Bleeding gastroduodenal ulcers: Improved outcome from a unified surgical approach. *Am. Surg.* **1994**, *60*, 313–315. [PubMed]
70. Mueller, X.; Rothenbuehler, J.M.; Amery, A.; Meyer, B.; Harder, F. Outcome of peptic ulcer hemorrhage treated according to a defined approach. *World J. Surg.* **1994**, *18*, 406–409; discussion 409–410. [CrossRef] [PubMed]
71. Poxon, V.A.; Keighley, M.R.; Dykes, P.W.; Heppinstall, K.; Jaderberg, M. Comparison of minimal and conventional surgery in patients with bleeding peptic ulcer: A multicentre trial. *Br. J. Surg.* **1991**, *78*, 1344–1345. [CrossRef]
72. Caragher, S.; Wang, D.; Moonsamy, P.; Fagenholz, P. Hepatic arterial haemorrhage caused by duodenal ulcer. *BMJ Case Rep.* **2022**, *15*, e249523. [CrossRef] [PubMed]
73. Eriksson, L.G.; Sundbom, M.; Gustavsson, S.; Nyman, R. Endoscopic marking with a metallic clip facilitates transcatheter arterial embolization in upper peptic ulcer bleeding. *J. Vasc. Interv. Radiol.* **2006**, *17*, 959–964. [CrossRef] [PubMed]
74. Fukamatsu, F.; Yamada, K.; Takekoshi, D.; Aonuma, T.; Oyama, K.; Yanagisawa, S.; Yamada, A.; Shimizu, A.; Fujinaga, Y. Embolization using both n-butyl cyanoacrylate and gelatin sponges in a patient with a posterior superior pancreaticoduodenal artery pseudoaneurysm that ruptured and bled into the drain tube. *Radiol. Case Rep.* **2023**, *19*, 876–880. [CrossRef] [PubMed]
75. Ripoll, C.; Bañares, R.; Beceiro, I.; Menchén, P.; Catalina, M.V.; Echenagusia, A.; Turegano, F. Comparison of transcatheter arterial embolization and surgery for treatment of bleeding peptic ulcer after endoscopic treatment failure. *J. Vasc. Interv. Radiol.* **2004**, *15*, 447–450. [CrossRef]

life

MDPI

Article

Surgical Repair of Bile Duct Injuries Due to Cholecystectomy—An Experience from a Referral Center in Slovenia

Irena Plahuta [1,2], Špela Turk [1], Barbara Lovrenčič Petreski [1], Tomislav Magdalenić [1], Stojan Potrč [1,2] and Arpad Ivanecz [1,2,*]

[1] Clinical Department of Abdominal and General Surgery, University Medical Centre Maribor, Ljubljanska Ulica 5, 2000 Maribor, Slovenia
[2] Department of Surgery, Faculty of Medicine, University of Maribor, Taborska Ulica 8, 2000 Maribor, Slovenia
* Correspondence: arpad.ivanecz@ukc-mb.si

Abstract: Background: Bile duct injury (BDI) during (laparoscopic) cholecystectomy has an incidence of up to 1.5%. This retrospective study aimed to report the outcomes of surgical repair of BDI due to these procedures at a tertiary referral center. Methods: A retrospective review of patients' records was conducted. The BDI's clinical presentations, Strasberg classification, surgical repairs, and outcomes were reported. Results: From 2003 to 2024, 47 BDIs were identified. In total, 34.0% were recognized intraoperatively. The BDI types included Strasberg types B (2, 4.3%), C (5, 10.6%), D (11, 23.4%), E1 (4, 8.5%), E2 (12, 25.5%), E3 (5, 10.6%), E4 (3, 6.4%), and E5 (5, 10.6%). The T-tube group included 6 (12.8%) patients, the primary repair and T-tube group included 10 (21.3%) patients, and the Biliodigestive anastomosis group included 31 (65.9%) patients. The overall morbidity rate was 40.4%, the major morbidity rate was 21.3%, and the mortality rate was 4.3%. Grade A patency was achieved in 95.6% of patients. In the Biliodigestive anastomosis group, the actuarial 1-, 5- and 10-year grade A patency rates were 77.0%, 70.0%, and 70.0%, respectively. Conclusion: The rate of BDI remains stable. The outcomes of repairs in terms of complications and patency rates are comparable to those in other reports.

Keywords: cholecystectomy; bile duct injury; biliodigestive anastomosis; patency; morbidity; mortality

1. Introduction

The first cholecystectomy was performed by Carl Johann August Langenbuch in 1882 in Berlin, and the first laparoscopic cholecystectomy was performed in 1985 by Erich Mühe in Böblingen, Germany [1,2]. Since then, cholecystectomy has been one of the most routinely performed procedures in surgery, and the laparoscopic approach is the gold standard for patients with symptomatic cholecystolithiasis [3].

Bile duct injuries (BDIs) still occur during these procedures, with an incidence of up to 1.5% [3]. Risk factors have been divided into three categories: factors dependent on the surgeon (false visual perception, surgical technique, and learning curve), the patient (anatomical variants, inflammatory processes, obesity), and the institution (equipment and availability of fluoroscopy) [4,5].

A critical view of safety (CVS) was introduced in 1995 to improve the safety of laparoscopic cholecystectomies [6,7]. It failed only 1 in 300 times, which means it worked 299 out of 300 times [7,8]. About 20% of surgeons accepted the core CVS principles but

 https://doi.org/10.3390/life15060874

struggled to meet all three criteria [6]. In addition to identifying the hepatocystic triangle and creating two "windows" in it, it is pivotal to mobilize the lower part of the gallbladder from the cystic plate [3]. The surgeon can confirm that the dissected structures enter the gallbladder wall and not the liver parenchyma [3,6]. In addition to the operative notes, it is important to use a high-quality imaging method to document the CVS [3,6]. Furthermore, Rouviere's sulcus (or *incisura hepatis dextra* or *Gans incisura*) is an anatomical landmark present in at least 80% of people [9]. Identifying Rouviere's sulcus and preparing structures delineating Calot's triangle above the level of that sulcus contributes to performing a safer cholecystectomy [10,11].

BDIs can endanger patients or significantly impair their quality of life; therefore, selecting the most effective treatment option for BDI is crucial [3,12,13]. BDIs are often unnoticed during index surgery [14]. When the injury is detected intraoperatively, immediately reconstructing bile ducts is sometimes possible [15]. When injury is suspected in the postoperative period, the type of injury must be identified using magnetic resonance cholangiopancreatography (MRCP), percutaneous transhepatic cholangiography, or endoscopic retrograde cholangiopancreatography (ERCP) [14]. In patients undergoing bile duct reconstruction due to BDI, preoperative or intraoperative Doppler ultrasonography can help to determine if arterial reconstruction is needed. Vascular continuity can also be assessed using magnetic resonance or computed tomography angiography [16].

Simple postoperative leaks can be managed through either drainage alone or combining drainage with the ERCP placement of biliary stents [14]. Some advanced centers, equipped with skilled gastroenterologists, treat selected patients with complex injuries through percutaneous–endoscopic rendezvous procedures, showing promising long-term outcomes [14]. Biliodigestive anastomosis (BDA) is the gold standard for treating severe and complete transection of bile ducts [17–19].

This retrospective study aimed to report the outcomes of the surgical repair of BDI due to (laparoscopic) cholecystectomy at a tertiary referral center.

2. Materials and Methods

A retrospective review of a database of patients who underwent treatment for BDI at our tertiary referral center from January 2003 to December 2024 was performed. Our department is one of two tertiary referral centers in Slovenia that surgically repair major BDI. We perform about 300 elective and emergency cholecystectomies yearly. Additionally, our dedicated hepato-pancreato-biliary team consists of five surgeons performing about 130 resections annually, including 30 pancreaticoduodenectomies [20,21].

All patients who underwent surgical repair for BDI due to the cholecystectomy were included in the research. Patients who endured BDI during ERCP and surgeries other than cholecystectomy (bile duct resections for cysts, neoplasms, and choledocholithiasis; liver resections for liver tumors and abscess drainages; surgery for gallbladder or perihilar cholangiocarcinoma; and pancreaticoduodenectomies) were excluded. Patients whose BDIs were repaired via ERCP were also excluded, as suggested by Cho et al. [22].

The patients' demographics, preoperative clinical characteristics, intraoperative details, and postoperative outcomes were retrieved from the database.

Surgical repair was always performed through an open approach. The following repairs were performed:

- T-tube placement.
- Primary sutures of the bile ducts with a T-tube placement.
- BDA was performed in a Roux-en-Y manner for complete transections of the bile ducts. The surgical technique was applied as described by the reference [23].

BDI was graded according to the Strassberg classification, as proposed by the World Society of Emergency Surgery [3,24]. Cholangitis was defined according to the Tokyo Guidelines 2018 [25].

The time frame of the repair was reported during the index surgery, as well as in the early (days 1–7), intermediate (1–6 weeks), and late (>6 weeks) periods post-surgery [15].

Postoperative morbidity was graded according to the Clavien–Dindo classification [26]. The most severe complication was taken into account [26]. Grades 1 and 2 indicate minor complications that require medical therapies for treatment. Severe complications encompassed grades $\geq$ 3a. Grade 3a means that interventional radiological or endoscopic procedures without general anesthesia are needed. Grade 3b necessitates the aforementioned and surgical procedures under general anesthesia. Grades 4a and 4b involve organ support, and grade 5 signifies mortality [26].

The primary endpoint was primary patency after BDI repair. "Patency" is defined as an open, functional biliary tree on the 90th day after surgical repair [22]. An open functional biliary tree means that it lacks stents and the need for invasive interventions. This definition applies to a patient who, after completing treatment, has no episodes of jaundice, cholangitis, external biliary fistula, or liver abscesses [22]. The grading of patency, its actual rates, and its actuarial duration were calculated as proposed by Cho et al. [22,27].

The secondary endpoints were postoperative outcomes (overall morbidity, severe morbidity, mortality).

IBM SPSS for Windows Version 29.0.0.0 (IBM Corporation, Armonk, NY, USA) was used for conducting statistical computations. Percentages were reported to one decimal place.

Categorical variables were displayed as numbers (percentages). Continuous variables were expressed as medians (interquartile range) [28].

Patients underwent check-ups according to their clinical state. This study was concluded on 31 December 2024 or upon the patient's death. The median follow-up period was calculated using the reverse Kaplan–Meier method and expressed as months (confidence interval). The Kaplan–Meier curves show the primary patency intervals, and the Survival Tables were used to calculate the 1-, 3-, 5-, and 10-year actuarial patencies [22,29].

The Institutional Ethics Committee approved this study (UKC-MB-KME-42/24). Before undergoing surgery, patients consented to their anonymous data being used for research. Their records were anonymized and deidentified before analysis. Informed consent for publication was obtained from all identifiable human participants. All methods were performed following the relevant guidelines and regulations.

3. Results

Patient data were retrieved from various sources, and there were inconsistent reporting and coding of diseases, complications, and procedures. Therefore, the search was conducted following the method shown in Figure 1.

From 2003 to 2024, 94 patients with BDIs were treated at our department. They were either operated on by us or referred to us by various gastroenterology departments and four secondary-level hospitals.

A total of 63 patients with BDIs due to cholecystectomy were identified. Six patients whose surgical treatment could not be assigned to any of the groups were excluded from further analysis (Figure 1). In addition, ten patients whose BDIs were resolved via ERCP were excluded on the basis of their injuries being resolved non-surgically [22].

A total of 47 patients with BDIs caused during cholecystectomy were further analyzed. Of these, 25 injuries (53.2%) occurred within our department, while other hospitals referred 22 patients (46.8%) to us, and 16 (72.2%) of them needed BDA.

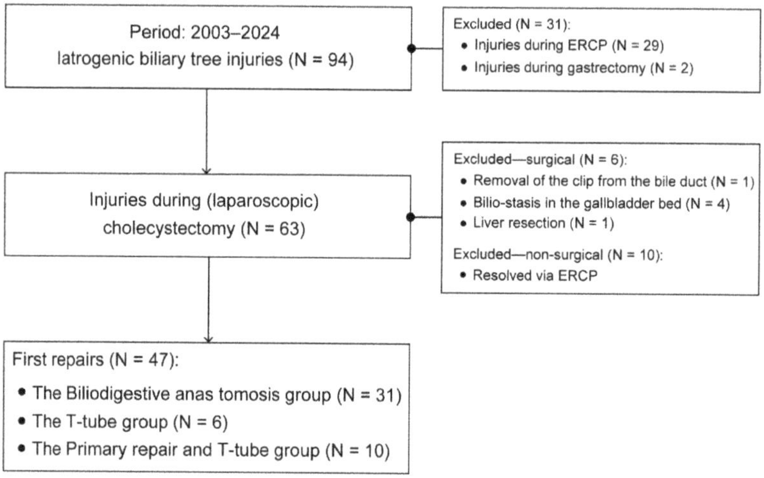

Figure 1. A study flow chart. The search excluded bile duct resections for cysts, neoplasms, and choledocholithiasis; liver resections for liver tumors and abscess drainages; surgery for gallbladder or perihilar cholangiocarcinoma; and pancreaticoduodenectomies. ERCP: Endoscopic retrograde cholangiopancreatography.

The incidence of BDI in our department was tracked from 2012 to 2024. During this period, we performed 3724 open or laparoscopic cholecystectomies, which resulted in 29 cases of BDI, 10 of which required surgical reconstruction (6 BDAs and 4 primary repairs). That gave an overall incidence of 0.8% and an incidence of major injuries of 0.3%.

These 47 patients were categorized into three groups based on the type of primary repair for BDI. The T-tube group included 6 (12.8%) patients, the primary repair and T-tube group included 10 (21.3%) patients, and the Biliodigestive anastomosis group included 31 (65.9%) patients. Their basic characteristics are detailed in Table 1.

Table 1. Basic characteristics of patients who endured bile duct injury during cholecystectomy.

Variable	Total (N = 47)	BDA Group (N = 31)	T-Tube Group (N = 6)	Primary Repair and T-Tube Group (N = 10)
Male sex	23 (48.9)	17 (54.8)	3 (50.0)	3 (30.0)
Age [years]	65 (18)	60 (20)	69 (16)	68 (13)
BMI [kg/m^2]	29 (7)	29 (5)	36 (3)	28 (2)
ASA 3 and 4	14 (29.8)	10 (32.3)	2 (33.3)	2 (20.0)
Method				
open	7 (15.0)	4 (12.9)	1 (16.7)	2 (20.0)
laparoscopic	20 (42.5)	13 (41.9)	3 (50.0)	4 (40.0)
conversion	20 (42.5)	14 (45.2)	2 (33.3)	4 (40.0)
Elective surgery	30 (63.8)	19 (61.3)	4 (66.7)	7 (70.0)

ASA: American Society of Anesthesiologists Score; BDA: Biliodigestive anastomosis; BMI: body mass index.

The indications for surgery were acute cholecystitis in 14 (29.8%) cases, persistent biliary colic in 3 (6.4%) cases, symptomatic cholecystolithiasis in 12 (25.5%) cases, and chronic cholecystitis in 18 (38.3%) cases.

Operative reports were available in only 25 (53.2%) cholecystectomy cases. Among them, Calot's triangle was dissected first in 16 cases, the cystic duct was identified as such in 21 cases, and the cystic artery was identified as such in 11 cases. A CVS was mentioned in 14 cases.

Table 2 shows the clinical presentations of BDI and the time frame of the repair. In total, 34.0% of BDIs were identified during cholecystectomy. Jaundice was the second-most common symptom, occurring in a quarter of cases, followed by bile in drain (23.4%) and biliary peritonitis (14.9%). BDI was recognized due to a concomitant lesion of the right hepatic artery in one (2.1%) patient. Three patients in the late repair period were operated on several months (9, 26, and 173) after cholecystectomy due to stenosis of the common bile duct.

Table 2. The clinical presentations of bile duct injuries and the time frame of the repair in 47 patients.

Clinical Presentation	Total (N = 47)	BDA Group (N = 31)	T-Tube Group (N = 6)	Primary Repair and T-Tube Group (N = 10)
During index surgery	16 (34.0)	9 (29.0)	2 (33.3)	5 (50.0)
Icterus/holangitis	12 (25.5)	12 (38.7)	0 (0.0)	0 (0.0)
Bile in drain	11 (23.4)	7 (22.6)	3 (50.0)	1 (10.0)
Biliary peritonitis	7 (14.9)	2 (6.5)	1 (16.7)	4 (40.0)
Hemorrhagic shock	1 (2.1)	1 (3.2)	0 (0.0)	0 (0.0)
Time of the repair				
During index surgery	16 (34.0)	9 (29.0)	2 (33.3)	5 (50.0)
Early (day 1–7)	15 (31.9)	10 (61.3)	4 (66.7)	1 (10.0)
Intermediate (1–6 weeks)	10 (21.3)	6 (19.4)		4 (40.0)
Late (>6 weeks)	6 (12.7)	6 (19.4)		

BDA: Biliodigestive anastomosis.

Injuries were graded according to the Strassberg classification (Table 3) [24]. Concomitant vascular injury was present in nine (19.1%) cases, a cystic artery was injured in one case (11.1%), and a right hepatic artery was injured in eight (88.9%) cases.

Table 3. Grading of injuries according to the Strassberg classification.

Grade of Injury	Total (N = 47)	BDA Group (N = 31)	T-Tube Group (N = 6)	Primary Repair and T-Tube Group (N = 10)
B	2 (4.3)	2 (6.5)		
C	5 (10.6)			5 (50.0)
D	11 (23.4)		6 (100.0)	5 (50.0)
E1	4 (8.5)	4 (12.9)		
E2	12 (25.5)	12 (38.7)		
E3	5 (10.6)	5 (16.1)		
E4	3 (6.4)	3 (9.7)		
E5	5 (10.6)	5 (16.1)		

B: occluded right posterior sectoral duct; C: bile leak from divided right posterior sectoral duct; D: bile leak from main bile duct without major tissue loss; E1 and E2: transected main bile duct with a stricture more than 2 cm from the hilus (E1) or less than 2 cm from the hilus (E2); E3 and E4: stricture of the hilus with right and left duct in communication (E3) or without communication (E4); E5: stricture of the main bile duct and the right posterior sectoral duct [24]. BDA: Biliodigestive anastomosis.

Repairs were BDA in 31 cases, T-tube placement in 6 cases, and primary repair of a bile duct and a T-tube placement in 10 cases. The cystic artery was properly ligated, and the right hepatic artery was reconstructed in all cases. The complications of the repairs according to the Clavien–Dindo classification are given in Table 4.

Table 4. The grading of complications according to the Clavien–Dindo classification.

Grade of Injury	Total (N = 47)	BDA Group (N = 31)	T-Tube Group (N = 6)	Primary Repair and T-Tube Group (N = 10)
CD 1	2 (4.3)	2 (6.5)		
CD 2	7 (14.9)	5 (16.1)		2 (20.0)
CD 3a	2 (4.3)	1 (3.2)	1 (16.7)	
CD 3b	2 (4.3)	2 (6.5)		
CD 4a	1 (2.1)	1 (3.2)		
CD 4b	3 (6.4)	2 (6.5)		1 (10.0)
CD 5	2 (4.3)	1 (3.2)		1 (10.0)
Overall morbidity	19 (40.4)	14 (45.2)	1 (16.7)	4 (40.0)
Severe morbidity ≥ CD 3a	10 (21.3)	7 (22.6)	1 (16.7)	2 (20.0)

BDA: Biliodigestive anastomosis; CD: Clavien–Dindo classification.

The description of severe morbidity is as follows: Clavien–Dindo grade 3a complications were percutaneous drainages of intra-abdominal fluid collections. One patient was reoperated on because of laparotomy dehiscence and another for the surgical lavage of biliary peritonitis (grade 3b). One patient was admitted to the intensive care unit due to respiratory insufficiency (grade 4a). One patient was admitted due to hemorrhagic shock, and two patients were admitted due to septic shock (grade 4b). One patient from the BDA group died of multiple organ dysfunction syndrome, and one patient from the primary repair and T-tube group died of pneumonia.

Table 5 shows severe morbidity (Clavien–Dindo ≥ 3a) according to the time frame of the repair.

Table 5. The rates and grading of severe morbidity (Clavien–Dindo ≥ 3a) according to the time frame of the repair.

Time Frame	Total (N = 47)	BDA Group (N = 31)	T-Tube Group (N = 6)	Primary Repair and T-Tube Group (N = 10)
During index surgery	1 (6.25%)	11.1% 3b		
Early (day 1–7)	5 (33.3%)	30.0% 3b, 2 pts 4b	25.0% 3a	20.0% 5
Intermediate (1–6 weeks)	3 (30.0%)	50.0% 3a, 4a, 5		25.0% 4b
Late (>6 weeks)				

BDA: Biliodigestive anastomosis.

When short-term outcomes were compared according to whether the cholecystectomy was elective or emergency, the Clavien–Dindo ≥ 3a grades after repairs were 16.7% and 29.4%, respectively. Two patients who died came from both groups.

The patency results after the BDI repairs are shown in Figure 2 [22].

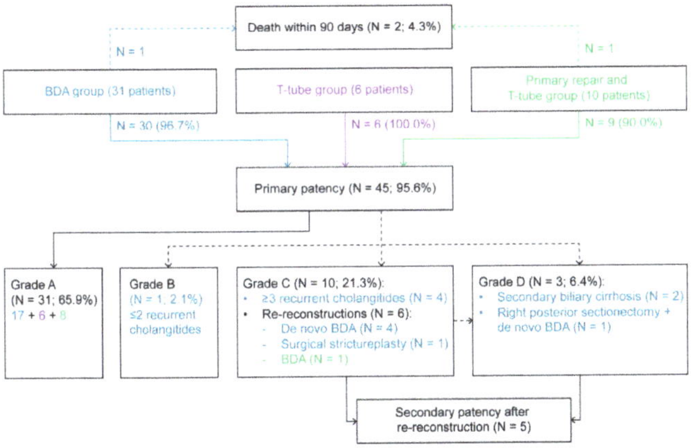

Figure 2. Patency of repairs of bile duct injuries. BDA: Biliodigestive anastomosis. Blue: BDA group; Purple: T-tube group; Green: Primary repair and T-tube group.

Two patients never reached primary patency because they died within 90 days after the surgical repair of BDI. Four patients with recurrent cholangitis were frequently treated with antibiotics.

One patient had a surgical strictureplasty and six patients underwent re-reconstructions of bile ducts. In the patient from the primary repair and T-tube group, BDA was created after ten endoscopic retrograde cholangiopancreatography procedures. In four cases, BDA was resected and created de novo. One patient underwent a concomitant posterior sectionectomy due to limited secondary liver cirrhosis. Of these seven patients, five achieved secondary patency and had no issues. Two patients developed secondary liver cirrhosis. The median gamma-glutamyl transferase and alkaline phosphatase values of patients with secondary biliary cirrhosis were 3.17 ukat/L and 2.52 ukat/L, respectively. One patient died of heart failure, and one patient remained on the waiting list for liver transplantation.

The median follow-up period was 94 (confidence interval 57.6–130.5) months. Figure 3 shows a Kaplan–Meier graph of actuarial primary patency dependent on time.

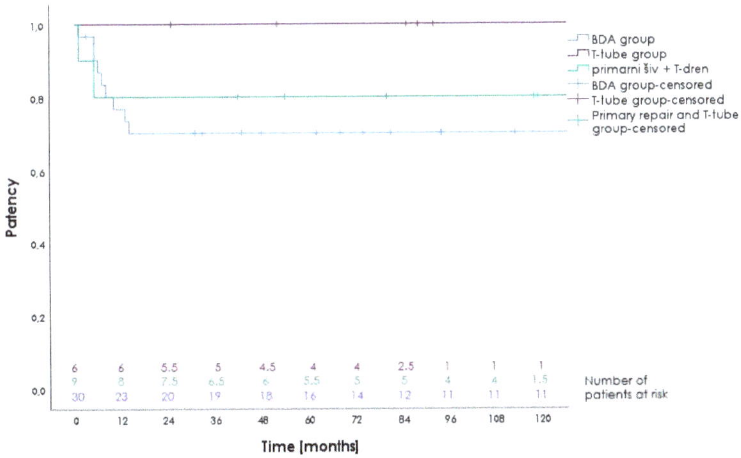

Figure 3. Kaplan–Meier curves of actuarial primary patency dependent on time. BDA: Biliodigestive anastomosis.

Table 6 shows the actuarial primary patency rates 1, 3, 5, and 10 years after repairs.

Table 6. The actuarial primary patency rates 1, 3, 5, and 10 years after repairs.

	BDA Group (N = 31)	T-Tube Group (N = 6)	Primary Repair and T-Tube Group (N = 10)
1 year	77.0%	100.0%	80.0%
3 years	70.0%	100.0%	80.0%
5 years	70.0%	100.0%	80.0%
10 years	70.0%	100.0%	80.0%

BDA: Biliodigestive anastomosis.

Five patients achieved secondary patency after re-reconstruction; its median duration was 106 months.

4. Discussion

This study analyzed 47 patients who underwent surgical repair of BDI due to cholecystectomy. The 90-day overall morbidity rate was 40.4%, the major morbidity rate was 21.3%, and the mortality rate was 4.3%. Grade A patency was achieved in 95.6% of patients. A total of 65.9% of patients remained in that grade, while 2.1% of patients slid into grade B, 21.3% of patients were reassigned to grade C, and 6.4% were reassigned to grade D. In the BDA group, the actuarial 1-, 5- and 10-year grade A patency rates were 77.0%, 70.0%, and 70.0%, respectively.

The majority of BDIs are iatrogenic, and they occur during abdominal surgeries or interventions such as endoscopic or percutaneous cannulation of the biliary tree [30,31]. In the last 21 years, our department has treated at least 94 iatrogenic BDIs, and 63 of them were due to cholecystectomy (Figure 1). A similar case series showed that most BDI referrals to a tertiary center were usually very serious complications [32,33]. In this study, 72.2% of referred patients needed BDA. Patients with BDI must be referred immediately to a surgeon experienced in managing BDI at a facility with a hepatobiliary multispecialty team. If a timely referral is not feasible, consultation with a surgeon experienced in managing BDI should be carried out [3,12].

The incidence of BDI was low (0.1–0.2%) during the era of open cholecystectomy, but this rate has tripled (0.4–0.6%) following the global implementation of the laparoscopic approach [34]. The incidence of major BDI in our department between 2012 and 2024 was 0.3%, and the overall incidence was 0.8%. That aligns with nationwide prospective databases that indicate figures of up to 1.5% [3,6,33–35].

Evaluating the risk factors for BDIs within our cohort presents certain challenges, particularly given the diversity of the five hospitals and various surgical teams involved. Among the patients, more than half were female, with a median age of 65 and a median body mass index of 29 kg/m^2. Chronic cholecystitis was the most common indication for surgery, accounting for 38.3% of cases. Additionally, two-thirds of the cholecystectomies were performed on an elective basis. Approximately 85.0% of these procedures were started laparoscopically (Table 1).

The most common etiological factor for BDI is misidentifying the common bile duct as the cystic duct; aberrant anatomy and difficult pathology are less commonly responsible for BDI [34]. This was also true in our case series, where the common bile duct was identified as the cystic duct in 29 cases (61.7%) (Strasberg type E injuries). In six (12.8%) cases, the right posterior sectoral duct was identified as the cystic duct (Strasberg type B and C injuries). A bile duct variation in the right posterior sector duct connecting directly to the cystic duct was present only in one patient (2.1%). However, out of our study's 25 available operative reports, CVS was only mentioned in 14 cases, although implementing that rule significantly decreases the rate of BDI [3].

Performing a cholecystectomy with two surgeons present is often not feasible in many settings. However, having a second surgeon can be beneficial, especially when the dissection is stalled, the anatomy is unclear, or the operating conditions are deemed "difficult". Consulting a more experienced surgeon can provide a critical moment in preventing BDI or its early recognition [3,12].

Intraoperative cholangiography (IOC) is an imaging technique used during cholecystectomy to identify choledocholithiasis and clarify the anatomy of the bile ducts [3]. However, routine use of IOC is not recommended, as it does not significantly reduce the risk of BDI [3,35]. Additionally, BDI can still occur after IOC due to misinterpreting the cholangiogram [3]. IOC is advisable in certain situations, particularly when the anatomy of the bile ducts is unclear. It may also be beneficial for patients with acute cholecystitis or a history of it, even though it may prolong the duration of surgery [3,35]. If there is concern about a potential BDI, performing IOC can assist in diagnosing and treating it on time [3]. Another technique is indocyanine green fluorescence cholangiography [36]. This method involves injecting a dye to visualize the bile duct structures without using X-rays [36]. Studies suggest that this technique may help to prevent BDI and is effective for acute and chronic gallbladder issues, especially when IOC cannot be performed [3,36].

Table 2 shows the clinical presentation and time frame of the repair of BDI. One-third of the injuries were recognized during cholecystectomy. Rates of intraoperatively recognized BDI ranged from 16% to 46% [34,37]. There was a low rate of biliary peritonitis in the BDA group (6.5%) and a high rate (40.0%) in the primary repair and T-tube group. In that group, biliary peritonitis was present in 40% of cases, and the repairs were completed after 7 days. When BDI is suspected in the postoperative period, a computed tomography scan of the abdomen should be conducted, and in cases of significant peritoneal fluid accumulation, percutaneous drainage should be carried out [14]. Then, a work-up with MRCP or ERCP must be carried out to delineate the anatomy to plan the repair [14].

The ERCP with stenting is a viable approach for treating BDI, but we excluded patients who underwent this repair, as proposed by Cho et al. [22]. Namely, patients who can only receive surgical treatment should be reported in the surgical case series. Those eligible only for non-surgical treatment can be included in case series that study endoscopic or interventional radiology methods [22]. However, mixing these patients in studies that compare surgical and non-surgical techniques is not appropriate [22]. That does not mean that we overlooked the fact that some complex injuries can only be treated with surgery and that there are patients who, while not suitable for surgery, can still be compatible with non-surgical options [22]. However, including these patients in comparative studies would make the results difficult to interpret [15].

The delayed recognition of BDI, injuries of the right hepatic artery (eight cases, or 88.9% of concomitant vascular injuries), and complications in repair contributed to the overall severe morbidity (Clavien–Dindo grade $\geq$ 3a) of 21.3% and mortality of 4.3% (Table 4) [15]. Reported rates of severe morbidity were as high as 43.0%, and mortality was as high as 4.6% [3,19,27,38].

The treatment of these injuries after the index operation depends on the severity of the injury, the time of diagnosis, and the patient's general condition. Late detection of the injury is associated with reduced survival [39]. In our study, the severe morbidity rate was 6.25% when the repair was performed during index surgery and increased upon early (33.3%) and intermediate repair (30%) (Table 5). Especially in the BDA group, the rates of complications skyrocketed from 11.1% to 30.0% and up to 50% in the intermediate time frame of the repair. On the contrary, the multicenter study showed that the timing of biliary reconstruction with hepaticojejunostomy does not have any impact on severe postoperative complications [15].

Surgical repairs in our institution were always carried out via an open approach. Currently, it is too early to recommend using laparoscopic and robotic tools for BDA in BDI repair [13]. However, the perspectives of minimally invasive repairs are quite promising for patients' quality of life [13].

Classification systems based on the biliary injury location include the first one published by Bismuth in 1982, that of Strasberg published in 1995, and others [3,24]. In 2013, the European Association for Endoscopic Surgery proposed the ATOM (Anatomic, Time Of detection, Mechanism) classification [3,40]. It covers all possible injuries by combining bile tract anatomical damage, vascular injury, the timing of detection, and damage mechanism. The intention was to standardize BDI definitions and facilitate data collection to develop preventive measures [40]. The main disadvantage of ATOM is that it may be too intricate and time-consuming for routine clinical practice [3]. We reported BDI according to the Strasberg classification (Table 3), as proposed by the World Society of Emergency Surgery [3]. Furthermore, we found this classification more useful than ATOM because we often classified BDI retrospectively according to the repair performed.

Figure 2 shows the results of actual patency. As expected, minor injuries repaired by a T-tube placement had an excellent outcome [3]. The results from the primary repair and T-tube group were less favorable, where one patient needed BDA. In the BDA group, 96.7% of patients attained primary patency, but only 56.6% remained in that grade.

Actuarial primary patency rates in the BDA group were 77.0%, 70.0%, and 70.0% at 1, 5, and 10 years, respectively (Figure 3 and Table 6). In the study by Cho et al., primary patency was achieved at 94.0%, and the 5- and 10-year rates were 92% [22]. Martínez–Mier reported a primary patency of 93.4%. The 1-, 5-, and 10-year rates were 91.2%, 53.9%, and 53.9%, respectively [41]. Lindemann et al. found a primary patency at 98.1%. The 1-, 5-, and 10-year retention rates were 96.4%, 90.6%, and 81.5% [42]. Otto et al. reported that actuarial grade A patency rates at 5 and 10 years were 88% and 74%, respectively [27].

The limitation of this study was the notably low number of patients, which precluded the use of advanced multivariate models and calculations. Another limitation was the retrospective nature of the study, with confined access to the patients' documentation. A useful future research direction would be to establish a nationwide registry of cholecystectomies to study their feasibility and safety in our country [12].

To conclude, the rate of BDI remains stable, and our center encourages colleagues to refer patients with confirmed or suspected BDI to a tertiary center. The outcomes in terms of complications and patency rates are comparable to those in other reports.

Author Contributions: Conceptualization: I.P. and A.I.; methodology: I.P., A.I. and Š.T.; software: I.P.; validation: A.I.; formal analysis: I.P.; investigation: B.L.P. and T.M.; resources: I.P., Š.T. and T.M.; data curation: S.P. and I.P.; writing—original draft preparation: I.P. and A.I.; writing—review and editing: I.P., Š.T., A.I., B.L.P. and S.P.; visualization: I.P.; supervision: S.P.; project administration: A.I.; funding acquisition: Š.T., A.I. and I.P. All authors have read and agreed to the published version of the manuscript.

Funding: The University Medical Centre Maribor funded the article processing charge, IRP-2023/02-10.

Institutional Review Board Statement: This study was conducted according to the guidelines of the Declaration of Helsinki and approved by the Institutional Ethics Committee of the University Medical Center Maribor (UKC-MB-KME-42/24, 25 September 2024).

Informed Consent Statement: Informed consent was obtained from all subjects involved in this study.

Data Availability Statement: Due to the patients' privacy, the data presented in this study are available upon request from the corresponding author.

Conflicts of Interest: The authors declare no conflicts of interest. The sponsor had no role in the design, execution, interpretation, or writing of this study.

References

1. Sparkman, R.S. 100th Anniversary of the First Cholecystectomy: A Reprinting of the 50th Anniversary Article From the Archives of Surgery, July 1932. *Arch. Surg.* **1982**, *117*, 1525. [CrossRef] [PubMed]
2. Blum, C.A.; Adams, D.B. Who did the first laparoscopic cholecystectomy? *J. Minim. Access Surg.* **2011**, *7*, 165–168. [CrossRef] [PubMed]
3. de'Angelis, N.; Catena, F.; Memeo, R.; Coccolini, F.; Martínez-Pérez, A.; Romeo, O.M.; De Simone, B.; Di Saverio, S.; Brustia, R.; Rhaiem, R.; et al. 2020 WSES guidelines for the detection and management of bile duct injury during cholecystectomy. *World J. Emerg. Surg.* **2021**, *16*, 30. [CrossRef] [PubMed]
4. Way, L.W.; Stewart, L.; Gantert, W.; Liu, K.; Lee, C.M.; Whang, K.; Hunter, J.G. Causes and prevention of laparoscopic bile duct injuries: Analysis of 252 cases from a human factors and cognitive psychology perspective. *Ann. Surg.* **2003**, *237*, 460–469. [CrossRef]
5. Pekolj, J. Introduction. In *Fundamentals of Bile Duct Injuries: From Prevention to Multidisciplinary Management*; Pekolj, J., Ardiles, V., Glinka, J., Eds.; Springer International Publishing: Cham, Switzerland, 2022; pp. 1–5.
6. Manatakis, D.K.; Antonopoulou, M.I.; Tasis, N.; Agalianos, C.; Tsouknidas, I.; Korkolis, D.P.; Dervenis, C. Critical View of Safety in Laparoscopic Cholecystectomy: A Systematic Review of Current Evidence and Future Perspectives. *World J. Surg.* **2023**, *47*, 640–648. [CrossRef]
7. Strasberg, S.M. A perspective on the critical view of safety in laparoscopic cholecystectomy. *Ann. Laparosc. Endosc. Surg.* **2017**, *2*, 91. [CrossRef]
8. Daly, S.C.; Deziel, D.J.; Li, X.; Thaqi, M.; Millikan, K.W.; Myers, J.A.; Bonomo, S.; Luu, M.B. Current practices in biliary surgery: Do we practice what we teach? *Surg. Endosc.* **2016**, *30*, 3345–3350. [CrossRef]
9. Dahmane, R.; Morjane, A.; Starc, A. Anatomy and surgical relevance of Rouviere's sulcus. *Sci. World J.* **2013**, *2013*, 254287. [CrossRef]
10. Lockhart, S.; Singh-Ranger, G. Rouviere's sulcus-Aspects of incorporating this valuable sign for laparoscopic cholecystectomy. *Asian J. Surg.* **2018**, *41*, 1–3. [CrossRef]
11. Basukala, S.; Thapa, N.; Tamang, A.; Shah, K.B.; Rayamajhi, B.B.; Ayer, D.; Karki, S.; Basukala, B.; Sharma, S.; Dhakal, S. Rouviere's sulcus—An anatomical landmark for safe laparoscopic cholecystectomy: A cross-sectional study. *Ann. Med. Surg.* **2022**, *75*, 103404. [CrossRef]
12. Brunt, L.M.; Deziel, D.J.; Telem, D.A.; Strasberg, S.M.; Aggarwal, R.; Asbun, H.; Bonjer, J.; McDonald, M.; Alseidi, A.; Ujiki, M.; et al. Safe Cholecystectomy Multi-society Practice Guideline and State of the Art Consensus Conference on Prevention of Bile Duct Injury During Cholecystectomy. *Ann. Surg.* **2020**, *272*, 3–23. [CrossRef] [PubMed]
13. Marichez, A.; Adam, J.P.; Laurent, C.; Chiche, L. Hepaticojejunostomy for bile duct injury: State of the art. *Langenbecks Arch. Surg.* **2023**, *408*, 107. [CrossRef] [PubMed]
14. Bonds, M.; Rocha, F. Cholecystectomy techniques and postoperative problems. In *Blumgart's Surgery of the Liver, Biliary Tract, and Pancreas*, 7th ed.; Jarnagin, W.R., Allen, P.J., Chapman, W.C., D'Angelica, M.I., DeMatteo, R.P., Do, R.K.G., Vauthey, J.-N., Blumgart, L.H., Eds.; Elsevier: Philadelphia, PA, USA, 2023; pp. 494–504.
15. Post cholecystectomy bile duct injury: Early, intermediate or late repair with hepaticojejunostomy—An E-AHPBA multi-center study. *HPB* **2019**, *21*, 1641–1647. [CrossRef]
16. Atay, A.; Gungor, F.; Sur, Y.; Gunes, O.; Dilek, F.H.; Karasu, Ş.; Dilek, O.N. Management of hepatic artery trauma during hepato-pancreato-biliary procedures: Evolving approaches, clinical outcomes, and literature review. *Ulus. Travma Acil Cerrahi Derg.* **2022**, *28*, 1549–1557. [CrossRef]
17. Perera, M.T.; Silva, M.A.; Hegab, B.; Muralidharan, V.; Bramhall, S.R.; Mayer, A.D.; Buckels, J.A.; Mirza, D.F. Specialist early and immediate repair of post-laparoscopic cholecystectomy bile duct injuries is associated with an improved long-term outcome. *Ann. Surg.* **2011**, *253*, 553–560. [CrossRef]
18. de Reuver, P.R.; Grossmann, I.; Busch, O.R.; Obertop, H.; van Gulik, T.M.; Gouma, D.J. Referral pattern and timing of repair are risk factors for complications after reconstructive surgery for bile duct injury. *Ann. Surg.* **2007**, *245*, 763–770. [CrossRef]
19. Stilling, N.M.; Fristrup, C.; Wettergren, A.; Ugianskis, A.; Nygaard, J.; Holte, K.; Bardram, L.; Sall, M.; Mortensen, M.B. Long-term outcome after early repair of iatrogenic bile duct injury. A national Danish multicentre study. *HPB* **2015**, *17*, 394–400. [CrossRef]
20. Plahuta, I.; Šarenac, Ž.; Golob, M.; Turk, Š.; Ilijevec, B.; Magdalenić, T.; Potrč, S.; Ivanecz, A. Laparoscopic and Open Distal Pancreatectomy-An Initial Single-Institution Experience with a Propensity Score Matching Analysis. *Life* **2025**, *15*, 97. [CrossRef]

21. Ivanecz, A.; Plahuta, I.; Mencinger, M.; Perus, I.; Magdalenic, T.; Turk, S.; Potrc, S. The learning curve of laparoscopic liver resection utilising a difficulty score. *Radiol. Oncol.* **2021**, *56*, 111–118. [CrossRef]
22. Cho, J.Y.; Baron, T.H.; Carr-Locke, D.L.; Chapman, W.C.; Costamagna, G.; de Santibanes, E.; Dominguez Rosado, I.; Garden, O.J.; Gouma, D.; Lillemoe, K.D.; et al. Proposed standards for reporting outcomes of treating biliary injuries. *HPB* **2018**, *20*, 370–378. [CrossRef]
23. Bredbeck, B.C.; Cho, C.S. Bile duct exploration and biliary-enteric anastomosis. In *Blumgart's Surgery of the Liver, Biliary Tract, and Pancreas*, 7th ed.; Jarnagin, W.R., Allen, P.J., Chapman, W.C., D'Angelica, M.I., DeMatteo, R.P., Do, R.K.G., Vauthey, J.-N., Blumgart, L.H., Eds.; Elsevier: Philadelphia, PA, USA, 2023; pp. 459–470.
24. Strasberg, S.M.; Hertl, M.; Soper, N.J. An analysis of the problem of biliary injury during laparoscopic cholecystectomy. *J. Am. Coll. Surg.* **1995**, *180*, 101–125. [PubMed]
25. Miura, F.; Okamoto, K.; Takada, T.; Strasberg, S.M.; Asbun, H.J.; Pitt, H.A.; Gomi, H.; Solomkin, J.S.; Schlossberg, D.; Han, H.S.; et al. Tokyo Guidelines 2018: Initial management of acute biliary infection and flowchart for acute cholangitis. *J. Hepatobiliary Pancreat. Sci.* **2018**, *25*, 31–40. [CrossRef] [PubMed]
26. Clavien, P.A.; Barkun, J.; de Oliveira, M.L.; Vauthey, J.N.; Dindo, D.; Schulick, R.D.; de Santibanes, E.; Pekolj, J.; Slankamenac, K.; Bassi, C.; et al. The Clavien-Dindo classification of surgical complications: Five-year experience. *Ann. Surg.* **2009**, *250*, 187–196. [CrossRef]
27. Otto, W.; Sierdziński, J.; Smaga, J.; Kornasiewicz, O.; Dudek, K.; Zieniewicz, K. Actuarial Patency Rates of Hepatico-Jejunal Anastomosis after Repair of Bile Duct Injury at a Reference Center. *J. Clin. Med.* **2022**, *11*, 3396. [CrossRef]
28. Habibzadeh, F. Statistical Data Editing in Scientific Articles. *J. Korean Med. Sci.* **2017**, *32*, 1072–1076. [CrossRef]
29. Bewick, V.; Cheek, L.; Ball, J. Statistics review 12: Survival analysis. *Crit. Care* **2004**, *8*, 389. [CrossRef]
30. Molinari, M. Traumatic Bile Duct Injuries. In *Actual Problems of Emergency Abdominal Surgery*; Garbuzenko, D.V., Ed.; IntechOpen: Rijeka, Croatia, 2016.
31. Breznik, S.; Slanič, A.; Ivanecz, A.; Lučev, J. Bilhemia After Percutaneous Liver Tumor Core Biopsy With the Percutaneous Embolization of Bilio-venous Fistula With Coils and Onyx. *Cureus* **2024**, *16*, e61414. [CrossRef] [PubMed]
32. Bektas, H.; Schrem, H.; Winny, M.; Klempnauer, J. Surgical treatment and outcome of iatrogenic bile duct lesions after cholecystectomy and the impact of different clinical classification systems. *Br. J. Surg.* **2007**, *94*, 1119–1127. [CrossRef]
33. Šileikis, A.; Žulpaitė, R.; Šileikytė, A.; Lukšta, M. Postcholecystectomy bile duct injuries: Evolution of surgical treatment. *Pol. Prz. Chir.* **2019**, *91*, 14–21. [CrossRef]
34. Kapoor, V.K. (Ed.) *Post-Cholecystectomy Bile Duct Injury*; Springer: Singapore, 2020; p. 264.
35. Törnqvist, B.; Strömberg, C.; Akre, O.; Enochsson, L.; Nilsson, M. Selective intraoperative cholangiography and risk of bile duct injury during cholecystectomy. *Br. J. Surg.* **2015**, *102*, 952–958. [CrossRef]
36. Goldstein, S.D.; Lautz, T.B. Fluorescent Cholangiography During Laparoscopic Cholecystectomy: Shedding New Light on Biliary Anatomy. *JAMA Surg.* **2020**, *155*, 978–979. [CrossRef] [PubMed]
37. Durowicz, S.; Kozicki, I.; Ciesielski, A.; Tarnowski, W. Excision of a part of the bile duct as an iatrogenic injury typical for laparoscopic cholecystectomy—Characteristics, treatment and long-term results, based on own material. *Wideochir. Inne Tech. Maloinwazyjne* **2020**, *15*, 70–79. [CrossRef] [PubMed]
38. Barbier, L.; Souche, R.; Slim, K.; Ah-Soune, P. Long-term consequences of bile duct injury after cholecystectomy. *J. Visc. Surg.* **2014**, *151*, 269–279. [CrossRef] [PubMed]
39. Törnqvist, B.; Strömberg, C.; Persson, G.; Nilsson, M. Effect of intended intraoperative cholangiography and early detection of bile duct injury on survival after cholecystectomy: Population based cohort study. *BMJ* **2012**, *345*, e6457. [CrossRef]
40. Fingerhut, A.; Dziri, C.; Garden, O.J.; Gouma, D.; Millat, B.; Neugebauer, E.; Paganini, A.; Targarona, E. ATOM, the all-inclusive, nominal EAES classification of bile duct injuries during cholecystectomy. *Surg. Endosc.* **2013**, *27*, 4608–4619. [CrossRef]
41. Martínez-Mier, G.; Moreno-Ley, P.I.; Mendez-Rico, D. Factors associated with patency loss and actuarial patency rate following post-cholecystectomy bile duct injury repair: Long-term follow-up. *Langenbecks Arch. Surg.* **2020**, *405*, 999–1006. [CrossRef]
42. Lindemann, J.; Krige, J.E.J.; Kotze, U.; Jonas, E. Factors leading to loss of patency after biliary reconstruction of major laparoscopic cholecystectomy bile duct injuries: An observational study with long-term outcomes. *HPB* **2020**, *22*, 1613–1621. [CrossRef]

life

MDPI

Case Report

Rectal Administration of Rifampicin and Isoniazid Suppositories: An Alternative Approach for the Treatment of Tuberculosis in a Patient with Multiple Comorbidities

Ioana Munteanu [1,2], Beatrice Burdușel [2,*], Catalin Constantin Coca [2], Dănuț Zisu [2], Constantin Gheorghevici [2], George Alexandru Diaconu [2], Diana Georgiana Stan [2], Nicolae Feraru [2], Andrei Tivda [2], Cristian George Popa [2], Florin Dumitru Mihălțan [2,3] and Corina Marginean [4]

1 Faculty of Medicine, Titu Maiorescu University, 040441 Bucharest, Romania; ioana.munteanu2015@yahoo.ro
2 "Marius Nasta" Institute of Pneumophtisiology, 050159 Bucharest, Romania
3 Faculty of Medicine, Carol Davila University of Medicine and Pharmacy, 050474 Bucharest, Romania
4 Faculty of Medicina, George Emil Palade University of Medicine and Pharmacy, Science and Technology, 540142 Târgu Mureș, Romania; corina.marginean@umf-st.ro
* Correspondence: beatriceciuchilan@gmail.com

Abstract: This article reports the case of a patient with a gastric neoplasm and total gastrectomy, presenting with severe digestive intolerance, who developed peritoneal and pulmonary tuberculosis. Standard treatment could not be administered. Therefore, treatment was initiated with isoniazid and rifampicin suppositories, and intravenous levofloxacin and amikacin, with significant remission of the digestive symptomatology. Although treatment with rifampicin suppositories has demonstrated efficacy in tuberculosis, it is rarely used in practice. This case highlights the importance of individualizing tuberculosis treatment and demonstrates that rectal administration of isoniazid and rifampicin suppositories, combined with intravenous levofloxacin and amikacin, was successfully used to treat tuberculosis in a patient with severe digestive intolerance, highlighting a potential alternative regimen when standard oral therapy is not feasible.

Keywords: tuberculosis; rectal suppositories; rifampicin; isoniazid; peritoneal

1. Introduction

Tuberculosis (TB) is a chronic infectious disease caused by the primary etiological agent *Mycobacterium tuberculosis*, with a predominant pulmonary tropism. The disease can manifest in various forms, ranging from latent infection to active disease, with a variable clinical presentation and the potential to develop severe complications [1]. Although mostly treatable, tuberculosis reemerged as the leading cause of death due to an infectious agent in 2023, after being surpassed by COVID-19 for three years, according to the WHO [2].

Treatment of active tuberculosis is most often carried out using standardized regimens; however, the individualization of antituberculosis therapy is justified in some cases. The most common route of drug administration is oral, including syrups for children, followed by intravenous administration [3]. Non-inferiority of rifampicin has been demonstrated with suppository administration [4], although this option is rarely used.

2. Case Presentation

We present the case of a 51-year-old male, a former smoker (40 pack-years, abstinent for 10 years), diagnosed with gastric neoplasm (poorly cohesive carcinoma with "signet ring" cells) one year prior to presentation to our service. The patient underwent a total gastrectomy and Roux-en-Y esophagojejunostomy and was undergoing chemotherapy. His medical history included arterial hypertension, previous myocardial infarction (severe single-vessel disease, treated with primary percutaneous coronary intervention with a stent on the left anterior descending artery), cardiorespiratory arrest due to ventricular fibrillation (resuscitated), and major right bundle branch block.

The patient was referred to the pulmonology department following combined imaging exploration (computed tomography—CT; positron emission tomography—PET) which revealed multiple pulmonary micro- and macronodular lesions with diffuse contours, located in the segments of both upper lobes and the right Fowler segment, with varying degrees of metabolic activity (Figure 1). Additionally, a flat, moderately enhancing lesion was located on the left lateral pleura, along with left pleurisy. There were also flat, metabolically active lesions at the level of the inner surface of the diaphragmatic domes and large-volume ascites.

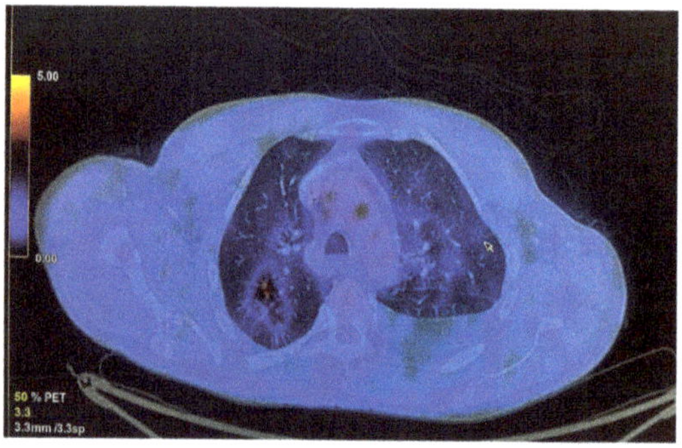

Figure 1. Metabolic activity in the posterior segment of the right upper lobe (RUL).

The patient's general condition was poor, with inappetence and a marked limitation of physical activity, with activities such as moving to the toilet being strenuous. Clinically, the patient was malnourished (BMI = 16 kg/m^2), inappetent, and dehydrated, presenting with abdominal distension and mild diffuse tenderness on palpation. Anamnestically, the patient reported daily vomiting (fasting and postprandial) for several weeks and the absence of bowel movements for 10 days, although the patient was passing flatus.

Vital signs were within normal limits. Laboratory findings showed leukocytosis ($14.91 \times 10^3/\mu L$) with neutrophilia (79.6%), thrombocytosis ($957 \times 10^3/\mu L$), an altered ionogram with hypochloremia (77 mmol/L), hyponatremia (120 mmol/L), and elevated serum urea (97 mg/dL).

3. Investigations

Induced sputum and GeneXpert TB testing revealed traces of *Mycobacterium tuberculosis*, though rifampicin resistance could not be assessed. Despite difficulties related to vomiting, repeated bronchoscopy attempts were made until an adequate bronchial sample was obtained, confirming a positive GeneXpert result without evidence of drug resistance.

The CT scan performed at the initiation of treatment revealed micronodular "tree-in-bud" infiltration predominantly in the upper half (Figure 2), bilaterally, with left-sided pleural effusion and large-volume fluid in the abdominopelvic cavity.

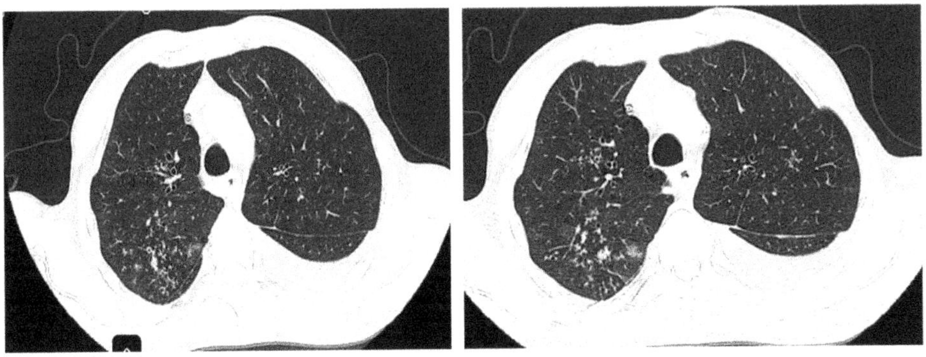

Figure 2. "Tree-in-bud" infiltration in the posterior segment of the right upper lobe (RUL) before treatment.

Regarding the large-volume ascites and suspicion of peritoneal tuberculosis, the cytological examination revealed rare mesothelial cells and lymphocytes and very rare neutrophils, without neoplastic cellularity. Therapeutic paracentesis was performed during the first two weeks prior to starting antituberculosis treatment.

For a definitive diagnosis, invasive diagnostic investigations are necessary, with the gold standard being peritoneal biopsy. However, given the patient's altered general condition and the positive result of the GeneXpert TB test at the pulmonary level, this procedure was not feasible, as our hospital does not have a general surgery department. Furthermore, transferring the patient to a surgery department of another hospital was not feasible in the context of a positive pulmonary GeneXpert test.

4. Treatment and Evolution

At the onset of therapy, the patient presented with persistent emetic episodes, with intolerance to orally administered medication. The attempt to place a nasogastric tube was complicated by esophageal mucosal laceration and self-limited hemorrhage, which required its removal. Subsequently, parenteral nutrition was initiated, and the patient maintained digestive intolerance, despite the administration of antiemetics or therapeutic combinations (metoclopramide, drotaverine, ondansetron, and octreotide).

In this case, standard therapeutic regimens for the treatment of tuberculosis, including isoniazid, rifampicin, pyrazinamide, and ethambutol, could not be administered due to the unavailability of injectable forms in our clinic and the intolerance to per os administration, i.e., an oral administration. Standard treatment protocols for tuberculosis recommend isoniazid dosages ranging from 4 to 6 mg/kg body weight and rifampicin doses between 8 and 12 mg/kg body weight [5]. Consequently, for the patient presented in this case, weighing approximately 45 kg, the indicated daily dosage corresponds to 180–270 mg of isoniazid and 360–540 mg of rifampicin. The therapeutic efficacy of antituberculosis regimens is enhanced through the utilization of fixed-dose combinations (FDCs). Within Romania, the sole FDC currently available integrates 150 mg of isoniazid with 300 mg of rifampicin [5]. This specific fixed-dose combination was selected for administration via suppositories in this case. For the formulation of the rectal suppositories, a prefabricated base composed of fatty acids and glycerol was used. After melting the base, the active pharmaceutical ingredients—isoniazid 150 mg and rifampicin 300 mg—were uniformly dispersed, and the resulting mixture was poured into molds for solidification. The treatment was supplemented by intravenous medication with levofloxacin 750 mg and amikacin 500 mg—corresponding to 10 mg/kg body weight—considering the possibility of toxicity at higher doses of amikacin and studies showing the efficacy of this dose in the treatment of tuberculosis [6].

Given that hepatotoxicity is a significant potential adverse effect of both isoniazid and rifampicin, hepatic function was monitored consistently throughout the treatment period, with results remaining within normal limits (Table 1). To mitigate the risk of isoniazid-induced peripheral neuropathy, vitamin B6 (pyridoxine) supplementation was concurrently administered. Furthermore, renal function was frequently assessed due to the potential nephrotoxicity associated with amikacin; however, no significant alterations were observed during therapy (Table 1).

Table 1. Laboratory blood investigations conducted at different time points during therapy.

Blood Parameters	Initiation of Treatment	1 Month of Treatment	2 Months of Treatment
Serum creatinine RR (reference range): 0.7–1.2 mg/dL	1.29 mg/dL	0.52 mg/dL	0.554 mg/dL
Serum urea RR: 17–43 mg/dL	97.9 mg/dL	21 mg/dL	27.3 mg/dL
Alanine transaminase RR: 0–50 U/L	15.6 U/L	12.6 U/L	41.9 U/L
Aspartate transaminase RR: 0–50 U/L	16.3 U/L	19.1 U/L	27.8 U/L
Hemoglobin RR: 13.5–16.9 g/dL	13.4 g/dL	9 g/dL	11.5 g/dL
Platelet count RR: 166–368 $\times$ 10^3 cells/μL	957 $\times$ 10^3 cells/μL	491 $\times$ 10^3 cells/μL	413 $\times$ 10^3 cells/μL
Erythrocyte sedimentation rate RR: 2–20 mm/h	23 mm/h	30 mm/h	10 mm/h

Regarding parenteral nutrition, total parenteral nutrition (TPN) was administered during the initial week. However, due to its subsequent unavailability from the pharmacy, the regimen was transitioned to an intravenous administration of 500 mL of 10% glucose solution twice daily, supplemented with 500 mL of physiological saline solution per day for the following period. Oral nutritional supplementation was not tolerated by the patient prior to the initiation of antituberculosis therapy. Approximately two to three weeks after initiating the treatment, the patient gradually resumed enteral feeding, which subsequently allowed for the tapering of the intravenous glucose solution.

Two months after the initiation of treatment (Figure 3), regression of interstitial densities, "tree-in-bud" micronodules, and the regression of ascites were noted. Although the lesions probably associated with tuberculosis were ameliorated, new pulmonary nodular lesions were detected, as well as an increase in a pre-existing nodule (Figure 4), most likely in the context of the underlying neoplastic pathology, whose treatment was interrupted during tuberculosis treatment.

Under the instituted treatment, the patient's condition improved, resuming oral feeding and completing the first two months of treatment with the mentioned combination. The patient was discharged and continued at-home treatment with isoniazid and rifampicin, following the completion of the initial two-month, four-antibiotic regimen.

Although the clinical evolution regarding abdominal tuberculosis was impressive, regarding the suspicion of pulmonary tuberculosis, cultures at two months from induced sputum, on a Lowenstein–Jensen solid medium, as well as the culture from bronchial aspirate, were negative.

At the end of the 3-month hospitalization period, the patient presented a weight gain of approximately 15 kg, resolution of ascites without recurrence, significant improvement in appetite, and improvement in general condition with the resumption of physical activity, including walks and daily bicycle exercises. This favorable clinical outcome retrospectively confirmed the correctness of the therapeutic decision.

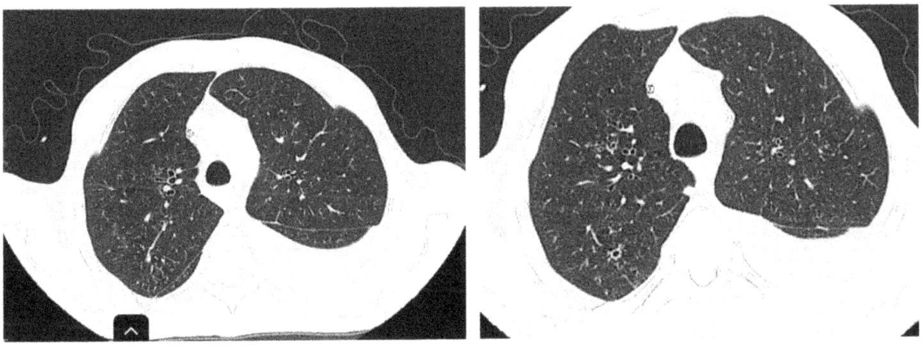

Figure 3. Improvement in "tree-in-bud" infiltration in the posterior segment of the right upper lobe (RUL) after 2 months of treatment.

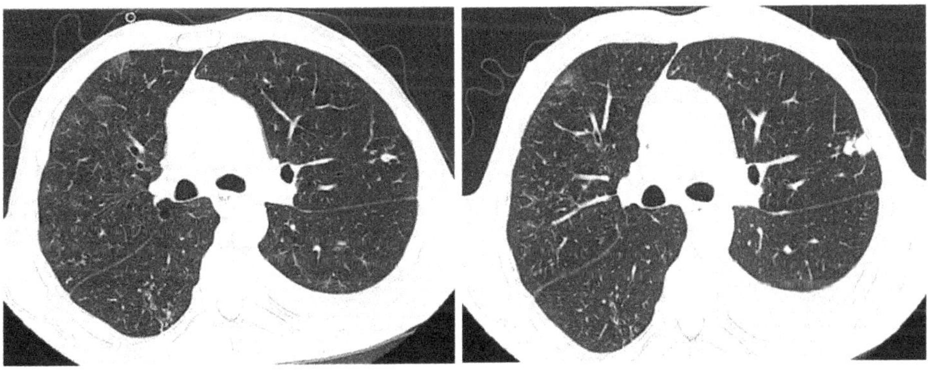

Figure 4. Enlargement of the pre-existing nodule and appearance of a new nodular formation at the superior lingular level.

5. Discussions

The diagnosis of peritoneal tuberculosis can be difficult, given its nonspecific presentation and the limitations of current diagnostic methods. A high degree of suspicion, especially in patients with risk factors for tuberculosis, is crucial. For diagnosis, a combination of clinical, laboratory, imaging, and histopathological elements is often required, and sometimes, empirical treatment may be necessary in cases with high clinical suspicion but negative test results [7]. In the context of our case, a definitive diagnosis via a peritoneal biopsy was precluded by several factors. As our institution is a single-specialty pneumophthisiology clinic without surgical capabilities, the procedure could not be performed on-site. Furthermore, transfer to a surgical department at another facility was contraindicated due to the patient's positive pulmonary GeneXpert result, posing an infectious risk, alongside concerns raised by the consulting surgeon regarding the patient's significant perioperative risk. Nevertheless, retrospectively, we can infer that the diagnosis of peritoneal tuberculosis was likely correct, given the patient's positive response to the instituted antituberculosis therapy, manifested by the resolution of ascites and improvement in symptoms.

The diagnosis and treatment of tuberculosis in patients with multiple comorbidities and poor nutritional status represent a challenge. In the presented case, the diagnosis was difficult to establish, given the complex clinical picture and the lack of conclusive bacteriological evidence for peritoneal tuberculosis.

The most common route of administration for antituberculosis treatment is oral. In particular situations, the administration of pharmaceutical preparations in the form of injectable solutions, infusions, or syrups may be used. The administration of syrups is especially recommended for pediatric patients under 6 years of age [3]. The option of rifampicin and/or isoniazid suppositories is rarely used but has been described. Also, considering that tuberculosis prophylaxis is carried out with isoniazid, the in vitro release of isoniazid from suppositories was studied in order to optimize the suppository dosage and form for this indication [8].

In a 2017 study on the treatment of tuberculosis, Noriyuki and Shigeatsu mentioned that they did not find significant differences between the group treated with rifampicin suppositories and the oral administration group regarding the time required for culture and smear negativity. These findings suggest that rifampicin suppositories could represent a viable therapeutic alternative for tuberculosis patients who cannot tolerate the oral administration of standard medication [4].

Given that rifampicin has low oral bioavailability and hepatotoxicity, although it is a first-line drug, mucoadhesive rectal gel was evaluated in a 2021 study on rabbits, as a tool for rifampicin administration, which significantly improved rifampicin bioavailability compared to oral suspension and solid rectal suppositories in rabbits. In addition, toxicity studies have demonstrated the ability of in situ mucoadhesive rectal gel to minimize rifampicin-induced hepatotoxicity, so studies on other routes of administration are important [9].

In our patient's case, digestive intolerance and the impossibility of administering standardized therapy required an atypical therapeutic approach. The use of isoniazid and rifampicin suppositories, although less conventional, proved effective in this context, allowing the patient to tolerate treatment and achieve significant clinical improvement.

Although assessing serum rifampicin levels would provide valuable pharmacokinetic data regarding absorption from suppositories, the unavailability of this assay within Romania's public healthcare system precluded such measurements. This aspect represents a significant limitation in the context of our case.

6. Conclusions

Although there are few reports of similar cases in the literature, there is evidence supporting the use of isoniazid and rifampicin suppositories as a viable therapeutic option in patients with digestive intolerance and contraindications for other forms of antituberculosis drug administration [4].

This case illustrates the complexity of therapeutic management in such situations and suggests that the administration of isoniazid and rifampicin suppositories can be a viable alternative when other routes of administration cannot be utilized.

Regarding peritoneal tuberculosis, its diagnosis can be challenging, given its nonspecific presentation and the limitations of current diagnostic modalities. A high degree of suspicion, particularly in patients with risk factors for tuberculosis, is crucial. For diagnosis, a combination of clinical, laboratory, imaging, and histopathological elements is often required, and sometimes, empirical treatment may be necessary in cases with high clinical suspicion but negative test results [7,10,11].

In this complex case, a treatment regimen combining the rectal administration of isoniazid and rifampicin suppositories with intravenous levofloxacin and amikacin resulted in a successful clinical outcome for tuberculosis despite severe digestive intolerance. This supports the consideration of rectally administered isoniazid and rifampicin as a viable component of therapy when standard routes are contraindicated.

Funding: This research received no external funding.

Institutional Review Board Statement: The study was conducted in accordance with the Declaration of Helsinki and approved by the Ethics Committee of the "Marius Nasta" Institute of Pneumophtisiology (no. 4522; approval date: 7 March 2025).

Informed Consent Statement: Informed consent was obtained from all subjects involved in the study.

Data Availability Statement: Data used to support the findings of this article are available from the corresponding author upon request.

Conflicts of Interest: The authors declare no conflicts of interest.

Abbreviations

The following abbreviations are used in this manuscript:

BMI	Body Mass Index
CT	Computed Tomography
FDCs	Fixed-Dose Combinations
GeneXpert TB	Refers to the Specific Diagnostic Test For Mycobacterium Tuberculosis
PET	Positron Emission Tomography
RUL	Right Upper Lobe
TB	Tuberculosis
TPN	Total Parenteral Nutrition
WHO	World Health Organization
COVID-19	Coronavirus Disease 2019
RR	Reference Range

References

1. Socaci, A.; Nini, G.; Marica, C. *Epidemiologia Tuberculozei. Tuberculoza de la Diagnostic la Tratament*; Partos: Timişoara, Romania, 2013; pp. 8–9.
2. Global Tuberculosis Report. World Health Organization: Geneva, Switzerland, 2024. Available online: https://www.who.int/teams/global-tuberculosis-programme/tb-reports/global-tuberculosis-report-2024 (accessed on 7 March 2025).
3. Fildan, A.P.; Homorodean, D.; Mahler, B.; Nedelcu, R.E.; Popa, C.G.; Popescu, G.G. Tratamentul tuberculozei. In *Tuberculoza Manual Pentru Profesioniștii din Sănătate*; Institutul de Pneumoftiziologie „Marius Nasta": Bucharest, Romania, 2022; pp. 152–154. Available online: https://marius-nasta.ro/wp-content/uploads/2022/07/Manual-TB-FINAL_A-1.pdf (accessed on 7 March 2025).
4. Tsubota, N.; Tanimukai, S. A clinical experience of rifampicin suppository for the treatment of pulmonary tuberculosis. *Kekkaku* **2015**, *90*, 543–547. [PubMed]
5. Munteanu, I.; Arghir, O.C.; Balta, M.; Balteanu, M.; Cazacu, A.C.; Ciomaga, M.; Cioran, N.V.; Coriu, R.; Dantes, E.; Dinca, M.; et al. *GHID METODOLOGIC DE IMPLEMENTARE A PROGRAMULUI NAŢIONAL DE PREVENIRE, SUPRAVEGHERE ȘI CONTROL AL TUBERCULOZEI ȘI ALTOR MICOBACTERIOZE*; Bucharest, Romania. 2023, pp. 39–40, ISBN 978-973-0-38231-0. Available online: https://marius-nasta.ro/wp-content/uploads/2023/04/Ghid%20metodologic%20TB.pdf (accessed on 7 March 2025).
6. Sabur, N.F.; Brar, M.S.; Wu, L.; Brode, S.K. Low-dose amikacin in the treatment of Multidrug-resistant Tuberculosis (MDR-TB). *BMC Infect. Dis.* **2021**, *21*, 254. [CrossRef] [PubMed]
7. Koff, A.; Azar, M.M. Diagnosing peritoneal tuberculosis. *BMJ Case Rep.* **2020**, *13*, e233131. [CrossRef] [PubMed] [PubMed Central]
8. Hudson, K.C.; Asbill, C.S.; Webster, A.A. Isoniazid release from suppositories compounded with selected bases. *Int. J. Pharm. Compd.* **2007**, *11*, 433–437. [PubMed]

9. Al-Joufi, F.; Elmowafy, M.; Alruwaili, N.K.; Alharbi, K.S.; Shalaby, K.; Alsharari, S.D.; Ali, H.M. Mucoadhesive In Situ Rectal Gel Loaded with Rifampicin: Strategy to Improve Bioavailability and Alleviate Liver Toxicity. *Pharmaceutics* **2021**, *13*, 336. [CrossRef] [PubMed]
10. Sen, D.; Brunton, J.; Melchior, L.; Klein, D.; Levy, G.H.; Wainscoat, B.; Chuang, L. Peritoneal tuberculosis: A case report on a rare cause of tumor marker elevation. *Case. Rep. Womens Health.* **2020**, *28*, e00264. [CrossRef] [PubMed] [PubMed Central]
11. Uygur-Bayramiçli, O.; Dabak, G.; Dabak, R. A clinical dilemma: Abdominal tuberculosis. *World J. Gastroenterol.* **2003**, *9*, 1098–1101. [CrossRef] [PubMed]

life

MDPI

Article

Impact of Depression on Health-Related Quality of Life in Ulcerative Colitis Patients—Are We Doing Enough? A Single Tertiary Center Experience

Dunja Jaksic [1,*], Sasa Vuksanovic [2], Aleksandar Toplicanin [2], Jelena Spiric-Milovancevic [2], Gorica Maric [3] and Aleksandra Sokic-Milutinovic [2,4]

[1] Department of Gastroenterology and Hepatology, Clinic for Internal Medicine, Clinical Hospital Center Zemun, 11 000 Belgrade, Serbia
[2] Clinic for Gastroenterology and Hepatology, University Clinical Center of Serbia, 11000 Belgrade, Serbia; sashavuksanovic9@gmail.com (S.V.); aleksandartoplicanin4@gmail.com (A.T.); spiricjelena77@gmail.com (J.S.-M.); asokicmilutinovic@gmail.com (A.S.-M.)
[3] Institute of Epidemiology Faculty of Medicine, University of Belgrade, 11000 Belgrade, Serbia; goricamaric87@gmail.com
[4] Faculty of Medicine, University of Belgrade, 11000 Belgrade, Serbia
* Correspondence: dunja1510@yahoo.co.uk

Abstract: Ulcerative colitis (UC) significantly impacts patients' health-related quality of life (HRQOL). This study aimed to evaluate HRQOL and the factors affecting it, and the prevalence of anxiety, depression and alexythimia in patients with UC. This cross-sectional study included 248 UC patients (21 with proctitis, 63 with left-sided UC and 164 with extensive colitis). Data were collected using standardized self-administered questionnaires [a socio-demographic questionnaire, General Anxiety Disorder-7 (GAD-7), the Patient Health Questionnaire-9 (PHQ-9), the Toronto Alexithymia Scale (TAS-20) and the Short Inflammatory Bowel Disease Questionnaire (SIBDQ)]. Clinical data on remission status, extraintestinal manifestations, comorbidities and the use of advanced therapies were also collected. Hierarchical regression analysis of variables predicting SIBDQ score was done. Clinical and laboratory remission was present in 95.6% of the patients. The prevalences of depression, anxiety and alexithymia were 44.7%, 34.3% and 30.2%, respectively. There were no differences in the PHQ-9, GAD-7 and TAS-20 scores in relation to remission status. The average SIBDQ score was 56.5. The patients in remission reported better SIBDQ scores compared to the symptomatic patients ($p = 0.002$). The hierarchical regression analysis showed that remission of disease and a higher depression score influenced HRQOL in the UC patients. The prevalence of depression, anxiety and alexithymia in the UC patients was high. Remission of disease and a high depression score were the main factors related to HRQOL.

Keywords: ulcerative colitis; depression; anxiety; alexithymia; health-related quality of life; remission

1. Introduction

Chronic inflammatory bowel diseases (IBD)—ulcerative colitis (UC) and Crohn's disease (CD)—are characterized by chronic gastrointestinal inflammation and a relapsing–remitting course [1]. The exact pathophysiology of IBD remains unclear. It is understood as a multifactorial interplay involving disturbance in gastrointestinal physiology, intestinal microbiome, immunology, and genetics [2]. At the beginning of the 21st century, the global incidence and prevalence of IBD were rising. The prevalence is rising in Western Europe, North America and Oceania, while the incidence is increasing in Latin America, Asia and Africa [3]. UC is characterized by diffuse inflammation affecting the rectal mucosa and extending to proximal segments of the colon. UC most commonly presents with diarrhea, which may contain blood and mucus. Fever and abdominal pain may also occur, as well as extraintestinal manifestations. The therapeutic options for UC patients include mesalazine, corticosteroids, immunosuppressants, advanced therapies (monoclonal antibodies and small molecules) and surgery.

Health-related quality of life (HRQOL) comprises the aspects of well-being that are related to or affected by the presence of disease or its treatment, as perceived by the patient [4]. A diagnosis of an IBD affects the HRQOL of patients due to their chronic symptoms, early-life onset, unpredictable course, the severity of the symptoms, as well as the side effects of conservative and surgical treatments, which interfere with daily activities and alter the patient's lifestyle [5]. Short-term and long-term therapeutic goals in UC have evolved from initially controlling the symptoms to healing the mucosa and restoring a normal quality of life. The STRIDE II recommendations, issued by the International Organization for IBD in 2021, state that the ultimate treatment goal is to maintain a normal HRQOL and prevent disability [6].

Psychological symptoms may worsen the HRQOL in outpatients with an IBD [7,8]. The incidence and prevalence of depression and anxiety are higher in IBD patients compared with populations without an IBD [9]. Based on a systematic review of 48 studies, the prevalence of anxiety disorders ranges from 3.8% to 25% in the general population, while in patients with chronic diseases, it is estimated to be as high as 70% [10]. The average prevalence of depression in Europe is 7%, which varies between regions [11]. In patients with an IBD, the prevalence of anxiety is 20.5% and the prevalence of depression is 21.2%, which are higher than those of healthy controls [12,13]. A systematic review and meta-analysis by Barberio et al., which included 30,118 patients, showed that one-third of IBD patients are anxious and a quarter are depressed. During the active phase of the disease, one in two patients is either anxious or depressed [14].

A meta-analysis by Bisgaard et al. revealed that all IBD patients, both adult and pediatric, are at a 1.5-times higher risk of anxiety and depression [15].

The relationship between IBDs and depression and anxiety seems to be bidirectional [15]. The mechanisms behind this relationship include increased levels of pro-inflammatory cytokines, vagal nerve signaling, gut dysbiosis, and changes in brain signaling and morphology [16]. The intestinal microbiota has recently been recognized as an integral part of the brain–gut axis, which can potentially modulate behavioral and cognitive functioning through endocrine, neural and metabolic signaling. This led to a change in terminology and some authors now refer to it as brain–gut–microbiota axis [17–19]. Patients who experience depression or anxiety tend to report more frequent disease relapses and a worse general well-being, as the emotional burden exacerbates their physical symptoms [20–23]. Relapses may worsen anxiety and depression and can make it harder for patients to adhere to treatment regimens or to seek care.

Certain researchers consider IBDs as examples of a psychosomatic disorder [24]. Alexithymia ("no words for feelings") is a personality feature characterized by difficulties in identifying, analyzing and verbalizing feelings, restricted imaginal capacities and a limited emotional experience [25]. Alexithymia is considered to be a risk factor for various psychiatric and psychosomatic disorders and its presence positively correlates with anxiety and depression in patients with an IBD [26–28]. The co-occurrence of depression, anxiety and alexithymia in IBD patients often creates a vicious cycle.

Patients with UC should be screened for co-existing anxiety and depressive disorders, and, once diagnosed, the patients should be provided with resources to address these conditions [29]. Despite the known impact of these mental health conditions on patients' morbidity and quality of life, they often go unrecognized and untreated. Addressing this gap requires increased awareness and routine mental health screening to improve the overall outcomes for IBD patients.

This study aimed to evaluate HRQOL using the SIBDQ and the possible factors affecting it, and the prevalence of anxiety, depression and alexithymia in patients with UC. The majority of the previously published studies focused on the prevalence of anxiety, depression and alexithymia in all IBD patients and the data focusing solely on UC patients are limited.

2. Materials and Methods

2.1. Study Design and Settings

This cross-sectional study was conducted at the Clinic for Gastroenterology and Hepatology, University Clinical Center of Serbia, in Belgrade, from January 2023 to February 2024. All participants gave written informed consent before participating in this study. The study was conducted in accordance with the 1964 Declaration of Helsinki and its later amendments and all applicable Serbian laws and guidelines. The study was approved by the Ethics Committee of the Faculty of Medicine, University of Belgrade (approval number: 17/I-12; date: 12 January 2023) prior to the start of the study, before the enrolment of the first patient.

2.2. Selection of Participants

Consecutive outpatients with a confirmed UC diagnosis, treated in the Clinic for Gastroenterology and Hepatology during the study period, were evaluated for inclusion in the study. UC was diagnosed according to clinical, laboratory, endoscopic and pathohistological findings [30].

The inclusion criteria were age > 18 years, provided signed informed consent, completed all questionnaires, and had a confirmed UC diagnosis.

The exclusion criteria were refusal to participate in study, inability to complete questionnaires due to cognitive deficit or language issues, or had an unconfirmed UC diagnosis.

2.3. Instruments

The collection of data on the socio-demographic and clinical characteristics of the participants (HRQOL, symptoms of anxiety, depression and alexithymia) was carried out using questionnaires. The questionnaires used in this study were as follows: a socio-demographic questionnaire, the Short Inflammatory Bowel Disease Questionnaire (SIBDQ), the Patient Health Questionnaire-9 (PHQ-9), General Anxiety Disorder-7 (GAD-7) and the Toronto Alexithymia Scale (TAS-20). The licensed Serbian translation of the SIBDQ was used. The PHQ-9, GAD-7 and TAS-20 were translated and validated in the Serbian language. All the questionnaires contain questions that are closed-ended. The questionnaires were completed by the patients in writing.

The patients with psychological scores suggesting depression and anxiety were advised to consult with a mental health professional.

2.4. Questionnaire on Socio-Demographic Characteristics

A standardized questionnaire was used to collect the following information: name and surname, sex, year of birth, education level, occupation, marital and employment statuses, income level, smoking status and alcohol consumption level. This section was completed by the patient. The next section of this questionnaire, which describes the clinical characteristics of the disease, was completed by the treating physician and was used to collect the following information: extent of the disease according to the Montreal classification, year of diagnosis, laboratory parameters (CRP, Hgb, Fe, ferritin, and fecal calprotectin), presence of extraintestinal manifestations, surgeries, comorbidities, allergies, presence of clinical (S0 according to Montreal classification) and laboratory remission and the ongoing therapy for UC [31]. Data on the clinical parameters of the patients with an IBD were obtained from their medical records.

2.5. Laboratory Analyses

Laboratory analyses were conducted within a few days of completing the questionnaire. The presence of laboratory remission was defined as unaltered levels of biomarkers, CRP and fecal calprotectin, and the absence of disease-related anemia.

2.6. Quality of Life Assessment (SIBDQ)

The SIBDQ is a questionnaire that is used to specifically assess the HRQOL of patients with an IBD [32]. It contains 10 questions covering 4 domains of quality of life: bowel, systemic, social and emotional. Each question offers 7 response options on a Likert scale, ranging from 1 (a severe problem) to 7 (not a problem at all), giving a total SIBDQ score ranging from 10 (poor HRQOL) to 70 (optimal HRQOL). There are no validated cut-offs for the different dimensions' scores. A SIBDQ score below 50 was considered as poor HRQOL.

2.7. Depression Symptom Score Assessment (PHQ-9)

The PHQ-9 is a self-assessment questionnaire that diagnoses and determines the severity of depression based on 9 major depressive criteria. The responses are scored 0 (never) to 3 (every day) [33]. The score ranges from 0 to 27, with a higher score indicating a greater degree of depression. Scores of 5, 10, 15, and 20 represent the cut-offs for mild, moderate, moderately severe, and severe depression, respectively. A PHQ-9 score > 9 had a sensitivity of 88% and a specificity of 88% for major depression compared with a structured psychiatric interview as the diagnostic gold standard [33].

2.8. Anxiety Symptom Score Assessment (GAD-7)

The GAD-7 is a self-assessment questionnaire for the intensity of symptoms of generalized anxiety disorder [34]. It consists of seven statements related to the core symptoms of the disorder (e.g., "I worry too much about different things"). Respondents are asked to indicate how often they experienced any of the listed symptoms over the previous two weeks. The responses are given on a Likert scale from 0 ("not at all") to 3 ("nearly every day"). The total score from the questionnaire indicates the intensity of the symptoms of generalized anxiety disorder. The results are categorized into four levels based on the intensity of anxiety symptoms: a score of 0 to 4 indicates minimal anxiety, 5 to 9 indicates mild anxiety, 10 to 14 indicates moderate anxiety, and 15 to 21 indicates a high anxiety symptom intensity. Using the threshold score of 10, the GAD-7 sensitivity is 89% and specificity is 82% compared to a structured psychiatric interview as the diagnostic gold standard [35].

2.9. Alexithymia Assessment (TAS-20)

The TAS-20 has 20 questions divided into 3 domains: difficulties in identifying emotions, difficulties in expressing emotions and externally oriented thinking (the tendency to focus attention outward) [36]. A score of up to 51 indicates no alexithymia, 52–60 indicates possible alexithymia, while a score above 60 indicates its presence. The test is devised not only to calculate total scores, but also to associate a score with each one of the aforementioned three dimensions.

2.10. Statistical Processing and Data Analysis

The data were analyzed using IBM SPSS 17.0 software package for Windows. Descriptive statistical methods were used to describe the socio-demographic characteristics of the patients. Parametric data are expressed as means and standard deviations, while non-parametric data are expressed as medians. The prevalences of anxiety, depression and alexithymia were calculated as the proportion of individuals with an IBD who have specific mental disorders out of all the individuals in the sample. Hierarchical regression analysis was performed to identify the factors associated with HRQOL in UC. The possible confounding variables identified in our study included age, sex, presence of comorbidities, previously diagnosed mental disorders and effects of medication, particularly corticosteroids. The effects of possible covariates were excluded using hierarchical regression analysis. The dependent variable was HRQOL, expressed as the SIBDQ score. Model 1 includes sex and age as independent variables or predictors. Model 2 adds disease duration, remission status, extraintestinal manifestations and advanced therapy treatment. Model 3 incorporates measures of depression, anxiety and alexithymia (PHQ-9, GAD-7 and TAS-20 total scores, respectively). A p value < 0.05 was considered statistically significant.

3. Results

3.1. Demographic Characteristics of Patients

This cross-sectional study included 248 patients with UC, of whom, 21 (8.5%) had proctitis, 63 (25.4%) had left-sided UC and 164 (66.1%) had extensive colitis. The demographic characteristics of the participants are described in Table 1. The mean age of our patients was 45 ± 15 years, with the majority having a secondary school-level education(52.4%) and were employed (64.0%), married (52%) and had a monthly income between RSD 50,000 and 100,000 (51.9%). In terms of life habits, 62.9% were non-smokers and 50% had never consumed alcohol.

Table 1. Demographic characteristics of patients with ulcerative colitis.

Variable	Frequency (%)
Sex (%)	
Male	117 (47.2)
Female	131 (52.8)
Age (years, mean ± SD)	45 ± 15
Educational level (%)	
Primary school	12 (4.8)
Secondary school	130 (52.4)
College	31 (12.5)
Faculty	75 (30.2)
Working status (%)	
Permanent job	137 (55.5)
Temporary job	21 (8.5)
Unemployed	45 (18.2)
Retired	44 (17.8)
Marital status (%)	
Married	129 (52.0)
Extramarital union	16 (6.5)
Widowed	14 (5.6)
Divorced	21 (8.5)
Single	68 (27.4)

Table 1. *Cont.*

Variable	Frequency (%)
Income level (%)	
<RSD 50,000	97 (39.9)
RSD 50–100,000	126 (51.9)
>RSD 100,000	20 (8.2)
Smoking status (%)	
Non-smoker	156 (62.9)
Smoker	50 (20.2)
Ex-smoker	42 (16.9)
Alcohol consumption (%)	
Never	124 (50.0)
Up to 1 glass/day	4 (1.6)
On occasion	120 (48.4)

SD—standard deviation; RSD—Serbian dinar.

3.2. *Clinical Characteristics of Patients with Ulcerative Colitis*

The clinical characteristics of the study population are described in Table 2. The mean age at UC diagnosis was 36 ± 14 years. The average disease duration was 9.3 ± 7.4 years. The average CRP value was 1.7 g/L (range 0–298.7). At the time the study was conducted, 95.6% of the patients were in clinical and laboratory remission. Extraintestinal manifestations were present in 22.6% of the patients, while 23.4% had a comorbidity. When it came to treatment, 49.6% of the participants were on mesalazine, 4.0% received corticosteroid treatment in the year before they enrolled in the study, 52% were on immunosuppressants and 79.8% were treated with advanced therapies (biologic drugs or small molecules). None of the patients were using corticosteroid therapy at the time the study was conducted.

Table 2. Clinical characteristics of patients.

Variable	Value	Accepted Normal Range
Age at diagnosis (years)	36 ± 14	
Age at diagnosis (%)		
<16 years of age	12 (4.8)	
17–40 years of age	161 (64.9)	
>40 years of age	75 (30.2)	
Disease duration (years)	9.3 ± 7.4	
CRP (g/L) (median, range)	1.7 (0–298.7)	0–5
Hemoglobin (g/L)	139.7 ± 17.3	120–160
Iron (μmolL)	14.9 ± 7.6	11–32
Ferritin (μgL) (median, range)	48.5 (0.9–580)	30–100
Calprotectin (μg/g) (median, range)	81.45 (0–2000)	0–100
In remission at the time of the study (%)		
Yes	237 (95.6)	
No	11 (4.4)	
Extraintestinal manifestations of disease (%)		
Yes	56 (22.6)	
No	192 (77.4)	
Presence of comorbidity (%)		
Yes	58 (23.4)	
No	190 (76.6)	
Prior mental disorder (%)		
Yes	1 (0.4)	
No	247 (99.6)	

Table 2. *Cont.*

Variable	Value	Accepted Normal Range
IBD therapy (%)		
Mesalazine	123 (49.6)	
Corticosteroid treatment in last year	10 (4.0)	
Immunosuppressants	129 (52.0)	
Azathioprine	115	
Methotrexate	14	
Advanced therapies	198 (79.8)	
Infliximab	23	
Infliximab biosimilar	83	
Adalimumab	34	
Adalimumab biosimilar	2	
Vedolizumab	52	
Tofacitinib	4	

3.3. HRQOL and Prevalence of Depression, Anxiety and Alexithymia

The patients' scores on the PHQ-9, GAD-7, TAS-20 and SIBDQ are shown in Table 3. The average SIBDQ score was 56.5 ± 10.9 (range 16–70). Poor HRQOL (SIBDQ < 50) was observed in 61 participants (24.6%). The average SIBDQ score in the UC patients in remission was 56.9, while those with active disease had an average SIBDQ score of 46.8.

Table 3. SIBDQ, PHQ-9, GAD-7 and TAS-20 scores in patients with UC.

Variable	Value	Score Range
SIBDQ (range)	56.5 ± 10.9 (16–70)	10–70
SIBDQ categories (%)		
Poor HRQOL	61 (24.6)	SIBDQ < 50
Optimal HRQOL	187 (75.4)	SIBDQ ≥ 50
PHQ-9 total score (range)	5.2 ± 4.5 (0–27)	0–27
PHQ-9 categories (%)		
None–minimal depression	137 (55.2)	0–4
Mild depression	75 (30.2)	5–9
Moderate depression	25 (10.1)	10–14
Moderately severe depression	9 (3.6)	15–19
Severe depression	2 (0.8)	20–27
GAD-7 total score (range)	4.3 ± 4.7 (0–21)	0–21
GAD-7 categories (%)		
Minimal anxiety	163 (65.7)	0–4
Mild anxiety	51 (20.6)	5–9
Moderate anxiety	21 (8.5)	10–14
Severe anxiety	13 (5.2)	15–21
TAS-20 total score (range)	46.7 ± 12.3 (20–94)	20–100
TAS-20 categories (%)		
No alexithymia	173 (69.8)	20–51
Possible alexithymia	41 (16.5)	52–60
Alexithymia present	34 (13.7)	61–100

The prevalence of depression, assessed using the PHQ-9 symptom score and a cut-off of 5 (including patients with mild depression), was 44.7%. If a PHQ-9 threshold score of 10 (excluding patients with mild depression) was used, the prevalence of depression was 14.5%.

Based on GAD-7, the prevalence of anxiety was 34.3%. A total of 30.2% of the participants had possible alexithymia, and 13.7% had alexithymia.

Figure 1 shows the SIBDQ, TAS-20, GAD-7 and PHQ-9 score distributions according to the localization of the UC. None of the scales reached statistical significance (for SIBDQ: F = 1.668, p = 0.191; for TAS-20: F = 0.041, p = 0.960; for GAD-7: F = 0.928, p = 0.397; for PHQ-9: F = 0.897, p = 0.409). When the participants were compared in terms of treatment with advanced therapy, none of the scores differed (PHQ-9: p = 0.565; GAD-7: p = 0.891; TAS-20: p = 0.874; SIBDQ: p = 0.117).

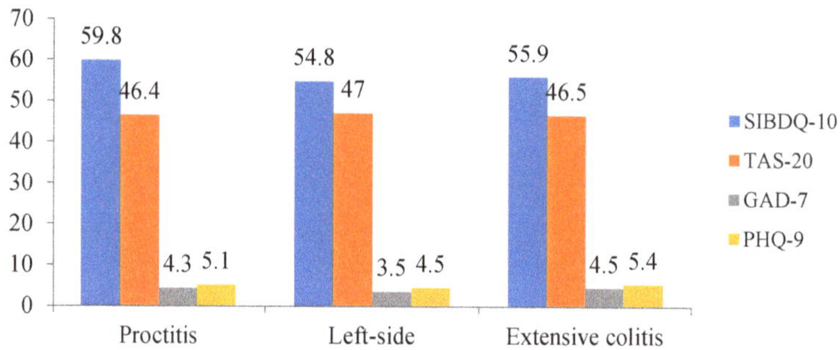

Figure 1. SIBDQ, TAS-20, GAD-7 and PHQ-9 score distributions according to UC localization.

Figure 2 shows the SIBDQ, TAS-20, GAD-7 and PHQ-9 score distributions between the patients in remission and the patients with active UC. The remission group had a statistically significant higher SIBDQ score (F = 0.667, p = 0.002). The scores for the mental health scales of the patients with active disease and those in remission did not differ significantly (for TAS-20: F = 0.001, p = 0.550; for GAD-7: F = 0.330, p = 0.972; for PHQ-9: F = 1.237, p = 0.294).

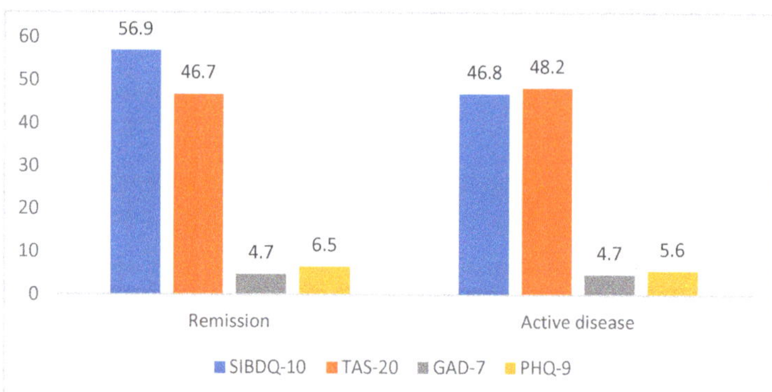

Figure 2. SIBDQ, TAS-20, GAD-7 and PHQ-9 score distributions between UC patients in remission and patients with active disease.

Table 4 presents the SIBDQ score distribution according to the level of depression, anxiety and alexithymia. All the scale scores including the PHQ-9, GAD-7 and TAS-20 scores were associated with the HRQOL of the UC patients, as measured by the SIBDQ score. The strongest correlation was observed between depression severity, measured by the PHQ-9 score and SIBDQ score (r = −0.584, $p < 0.001$), which was negative, indicating that a higher depression score among the UC patients correlated with worse HRQOL. Similarly, anxiety level moderately and negatively correlated with SIBDQ scores (r = −0.398,

$p < 0.001$), indicating an association between a higher anxiety level and impaired HRQOL in UC patients. The relationship between the TAS-20 and SIBDQ scores was also negative but it was weak-to-moderate in strength (r = −0.339, $p < 0.001$), showing that an increase in the alexithymia score significantly deteriorates the HRQOL of UC patients.

Table 4. SIBDQ score values according to level of depression, anxiety and alexithymia.

Variable	Value	
	Score	Correlation with SIBDQ
PHQ-9 categories		
None–minimal depression	61.6 ± 7.2	
Mild depression	53.7 ± 9.4	r = −0.584
Moderate depression	46.1 ± 11.6	$p < 0.001$
Moderate-severe depression	37.1 ± 8.5	
Severe depression	29.0 ± 5.7	
GAD-7 categories		
Minimal anxiety	59.4 ± 8.7	
Mild anxiety	54.8 ± 11.0	r = −0.398
Moderate anxiety	50.2 ± 9.4	$p < 0.001$
Severe anxiety	36.4 ± 11.3	
TAS-20 categories		
No alexithymia	58.6 ± 10.0	r = −0.339
Possible alexithymia	54.2 ± 11.0	$p < 0.001$
Alexithymia present	48.2 ± 10.8	

3.4. *Regression Analysis of Factors Associated with SIBDQ Score*

In Table 5, the results of the hierarchical regression analysis of factors influencing the SIBDQ score in the UC patients is shown. In model 1 and model 2, the effect of sex was positive, but very small and non-significant (β = 0.03 and 0.04, respectively). In model 3, the relationship became slightly negative (β = −0.06) but remained non-significant. Across all the models, age had a minimal effect, with consistently non-significant β values (close to 0). In model 2 and model 3, disease duration showed negligible effects (β = −0.01 and 0.03, respectively), indicating no meaningful relationship. In model 2, remission had a significant positive effect (β = 0.20, $p < 0.01$), indicating that the patients in remission tended to have higher SIBDQ scores. In model 3, this remained significant, but the effect slightly decreased in strength (β = 0.17, $p < 0.01$). In model 2, extraintestinal manifestations had a significant negative effect (β = −0.13, $p < 0.05$), indicating worse scores for those with extraintestinal manifestations. In model 3, this effect became non-significant (β = −0.02). Advanced therapy treatment, in model 2 and model 3, had no significant effect (β close to 0). The PHQ-9 score, in model 3, had a strong negative effect (β = −0.62, $p < 0.01$), which indicates that higher depression scores were significantly associated with worse outcome scores. The GAD-7 score, in model 3, had no significant effect (β = −0.06), suggesting that anxiety had little additional influence when controlling for other variables. The TAS-20 score, in model 3, had no significant effect (β = 0.01), indicating alexithymia was not a key predictor in this model. Remission status was consistently associated with higher scores, indicating better outcomes for patients in remission. Extraintestinal manifestations negatively affected the SIBDQ scores, but this effect diminished after controlling for psychological variables. The depression symptom (PHQ-9) score was the strongest predictor in model 3. The anxiety symptom (GAD-7) score and alexithymia (TAS-20) score did not contribute much when depression was included in the model. Overall, the variables in the first model (age and sex) explained 0.4% of the variance in the SIBDQ scores (F for change in $R^2 = 0.525$, $p > 0.05$). Adding remission status, presence of extraintestinal manifestations and treatment with advanced therapies explained another 5.3% of the variance (F for change in R^2 = 2.904, $p < 0.05$). Finally, including the PHQ-9, GAD-7 and TAS-20 total scores resulted in 40.6% of the variance being explained (F for change in R^2 = 25.776, $p < 0.01$). This means that all the variables in the three models explained a total of 46.3% of the difference in SIBDQ scores in the patients with UC.

Table 5. Factors associated with SIBDQ score in UC patients—hierarchical regression analysis.

Variable	Model 1			Model 2			Model 3		
	B	**SE (B)**	**β**	**B**	**SE (B)**	**β**	**B**	**SE (B)**	**β**
Sex	0.64	1.39	0.03	0.81	1.37	0.04	−1.24	1.05	−0.06
Age	0.04	0.05	0.06	0.04	0.05	0.06	−0.01	0.04	−0.01
Disease duration				−0.01	0.10	−0.01	0.04	0.08	0.03
Remission yes vs. no				9.62	3.32	0.20	9.10	2.53	0.17
Extraintestinal manifestations yes vs. no				−3.28	1.63	−0.13	−0.54	1.26	−0.02
Advanced therapy treatment yes vs. no				−0.55	1.86	−0.02	0.65	1.42	0.02
PHQ-9 total score							−1.47	0.19	−0.62
GAD-7 total score							−0.13	0.18	−0.06
TAS-20 total score							0.01	0.05	0.01
R^2		0.004			0.057			0.463	
F for change in R^2		0.525			2.904			25.776	

4. Discussion

4.1. Demographic and Clinical Data

This cross-sectional study included 248 patients diagnosed with UC, of whom, 21 (8.5%) had proctitis, 63 (25.4%) had left-sided UC and 164 (66.1%) had extensive colitis. The mean age of our patients was 45 ± 15 years. The mean age at UC diagnosis was 36 ± 14 years, which is consistent with previously published results [37]. The average disease duration was 9.3 ± 7.4 years (range 0–49 years). The gender distribution was equal, with a slight female predominance since we included 131 (52.8%) females and 117 (47.2%) males, which is in agreement with the majority of studies describing an equal distribution of UC between genders [37].

Age and gender did not impact the HRQOL in our patients, which was shown by the regression analysis. The majority of the UC patients in our study had a secondary-level education (52.4%), were married (52%) and employed (64.0%), with a moderate monthly income (51.9%). The Global Burden of Disease study suggested higher IBD rates in individuals with a higher socioeconomic status, while our findings revealed that only 8.2% patients had a high monthly income [38].

In terms of life habits, 62.9% of the patients had never smoked, 20% were active smokers and 16.9% were ex-smokers, which is consistent with the previously reported possible protective role of smoking in UC patients [37]. Nevertheless, the data from a recent study revealed that current smokers had a 2.3-fold higher risk of UC in prospective analyses vs. those who have never smoked [39]. The smoking status after diagnosis, according to published data, does not affect the disease course or clinical outcomes [40].

At the time the study was conducted, 95.6% of the participants were in clinical and laboratory remission, resulting in normal average values for their laboratory parameters. Extraintestinal manifestations were present in 22.6% patients, while 23.4% had a comorbidity. Only one (0.4%) participant had a previously diagnosed depressive disorder.

In the hierarchical regression analysis, extraintestinal manifestations negatively affected the SIBDQ score, but this effect disappeared after controlling for psychological variables.

Half of the participants were treated with mesalazine and 52% were on immunosuppressants. Ten patients (4%) were treated with corticosteroids in the year before the study, but none of the patients were taking corticosteroids during the study period. The majority of patients (79.8%) were treated with advanced therapies (biologic drugs or small molecules) since our study was conducted at a tertiary referral center. The high percentage of patients using advanced therapy may not be reflective of a broader UC population, but it includes UC patients with severe form of disease in whom low HRQOL and psychological disorders are to be expected.

4.2. Health-Related Quality of Life

The average SIBDQ score was 56.5 ± 10.9. Poor HRQOL (SIBDQ < 50) was observed in 61 of the UC patients (24.6%). The patients in remission, as expected, had better SIBDQ scores compared to those experiencing active symptoms (56.9 vs. 46.8, respectively, $p = 0.002$). The results of the hierarchical regression analysis showed that remission of disease and a higher depression score were the main factors influencing HRQOL in the UC patients.

In previously published studies, disease activity was found to be the most important predictor of HRQOL [41,42]. A prospective observational study on 115 patients with an IBD found that clinical remission normalized the HRQOL in 82% of the patients with UC, which, importantly, was not related to the type of treatment [43]. In a group of IBD patients in remission, the low HRQOL was significantly associated with surgery, disease duration, sleep disturbance, anxiety/depression and high illness perception [44]. Anxiety, depression, fatigue and IBS symptoms were all independently associated with a lower HRQOL in patients with an inactive IBD [45]. Psychological symptoms of emotional disorders appear to be associated with a lower HRQOL in IBD patients [46].

We found no differences in HRQOL regarding the use of advanced therapies. Among UC patients in a real-world setting, the patients on advanced therapies were less likely to be in remission, and had more moderate-to-severe disease and worse patient reported outcome (PROs) than patients on mesalazine therapy [47]. The results of a meta-analysis suggested that biologics have the potential to improve the HRQOL of UC patients [48]. High-quality evidence suggests that infliximab provides a clinically meaningful improvement in HRQOL in UC patients receiving induction therapy. Moderate-quality evidence suggests that vedolizumab provides a clinically meaningful improvement in HRQOL in UC patients receiving maintenance therapy. Biological therapies have shown improvement in the HRQOL of patients with ulcerative colitis during the induction phase, with benefits that are maintained during maintenance treatment [48,49]. Studies have indicated that small molecules can improve HRQOL [49,50].

4.3. Depression, Anxiety and Alexithymia in UC Patients

The instruments used for the assessment of HRQOL, depression, anxiety and alexithymia in UC vary among studies [51]. In our study, the prevalence of depression, anxiety and alexithymia was 44.7%, 34.3% and 30.2%, respectively, which is consistent with previously published data [8,14,15,52]. There were no differences in the PHQ-9, GAD-7 and TAS-20 scores in relation to remission status ($p > 0.05$).

It was previously reported that during the active phase of the disease, one in two patients is either anxious or depressed [14]. Prior investigations revealed that in patients newly diagnosed with moderate-to-severe UC, the prevalence of depression was 41.8% and that of anxiety was 33.7% in the first four weeks after diagnosis [8]. A Chinese cross-sectional study showed that 58% of patients with active UC had depression, while 50% had anxiety [52].

A retrospective study of 327 outpatient IBD patients showed that the prevalence of anxiety was 21.2% and that of depression was 25.8% [53]. In that study, the presence of depression and/or anxiety was determined using the PHQ-9 and GAD-7 self-report questionnaires or by diagnosis through a psychiatric interview.

A prospective cohort study from Manitoba, which included 363 participants, found that the prevalence of depression was twice as high in the IBD group compared to the control group, with 27.2% of the IBD patients and 12.3% of the controls being affected [9]. The IBD subtype (CD or UC) was unrelated to a psychiatric diagnosis. The strength of the Manitoba study is that they used a psychiatric interview, the composite international diagnostic interview, based on diagnostic criteria from the *Diagnostic and Statistical Manual of Mental Disorders (DSM-IV)* published by the American Psychiatric Association, which is the gold standard for diagnosing depression [54].

In one study, 33% of IBD patients had symptoms of anxiety and 16.5% had symptoms of depression [55]. They found that exposure to more than one biologic therapy, fatigue and symptoms of anxiety were associated with a lower HRQOL in the multivariate analysis.

A review of seven studies found that the incidence of depression was 3.6–26.9/1000 person-years in IBD patients, compared to 2.5–12.2/1000 person-years in the reference population [15]. The incidence of anxiety in the IBD patients was 4.0–25.0/1000 person-years, while in the controls, it was 3.0–16.3/1000 person-years. A meta-analysis of five studies examining the risk of anxiety and depression after an IBD diagnosis showed that IBD patients had an increased risk of anxiety (HR: 1.48; 95% CI: 1.29–1.70) and depression (HR: 1.55; 95% CI: 1.35–1.78) [15].

We did not find an association between mental disorders and the use of biological therapy, which is consistent with the results of a study with a similar methodology [23].

The prevalence of psychological disturbances in IBDs varies across studies, owing to heterogeneity in the study populations, time of assessment (whether it is across the lifespan or over a single period of life, usually the first year after the IBD diagnosis) or assessment tools for depression and anxiety.

The prevalence of alexithymia in our study was 30.2%, which is consistent with the literature data [27,56,57]. The mean TAS-20 score was 46.7 ± 12.3.

A total of 41 patients (16.5%) had possible alexithymia and 34 patients (13.7%) had a TAS-20 score >61, indicating they had alexithymia. In one systematic review, the mean alexithymia score ranged from 39 to 53.2, thus mostly falling in the normal range and indicating no alexithymia and the authors concluded that IBD patients cannot be considered alexithymic to a clinically significant extent [27]. They are more alexithymic compared to healthy participants, similar to patients with irritable bowel syndrome, and less alexithymic than patients with major depressive disorder. In the aforementioned study, there was an association between the level of alexithymia and other relevant psychological variables, such as anxiety and depression, but that was not confirmed in our study [27].

4.4. *Influence of Depression, Anxiety and Alexithymia on HRQOL*

A higher depression symptom score was one of the main factors influencing HRQOL in the UC patients. Our results are consistent with the results in the literature [8,44,58]. A Korean nationwide prospective cohort study highlighted that the presence of either significant anxiety or depression had a strong negative impact on both disease-specific and generic HRQOL [8]. The prospective study showed that anxiety and/or depression, particularly anxiety, present at the time of UC diagnosis did not influence long-term clinical outcomes (remission rates, response rates or hospitalization rates), but they persistently impaired HRQOL [7]. In one cross-sectional study, a low HRQOL, measured by the SIBDQ score, was associated with UC but not CD, IBD surgery, disease duration, sleep disturbance or anxiety/depression [44].

4.5. Other Factors Influencing HRQOL—Possible Role of Gut–Brain Axis and Genetic Factors?

The absence of differences in the PHQ-9 and GAD-7 scores of patients in remission and those with active disease suggests that psychological disorders are not solely caused by the presence of an IBD. Anxiety and depression persisted in the UC patients even during remission.

The gut–brain–microbiota axis establishes a connection between the brain and the vast community of bacteria in the intestinal tract [18]. Recent studies have shown that the gut microbiome influences brain processes [19]. The ability of the gut microbiota to affect central nervous system (CNS) activities is mainly mediated trough neurological (autonomic nervous system), hormonal (hypothalamus–pituitary–adrenal axis) and immunological (cytokine and chemokine) processes, all of which are interrelated [59]. The gut microbiome synthesizes various molecules that can impact brain function, including neurotransmitters (dopamine, serotonin, GABA, short chain fatty acids (SCFAs) and tryptophan). Psychological disorders are related to reduced gut microbiota richness and diversity. Compared to UC patients without depression and or anxiety, those with these conditions exhibit lower microbial diversity, a decrease in anti-inflammatory SCFA (butyrate)-producing bacteria, an increase in lactic acid-producing bacteria and higher levels of bacteria associated with glutamate and GABA metabolism [52,60,61].

Recent Mendelian randomization studies suggested a genetic predisposition to depression increases the risk of IBDs (both CD and UC). Also, the authors suggested that genetic susceptibility to UC is associated with anxiety, but not vice versa [62,63].

4.6. Strengths and Limitations of the Study

The strengths of our study are as follows:

- The study focused on an important clinical issue: the psychological burden of UC and its effects on HRQOL.
- We simultaneously investigated HRQOL and anxiety/depression status, along with the clinical and demographic characteristics of a large group of UC patients.

The limitations of the study are as follows:

- The institution where the study was conducted is a tertiary center and mainly treats patients with more severe and complex disease behaviors. A multicenter study, with a larger number of patients and more patients on conventional therapy, would provide a more accurate assessment of HRQOL, as well as the prevalence of anxiety, depression and alexithymia in the population of patients with UC as a whole.
- A cross-sectional study design cannot reveal the direction of causal relationships between psychological disorders, UC and HRQOL and the long-term impact of psychological factors on disease progression and HRQOL.
- In this study, self-administered questionnaires were used, which were completed by the participant on their symptoms of anxiety, depression, and alexithymia at the time of assessment.
- Questionnaires are not used for diagnosing psychiatric disorders, but they can be used for screening and identifying patients who require further psychiatric evaluation. The gold standard for diagnosing these disorders remains a psychiatric interview.

5. Conclusions

The prevalence of depression, anxiety and alexithymia in UC patients was high, even if the disease was in remission. Remission of disease and a high depression score were the main factors related to HRQOL. Depression adversely affected HRQOL in the UC patients, highlighting the need for psychological screening and mental health support for all UC patients.

We strongly recommend, based on our study results, routine mental health screening for all UC patients and referrals to mental health specialists if needed.

Author Contributions: Conceptualization, A.S.-M.; methodology, A.S.-M. and G.M.; formal analysis, G.M.; investigation, S.V., A.T. and J.S.-M.; resources A.S.-M.; data curation D.J.; writing—original draft preparation, D.J.; writing—review and editing, D.J.; supervision, A.S.-M. and G.M.; project administration, A.S.-M. All authors have read and agreed to the published version of the manuscript.

Funding: This research received no external funding.

Institutional Review Board Statement: The study was conducted in accordance with the 1964 Declaration of Helsinki and its later amendments and all applicable Serbian laws and guidelines. The study was approved by the Ethics Committee of Faculty of Medicine, University of Belgrade (approval number 17/I-12 date: 12 January 2023), prior to the start of the study, before the enrolment of the first patient.

Informed Consent Statement: Written informed consent was obtained from the patients for participation in this research and the subsequent use of the obtained data.

Data Availability Statement: The raw data supporting the conclusions of this article will be made available by the authors on request.

Conflicts of Interest: The authors declare no conflicts of interest.

Abbreviations

The following abbreviations are used in this manuscript:

IBD	Inflammatory bowel disease
UC	Ulcerative colitis
CD	Crohn's disease
SIBDQ	Short Inflammatory Bowel Disease Questionnaire
PHQ- 9	Patient Health Questionnaire-9
GAD-7	General Anxiety Disorder-7
TAS-20	Toronto Alexithymia Scale

References

1. Liu, D.; Saikam, V.; Skrada, K.A.; Merlin, D.; Iyer, S.S. Inflammatory bowel disease biomarkers. *Med. Res. Rev.* **2022**, *42*, 1856–1887. [CrossRef]
2. Mulder, D.J.; Noble, A.J.; Justinich, C.J.; Duffin, J.M. A tale of two diseases: The history of inflammatory bowel disease. *J. Crohns Colitis.* **2014**, *8*, 341–348. [CrossRef] [PubMed]
3. Kaplan, G.; Hracs, L.; Windsor, J.; Gorospe, J.; Cummings, M.; Coward, S.; Buie, M.; Quan, J.; Goddard, Q.; Caplan, L.; et al. The Global Evolution of Inflammatory Bowel Disease across Four Epidemiologic Stages. *Res. Sq.* 2024; *preprint*. [CrossRef]
4. Karimi, M.; Brazier, J. Health, health-related quality of life, and quality of life: What is the difference? *Pharmacoeconomics* **2016**, *34*, 645–649. [CrossRef]
5. Nugent, Z.; Singh, H.; Targownik, L.; Strome, T.; Snider, C.; Bernstein, C.N. Predictors of emergency department use by persons with inflammatory bowel diseases: A population-based study. *Inflamm. Bowel Dis.* **2016**, *22*, 2907–2916. [CrossRef]
6. Turner, D.; Ricciuto, A.; Lewis, A.; D'amico, F.; Dhaliwal, J.; Griffiths, A.M.; Bettenworth, D.; Sandborn, W.J.; Sands, B.E.; Reinisch, W.; et al. International Organization for the Study of IBD. STRIDE-II: An Update on the Selecting Therapeutic Targets in Inflammatory Bowel Disease (STRIDE) Initiative of the International Organization for the Study of IBD (IOIBD): Determining Therapeutic Goals for Treat-to-Target strategies in IBD. *Gastroenterology* **2021**, *160*, 1570–1583. [CrossRef] [PubMed]

7. Oh, S.J.; Choi, C.H.; Jung, S.A.; Song, G.A.; Kim, Y.J.; Koo, J.S.; Shin, S.J.; Seo, G.S.; Lee, K.M.; Jang, B.I.; et al. Anxiety and Depression Are Associated with Poor Long-term Quality of Life in Moderate-to-Severe Ulcerative Colitis: Results of a 3-Year Longitudinal Study of the MOSAIK Cohort. *Gut Liver* **2024**, *19*, 253–264. [CrossRef]
8. Moon, J.R.; Lee, C.K.; Hong, S.N.; Im, J.P.; Ye, B.D.; Cha, J.M.; Jung, S.A.; Lee, K.M.; Park, D.I.; Jeen, Y.T.; et al. MOSAIK study group of the Korean Association for Study of Intestinal Diseases. Unmet Psychosocial Needs of Patients with Newly Diagnosed Ulcerative Colitis: Results from the Nationwide Prospective Cohort Study in Korea. *Gut Liver* **2020**, *14*, 459–467, Erratum in *Gut Liver* **2021**, *15*, 146–147. [CrossRef]
9. Walker, J.R.; Ediger, J.P.; Graff, L.A.; Greenfeld, J.M.; Clara, I.; Lix, L.; Rawsthorne, P.; Miller, N.; Rogala, L.; McPhail, C.M.; et al. The Manitoba IBD cohort study: A population-based study of the prevalence of lifetime and 12-month anxiety and mood disorders. *Am. J. Gastroenterol.* **2008**, *103*, 1989–1997. [CrossRef]
10. Remes, O.; Brayne, C.; van der Linde, R.; Lafortune, L. A systematic review of reviews on the prevalence of anxiety disorders in adult populations. *Brain Behav.* **2016**, *6*, e00497. [CrossRef]
11. Arias-de la Torre, J.; Vilagut, G.; Ronaldson, A.; Serrano-Blanco, A.; Martín, V.; Peters, M.; Valderas, J.M.; Dregan, A.; Alonso, J. Prevalence and variability of current depressive disorder in 27 European countries: A population-based study. *Lancet Public Health* **2021**, *6*, e729–e738. [CrossRef] [PubMed]
12. Torres, J.; Ellul, P.; Langhorst, J.; Mikocka-Walus, A.; Acosta, M.B.-D.; Basnayake, C.; Ding, N.J.S.; Gilardi, D.; Katsanos, K.; Moser, G.; et al. European Crohn's and Colitis Organisation Topical Review on Complementary Medicine and Psychotherapy in Inflammatory Bowel Disease. *J. Crohn's Colitis.* **2019**, *13*, 673–685e. [CrossRef]
13. Irving, P.; Barrett, K.; Nijher, M.; de Lusignan, S. Prevalence of depression and anxiety in people with inflammatory bowel disease and associated healthcare use: Population-based cohort study. *BMJ Ment. Health* **2021**, *24*, 102–109. [CrossRef]
14. Barberio, B.; Zamani, M.; Black, C.J.; Savarino, E.V.; Ford, A.C. Prevalence of symptoms of anxiety and depression in patients with inflammatory bowel disease: A systematic review and meta-analysis. *Lancet Gastroenterol. Hepatol.* **2021**, *6*, 359–370. [CrossRef]
15. Bisgaard, T.H.; Allin, K.H.; Elmahdi, R.; Jess, T. The bidirectional risk of inflammatory bowel disease and anxiety or depression: A systematic review and meta-analysis. *Gen. Hosp. Psychiatry.* **2023**, *83*, 109–116. [CrossRef]
16. Bisgaard, T.H.; Allin, K.H.; Keefer, L.; Ananthakrishnan, A.N.; Jess, T. Depression and anxiety in inflammatory bowel disease: Epidemiology, mechanisms and treatment. *Nat. Rev. Gastroenterol. Hepatol.* **2022**, *19*, 717–726. [CrossRef]
17. Peppas, S.; Pansieri, C.; Piovani, D.; Danese, S.; Peyrin-Biroulet, L.; Tsantes, A.G.; Brunetta, E.; Tsantes, A.E.; Bonovas, S. The Brain-Gut Axis: Psychological Functioning and Inflammatory Bowel Diseases. *J. Clin. Med.* **2021**, *10*, 377. [CrossRef] [PubMed]
18. Cryan, J.F.; O'Riordan, K.J.; Cowan, C.S.M.; Sandhu, K.V.; Bastiaanssen, T.F.S.; Boehme, M.; Codagnone, M.G.; Cussotto, S.; Fulling, C.; Golubeva, A.V.; et al. The Microbiota-Gut-Brain Axis. *Physiol. Rev.* **2019**, *99*, 1877–2013. [CrossRef]
19. Arzani, M.; Jahromi, S.R.; Ghorbani, Z.; Vahabizad, F.; Martelletti, P.; Ghaemi, A.; Sacco, S.; Togha, M.; School of Advanced Studies of the European Headache Federation (EHF-SAS). Gut-brain Axis and migraine headache: A comprehensive review. *J. Headache Pain.* **2020**, *21*, 15. [CrossRef]
20. Jordi, S.B.U.; Lang, B.M.; Auschra, B.; von Känel, R.; Biedermann, L.; Greuter, T.; Schreiner, P.; Rogler, G.; Krupka, N.; Sulz, M.C.; et al. Depressive symptoms predict clinical recurrence of inflammatory bowel disease. *Inflamm. Bowel Dis.* **2022**, *28*, 560–571. [CrossRef]
21. Fairbrass, K.M.; Gracie, D.J.; Ford, A.C. Relative Contribution of Disease Activity and Psychological Health to Prognosis of Inflammatory Bowel Disease During 6.5 Years of Longitudinal Follow-Up. *Gastroenterology* **2022**, *163*, 190–203. [CrossRef] [PubMed]
22. Narula, N.; Pinto-Sanchez, M.I.; Calo, N.C.; Ford, A.C.; Bercik, P.; Reinisch, W.; Moayyedi, P. Anxiety but Not Depression Predicts Poor Outcomes in Inflammatory Bowel Disease. *Inflamm. Bowel Dis.* **2019**, *25*, 1255–1261. [CrossRef] [PubMed]
23. Lontai, L.; Elek, L.P.; Balogh, F.; Angyal, D.; Pajkossy, P.; Gonczi, L.; Lakatos, P.L.; Iliás, Á. Burden of Mental Health among Patients with Inflammatory Bowel Disease—A Cross-Sectional Study from a Tertiary IBD Center in Hungary. *J. Clin. Med.* **2024**, *13*, 2002. [CrossRef]
24. La Barbera, D.; Bonanno, B.; Rumeo, M.V.; Alabastro, V.; Frenda, M.; Massihnia, E.; Morgante, M.C.; Sideli, L.; Craxì, A.; Cappello, M.; et al. Alexithymia and personality traits of patients with inflammatory bowel disease. *Sci. Rep.* **2017**, *7*, 41786. [CrossRef]
25. Sifneos, P.E. The prevalence of 'alexithymic' characteristics in psychosomatic patients. *Psychother. Psychosom.* **1973**, *22*, 255–262. [CrossRef]
26. van der Velde, J.; Servaas, M.N.; Goerlich, K.S.; Bruggeman, R.; Horton, P.; Costafreda, S.G.; Aleman, A. Neural correlates of alexithymia: A meta-analysis of emotion processing studies. *Neurosci. Biobehav. Rev.* **2013**, *37*, 1774–1785. [CrossRef]
27. Martino, G.; Caputo, A.; Schwarz, P.; Bellone, F.; Fries, W.; Quattropani, M.C.; Vicario, C.M. Alexithymia and Inflammatory Bowel Disease: A Systematic Review. *Front. Psychol.* **2020**, *11*, 1763. [CrossRef] [PubMed]
28. Scaldaferri, F.; D'Onofrio, A.M.; Calia, R.; Di Vincenzo, F.; Ferrajoli, G.F.; Petito, V.; Maggio, E.; Pafundi, P.C.; Napolitano, D.; Masi, L.; et al. Gut Microbiota Signatures Are Associated with Psychopathological Profiles in Patients with Ulcerative Colitis: Results from an Italian Tertiary IBD Center. *Inflamm. Bowel Dis.* **2023**, *29*, 1805–1818. [CrossRef]

29. Rubin, D.T.; Ananthakrishnan, A.N.; Siegel, C.A.; Sauer, B.G.; Long, M.D. ACG Clinical Guideline: Ulcerative Colitis in Adults. *Am. J. Gastroenterol.* **2019**, *114*, 384–413. [CrossRef]
30. Maaser, C.; Sturm, A.; Vavricka, S.R.; Kucharzik, T.; Fiorino, G.; Annese, V.; Calabrese, E.; Baumgart, D.C.; Bettenworth, D.; Borralho Nunes, P.; et al. ECCO-ESGAR guideline for diagnostic assessment in IBD Part 1: Initial diagnosis, monitoring of known IBD, detection of complications. *J. Crohn's Colitis* **2019**, *13*, 144–164. [CrossRef]
31. Silverberg, M.S.; Satsangi, J.; Ahmad, T.; Arnott, I.D.; Bernstein, C.N.; Brant, S.R.; Caprilli, R.; Colombel, J.F.; Gasche, C.; Geboes, K.; et al. Toward an integrated clinical, molecular and serological classification of inflammatory bowel disease: Report of a Working Party of the 2005 Montreal World Congress of Gastroenterology. *Can. J. Gastroenterol.* **2005**, *19*, 5A–36A. [CrossRef]
32. Irvine, E.J.; Zhou, Q.; Thompson, A.K. The Short Inflammatory Bowel Disease Questionnaire: A quality of life instrument for community physicians managing inflammatory bowel disease. CCRPT Investigators. Canadian Crohn's Relapse Prevention Trial. *Am. J. Gastroenterol.* **1996**, *91*, 1571–1578.
33. Kroenke, K.; Spitzer, R.L.; Williams, J.B. The PHQ-9: Validity of a brief depression severity measure. *J. Gen. Intern. Med.* **2001**, *16*, 606–613. [CrossRef]
34. Löwe, B.; Decker, O.; Müller, S.; Brähler, E.; Schellberg, D.; Herzog, W.; Herzberg, P.Y. Validation and standardization of the Generalized Anxiety Disorder Screener (GAD-7) in the general population. *Med. Care.* **2008**, *46*, 266–274. [CrossRef] [PubMed]
35. Castro, C.M.; Mithal, A.; Deyhim, T.; Rabinowitz, L.G.; Olagoke, O.; Freedman, S.D.; Cheifetz, A.S.; Ballou, S.K.; Papamichael, K. Morning Salivary Cortisol Has a Positive Correlation with GAD-7 Scores in Patients with Ulcerative Colitis. *J. Clin. Med.* **2024**, *13*, 6707. [CrossRef] [PubMed]
36. Bagby, R.M.; Parker, J.D.; Taylor, G.J. The twenty-item Toronto Alexithymia Scale--I. Item selection and cross-validation of the factor structure. *J. Psychosom. Res.* **1994**, *38*, 23–32. [CrossRef]
37. da Silva, B.C.; Lyra, A.C.; Rocha, R.; Santana, G.O. Epidemiology, demographic characteristics and prognostic predictors of ulcerative colitis. *World J. Gastroenterol.* **2014**, *20*, 9458–9467. [CrossRef] [PubMed]
38. Li, C.J.; Wang, Y.K.; Zhang, S.M.; Ren, M.D.; He, S.X. Global burden of inflammatory bowel disease 1990–2019: A systematic examination of the disease burden and twenty-year forecast. *World J. Gastroenterol.* **2023**, *29*, 5751–5767. [CrossRef]
39. Pedersen, K.M.; Çolak, Y.; Vedel-Krogh, S.; Kobylecki, C.J.; Bojesen, S.E.; Nordestgaard, B.G. Risk of ulcerative colitis and Crohn's disease in smokers lacks causal evidence. *Eur. J. Epidemiol.* **2022**, *37*, 735–745. [CrossRef]
40. Caron, B.; Honap, S.; Peyrin-Biroulet, L. Epidemiology of Inflammatory Bowel Disease across the Ages in the Era of Advanced Therapies. *J. Crohns Colitis.* **2024**, *18* (Suppl. S2), ii3–ii15. [CrossRef]
41. Janke, K.H.; Klump, B.; Gregor, M.; Meisner, C.; Haeuser, W. Determinants of life satisfaction in inflammatory bowel disease. *Inflamm. Bowel Dis.* **2005**, *11*, 272–286. [CrossRef] [PubMed]
42. Irvine, E.J. Quality of life of patients with ulcerative colitis: Past, present, and future. *Inflamm. Bowel Dis.* **2008**, *14*, 554–565. [CrossRef]
43. Casellas, F.; Barreiro de Acosta, M.; Iglesias, M.; Robles, V.; Nos, P.; Aguas, M.; Riestra, S.; de Francisco, R.; Papo, M.; Borruel, N. Mucosal healing restores normal health and quality of life in patients with inflammatory bowel disease. *Eur. J. Gastroenterol. Hepatol.* **2012**, *24*, 762–769. [CrossRef] [PubMed]
44. Larussa, T.; Flauti, D.; Abenavoli, L.; Boccuto, L.; Suraci, E.; Marasco, R.; Imeneo, M.; Luzza, F. The Reality of Patient-Reported Outcomes of Health-Related Quality of Life in an Italian Cohort of Patients with Inflammatory Bowel Disease: Results from a Cross-Sectional Study. *J. Clin. Med.* **2020**, *9*, 2416. [CrossRef]
45. Nazarian, A.; Bishay, K.; Gholami, R.; Scaffidi, M.A.; Khan, R.; Cohen-Lyons, D.; Griller, N.; Satchwell, J.B.; Baker, J.P.; Grover, S.C.; et al. Factors Associated with Poor Quality of Life in a Canadian Cohort of Patients with Inflammatory Bowel Disease: A Cross-sectional Study. *J. Can. Assoc. Gastroenterol.* **2020**, *4*, 91–96. [CrossRef]
46. Mitropoulou, M.A.; Fradelos, E.C.; Lee, K.Y.; Malli, F.; Tsaras, K.; Christodoulou, N.G.; Papathanasiou, I.V. Quality of Life in Patients with Inflammatory Bowel Disease: Importance of Psychological Symptoms. *Cureus* **2022**, *14*, e28502. [CrossRef]
47. Cross, R.K.; Naegeli, A.N.; Harrison, R.W.; Moore, P.C.; Mackey, R.H.; Crabtree, M.M.; Lemay, C.A.; Arora, V.; Morris, N.; Sontag, A.; et al. Disease Burden and Patient-Reported Outcomes Among Ulcerative Colitis Patients According to Therapy at Enrollment into CorEvitas' Inflammatory Bowel Disease Registry. *Crohns Colitis* **2022**, *4*, otac007. [CrossRef]
48. LeBlanc, K.; Mosli, M.H.; Parker, C.E.; MacDonald, J.K. The impact of biological interventions for ulcerative colitis on health-related quality of life. *Cochrane Database Syst. Rev.* **2015**, *2015*, CD008655. [CrossRef]
49. Armuzzi, A.; Liguori, G. Quality of life in patients with moderate to severe ulcerative colitis and the impact of treatment: A narrative review. *Dig. Liver Dis.* **2021**, *53*, 803–808. [CrossRef]
50. Panés, J.; Vermeire, S.; Lindsay, J.O.; Sands, B.E.; Su, C.; Friedman, G.; Zhang, H.; Yarlas, A.; Bayliss, M.; Maher, S.; et al. Tofacitinib in Patients with Ulcerative Colitis: Health-Related Quality of Life in Phase 3 Randomised Controlled Induction and Maintenance Studies. *J. Crohns Colitis.* **2018**, *12*, 145–156, Erratum in *J. Crohns Colitis* **2019**, *13*, 139–140. [CrossRef]
51. Mikocka-Walus, A.; Knowles, S.R.; Keefer, L.; Graff, L. Controversies revisited: A systematic review of the comorbidity of depression and anxiety with inflammatory bowel diseases. *Inflamm. Bowel Dis.* **2016**, *22*, 752–762. [CrossRef] [PubMed]

52. Yuan, X.; Chen, B.; Duan, Z.; Xia, Z.; Ding, Y.; Chen, T.; Liu, H.; Wang, B.; Yang, B.; Wang, X.; et al. Depression and anxiety in patients with active ulcerative colitis: Crosstalk of gut microbiota, metabolomics and proteomics. *Gut Microbes* **2021**, *13*, 1987779. [CrossRef]
53. Byrne, G.; Rosenfeld, G.; Leung, Y.; Qian, H.; Raudzus, J.; Nunez, C.; Bressler, B. Prevalence of Anxiety and Depression in Patients with Inflammatory Bowel Disease. *Can. J. Gastroenterol. Hepatol.* **2017**, *2017*, 6496727. [CrossRef]
54. American Psychiatric Association. *Diagnostic and statistical manual of mental disorders: DSM-IV-TR*, 4th ed.; text rev; American Psychiatric Association: Washington, DC, USA, 2000.
55. Stroie, T.; Preda, C.; Meianu, C.; Croitoru, A.; Gheorghe, L.; Gheorghe, C.; Diculescu, M. Health-Related Quality of Life in Patients with Inflammatory Bowel Disease in Clinical Remission: What Should We Look For? *Medicina* **2022**, *58*, 486. [CrossRef]
56. Porcelli, P.; Zaka, S.; Leoci, C.; Centonze, S.; Taylor, G.J. Alexithymia in inflammatory bowel disease. A case-control study. *Psychother. Psychosom.* **1995**, *64*, 49–53. [CrossRef] [PubMed]
57. Iglesias-Rey, M.; Barreiro-de Acosta, M.; Caamaño-Isorna, F.; Vázquez Rodríguez, I.; Lorenzo González, A.; Bello-Paderne, X.; Domínguez-Muñoz, J.E. Influence of alexithymia on health-related quality of life in inflammatory bowel disease: Are there any related factors? *Scand. J. Gastroenterol.* **2012**, *47*, 445–453. [CrossRef]
58. Takahashi, M.; Nunotani, M.; Aoyama, N. Construction of an Explanatory Model for Quality of Life in Outpatients with Ulcerative Colitis. *Inflamm. Intest. Dis.* **2023**, *8*, 23–33. [CrossRef] [PubMed]
59. Luqman, A.; He, M.; Hassan, A.; Ullah, M.; Zhang, L.; Rashid Khan, M.; Din, A.U.; Ullah, K.; Wang, W.; Wang, G. Mood and microbes: A comprehensive review of intestinal microbiota's impact on depression. *Front. Psychiatry* **2024**, *15*, 1295766. [CrossRef]
60. Xu, L.; Li, Y.; He, Y. The variation characteristics of fecal microbiota in remission UC patients with anxiety and depression. *Front. Microbiol.* **2023**, *14*, 1237256. [CrossRef]
61. McGuinness, A.J.; Davis, J.A.; Dawson, S.L.; Loughman, A.; Collier, F.; O'Hely, M.; Simpson, C.A.; Green, J.; Marx, W.; Hair, C.; et al. A systematic review of gut microbiota composition in observational studies of major depressive disorder, bipolar disorder and schizophrenia. *Mol. Psychiatry* **2022**, *27*, 1920–1935. [CrossRef]
62. Luo, J.; Xu, Z.; Noordam, R.; van Heemst, D.; Li-Gao, R. Depression and Inflammatory Bowel Disease: A Bidirectional Two-sample Mendelian Randomization Study. *J. Crohns Colitis.* **2022**, *16*, 633–642. [CrossRef] [PubMed]
63. He, Y.; Chen, C.L.; He, J.; Liu, S.D. Causal associations between inflammatory bowel disease and anxiety: A bidirectional Mendelian randomization study. *World J. Gastroenterol.* **2023**, *29*, 5872–5881. [CrossRef] [PubMed]

life

Review

Backwash Ileitis—From Pathogenesis to Clinical Significance: Literature Review

Alina-Ecaterina Jucan [1,2], Otilia Nedelciuc [1,2,*], Vasile-Claudiu Mihai [3], Mihaela Dranga [1,2], Mihaela-Cristiana Andronic [1], Simona-Stefania Juncu [1,2], Georgiana-Elena Sarbu [1,2], Ioana-Ruxandra Mihai [4], Andrei Andronic [5], Irina Ciortescu [1,2], Vasile Drug [1,2], Cristina Cijevschi Prelipcean [2] and Catalina Mihai [1,2]

1 Department of Gastroenterology, "Grigore T. Popa" University of Medicine and Pharmacy, 700115 Iasi, Romania; ghiata.alina-ecaterina@d.umfiasi.ro (A.-E.J.); mihaela_dra@yahoo.com (M.D.); andronic_mihaela-cristiana@d.umfiasi.ro (M.-C.A.); juncu_simona-stefania@d.umfiasi.ro (S.-S.J.); georgiana_ciobanu23@yahoo.com (G.-E.S.); irinaciortescu@yahoo.com (I.C.); vasidrug@email.com (V.D.); catalina.mihai@umfiasi.ro (C.M.)

2 Department of Gastroenterology, Saint Spiridon County Hospital, 700111 Iasi, Romania; cristina.cijevschi.prelipcean@umfiasi.ro

3 Department of Radiology, Faculty of Medicine, "Grigore T. Popa" University of Medicine and Pharmacy, 700115 Iasi, Romania; mihai_vasile-claudiu@d.umfiasi.ro

4 Department of Rheumatology and Rehabilitation, Faculty of Medicine, "Grigore T. Popa" University of Medicine and Pharmacy, 700115 Iasi, Romania; ioana-ruxandra_mihai@umfiasi.ro

5 Discipline of Medical Semiology, Medical Department I, "Grigore T. Popa" University of Medicine and Pharmacy, 700115 Iasi, Romania; andrei.andronic@umfiasi.ro

* Correspondence: otilianedelciuc@yahoo.com

Abstract: Backwash ileitis (BWI) refers to inflammation in the distal ileum in patients with extensive ulcerative colitis (UC) that is thought to be caused by a "reflux" or "backwash" of colonic contents. In the absence of well-defined diagnostic criteria for BWI, more recently, the term UC-associated ileitis was proposed in favor of the backwash theory, which questions the existence of backwash ileitis as a distinct disease-specific subset of patients. Moreover, distinguishing UC-associated BWI from terminal ileitis of Crohn's disease or other conditions could be a diagnostic challenge and significantly affect treatment management. Therefore, clinical, endoscopic, histologic, and imagistic diagnostic features may aid in making this distinction. This literature review related to BWI outlines the hypothesis that the ileum may also become involved in UC as a primary manifestation of UC based on recent findings. This study also highlights the possibility that associated ileitis in UC patients may represent a potential risk factor for neoplasia, a positive association with primary sclerosing cholangitis, and a higher risk for the subsequent development of pouchitis after restorative proctocolectomy. It synthesizes recent key findings and highlights areas for further research.

Keywords: backwash ileitis; ulcerative colitis; primary sclerosing cholangitis; proctocolectomy; colorectal cancer

1. Introduction

Ulcerative colitis (UC) and Crohn's disease (CD) are chronic relapsing and recurring inflammatory bowel diseases of the gastrointestinal tract. According to the European Crohn's and Colitis Organization (ECCO) guidelines, the quality of the diagnosis of CD and UC was improved by the recent ECCO consensus position statements based on clinical, biochemical, endoscopic, and recent histological features [1,2].

UC is a disease that begins in the rectum and may extend proximally, in continuity, involving a variable colon length. Most patients with UC do not have an extension of the inflammatory process into the terminal ileum (TI), and the involvement of TI would generally raise suspicion for CD. The original interpretation of the term commonly known as backwash ileitis (BWI) was given by the extension of inflammation and injury to the terminal portion of the ileum in patients with extensive UC resulting from a reaction to reflux of colonic contents [3]. Due to recent evidence regarding this concept, the controversy over whether backwash ileitis is a misnomer or considered a primary manifestation of UC involving the ileum is still debatable [4].

Associated BWI in UC patients is not necessarily a benign phenomenon; it seems to influence the natural course of UC and appears to predispose patients to a more refractory course of the disease. Findings show a strong association between BWI and primary sclerosing cholangitis (PSC) in UC patients [5]. Recent findings also substantiate the link between BWI and an increased risk of colorectal cancer in proctocolectomy specimens. Moreover, an extensive UC BWI was reported as a risk factor for pouchitis [6,7].

Therefore, this literature review aims to systematically highlight the evidence regarding the contemporary and revised definition of BWI by distinguishing BWI from CD or other ileitis, including clinical, endoscopic, histological, and imaging data. The presence of BWI, PSC, and pouchitis concurrently could underline that immunologic, metabolic, or genetic disorders represent the vital cause of these abnormal changes.

2. Contemporary Definition and Etiopathogenesis—The State of the Art

This work was performed on a survey of articles collected by exploring the PubMed, GoogleScholar, EMBASE, and MEDLINE databases utilizing the following keywords: "backwash ileitis", "terminal ileitis", "ulcerative colitis", "UC-associated ileitis", "primary sclerosing cholangitis", "colonic neoplasia", "pouchitis", and "proctocolectomy" in all possible combinations. A retrospective search was carried out to find relevant studies in the field. We extracted information regarding a complete diagnosis (clinical, endoscopic, histopathological, and imaging features) of BWI. We summarized current knowledge related to the topic to promote further research that can improve understanding and help develop clinical practice guidelines for better disease management and control.

The term "backwash" was described in the literature as early as 1936 by Crohn and Rosenak, suggesting that the ileal inflammation observed in severe colitis is due to retrograde colonic contents secondary to the destruction of the ileocecal valve (ICV). The study indicated that these changes were found in some patients with a possible previously undescribed "combined form of ileitis and colitis" [8]. The exact mechanism of this condition was never clearly explained. The hypothetical pathophysiology for this phenomenon suggests that severe inflammation of the proximal cecum/ileocecal mucosa may lead to the malfunction of the ICV that retrogrades colonic material into the distal terminal ileum and, consequently, ileitis [9].

However, despite lacking evidence for backwash as the primary etiopathogenesis for this condition, the term "backwash" ileitis has become notorious in the literature [10,11]. Recent evidence suggests the presence of BWI in up to 35% of patients with UC [12]. Over time, different definitions of BWI have been described depending on the length of ileal involvement (any length from 0.5 cm above the ileocecal valve) [13]. According to recent evidence against BWI theory in UC in favor of primary UC involvement, an updated definition of BWI in the context of a more precise distinction of BWI from CD or other ileitis is needed.

More recently, Patil et al. [12] proposed in their study that the term "UC-associated ileitis" be used instead of BWI, as evidence of primary small bowel/ileal involvement in

UC has been increasingly documented. However, studies to date do not provide solid evidence regarding the change in nomenclature of the original terminology. Therefore, further research is needed. Table 1 presents the controversial studies that could change the perspective of the proposed initial "backwash" theory. Initially, we found 10 studies for interpretation. In total, 1/10 had no pathological evaluation to confirm the diagnosis, and in 4/10 studies, patients were likely to have CD and not BWI. Finally, 5/10 studies referred to ileitis associated with UC as the primary UC involvement against the backwash theory of ileitis in UC.

In addition, as many of the UC patients with the initial diagnosis of "BWI" had changed the diagnosis to CD over time [14], the existence of BWI as a distinct disorder has been questioned since its initial description. Also, there is no clear or convincing evidence that ileocecal reflux produces disease in the ileum, either in regular patients or in those with IBD.

Table 1. The controversial studies that could change the perspective of the proposed initial "backwash" theory.

Study	Type of Study	No. of Patients	Characteristics Against "BWI"	Study Conclusion
Abdelrazeq [9] (2005)	Prospective	100	- In total, 22 of the patients had ileal involvement - The presence of "BWI" did not correlate with the severity of colitis	- Total proctocolectomy with ileal-pouch anal anastomosis; all patients had pancolitis - Likely primary involvement of UC in the ileum
Haskell [4] (2005)	Retrospective	200	- All patients had a colectomy for medically refractory disease - In total, 34 of the patients had ileal inflammation - In total, 60% of patients with ileal inflammation did not have cecal involvement - In total, 46% of patients showed only mild to moderate activity in the colon	- The activity in the colon was not severe enough to induce incompetence of the ICV
Goldstein [15] (2006)	Retrospective	250 UC 100 CD	- In UC patients, the degree of inflammatory activity in the ileum correlated similarly with that in the colon - In total, 47 cases of UC patients showed quiescent or only mild inflammation of the cecum	- Ileitis in UC likely represents primary UC involvement - CD cohort had distinct features, including more activity in the ileum versus the colon
Yamamoto [16] (2008)	Prospective case control	50	- In patients with BWI and non-BWI, the levels of inflammatory cytokines (IL-1, IL-6, IL-8, and TNF-alfa) were significantly elevated compared with the control group - In total, 8 of 12 cases with ileal involvement had a completely normal cecum and were thought to represent "non-backwash" ileitis	Endoscopic aspect: - In total, 38 patients (76%) had normal TI - In total, 4 patients (8%)—BWI - In total, 8 patients (16%) had non-backwash ileitis (ileitis without cecum involvement) Reflux of colonic contents may not be the only mechanism contributing to the etiology of ileal inflammation in UC
Hamilton [17] (2016)	Prospective case control	72	- In total, 16 of the UC patients had ileitis, but only 6 had inflammation of the cecum, and none showed a dilated or patulous ICV	- Ileitis was not associated with NSAID use, UC-related - Medications, bowel preparation, or infection

BWI: backwash ileitis; UC: ulcerative colitis; CD: Crohn's disease.

3. Clinical Significance and Differential Diagnosis

Routine intubation of the TI is not necessary in mild to moderate UC. However, it should be performed as part of a complete colonoscopy when needed, not only for differential diagnosis but also for assessing disease management, complications, and prognosis in UC [18].

The first clue for diagnosing BWI is the endoscopic appearance of the ICV. The "fish-mouth" presentation of the ICV, associated with BWI, refers to a gaping appearance, likely caused by the loss of the normal ICV tone. A smooth, tubular ICV without stenosis or deformity, allowing easy endoscope passage, contrasts with the narrowed and irregular ICV seen in CD [13].

The macroscopic view of BWI, often observed in moderate-to-severe pancolitis, reveals a short, continuous segment of diffuse erythema, edema, granularity, and friability, with or without superficial erosions and loss of the vascular pattern, resembling the mucosa of the right colon [19]. Unlike CD ileitis, which typically presents with linear ulcerations, cobblestoning, deep ulcers, or strictures, BWI remains a superficial inflammation, confirmed by biopsy specimens [20].

Differentiating BWI from Crohn's ileitis is crucial, as the two conditions share overlapping clinical and endoscopic features but have distinct histopathological and radiological differences [15].

3.1. Endoscopic Findings

BWI typically presents as a continuous inflammation extending from the cecum into the terminal ileum, whereas CD ileitis often manifests with skip lesions and segmental involvement [21]. Endoscopically, BWI is associated with diffuse erythema, granularity, friability, and superficial ulceration without deep fissuring or strictures. Conversely, CD exhibits cobblestoning, aphthous ulcers, deep linear ulcerations, and luminal narrowing [22].

Additional endoscopic features distinguishing BWI from CD include a patulous ileocecal valve (ICV) in BWI, often accompanied by the reflux of colonic contents into the ileum [15]. In contrast, CD is more likely to present with stenosis of the ICV due to fibrosis and chronic inflammation, leading to a narrowed or ulcerated appearance [23]. Histologic confirmation is necessary for cases where endoscopic findings are inconclusive. In BWI, mucosal inflammation remains superficial and continuous, extending from the inflamed cecum, while CD often exhibits patchy involvement with areas of normal mucosa between affected segments [21].

Several other conditions may mimic BWI on endoscopy, including lymphoid hyperplasia, vasculitis, eosinophilic enteritis, NSAID-induced enteropathy, radiation enteritis, and infectious ileitis [24]. Lymphoid hyperplasia is often incidental but can sometimes lead to nodular mucosal changes resembling inflammatory disease. Vasculitic conditions, such as Henoch–Schönlein purpura or Behçet's disease, may present with ulceration and hemorrhagic necrosis of the ileal mucosa [24].

3.2. Histologic Findings

Histological examination plays a critical role in differentiating BWI from CD. BWI is characterized by superficial mucosal inflammation, villous atrophy, and increased lamina propria cellularity without transmural inflammation, granulomas, or neural hyperplasia [15]. In contrast, CD is associated with transmural inflammation, granulomas, pyloric metaplasia, and crypt architectural distortion, findings absent in BWI [22]. Additionally, mucous gland metaplasia and isolated ileal erosions are more characteristic of CD than BWI [15].

More recent histologic studies suggest that pattern recognition of inflammation and crypt architecture can aid in differentiating these conditions [23]. BWI is often linked to pancolitis and right-sided colonic involvement, whereas CD frequently exhibits focal crypt abscesses, fissuring ulcers, and transmural inflammation [21]. Moreover, cases of chronic

BWI may exhibit progressive crypt atrophy and mucosal distortion, which may overlap with early-stage CD [22].

Lymphoid hyperplasia, though often benign, can histologically resemble CD, necessitating careful evaluation of crypt distortion and granulomas to exclude IBD [24]. Additionally, vasculitis-related ileitis may show leukocytoclastic vasculitis and fibrinoid necrosis, which are absent in CD [25].

The histological pattern may suggest acute or chronic ileitis in both BWI and CD ileitis. In BWI, the inflammation is limited to the mucosa, with villous atrophy and scattered crypt abscesses. Still, transmural lymphoid aggregates, noncaseating granulomas, and fissuring ulcers indicate CD ileitis [15,22].

3.3. *Imagistic Findings*

Backwash ileitis (BWI) can be visualized on cross-sectional imaging, mainly in patients with pancolitis, as segmental inflammation of the terminal ileum. This aspect can complicate the diagnostic process and raise concerns about proper management. As most cases appear in the context of moderately to severely active UC, the imaging features that should raise suspicion about this condition include extensive inflammation of the entire colon with involvement of the terminal ileum [26–28].

Current practice in the field of IBD focuses on using non-invasive explorations for a complete evaluation of disease extension and follow-up of response to treatment. Abnormal parameters involving the bowel wall thickness (BWT), stratification (BWS), and vascularity can also be extrapolated for this condition. Although non-specific, the continuous colon inflammation, with no skip lesions, suggests UC; thus, terminal ileum involvement requires differentiation between BWI and terminal ileum involvement from CD. In some rare cases, ileitis was observed in patients with only left-sided colonic involvement, thus possibly delaying the correct diagnosis and proper treatment [27,29].

Historically, barium studies used to evaluate the digestive tract included small bowel follow-through and barium enema. The features of BWI, such as a widely patent ileocecal valve and persistent dilatation of the terminal ileum, lead to the hypothesis that the inflammation was caused by the reflux of colic content due to a pathologically enlarged ileocecal valve [27]. These studies have been replaced in the modern era by computed tomography (CT) and magnetic resonance enterography (MRE) due to their capability to assess the bowel wall and surrounding tissues.

Intestinal ultrasound (IUS) is an easily accessible, non-expensive, and non-radiating tool that can detect an increased BWT, color Doppler signal (as a sign of increased vascularity), and loss of the BWS. However, its accuracy for evaluating the terminal ileum depends on a series of factors, such as the patient's preparation and the experience of the clinician or radiologist. In addition, due to the low specificity of these parameters, more studies have focused on using MRI for a more appropriate disease characterization.

CT exploration of the bowel wall is highly dependent on bowel distension. It is usually performed only in acute clinical settings because of the radiation-associated risks, but it can offer valuable information, similar to MRE. Pathological findings are identical to those of IUS; the lead pipe appearance of the colon is highly suggestive of UC, which, in association with the clinical aspects and the presence of terminal ileum inflammation, should raise suspicion of BWI [30].

MRI is one of the best imaging methods available for evaluating patients with IBD, both in the initial phase to assess the extent of inflammation in the small bowel and for following up with the patients under treatment [31]. Only a few studies on the use of MRE for BWI have been published to date, suggesting the need for extensive research for this condition. Patient preparation is thorough and essential for obtaining diagnostic images, requiring complete patient cooperation. The proper bowel distention can be tested by obtaining a T2 sequence and supplementing the intraluminal fluid with additional contrast [32]. The specific differentiation of terminal ileum inflammation between UC and CD can only be made with a combination of ileocolonoscopy and clinical parameters. However, MRE can offer a series of parameters that are more suggestive of BWI than the terminal ileum involvement of CD. For instance, the BWT of the TI in patients with CD is significantly higher than in those with BWI, and the difference in the transmural nature of CD can explain it. In addition, eccentric thickening was observed in patients with CD compared to the circumferential involvement of BWI. The length of the diseased terminal ileum was also significantly longer in patients with CD. As mentioned before, the patency of the ICV can be evaluated by imaging: the gaping of this valve, measured as the distance between its lips, was significantly higher in those with BWI than those with terminal ileitis due to CD. The patency index, which is more accurate due to normalizing the ileocecal valve gaping to the intraluminal diameters of the terminal ileum or cecum, is also statistically significant when used to characterize BWI. Symmetrical enhancement of the inner wall of the terminal ileum is another feature of BWI that can differentiate it from CD. At the same time, no difference in the diffusion restriction at this level was observed between the two. Terminal ileum distension was observed more frequently in BWI, while the frequency of "comb sign" and lymph node involvement was significantly higher in those with CD [27,32].

3.4. Additional Diagnostic Modalities

Fluoroscopic small bowel follow-through and capsule endoscopy can further assist in differentiating these conditions. In BWI, imaging findings are localized to the terminal ileum, with no evidence of deep ulceration or fibrosis [15]. CD, however, frequently involves multiple segments of the small intestine, with characteristic cobblestone mucosa, strictures, and deep ulcerations [21]. MRE studies suggest that while BWI may be identified by ICV gaping and terminal ileum dilation, these features alone are unreliable differentiators from other causes of ileitis [27].

Backwash ileitis must be distinguished from CD, infectious ileitis, ischemic ileitis, NSAID-induced enteropathy, radiation enteritis, neoplastic conditions, lymphoid hyperplasia, and vasculitis. Histopathological findings, radiologic imaging, and endoscopic assessment provide key diagnostic clues, and a multimodal approach is essential for accurate differentiation. In cases where histopathology is inconclusive, molecular and microbiological testing should be considered to rule out infectious and neoplastic mimics [15].

A positive diagnosis of BWI in patients who are scheduled for proctocolectomy is considered a risk factor for developing postoperative Crohn's disease-like pouch complications. Although pre-operative CT or MRE does not influence the surgical results and the rate of complications [29], they can demonstrate the extent of the disease and other manifestations or complications, which is essential for a better understanding of the patient's condition.

4. The Relationship of BWI with CRC, PSC, and Pouchitis

Backwash ileitis in UC patients may represent a potential risk factor for neoplasia, a positive association with primary sclerosing cholangitis, and a higher risk for the subsequent development of pouchitis after restorative proctocolectomy; Figure 1 illustrates the link between these entities.

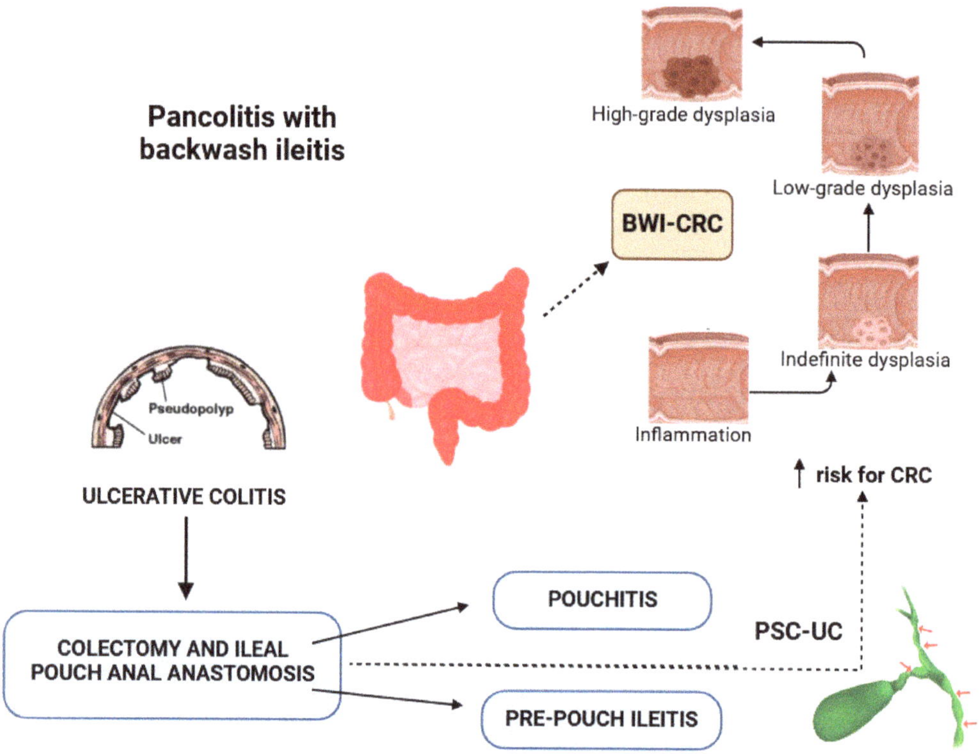

Figure 1. BWI-CRC: backwash ileitis–colorectal cancer; PSC-UC: primary sclerosing cholangitis–ulcerative colitis. ↑ risk for CRC = increased risk for colorectal cancer; ↑: multiple strictures of the biliary tree.

4.1. BWI and the Risk of CRC

The relationship between ileal inflammation in patients with UC and the risk of CRC development has been assessed in several studies in the literature. Still, the results of these studies are contradictory [4,33–35]. When first described, ileitis in UC patients was believed to be the consequence of extensive and severe disease that affected the ileocecal junction and led to the retrograde flow of colonic contents [36,37]. Considering this hypothesis, the association of BWI with CRC can be explained through the continuous cycle of inflammation, healing, and re-inflammation that can lead to dysplasia and cancer. It is well known that the long duration and extent of disease are the risk factors for malignant transformation in UC patients [38].

Research on the association of UC and BWI suggests that these increase the risk for CRC. One of these studies, by Heuschen et al. [33], reported a strong association between BWI and CRC that undergo proctocolectomy. This was a prospective study involving 590 consecutive UC patients with restorative proctocolectomy. CRC was found in 11.2% of all 590 patients. The frequency of CRC was significantly higher (29.0%) in the group of patients with pancolitis and BWI compared with patients with pancolitis without BWI (9.0%) and patients with left-sided colitis (1.8%). Additionally, CRC patients with pancolitis and BWI had significantly more multiple tumor growth (45.2%) than patients with pancolitis without BWI (24.2%) and left-sided colitis (0%). The data presented by Heuschen et al. were afterward questioned, considering that the number of patients previously diagnosed with CRC in the three study groups was not equal.

Another known risk factor for CRC in patients with UC is the presence of primary sclerosing cholangitis (PSC). In the study of Heuschen et al. [33], PSC was strongly associated with BWI, yet interestingly, it was not related to the development of CRC. However, in other studies, PSC has been considered a potential risk factor for malignancy transformation in patients with UC [39].

Alterations in the enterohepatic circulation of cholic acids are theorized to be implicated in the tumorigenesis of CRC [40]. The terminal ileum is the site of cholic acid absorption, which may indicate their potential involvement in the development of BWI in patients with UC. Likewise, the mucosal inflammation from BWI could also alter the enterohepatic circulation of cholic acids.

Another study that sustained the association between BWI and the risk of colonic neoplasia was conducted by Navaneethan et al. [34]. It was a prospective study that included 4198 UC patients who underwent colectomy. The results of this research revealed that endoscopic and histologic features (the grade of dysplasia) that predict colonic neoplasia were more frequent in BWI patients, suggesting that BWI may be a risk factor for CRC. Moreover, in the study mentioned above [34], PSC was found to be an independent risk factor for colonic neoplasia in UC patients with proctocolectomy. Despite this, BWI was not related to the malignant development of CCR when colon cancer alone was investigated (5.6% of patients with colon cancer in the BWI group compared to 3% in the control group, $p = 0.14$). In this study, there was also no difference in the frequency of multiple tumors between the BWI group and the control groups.

Other research from the literature failed to establish an actual connection between BWI and CRC. The study of Haskell et al. [4] showed a similar low rate of dysplasia and carcinoma in patients with BWI compared with the controls, suggesting that patients with BWI do not have an increased risk of developing colorectal neoplasia.

Furthermore, Rutter et al. [35] conducted a case-control study involving 204 UC patients in which cancer surveillance was evaluated. The results of his research showed no significant association between BWI and cancer risk in UC cases after 5 years of follow-up. BWI was found mainly in patients with chronic extensive disease that involved the ICV. Even though the odds ratio of neoplasia was 2.5 for patients with BWI, this result was not appreciated as significant because not all patients had terminal ileal intubation. Table 2 resumes the studies about BWI and CRC risk.

Table 2. Studies about UC-BWI and CRC.

Study	No. of UC Cases	BWI	CRC/Dysplasia in UC-BWI Patients	Study Conclusion
Heuschen et al. [33] (2001)	590	18.13%	29%	- Strong association between BWI and CRC in UC
Rutter et al. [35] (2004)	204	12% - Terminal ileal intubation had been achieved only in 70% of patients, of whom 12% had BWI	4.8% (result was not significant)	- Association between BWI and the risk of colonic neoplasia in the colectomy specimen - BWI was not related to the malignant development of CCR when colon cancer alone was investigated

Table 2. *Cont.*

Study	No. of UC Cases	BWI	CRC/Dysplasia in UC-BWI Patients	Study Conclusion
Haskell et al. [4] (2005)	200	17%	0%	- BWI in UC is not associated with an increased risk of cancer at UC
NavaNathan et al. [34] (2013)	4198	24.9%	18%	- BWI with extensive colitis was associated with the risk of identifying colon neoplasia but not cancer alone in the proctocolectomy specimen.

BWI: backwash ileitis; UC: ulcerative colitis; CRC: colorectal cancer.

4.2. BWI and PSC

BWI and PSC are considered to be two distinct conditions often associated with IBD, particularly with UC. The exact link between these conditions is not entirely understood. Although PSC-IBD shares specific common characteristics that could argue for the existence of a single condition, taken separately, none represent a solid argument.

PSC has an incidence of 0.07–1.3/100,000 people, and IBD is diagnosed in 70% of these cases (from which 75% are with UC). PSC is present in 2-14% of patients with IBD. UC associated with PSC has been considered to have a distinctive phenotype characterized by pancolitis, BWI, rectal sparing, and increased risk for CRC.

While several studies have shown an increased prevalence of BWI in patients with UC and PSC [41–44], others have not [45,46] (Table 3).

Table 3. The prevalence of BWI in PSC-UC patients.

Studies	PSC-IBD (No. of Cases)	BWI (%)
Loftus et al. [41] (2005), United States, Gut.	71	51
Sokol et al. [47] (2008), United States, World J Gastroenterol.	75	18.7
Joo et al. [42] (2009), Korea, Am J Surg Pathol.	40	35.7
Ye et al. [43] (2011) Korea, Inflamm Bowel Dis.	21	42.9
Jørgensen et al. [47] (2012), Norway, Inflamm Bowel Dis.	155	20
Boonstra et al. [45] (2012), Netherlands, Inflamm Bowel Dis.	80	5
Sinakos et al. [46] (2013), United States, Inflamm Bowel Dis.	129	11.6
Navaneethan et al. [34] (2013), United States, Dig Dis Sci.	31	17.4
Murasugi S et al. [44] (2020), Japan, Gastroenterol Res Pract.	35	37

UC: ulcerative colitis; BWI: backwash ileitis; PSC: primary sclerosing cholangitis.

Clinical features in PSC-IBD were first evaluated in 2005 in a paper by Loftus et al., who described a unique phenotype of IBD in these patients, characterized by a high frequency of pancolitis, rectal sparing, and BWI. In this study, BWI was more frequent in the PSC-IBD group (51%) than in the control group (7%) [41].

Subsequent studies were performed describing the distinctive phenotype of IBD with PSC. In 2008, Sokol et al. [48] confirmed that patients with PSC-IBD have a particular disease phenotype, BWI, which is found in 18.7% of patients. Although these patients had a milder form of the disease, they presented a higher risk of CRC.

PSC has been considered a potential risk factor for CRC in UC patients. The pathophysiological mechanism responsible for PSC alters the enterohepatic circulation of cholic acids. The same mechanism is considered to be a risk factor for the occurrence of CRC. Taking into account that the absorption of cholic acids takes place in the terminal ileum, they can be considered to be involved in the occurrence of BWI in patients with UC. On the other hand, ileal inflammation in BWI can also lead to alterations in the enterohepatic circulation of cholic acids [49].

In two studies from Korea (2009, 2011), BWI was more frequently described in PSC-UC patients (35.7% and 42.9%), and the risk of developing CRC was also higher in these patients [42,43]. Heuschen et al. [33] reported that BWI was frequent in PSC-UC patients (26.7%), but it was not associated with the development of CRC in these patients. Jørgensen et al. [47] reported that BWI was seen in 20% of PSC-UC patients. His study showed a significant difference between BWI's endoscopic and histologic findings. Ileal inflammation was found in 12% of cases in endoscopy and 20% of cases in histology. The right colon was also involved in patients with confirmed histologic ileal inflammation. The colonic inflammatory changes were considerably higher in these patients than those without BWI [47].

Disparities between endoscopic disease activity and clinical manifestations were described to be more frequent in patients with PSC-UC compared to UC alone. Some authors consider that the presence of BWI may be overestimated due to the frequent involvement of the right colon in PSC-UC compared to UC controls. As stated by the IPSCSG (International PSC Study Group) consensus panel on definitions, there are insufficient data to define BWI as a typical PSC-IBD phenomenon [50]. Another study reported a low prevalence of BWI in PSC-UC patients (6%), with no statistical differences between the control group (2%—UC without PSC) [45]. A more recent Korean study by Murasugi et al. reported more moderate/severe UC associated with PSC than previous studies. BWI was found in 37% of PSC-UC cases. Similar to earlier studies with the PSC-UC cases, patients presented pancolitis, occasionally with BWI and rectal sparing [44].

4.3. BWI and Ileoanal Pouch-Related Complications

The impact of BWI on the development of pouchitis after IPAA was first assessed in the study of Gustavsson et al. in 1987 [51]. This research included 131 patients with proctocolectomy and IPAA. Twenty patients were diagnosed with pouchitis after the intervention, and only 10% presented previous BWI. According to the results of this study, previous BWI did not influence the development of pouchitis.

The literature data regarding the relationship between BWI and pouchitis in patients with IPAA remain vague. Some studies reported higher rates of pouchitis in patients with BWI [29,52], while others have shown that BWI does not affect the outcome of patients with IPAA [53–55].

The study of Urquhart et al. investigated the incidence of pouch neoplasia in IBD patients following IPAA. From a total of 1319 patients, 95.2% had UC, and BWI was found in 14.4% of patients before IPAA. The presence of BWI, extensive colitis, and PSC before IPAA was identified as potential factors for the risk of pouch neoplasia [52].

Recent research by Freund et al. [29] reported that BWI is a predictive factor for later developing Crohn's disease-like pouch complications (CDLPCs).

Furthermore, Jillawar et al. reported that BWI was not among the risk factors that were statistically associated with complications after restorative proctocolectomy with IPAA [53]. White et al. prospectively compared the outcome of IPAA in colitis patients with BWI and without BWI. The reported results showed that the incidence of acute/chronic pouchitis and de novo Crohn's disease after IPAA did not differ significantly between patients with or without BWI [54]. Arrossi et al. [55] reported that BWI does not affect pouch outcomes in patients undergoing restorative proctocolectomy.

5. Current Therapy and Future Directions

Managing BWI requires medical therapies, lifestyle modifications, close monitoring, and, in some cases, surgical intervention. Given the fact that BWI appears in the context of UC, the treatment is similar but may require a more aggressive approach, depending on the severity of the disease and ileal involvement. There are no specific treatments for BWI. Regardless of the extension of the lesions in the colon associated with BWI, the treatment is similar to that of pancolitis. As described and mentioned above, therapy also focuses on related complications and associated diseases.

Severe UC with marked ileal inflammation describing BWI underscores the complexity and severity that UC can present when inflammation extends into the TI. In this condition, management of the disease focuses on controlled therapy of the extensive mucosal inflammation and close monitoring (laboratory tests, imaging, and endoscopic evaluations) to assess treatment efficacy. Accurate recognition and diagnosis of severe UC with BWI is critical for preventing complications and optimizing treatment.

In the literature are also mentioned two cases of BWI complicated by massive hemorrhage and perforation that required surgical intervention. In both cases, staged operation without sacrificing the involved area of the terminal ileum led to ileal pouch–anal anastomosis, with a favorable postoperative outcome [56].

Although laboratory tests alone cannot confirm BWI, they provide supportive evidence. Common inflammatory markers of active inflammation, such as elevated C-reactive protein and erythrocyte sedimentation rate, are not disease-specific [57]. Fecal Calprotectin appears to be the most popular and well-studied non-invasive biomarker in diagnosing and monitoring IBD patients [58]. Also, a Complete Blood Count may reveal anemia or leukocytosis in active disease. At present, no biomarker is accurate enough to replace endoscopy with biopsies. Although more assessments should focus on specific biomarkers, comparative studies and more clinical trials are also needed to establish the full potential of new biomarkers to impact clinical care.

Findings in the literature have changed the traditional dogma that UC affects only the colon, and inflammatory changes in the ileum have likely been described as primary UC involvement instead of the "backwash" theory (changes due to ICV incompetence). The term "UC-associated ileitis" proposed by Patil et al. [12] to be used instead of "BWI" needs validation; therefore, future research that contradicts the "backwash" theory and its clinical implications should be conducted using strict and uniform criteria.

The emphasis on TI intubation and colonoscopic surveillance should also be considered. Routine intubation of the TI should be performed as part of a complete colonoscopy, not only for differential diagnosis but also for assessing disease management, complications, and prognosis in UC.

6. Conclusions

In conclusion, the traditional dogma that the only mechanism causing BWI is the severe inflammation leading to ICV incompetence has been changed. Published evidence in the last decades considered BWI as a primary manifestation of UC involving the ileum. The controversy over whether BWI is a misnomer or considered ileitis likely with primary UC involvement needs to be clarified by further research in this field. Associated ileitis in UC patients predisposes them to a more refractory course of the disease; therefore, establishing a correct and complete diagnosis of the disease leads to better management of the disease, avoiding associated complications.

Author Contributions: Conceptualization, C.M. and A.-E.J.; methodology, O.N.; software, A.A.; validation, C.C.P., V.D. and I.C.; formal analysis, V.-C.M.; investigation, G.-E.S.; resources, M.-C.A.; data curation, M.D.; writing—original draft preparation, A.-E.J.; writing—review and editing, O.N.; visualization, S.-S.J.; supervision, C.M.; project administration, I.-R.M. All authors have read and agreed to the published version of the manuscript.

Funding: This research received no external funding.

Conflicts of Interest: The authors declare no conflicts of interest.

References

1. Feakins, R.; Borralho Nunes, P.; Driessen, A.; Gordon, I.O.; Zidar, N.; Baldin, P.; Christensen, B.; Danese, S.; Herlihy, N.; Iacucci, M.; et al. Definitions of Histological Abnormalities in Inflammatory Bowel Disease: An ECCO Position Paper. *J. Crohns Colitis* **2024**, *18*, 175–191. [CrossRef] [PubMed] [PubMed Central]
2. Cicerone, C.; D'Amico, F.; Allocca, M.; Zilli, A.; Parigi, T.L.; Danese, S.; Furfaro, F. A Comprehensive Multidisciplinary Approach to Diagnosing Chronic Inflammatory Bowel Diseases: Integration of Clinical, Endoscopic, and Imaging Modalities. *Diagnostics* **2024**, *14*, 1530. [CrossRef]
3. Lim, H.J.; Do Kim, H.; Soh, J.S.; Kim, S.Y.; Jung, Y.J.; Lim, H.; Kang, H.S.; Kim, J.H. Discrete terminal ileal ulcers in patients diagnosed with ulcerative colitis: Clinical significance and natural course. *BMC Gastroenterol.* **2021**, *21*, 285. [CrossRef] [PubMed] [PubMed Central]
4. Haskell, H.; Andrews, C.W.; I Reddy, S.; Dendrinos, K.; A Farraye, F.; Stucchi, A.F.; Becker, J.M.; Odze, R.D. Pathologic features and clinical signifcance of "backwash" ileitis in ulcerative colitis. *Am. J. Surg. Pathol.* **2005**, *29*, 1472–1481. [CrossRef] [PubMed]
5. Mertz, A.; Nguyen, N.A.; Katsanos, K.H.; Kwok, R.M. Primary sclerosing cholangitis and inflammatory bowel disease comorbidity: An update of the evidence. *Ann. Gastroenterol.* **2019**, *32*, 124–133. [CrossRef] [PubMed] [PubMed Central]
6. Fadel, M.G.; Geropoulos, G.; Warren, O.J.; Mills, S.C.; Tekkis, P.P.; Celentano, V.; Kontovounisios, C. Risks Factors Associated with the Development of Crohn's Disease After Ileal Pouch-Anal Anastomosis for Ulcerative Colitis: A Systematic Review and Meta-Analysis. *J. Crohns Colitis* **2023**, *17*, 1537–1548. [CrossRef] [PubMed] [PubMed Central]
7. Barnes, E.L.; Holubar, S.D.; Herfarth, H.H. Systematic Review and Meta-analysis of Outcomes After Ileal Pouch-anal Anastomosis in Primary Sclerosing Cholangitis and Ulcerative Colitis. *J. Crohns Colitis* **2021**, *15*, 1272–1278. [CrossRef] [PubMed]
8. Crohn, B.B.; Rosenak, B.D. A Combined form of Ileitis and Colitis. *JAMA* **1936**, *106*, 1–7. [CrossRef]
9. Abdelrazeq, A.S.; Wilson, T.R.; Leitch, D.L.; Lund, J.N.; Leveson, S.H. Ileitis in ulcerative colitis: Is it a backwash? *Dis. Colon Rectum* **2005**, *48*, 2038–2046. [CrossRef]
10. McCready, F.J.; Bargen, J.A.; Dockerty, M.B.; Waugh, J.M. Involvement of the ileum in chronic ulcerative colitis. *N. Engl. J. Med.* **1949**, *240*, 119–127. [CrossRef] [PubMed]
11. Morson, B.C.; Dawson, I.M. *Gastrointestinal Pathology*; Blackwell Scientific: Oxford, UK, 1979; pp. 316–317.
12. Patil, D.T.; Odze, R.D. Backwash Is Hogwash: The Clinical Significance of Ileitis in Ulcerative Colitis. *Am. J. Gastroenterol.* **2017**, *112*, 1211–1214. [CrossRef] [PubMed]
13. Shen, B. Indeterminate colitis and inflammatory bowel disease unclassified. *Atlas Endosc. Imaging Inflamm. Bowel Dis.* **2020**, *10*, 129–146. [CrossRef]
14. Everhov, Å.H.; Sachs, M.C.; Malmborg, P.; Nordenvall, C.; Myrelid, P.; Khalili, H.; Elmberg, M.; Ekbom, A.; Askling, J.; Jakobsson, G.; et al. Changes in inflammatory bowel disease subtype during follow-up and over time in 44,302 patients. *Scand. J. Gastroenterol.* **2019**, *54*, 55–63. [CrossRef] [PubMed]
15. Goldstein, N.; Dulai, M. Contemporary morphologic definition of backwash ileitis in ulcerative colitis and features that distinguish it from Crohn's disease. *Am. J. Clin. Pathol.* **2006**, *126*, 365–376. [CrossRef]

16. Yamamoto, T.; Maruyama, Y.; Umegae, S.; Matsumoto, K.; Saniabadi, A.R. Mucosal inflammation in the terminal ileum of ulcerative colitis patients: Endoscopic findings and cytokine profiles. *Dig. Liver Dis.* **2008**, *40*, 253–259. [CrossRef] [PubMed]
17. Hamilton, M.J.; Makrauer, F.M.; Golden, K.; Wang, H.; Friedman, S.; Burakoff, R.B.; Levine, J.S.; Joshi, P.; Banks, P.A.; Odze, R.D. Prospective evaluation of terminal ileitis in a surveillance population of patients with ulcerative colitis. *Inflamm. Bowel Dis.* **2016**, *22*, 2448–2455. [CrossRef] [PubMed]
18. Macrae, F.A.; Bhathal, P.S. Colonoscopy and biopsy. *Baillieres Clin. Gastroenterol.* **1997**, *11*, 65–82. [CrossRef] [PubMed]
19. Fausel, R.A.; Kornbluth, A.; Dubinsky, M.C. The First Endoscopy in Suspected Inflammatory Bowel Disease. *Gastrointest. Endosc. Clin. North Am.* **2016**, *26*, 593–610. [CrossRef]
20. Yantiss, R.K.; Odze, R.D. Diagnostic difficulties in inflammatory bowel disease pathology. *Histopathology* **2006**, *48*, 116–132. [CrossRef]
21. Levine, A.; de Bie, C.I.; Turner, D.; Cucchiara, S.; Sladek, M.; Murphy, M.S.; Escher, J.C. EUROKIDS Porto IBD Working Group of ESPGHAN. Atypical disease phenotypes in pediatric ulcerative colitis: 5-year analyses of the EUROKIDS Registry. *Inflamm. Bowel Dis.* **2013**, *19*, 370–377. [CrossRef]
22. Sahn, B.; De Matos, V.; Stein, R.; Ruchelli, E.; Masur, S.; Klink, A.J.; Baldassano, R.N.; Piccoli, D.A.; Russo, P.; Mamula, P. Histological features of ileitis differentiating pediatric Crohn disease from ulcerative colitis with backwash ileitis. *Dig. Liver Dis.* **2018**, *50*, 147–153. [CrossRef] [PubMed]
23. DeRoche, T.C.; Xiao, S.Y.; Liu, X. Histological evaluation in ulcerative colitis. *Gastroenterol. Rep.* **2014**, *2*, 178–192. [CrossRef]
24. Bojic, D.; Markovic, S. Terminal ileitis is not always Crohn's disease. *Ann. Gastroenterol.* **2011**, *24*, 271–275. [PubMed] [PubMed Central]
25. Dilauro, S.; Crum-Cianflone, N.F. Ileitis: When it is not Crohn's disease. *Curr. Gastroenterol. Rep.* **2010**, *12*, 249–258. [CrossRef] [PubMed]
26. Allocca, M.; Danese, S.; Laurent, V.; Peyrin-Biroulet, L. Use of Cross-Sectional Imaging for Tight Monitoring of Inflammatory Bowel Diseases. *Clin. Gastroenterol. Hepatol.* **2020**, *18*, 1309–1323. [CrossRef] [PubMed]
27. Erden, A.; Öz, D.K.; Çoruh, A.G.; Erden, I.; Ateş, F.S.Ö.; Törüner, M. Backwash ileitis in ulcerative colitis: Are there MR enterographic features that distinguish it from Crohn disease? *Eur. J. Radiol.* **2019**, *110*, 212–218. [CrossRef]
28. Saber, M.; Bell, D.; Morgan, M. Backwash Ileitis. Reference Article, Radiopaedia.org. Available online: https://radiopaedia.org/articles/6830 (accessed on 24 February 2025).
29. Freund, M.R.; Horesh, N.; Meyer, R.; Garoufalia, Z.; Gefen, R.; Emile, S.H.; Wexner, S.D. Can preoperative CT/MR enterography preclude the development of Crohn's disease-like pouch complications in ulcerative colitis patients undergoing J pouch surgery? *Colorectal. Dis.* **2023**, *25*, 1460–1468. [CrossRef] [PubMed]
30. Lee, S.B.; Kim, S.H.; Son, J.H.; Baik, J.Y. Evaluation of bowel distension and bowel wall visualization according to patient positions during administration of oral contrast media for CT enterography. *Br. J. Radiol.* **2017**, *90*, 20170352. [CrossRef]
31. Maaser, C.; Sturm, A.; Vavricka, S.R.; Kucharzik, T.; Fiorino, G.; Annese, V.; Calabrese, E.; Baumgart, D.C.; Bettenworth, D.; Borralho Nunes, P.; et al. European Crohn's and Colitis Organisation [ECCO] and the European Society of Gastrointestinal and Abdominal Radiology [ESGAR]. ECCO-ESGAR Guideline for Diagnostic Assessment in IBD Part 1: Initial diagnosis, monitoring of known IBD, detection of complications. *J. Crohns Colitis* **2019**, *13*, 144–164. [CrossRef] [PubMed]
32. Khosravi, B.; Salehnia, A.; Pak, N.; Montazeri, S.A.; Sima, A.R.; Vahedi, H.; Malekzadeh, R.; Radmard, A.R. A Practical Index to Distinguish Backwash Ileitis From Crohn's Terminal Ileitis in MR Enterography. *Inflamm. Bowel Dis.* **2023**, *5*, 42–50. [CrossRef] [PubMed]
33. Heuschen, U.A.; Hinz, U.; Allemeyer, E.H.; Stern, J.; Lucas, M.; Autschbach, F.; Herfarth, C.; Heuschen, G. Backwash ileitis is strongly associated with colorectal carcinoma in ulcerative colitis. *Gastroenterology* **2001**, *120*, 841–847. [CrossRef] [PubMed]
34. Navaneethan, U.; Jegadeesan, R.; Gutierrez, N.G.; Venkatesh, P.G.; Arrossi, A.V.; Bennett, A.E.; Rai, T.; Remzi, F.H.; Shen, B.; Kiran, R.P. Backwash ileitis and the risk of colon neoplasia in ulcerative colitis patients undergoing restorative proctocolectomy. *Dig. Dis. Sci.* **2013**, *58*, 2019–2027. [CrossRef] [PubMed]
35. Rutter, M.D.; Saunders, B.P.; Wilkinson, K.H.; Rumbles, S.; Schofield, G.; Kamm, M.A.; Williams, C.B.; Price, A.B.; Talbot, I.C.; Forbes, A. Cancer surveillance in longstanding ulcerative colitis: Endoscopic appearances help predict cancer risk. *Gut* **2004**, *53*, 1813–1816. [CrossRef] [PubMed]
36. Korelitz, B.I.; Shamah, S. The Ileitis of Ulcerative Colitis. Why Is It Not Crohn's Disease? *Inflamm. Bowel. Dis.* **2017**, *23*, E7–E8. [CrossRef] [PubMed]
37. Saltzstein, S.L.; Rosenberg, B.F. Ulcerative colitis of the ileum, and regional enteritis of the colon: A comparative histopathologic study. *Am. J. Clin. Pathol.* **1963**, *40*, 610–623. [CrossRef] [PubMed]
38. Porter, R.J.; Arends, M.J.; Churchhouse, A.M.D.; Din, S. Inflammatory Bowel Disease-Associated Colorectal Cancer: Translational Risks from Mechanisms to Medicines. *J. Crohns Colitis* **2021**, *15*, 2131–2141. [CrossRef] [PubMed] [PubMed Central]
39. Wang, R.; Leong, R.W. Primary sclerosing cholangitis as an independent risk factor for colorectal cancer in the context of inflammatory bowel disease: A review of the literature. *World J. Gastroenterol.* **2014**, *21*, 8783–8789. [CrossRef]

40. Liu, Y.; Zhang, S.; Zhou, W.; Hu, D.; Xu, H.; Ji, G. Secondary Bile Acids and Tumorigenesis in Colorectal Cancer. *Front. Oncol.* **2022**, *28*, 813745. [CrossRef]
41. Loftus, E.V., Jr.; Harewood, G.C.; Loftus, C.G.; Tremaine, W.J.; Harmsen, W.S.; Zinsmeister, A.R.; Jewell, D.A.; Sandborn, W.J. PSC-IBD: A unique form of inflammatory bowel disease associated with primary sclerosing cholangitis. *Gut* **2005**, *54*, 91–96. [CrossRef]
42. Joo, M.; Abreu-e-Lima, P.; Farraye, F.; Smith, T.; Swaroop, P.; Gardner, L.; Lauwers, G.Y.; Odze, R.D. Pathologic features of ulcerative colitis in patients with primary sclerosing cholangitis: A case-control study. *Am. J. Surg. Pathol.* **2009**, *33*, 854–862. [CrossRef]
43. Ye, B.D.; Yang, S.K.; Boo, S.J.; Cho, Y.K.; Yang, D.H.; Yoon, S.M.; Kim, K.J.; Byeon, J.S.; Myung, S.J.; Yu, C.S.; et al. Clinical characteristics of ulcerative colitis associated with primary sclerosing cholangitis in Korea. *Inflamm. Bowel Dis.* **2011**, *17*, 1901–1906. [CrossRef] [PubMed]
44. Murasugi, S.; Ito, A.; Omori, T.; Nakamura, S.; Tokushige, K. Clinical Characterization of Ulcerative Colitis in Patients with Primary Sclerosing Cholangitis. *Gastroenterol. Res. Pract.* **2020**, *2020*, 7969628. [CrossRef]
45. Boonstra, K.; van Erpecum, K.J.; van Nieuwkerk, K.M.; Drenth, J.P.; Poen, A.C.; Witteman, B.J.; Tuynman, H.A.; Beuers, U.; Ponsioen, C.Y. Primary sclerosing cholangitis is associated with a distinct phenotype of inflammatory bowel disease. *Inflamm. Bowel Dis.* **2012**, *18*, 2270–2276. [CrossRef] [PubMed]
46. Sinakos, E.; Samuel, S.; Enders, F.; Loftus, E.V.J.; Sandborn, W.I.; Lindor, K.D. Inflammatory bowel disease in primary sclerosing cholangitis: A robust yet changing relationship. *Inflamm. Bowel Dis.* **2013**, *19*, 1004–1009. [CrossRef]
47. Jørgensen, K.K.; Grzyb, K.; Lundin, K.E.; Clausen, O.P.; Aamodt, G.; Schrumpf, E.; Vatn, M.H.; Boberg, K.M. Inflammatory bowel disease in patients with primary sclerosing cholangitis: Clinical characterization in liver transplanted and nontransplanted patients. *Inflamm. Bowel Dis.* **2012**, *18*, 536–545. [CrossRef]
48. Sokol, H.; Cosnes, J.; Chazouilleres, O.; Beaugerie, L.; Tiret, E.; Poupon, R.; Seksik, P. Disease activity and cancer risk in inflammatory bowel disease associated with primary sclerosing cholangitis. *World J. Gastroenterol.* **2008**, *14*, 3497–3503. [CrossRef] [PubMed]
49. Shetty, K.; Rybicki, L.; Brzezinsky, A.; Carey, W.D.; Lashner, B.A. The risk of cancer or dysplasia in ulcerative colitis patients with primary sclerosing cholangitis. *Am. J. Gastroenterol.* **1999**, *94*, 1643–1649.
50. Ponsioen, C.Y.; Assis, D.N.; Boberg, K.M.; Bowlus, C.L.; Deneau, M.; Thorburn, D.; Aabakken, L.; Färkkilä, M.; Petersen, B.; Rupp, C.; et al. Defining primary sclerosing cholangitis: Results from an international primary sclerosing cholangitis study group consensus process. *Gastroenterology* **2021**, *161*, 1764–17675. [CrossRef]
51. Gustavsson, S.; Weiland, L.H.; Kelly, K.A. Relationship of backwash ileitis to ileal pouchitis after ileal pouch-anal anastomosis. *Dis. Colon Rectum* **1987**, *30*, 25–28. [CrossRef]
52. Urquhart, S.A.; Comstock, B.P.; Jin, M.F.; Day, C.N.; Eaton, J.E.; Harmsen, W.S.; Raffals, L.E.; Loftus, E.V., Jr.; Coelho-Prabhu, N. The Incidence of Pouch Neoplasia Following Ileal Pouch-Anal Anastomosis in Patients With Inflammatory Bowel Disease. *Inflamm. Bowel Dis.* **2024**, *30*, 183–189. [CrossRef]
53. Jillawar, N.; Bandla, V.; Galam, P.; Vajja, R.; Nirhale, D. Study of late complications of restorative proctocolectomy with ileal pouch-anal anastomosis for ulcerative colitis operated at a tertiary care center and factors affecting to that. *Ann. Afr. Med.* **2023**, *22*, 497–500. [CrossRef] [PubMed]
54. White, E.; Melmed, G.Y.; Vasiliauskas, E.A.; Dubinsky, M.; Berel, D.; Targan, S.R.; Fleshner, P.R. A prospective analysis of clinical variables, serologic factors, and outcome of ileal pouch-anal anastomosis in patients with backwash ileitis. *Dis. Colon Rectum* **2010**, *53*, 987–994. [CrossRef] [PubMed]
55. Arrossi, A.V.; Kariv, Y.; Bronner, M.P.; Hammel, J.; Remzi, F.H.; Fazio, V.W.; Goldblum, J.R. Backwash ileitis does not affect pouch outcome in patients with ulcerative colitis with restorative proctocolectomy. *Clin. Gastroenterol. Hepato.l* **2011**, *9*, 981–988. [CrossRef]
56. Okita, Y.; Miki, C.; Araki, T.; Inoue, M.; Otake, K.; Uchida, K.; Kusunoki, M. Ulcerative colitis with severe backwash ileitis successfully treated by staged operation without sacrificing any involved ileum. *J. Pediatr. Surg.* **2009**, *44*, 37–39.
57. Chen, P.; Zhou, G.; Lin, J.; Li, L.; Zeng, Z.; Chen, M.; Zhang, S. Serum Biomarkers for Inflammatory Bowel Disease. *Front. Med.* **2020**, *7*, 123. [CrossRef]
58. Langhorst, J.; Kairey, L.; Oberle, A.; Boone, J.; Dobos, G.; Juette, H.; Tannapfel, A.; Rueffer, A. Assessing Histological Inflammatory Activity in Patients With Ulcerative Colitis: A Diagnostic Accuracy Study Testing Fecal Biomarkers Lactoferrin and Calprotectin. *Crohn's Colitis 360* **2020**, *2*, otaa053. [CrossRef]

life MDPI

Case Report

A Case of a Neuroendocrine Tumor in a Liver Transplant Patient: Diagnostic and Management Difficulties

Carmen Colaci [1,*], Caterina Mercuri [2], Alessandro Corea [2], Rocco Spagnuolo [1] and Patrizia Doldo [2]

[1] Department of Health Sciences, University "Magna Graecia", 88100 Catanzaro, Italy; spagnuolo@unicz.it
[2] Department of Clinical and Experimental Medicine, University "Magna Graecia", 88100 Catanzaro, Italy; c.mercuri@unicz.it (C.M.); alessandro.coales@gmail.com (A.C.); doldo@unicz.it (P.D.)
* Correspondence: carmen.colaci@studenti.unicz.it

Abstract: Neuroendocrine tumors (NETs) of the liver are a rare entity. NETs are often poorly recognized, with diagnostic difficulties and differential challenges between primary tumors of the liver and metastases from other organs, mainly from the gastrointestinal tract. Multidisciplinary and multi-technical diagnosis is mandatory to properly treat these tumors. This case describes the complex history and the treatment course of a 68-year-old man with a history of NET onset after liver transplantation. Liver transplantation is the treatment of choice for patients with advanced liver disease or acute liver failure, but careful pre- and post-transplant patient monitoring is required. Liver transplant patients receive immunosuppressive therapy, and donor livers should be screened to exclude potential malignancies. This clinical case, in addition to emphasizing the diagnostic and therapeutic difficulty of hepatic NET, underlines the role of post-transplant immunosuppressive therapy and pre-transplant screening, which includes a thorough evaluation of donor and recipient history, physical examination, and laboratory tests. Moreover, post-transplant immunosuppressive therapy is essential to maintain the viability of the transplanted organ, but it is not free from potential risks, including an increased risk of cancer. Therefore, close monitoring of therapy is necessary to optimize long-term results and the patient's quality of life.

Keywords: NET; liver; immunosuppressive therapy; liver transplantation; HCC; holangiocarcinoma

1. Introduction

Neuroendocrine tumors arise from neuro-ectodermal cells, which are dispersed throughout the body. They are characterized by slow growth and the ability to secrete hormones or biogenic amines [1]. They often originate from the gastroenteropancreatic (GEP) tract (GEP-NET) and the bronchopulmonary tree. In addition, they present variable behavior and prognosis. In fact, their aggressiveness depends on the site of origin. For instance, NETs of the small intestine have a high malignant potential, whereas gastric and rectal NETs have a low tendency to metastasize but can progress rapidly once they become metastatic [2]. Despite being rare entities, the incidence and prevalence of NETs continue to increase globally, with the highest rates in the United States, Canada, and Norway [3]. Due to the indolent nature of the disease, its prevalence represents an imminent health crisis. It may come as a surprise that gastrointestinal NETs are now the second most prevalent gastrointestinal malignancy after colon cancer. The current prevalence of NETs in the United States amounts to approximately 170,000 patients [4]. GEP NETs are the most common subtype, accounting for 55–70% of all NETs. In comparison, primary hepatic neuroendocrine tumors (PHNETs) are extremely rare neoplasms, with only 94 documented cases as of 2009, first identified by Edmondson in 1958. Due to their rarity, it is crucial to exclude metastatic NETs and primary liver tumors, such as hepatocellular carcinoma (HCC) and cholangiocarcinoma (CCA), before diagnosing PHNETs [5]. A key role in the occurrence of post-liver transplant tumors could be played by immunosuppressive therapy [6]. The presented report is the first case in the literature of de novo PHNET on a liver transplant and is designed to focus on the diagnostic and therapeutic difficulties of managing the transplanted liver and on the importance of carefully monitoring the patient before and after the transplant.

2. Case Presentation

Here, we report the case of a 68-year-old male admitted to our Gastroenterology Unit in January 2024 after the report of a lesion of uncertain significance in the principal biliary duct.

Our patient was a former smoker and previous alcohol drinker, allergic to ceftriaxone. He had no family history of neoplastic diseases of the gastrointestinal tract and was hypertensive on furosemide treatment. In 2019, he underwent orthotopic liver transplantation for HCC, which occurred on alcoholic cirrhosis, and has been on immunosuppressive therapy with tacrolimus 3 mg 1 tablet daily since then. At the end of June 2023, following the appearance of hyperchromic urine and acholic stools, the patient underwent routine blood examinations with findings of increased liver indices of cytolysis and cholestasis. Therefore, in July 2023, he underwent magnetic resonance cholangiography (MR cholangiography) at another clinical center, which showed a stenosis of the main bile duct with dilatation of the intra- and extra-hepatic bile ducts and a lesion of approximately 40 mm surrounding the bile duct, portal vein, and common hepatic artery. On 14 August 2023, the patient arrived at the emergency room of the former hospital for generalized itching and abdominal pain. Blood tests confirmed increases in the cytolysis and cholestasis indices: total bilirubin—11.4 mg/dL (n.v. 0.3–1 mg/dL), AST—91 U/L (n.v. 5–40 U/L), ALT—138 U/L (n.v. 5–35 U/L), and GGT—495 U/L (n.v. 11–60 U/L). There were also increases in the tumor markers: carcinoembryonal antigen (CEA)—9.3 ng/mL (n.v. 0–4ng/mL), alpha fetal protein (AFP)—12.15 ng/mL (n.v. 0–7 ng/mL), and Ca—19.9 at 4000 U/mL (n.v. 0–37 U/mL).

An abdominal CT scan with contrast was also performed at admission, which confirmed a marked dilatation of the intrahepatic bile ducts in both hemispheres, recognizable up to a few mm downstream of the hepatic hilum, and the presence of hypodense tissue of suspected malignant significance surrounding the main bile duct (which was no longer recognizable), the portal vein, the proper hepatic artery, and the distal portion of the common hepatic artery, measuring 40 mm, similar to the previous MR cholangiography. No other liver nodules or abdominal organ changes were observed, nor were intraperitoneal or retroperitoneal fluid collections/effusions. In ordered to perform biopsies to determine the nature of the lesion found on the abdominal CT scan, the patient underwent percutaneous transhepatic cholangiography, which confirmed marked dilatation of the intrahepatic bile ducts and obstruction of the common hepatic duct, without contrast medium flow downstream. Due to the inability to pass through the obstruction, biopsies could not be taken. Therefore, an external biliary 8F caliber drain and a pig-tail tip placed at the level of the obstruction was inserted. Subsequently, 4 days later, the patient underwent a total-body positron emission tomography (PET) scan, which showed the presence of a hepatic hilar finding in the same area as the tissue component seen in the previous CT scan, characterized by high glycolytic metabolism of suspected heteroplastic nature. No other suspected heteroplastic lesions were found during the PET scan. On 4 September 2023, the patient underwent exploratory laparotomy with subsequent biliary–digestive anastomosis. Histological examination of the surgical specimen showed, at the level of the vegetating tissue of the biliary tract, biliary mucosa with papillary architecture and high-grade dysplasia. Meanwhile, in the common hepatic duct tract, fragments of biliary wall showed extensive fibrosclerosis and mild chronic phlogosis, limited by diathermocoagulative artefacts. On 29 September 2023, the patient had his first oncological visit to our hospital for suspected biliary cancer, given the strong radiological and laboratory evidence, despite the histological examination of the biopsies taken during the exploratory laparotomy being conclusive. Another abdominal MRI at our center confirmed the presence of a 40 mm formation, at the hepatic hilum, of heterogeneous nature, infiltrating the portal vein, bile ducts, and part of the common bile duct. Additionally, this lesion appeared to not be divisible from the head of the pancreas. A new repetitive 4 cm lesion was also identified in the VI hepatic segment. The presence of peritoneal fluid and signs of portal hypertension with splenomegaly were reported. In January 2024, the patient was admitted to our gastroenterology unit and underwent an ultrasound-guided liver biopsy of the VI hepatic segment lesion (Figure 1).

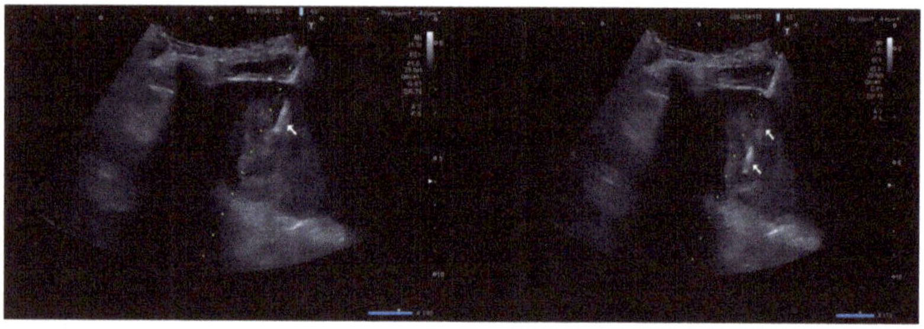

Figure 1. Ultrasound image of biopsied liver segment VI lesion. The arrow indicates the presence of the VI liver segment.

The histological examination of the biopsy showed the presence of poorly differentiated neuroendocrine carcinoma (NEC), whose immunophenotype was reported as CK 19+, CK7−, CK20−, CDX2+, synaptophysin+, Ki67 90%. During hospitalization, the patient underwent colonoscopy and gastroscopy, and F1 esophageal varices (Japan Research Society of Portal Hypertension—JRSPH) were shown (Figure 2). No other pathological findings were shown (Figure 3).

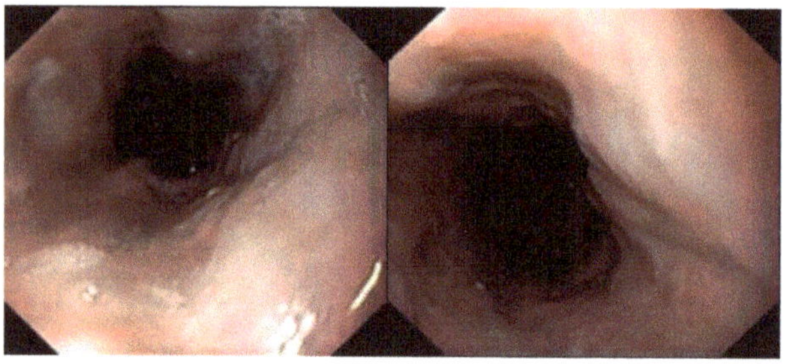

Figure 2. F1 esophageal varices in gastroscopy: the **left** image shows the portion of the middle esophagus; the **right** image shows the distal esophagus.

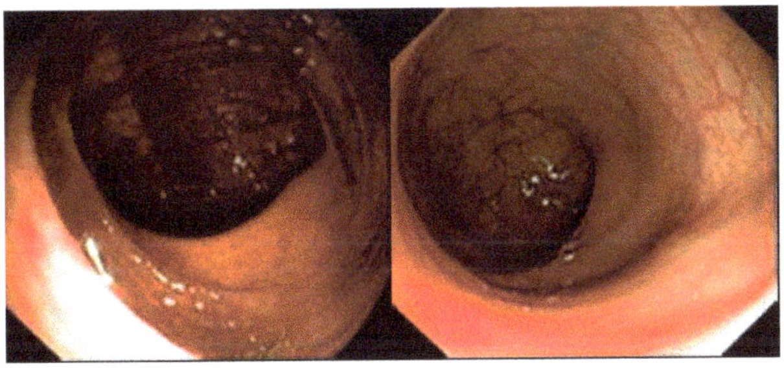

Figure 3. Normal colonoscopy findings: the **left** image shows the cecum; the **right** image shows the descending colon.

Then, systemic therapy with carboplatin and etoposide was initiated. On 15 February 2024, the patient started the first cycle of therapy, completed without any side effects. Further disease reassessment with a total body CT scan was postponed due to the patient's strong desire to return home. On 2 April 2024, the patient was scheduled for the second cycle of therapy, but due to Grade 1 thrombocytopenia, the treatment session was postponed. Since then, the patient has not received any systemic therapy due to persistent thrombocytopenia. On 3 June 2024, a follow-up total body CT scan confirmed the presence of the known hepatic hilar formation and the 4 cm repetitive lesion in the VI hepatic segment, but also multiple irregular hypodense formations with peripheral contrast enhancement in the right hepatic sections, suspected for nodules of HCC. The treatment of choice for the newly evidenced liver lesions was a combination of bevacizumab and atezolizumab, but due to the patient's history of liver transplantation and immunosuppressive therapy, no treatment was feasible at that time.

3. Discussion

Liver transplantation is the preferred treatment for patients with advanced liver disease or acute liver failure. From 1968 to 2018, a total of 80,000 transplants were performed worldwide. In 2023 alone, Italy conducted 39 liver transplants. It is estimated that survival rates have significantly improved over the last 25 years, reaching 96% and 71% at 1 and 10 years post-transplant, respectively [1]. Several observational studies have shown that the rate of de novo neoplasms in liver transplant patients increases 2-fold for malignant neoplasms of solid organs and 30-fold for lymphoproliferative neoplasms compared to the general population [2,3]. However, the rate of lymphoproliferative neoplasms in liver transplant recipients is lower than in recipients of other solid organ transplants, and the incidence of these neoplasms develops in the first 12–18 months post-transplant [7]. New malignancies of solid organs occur most commonly after the first year post-transplant and are associated with increasing age of the recipient. Liver transplant patients who have a history of alcoholic liver disease or primary sclerosing cholangitis present a higher risk [8]. The most frequent neoplasms include non-melanoma skin cancer and esophageal and colorectal neoplasms [8]. No data are available in the literature about NET development in liver transplant patients. The occurrence of PHNET is extremely rare in a liver transplant patient. Currently, our clinical case is the only one reported in the literature. Numerous risk factors are associated with the occurrence of NETs. Since they are rare entities, it is difficult to obtain clear data. Family history of malignancy, cigarette smoking, and alcohol consumption have been observed to increase the risk of developing NETs. A further relationship exists between liver diseases, such as cirrhosis and hepatitis, and the development of NETs. Such conditions can alter the normal metabolism of hormones and neurotransmitters, which can influence the growth of NETs. For example, cirrhosis can lead to increased levels of certain growth factors and cytokines that can promote tumor growth. In addition, liver dysfunction can impair the liver's ability to metabolize hormones produced by NETs, causing systemic effects and exacerbating symptoms [9]. Generally, NETs are asymptomatic, except for the eventual excessive production of certain hormones, which, depending on the substance produced, can cause diarrhea and facial flushing (carcinoid syndrome), hypoglycemia (insulinoma), heartburn, and vomiting (gastrinoma) [2]. PHNETs present unique clinical features, characterized by slow and often asymptomatic growth until advanced stages. They are often detected incidentally and may present as endocrinologically silent liver masses [10]. Notably, only 6.8% of PHNET cases are associated with the classic carcinoid syndrome related to liver metastases from extrahepatic NETs. The diagnosis is commonly made because of the mass effect in the liver or adjacent structures, which may lead to symptoms such as abdominal distension, non-specific pain, jaundice, and a palpable mass in the right upper quadrant [11]. In our case, the patient had no carcinoid syndrome but mainly cholestasis symptoms, such as generalized itching and abdominal pain with the appearance of acholic stools and hyperchromic urine. Diagnosing PHNETs is complex and often involves misdiagnosis as hepatocellular carcinoma (HCC) or cholangiocarcinoma (CCA) due to overlapping imaging features. CCA, while rare, is more common than PHNETs and presents various symptoms based on its type [2]. Over the past three decades, the incidence of CCA has reportedly increased, with higher rates observed in the United States and among Hispanic and Asian populations compared to African-American populations [11]. CCA is classified into three types based on the location of tumor development: intrahepatic CCA (iCCA), perihilar CCA (pCCA), and distal CCA (dCCA), corresponding to the intrahepatic bile duct, right and left bile ducts, common hepatic duct, and cystic duct, respectively. Patients with pCCA and dCCA typically present with jaundice and elevated cholestasis markers, while those with iCCA often exhibit non-specific symptoms [12]. In fact, given the increased indexes of cholestasis and the MRI imaging of a formation occupying the hepatic hilum, infiltrating the portal vein, the biliary tract, and part of the principal biliary duct, our first diagnostic hypothesis was CCA. For these reasons, in the context of our case, the initial diagnostic hypothesis was more than acceptable. The gross radiological features of PHNETs can be very varied. They can present as solid or cystic lesions, as well as diffuse or well-circumscribed in margins. In addition, as shown in the study of Wang et al., they are richly vascularized by the hepatic artery [13]. However, HCC and CCA also exhibit moderate vascularity, with HCC characterized by marked arterial enhancement and delayed washout during portal phases, while CCA progressively absorbs contrast during arterial and venous phases. Despite advances in imaging techniques, the risk of diagnostic errors and the challenges in obtaining a correct differential diagnosis remain high [14]. The diagnostic evaluation of PHNETs often requires additional examinations, such as PET scans, gastroscopy, colonoscopy, bronchoscopy, and octreotide scans [15]. In our patient, gastroscopy and colonoscopy were negative. Instead, the total body PET scan confirmed the hepatic hilar finding with features of high glycolytic metabolism.

Needle biopsies can help in the preoperative diagnosis of PHNETs, but their accuracy is often insufficient. Consequently, the diagnosis can only be confirmed after surgery [16]. Furthermore, immunohistochemical markers, such as neuron-specific enolase, chromogranin A, and synaptophysin, are used for their high sensitivity in the diagnosis of neuroendocrine tumors [17]. In our case, needle biopsies were sufficient for diagnosis. There are no guidelines for the treatment of PHNET, and surgical resection is the option of choice. Patients with PHNETs that are not candidates for surgery may undergo transarterial chemo embolization (TACE), which provides tumor mass reduction and symptoms control, but the current evidence is still limited [18]. The interesting point of this case is the occurrence de novo of the NET on a transplanted liver. The role of immunosuppressive therapy is essential for successful liver transplantation but carries a risk of toxicity. This therapy increases the likelihood of developing cancers, such as non-melanoma skin cancer, hepatocellular carcinoma (HCC) recurrence, non-Hodgkin lymphoma, and lung and renal cell cancers [19]. Calcineurin inhibitors are associated with a higher neoplastic risk, while mTOR inhibitors, particularly sirolimus, may reduce the risk of HCC recurrence and non-melanoma skin cancer. However, there are no data on the effects of mTOR inhibitors on other malignancies [20]. Because of the above, patients who are candidates for liver transplantation must be screened for the presence of any malignancy [21]. In addition, donors should also be carefully selected. In this regard, the literature reports a case of a PHNET in a patient who received a liver transplant from a donor. Immediately after the liver transplantation for alcoholic cirrhosis, a hypoechogenic lesion (15 mm) in the left hepatic lobe was found on abdominal ultrasonography, while liver biopsy confirmed it to be a PHNET [22]. Genetic analysis of the PHNET confirmed the donor origin of the neoplasm, although the donor had been screened for malignancies [23]. For our case, the transplant was performed in 2019, and since then, the patient has been receiving immunosuppressive treatment with tacrolimus. A genetic investigation was not performed to rule out the possibility that the new lesion could have originated from the donor liver. It seems unlikely that the PHNET is donor-derived, as no suspicious lesions had emerged in imaging checks prior to August 2023. There is no evidence regarding the development of PHNET in patients on immunosuppressive therapy with tacrolimus. On the contrary, sirolimus, an agent belonging to the mTOR inhibitors, such as tacrolimus, is now studied for the treatment of lung, pancreatic, and gastrointestinal NET [22].

4. Conclusions

This case report highlights the diagnostic and therapeutic challenges of PHNET in patients already undergoing liver transplantation. PHNET remains a poorly understood condition that must undergo differential diagnosis from metastatic NETs in other organs and major liver malignancies, such as HCC and cholangiocarcinoma. Moreover, the fact that it is a clinically silent lesion makes its detection mostly incidental. Despite their rarity, the incidence of these tumors is increasing, probably due to improved diagnostic techniques and increased awareness among healthcare professionals. It is crucial that healthcare professionals are vigilant in monitoring transplanted patients for the presence of these lesions to ensure timely and appropriate treatment. Overall, a personalized approach to the management of PHNET is crucial to improve the outcome and quality of life of these patients. Pre-transplant screening is a key element in optimizing outcomes and reducing complications. After transplantation, a further crucial role is played by immunosuppressive therapy in preventing organ rejection, but the latter must be carefully managed due to the risk of associated infectious and neoplastic complications. Research into the molecular mechanisms underlying neuroendocrine tumors of the liver is ongoing, with the hope of developing more effective therapeutic options.

Author Contributions: Conceptualization, C.C., A.C. and P.D.; methodology, C.C., A.C. and R.S.; software, C.M. and A.C.; validation, C.C., R.S. and P.D.; formal analysis, C.C., C.M. and A.C.; investigation, C.C., A.C. and R.S.; resources, C.C., A.C. and P.D.; data curation, C.C. and C.M.; writing—original draft preparation, C.C., C.M. and A.C.; writing—review and editing, A.C., R.S. and P.D.; visualization, C.C., C.M. and A.C.; supervision, R.S. and P.D. All authors have read and agreed to the published version of the manuscript.

Funding: This research received no external funding.

Institutional Review Board Statement: This study was conducted in accordance with the Declaration of Helsinki. Ethical approval was not requested due to the observational, retrospective, and anonymized nature of this study.

Informed Consent Statement: Written informed consent was obtained from the patient for the publication of this article (including the publication of images).

Data Availability Statement: No new data were created or analyzed in this study.

Conflicts of Interest: The authors declare no conflicts of interest.

References

1. Cives, M.; Strosberg, J. An Update on Gastroenteropancreatic Neuroendocrine Tumors. *Oncology* **2014**, *28*, 749–756, 758.
2. Cives, M.; Strosberg, J.R. Gastroenteropancreatic Neuroendocrine Tumors. *CA. Cancer J. Clin.* **2018**, *68*, 471–487. [CrossRef] [PubMed]
3. Leoncini, E.; Boffetta, P.; Shafir, M.; Aleksovska, K.; Boccia, S.; Rindi, G. Increased Incidence Trend of Low-Grade and High-Grade Neuroendocrine Neoplasms. *Endocrine* **2017**, *58*, 368–379. [CrossRef]
4. Chauhan, A.; Kohn, E.; Del Rivero, J. Neuroendocrine Tumors—Less Well Known, Often Misunderstood, and Rapidly Growing in Incidence. *JAMA Oncol.* **2020**, *6*, 21–22. [CrossRef] [PubMed]
5. Nomura, Y.; Nakashima, O.; Akiba, J.; Ogasawara, S.; Fukutomi, S.; Yamaguchi, R.; Kusano, H.; Kage, M.; Okuda, K.; Yano, H. Clinicopathological Features of Neoplasms with Neuroendocrine Differentiation Occurring in the Liver. *J. Clin. Pathol.* **2017**, *70*, 563–570. [CrossRef] [PubMed]
6. Aseni, P.; Vertemati, M.; De Carlis, L.; Sansalone, C.V.; Bonacina, E.; Minola, E.; Oreste, P.; Vizzotto, L.; Rondinara, G. De Novo Cancers and Post-Transplant Lymphoproliferative Disorder in Adult Liver Transplantation. *Pathol. Int.* **2006**, *56*, 712–715. [CrossRef]
7. Das, S.; Al-Toubah, T.; El-Haddad, G.; Strosberg, J. ^{177}Lu-DOTATATE for the Treatment of Gastroenteropancreatic Neuroendocrine Tumors. *Expert Rev. Gastroenterol. Hepatol.* **2019**, *13*, 1023–1031. [CrossRef]
8. Lokuhetty, D.; White, V.; Watanabe, R.; Cree, I. *WHO Classification of Tumours of the Digestive System*; International Agency for Research on Cancer: Lyon, France, 2018.
9. Leoncini, E.; Carioli, G.; La Vecchia, C.; Boccia, S.; Rindi, G. Risk factors for neuroendocrine neoplasms: A systematic review and meta-analysis. *Ann Oncol.* **2016**, *27*, 68–81. [CrossRef]
10. Tang, L.H.; Untch, B.R.; Reidy, D.L.; O'Reilly, E.; Dhall, D.; Jih, L.; Basturk, O.; Allen, P.J.; Klimstra, D.S. Well-Differentiated Neuroendocrine Tumors with a Morphologically Apparent High-Grade Component: A Pathway Distinct from Poorly Differentiated Neuroendocrine Carcinomas. *Clin. Cancer Res. Off. J. Am. Assoc. Cancer Res.* **2016**, *22*, 1011–1017. [CrossRef]
11. Jia, C.; Zhang, Y.; Xu, J.; Sun, K. Experience in Primary Hepatic Neuroendocrine Tumor. *Turk. J. Gastroenterol.* **2012**, *23*, 546–551. [CrossRef]
12. Andriani, J.; Budipramana, V.S.; Sadikin, C. Diagnostic Problem of Primary Hepatic Neuroendocrine Tumor in 18-Year-Old Woman: A Case Report. *Int. J. Surg. Case Rep.* **2022**, *95*, 107224. [CrossRef] [PubMed]
13. Kellock, T.; Tuong, B.; Harris, A.C.; Yoshida, E. Diagnostic Imaging of Primary Hepatic Neuroendocrine Tumors: A Case and Discussion of the Literature. *Case Rep. Radiol.* **2014**, *2014*, 156491. [CrossRef] [PubMed]
14. Wang, L.-X.; Liu, K.; Lin, G.-W.; Jiang, T. Primary Hepatic Neuroendocrine Tumors: Comparing CT and MRI Features with Pathology. *Cancer Imaging* **2015**, *15*, 13. [CrossRef] [PubMed]
15. Vilgrain, V. Staging Cholangiocarcinoma by Imaging Studies. *HPB* **2008**, *10*, 106–109. [CrossRef]
16. Tuan Linh, L.; Minh Duc, N.; Tu Minh, H.; Ngoc Cuong, N.; Thu Ha, V.; Luan, D.-T.; Tra My, T.-T.; Van Lenh, B. Primary Hepatic Neuroendocrine Tumor. *Endocrinol. Diabetes Metab. Case Rep.* **2021**, *2021*, 20–0220. [CrossRef]
17. Yu, W.-M.; Li, R.; Sun, B.-L.; Du, J.-K.; Tuo, H.-F. Primary Hepatic Neuroendocrine Tumour with Multiple Liver Metastases: A Case Report with Literature Review. *Int. J. Surg. Case Rep.* **2021**, *89*, 106590. [CrossRef]
18. Chen, N.; Slater, K. Primary Hepatic Neuroendocrine Tumours-Case Series of a Rare Malignancy. *Int. J. Surg. Case Rep.* **2019**, *55*, 145–148. [CrossRef]
19. Suzuki, A.; Maeda, Y.; Sakamoto, K.; Kamei, R.; Yamamoto, T. A Case of Resection of Primary Hepatic Neuroendocrine Tumor. *Gan To Kagaku Ryoho* **2022**, *49*, 1259–1262.
20. Tang, Y.; Chen, X.; Lu, X.; Yuan, Z.; Yang, Y.; Qiu, C.; Li, H. Case Report: Primary Hepatic Neuroendocrine Tumor: Two Cases Report with Literature Review. *Front. Oncol.* **2023**, *13*, 1225583. [CrossRef]
21. Engels, E.A.; Pfeiffer, R.M.; Fraumeni, J.F.; Kasiske, B.L.; Israni, A.K.; Snyder, J.J.; Wolfe, R.A.; Goodrich, N.P.; Bayakly, A.R.; Clarke, C.A.; et al. Spectrum of Cancer Risk Among US Solid Organ Transplant Recipients. *JAMA* **2011**, *306*, 1891. [CrossRef]

22. Mrzljak, A.; Kocman, B.; Skrtic, A.; Furac, I.; Popic, J.; Franusic, L.; Zunec, R.; Mayer, D.; Mikulic, D. Liver Re-Transplantation for Donor-Derived Neuroendocrine Tumor: A Case Report. *World J. Clin. Cases* **2019**, *7*, 2794–2801. [CrossRef] [PubMed]
23. Rodríguez-Perálvarez, M.; Tsochatzis, E.; Naveas, M.C.; Pieri, G.; García-Caparrós, C.; O'Beirne, J.; Poyato-González, A.; Ferrín-Sánchez, G.; Montero-Álvarez, J.L.; Patch, D.; et al. Reduced Exposure to Calcineurin Inhibitors Early after Liver Transplantation Prevents Recurrence of Hepatocellular Carcinoma. *J. Hepatol.* **2013**, *59*, 1193–1199. [CrossRef] [PubMed]

life

MDPI

Systematic Review

Efficacy of Dupilumab in the Treatment of Eosinophilic Esophagitis: A Systematic Review and Network Meta-Analysis of Randomized Controlled Trials

Szu-Hung Chu [1,†], Jeng-Jung Chen [1,2,†], Chung-Chu Chen [3,4], Wei-Te Lei [1,5,6], Chi-Hone Lien [1], Shung-Long Weng [2,5,7], Chun-Yan Yeung [1,5], Lawrence Yu-Ming Liu [3,5], Yu-Lin Tai [1], Ya-Ning Huang [1,8] and Chien-Yu Lin [1,5,*]

[1] Department of Pediatrics, Hsinchu Municipal MacKay Children's Hospital, Hsinchu 30070, Taiwan; 4525@mmh.org.tw (S.-H.C.)
[2] Department of Biological Science and Technology, National Yang Ming Chiao Tung University, Hsinchu 30010, Taiwan
[3] Department of Internal Medicine, Hsinchu MacKay Memorial Hospital, Hsinchu 30071, Taiwan
[4] Centers of Natural Science, Minghsin University of Science and Technology, Hsinchu 30401, Taiwan
[5] Department of Medicine, MacKay Medical College, New Taipei 25245, Taiwan
[6] Graduate Institute of Clinical Medical Sciences, College of Medicine, Chang Gung University, Taoyuan 33302, Taiwan
[7] Department of Obstetrics and Gynecology, Hsinchu Municipal MacKay Children's Hospital, Hsinchu 30070, Taiwan
[8] College of Public Health, National Taiwan University, Taipei 10055, Taiwan
* Correspondence: mmhped.lin@gmail.com
† These authors contributed equally to this work.

Abstract: Eosinophilic esophagitis (EoE) is a chronic, immune-mediated disorder of the esophagus with rising prevalence. Dupilumab (DUPI), a monoclonal antibody that targets the interleukin-4 receptor α, has shown promise as a treatment option. We conducted a systematic review and network meta-analysis of randomized controlled trials searching the PubMed/Medline database, the Cochrane Database of Systematic Reviews, the Cochrane Central Register of Controlled Trials (CENTRAL), and the medRxiv preprint server up to 31 July 2024, assessing DUPI's efficacy and optimal dosing in the treatment of EoE. Finally, three randomized-controlled trials comprising 470 participants, including 102 children under 12 years of age, were included in the qualitative synthesis. Both high-exposure (HE-DUPI, 300 mg weekly) and low-exposure (LE-DUPI, 300 mg biweekly) regimens achieved significant histologic remission relative to placebo (OR = 26.88, 95% CI 11.98–60.29 for LE-DUPI; OR = 29.15, 95% CI 13.68–62.12 for HE-DUPI). Although overall adverse events were comparable between groups, HE-DUPI was associated with a notable increase in serious adverse events. These findings suggest that DUPI is effective in promoting histologic remission in EoE, with LE-DUPI emerging as a preferred option for balancing efficacy and safety. This study highlights the efficacy and safety profiles of different dosing regimens and pediatric groups. Further studies are warranted to explore long-term outcomes and identify patient subgroups that may derive the greatest benefit from DUPI therapy.

Keywords: dupilumab; eosinophilic esophagitis; biological agents; monoclonal antibody

1. Introduction

Eosinophilic esophagitis (EoE) is a chronic, immune-mediated esophageal disease characterized clinically by symptoms related to esophageal dysfunction and histologically by eosinophil-predominant inflammation [1]. Since its first description as a distinct clinicopathological entity in 1993, the understanding of EoE has evolved significantly [1,2]. The estimated prevalence of EoE ranges from 0.5 to 1 case per 1000 people, with an apparent increasing incidence over the past few decades [3–5]. Recent data indicate that the incidence is particularly high in developed countries, with rates as high as 5–10 new cases per 100,000 person-years [6].

The cardinal symptoms of EoE vary with age and include dysphagia, food impaction, chest pain, abdominal pain, and feeding disorders in younger children [7]. The disease course is typically chronic with fluctuating symptoms, significantly impacting patients' quality of life through dietary restrictions, frequent medical visits, and psychological stress [8,9]. A strong association with atopic conditions has been observed, with studies reporting that 28 to 86% of adults and 42 to 93% of children with EoE have concurrent allergic diseases such as asthma, atopic dermatitis, or food allergies [10,11]. Recent genetic studies have identified several susceptibility loci, including variants in the TSLP/WDR36 and CAPN14 genes, suggesting a complex genetic architecture underlying the disease [12,13].

The diagnosis of EoE requires both clinical symptoms and histological findings, with a peak eosinophil count of $\geq$15 eosinophils per high-power field on esophageal biopsy a key diagnostic criterion [12,14]. Historically, dietary modifications and proton pump inhibitors have been the mainstay of treatment. However, the efficacy of these approaches is not always satisfactory, with studies showing response rates of 30–50% for proton pump inhibitors and varying success rates for dietary elimination strategies [8,15]. Given the underlying immune-mediated inflammatory nature of EoE, characterized by a type 2 inflammatory response with elevated levels of IL-4, IL-5, and IL-13, various immunomodulatory agents have been investigated as potential treatments [16]. Dupilumab (DUPI), a fully human monoclonal IgG4 antibody that blocks interleukin-4 receptor α and subsequent inflammatory cascades, has shown promise in treating several allergic diseases [17–19]. Its efficacy in reducing the clinical severity of conditions such as severe atopic dermatitis has been well documented, albeit with noted adverse effects including local reactions [20].

In May 2022, DUPI received approval from the US Food and Drug Administration for the treatment of EoE in adults and children older than 12 years [21]. This approval was based on phase 3 clinical trial data demonstrating significant improvements in both histological and clinical parameters [22]. Previous systematic reviews and meta-analyses of randomized controlled trials have demonstrated the clinical efficacy of DUPI in adults and adolescents [23]. Additionally, several real-world cohort studies have reported the promising efficacy of DUPI in the treatment of EoE, with no significant adverse events observed [24]. However, the efficacy and safety of DUPI in treating EoE in children under 12 years of age remain largely unclear. Moreover, following its approval, various dosing regimens have been implemented, yet the optimal therapeutic strategy remains to be determined. Furthermore, both randomized controlled trials (RCTs) and cohort studies are extensively utilized in clinical research, yet they differ significantly in study design, methodology, and application. RCTs are rigorously designed and carefully controlled to minimize confounding factors, thereby providing high-quality evidence on the efficacy and safety of investigational drugs [25]. To address these knowledge gaps, we conducted a systematic review and network meta-analysis of RCTs to comprehensively evaluate the clinical efficacy of DUPI in the treatment of EoE. By synthesizing data from randomized controlled trials, our study aims to provide an updated assessment of DUPI's role in EoE management, with a particular focus on its use in young children, and to determine the optimal dosing regimen.

2. Materials and Methods

2.1. Study Design and Literature Search

This study was conducted in accordance with the Preferred Reporting Items for Systematic Reviews and Meta-Analyses (PRISMA) guidelines [26], which ensures transparent and complete reporting of systematic reviews and meta-analyses. Informed consent was waived due to the anonymous nature of the systematic review, as approved by our institutional review board. The 'PICO' (Patient, Intervention, Comparison, Outcome) criteria, a fundamental framework for evidence-based medicine research, were systematically applied for the literature search (Supplementary Table S1). The P refers to the patient population, including individuals with confirmed eosinophilic esophagitis (EoE), defined as $\geq$15 eosinophils per high-power field on esophageal biopsy. The intervention (I) was treatment with dupilumab (DUPI), a fully human monoclonal antibody targeting the IL-4/IL-13 pathway. The comparison group (C) consisted of individuals receiving a placebo or different dosing regimens of DUPI in randomized controlled trials. Finally, the outcomes measured (O) were histologic remission (defined as $\leq$6 eosinophils per high-power field) and treatment-emergent adverse events. Since the assessment of clinical EoE symptoms may be less reliable in young children, we utilized objective pathological findings as the primary outcome measure.

We conducted a comprehensive search of electronic medical databases using the primary terms 'eosinophilic esophagitis' and 'dupilumab', along with related keywords, Boolean operators (AND, OR, NOT), and Medical Subject Headings (MeSH) terms. The complete search strategy included variations of these terms such as 'allergic esophagitis', 'anti-IL4 receptor alpha', and 'biologic therapy'. The databases searched included PubMed/Medline, the Cochrane Database of Systematic Reviews, the Cochrane Central Register of Controlled Trials (CENTRAL), and the medRxiv preprint server, with the search concluding on 31 July 2024. To maximize the capture of relevant studies, no restrictions were applied regarding language, publication year, or participant characteristics such as age, gender, or disease severity. Additionally, reference lists of included studies and relevant review articles were manually screened to identify any additional eligible studies. Two authors with expertise in systematic reviews conducted the literature search independently (JJ Chen and WT Lei) using standardized data extraction forms. Any disagreements or discrepancies in study selection or data extraction were resolved through discussion and consensus with a third author (SH Chu), who served as the arbitrator. The quality of included studies was assessed using the Cochrane risk of bias tool for randomized controlled trials.

2.2. Study Selection, Data Extraction, Systematic Review, and Meta-Analyses

We included randomized controlled trials (RCTs) that investigated the efficacy of DUPI in treating EoE. The exclusion criteria were as follows: duplicate publications from different databases, irrelevant articles (e.g., epidemiological studies or surveillance reports), studies that did not evaluate histologic remission or adverse events, case reports, animal studies, trials with no comparison arm, editorials, and review articles.

Different dosing regimens of DUPI for EoE were classified into high-exposure (HE-DUPI) and low-exposure (LE-DUPI) categories, based on study design. HE-DUPI referred to a weekly administration of 300 mg of DUPI, while LE-DUPI referred to a biweekly administration of 300 mg of DUPI for adults and adolescents. In children, HE-DUPI was designed to achieve steady-state trough concentrations similar to those from a weekly 300 mg administration in adults, while LE-DUPI corresponded to biweekly dosing [27].

The primary outcome was histologic remission of EoE, defined as a peak esophageal intraepithelial eosinophil count of $\leq$6 per high-power field ($\leq$20 per square millimeter) at week 16. Secondary outcomes included adverse events reported by the participants. Two authors independently assessed and extracted data from the selected articles, including the first author's name, study country, study type, participant population, age/gender, DUPI dosage, treatment interval, treatment duration, histologic outcomes, clinical outcomes, adverse events, and authors' conclusions.

The quality of the included studies was assessed using the revised Cochrane risk-of-bias tool for randomized trials (RoB 2) [28]. Two authors independently evaluated study quality, focusing on domains such as selection, ascertainment, causality, and reporting. Any disagreements were resolved by discussion with a third author.

We conducted network meta-analyses using random-effects models to assess the efficacy of DUPI under different dosing schedules. Subgroup analysis and sensitivity tests were performed.

2.3. Statistical Analyses

Given the inherent variability in effect sizes across clinical studies, we employed a sophisticated random-effects regression model for meta-analyses, which allows for heterogeneity between study populations and methodological approaches. The Lu and Ades network meta-analysis model was implemented to comprehensively integrate both direct and indirect comparative evidence, enabling a more nuanced assessment of treatment effects across different study designs [29,30]. This approach provides a robust methodology for synthesizing complex clinical data while accounting for potential inter-study variations. Heterogeneity was rigorously assessed using the τ^2 (tau-squared) statistic, a sophisticated measure that quantifies the variance in effect sizes between studies. The odds ratio (OR) was used to quantify the risk of incidence associated with exposure compared to placebo. To mitigate potential publication bias, a critical methodological concern in meta-analyses, we employed multiple complementary analytical techniques. Specifically, we utilized comparison-adjusted funnel plots, which offer a more refined visual representation of potential reporting biases compared to traditional funnel plot methods. Additionally, Egger's test was conducted to statistically evaluate asymmetry in the research landscape, providing a quantitative assessment of potential publication bias.

To address potential inconsistencies within our network meta-analysis, we implemented two advanced methodological approaches: the loop-specific approach and node-splitting models. These sophisticated analytical techniques allow for a comprehensive evaluation of potential discrepancies between direct and indirect evidence within the research network. Statistical significance was conservatively defined as a p-value less than 0.05. All statistical analyses were performed using MedCalc (MedCalc Software, Ostend, Belgium) v18 and R software version 4.4.3 (R Foundation for Statistical Computing, Vienna, Austria), leveraging the advanced statistical capabilities of these robust computational platforms. This methodological approach ensures a comprehensive, rigorous, and transparent analysis of the available clinical evidence, providing a nuanced understanding of treatment effects while mitigating potential sources of bias and methodological heterogeneity.

3. Results

3.1. Study Selection Process

A comprehensive search of electronic databases up to 31 July 2024 was conducted to identify studies investigating dupilumab (DUPI) treatment for eosinophilic esophagitis (EoE) (Figure 1). Articles were excluded based on predetermined criteria, including duplicate publications, cohort studies, irrelevant studies, and review articles. Ultimately, five RCTs examining different DUPI dosing regimens were included in our analysis [22,27,31–33]. However, the publications by Rothenberg et al. and Bredenoord et al. were a follow-up study and a subgroup analysis study from a phase 3 trial, respectively, and were therefore excluded from the meta-analysis [22,32,33]. The overall methodological quality of these studies was high, with a low risk of bias (Supplementary Table S2). One study was a phase 2 trial published in 2020, while the other two were phase 3 trials (Table 1). Both phase 3 trials consisted of multiple parts, with some portions of the trials still ongoing. These trials were conducted across the United States, Australia, Canada, and Europe. A total of 470 participants, including 102 children under 12 years of age, were ultimately included in the qualitative synthesis.

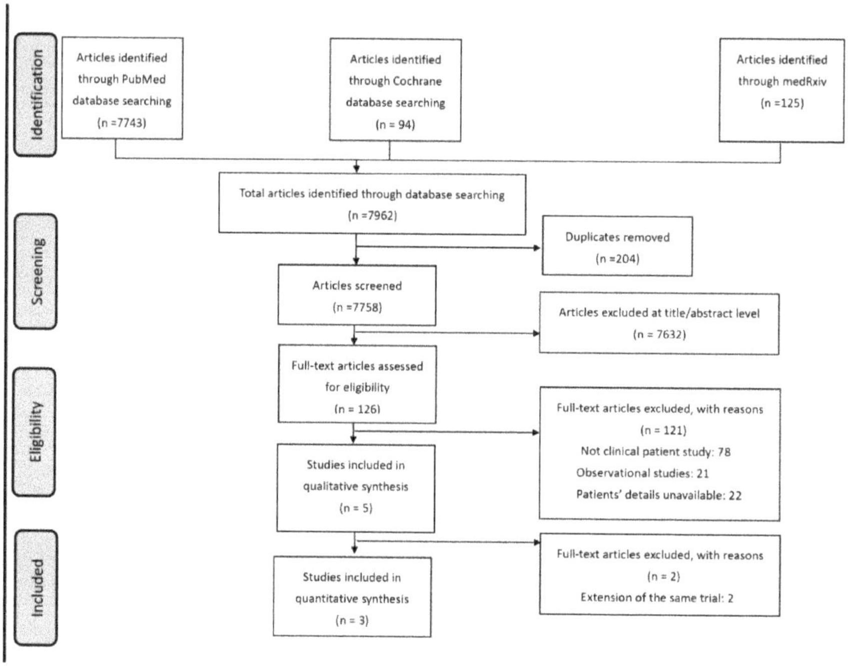

Figure 1. PRISMA flowchart of the literature search.

3.2. Histologic Remission Outcomes

Histologic remission, reported consistently across all included studies, served as our primary outcome measure. A network meta-analysis was performed to compare treatment efficacy (network graph, Supplementary Figure S1). This network graph demonstrates direct comparisons among the HE-DUPI, LE-DUPI, and placebo treatments. The numbers on the edges indicate the number of studies supporting each comparison. The analysis revealed a significantly lower rate of histologic remission in the placebo group compared to the DUPI treatment groups (Supplementary Figure S2). Specifically, both HE-DUPI and LE-DUPI demonstrated significantly higher rates of histologic remission compared to placebo (Figure 2). HE-DUPI demonstrated a non-significantly higher remission rate compared to LE-DUPI (OR = 1.07, 95% CI 0.63–1.82). Sensitivity analyses were performed by sequentially removing individual trials to assess the robustness of our findings. While variations in the odds ratio were observed, the overall conclusion remained unchanged, confirming the reliability of our results. Subgroup analyses stratified by adults, adolescents, and young children yielded consistent results.

Table 1. Characteristics of enrolled trials.

Study	Country	Part	Participants Number, Total (Each Group)	Age in Each Group (Years Old)	Gender in Each Group (M/F)	Intervention and Comparison Groups		Outcomes Extraction	Selected in Final Meta-Analysis
						Dose and Frequency	Duration		
Hirano 2020 [31]	United States		47 (23 + 24)	33.1, 36.1	13/10, 10/14	300 mg weekly vs. placebo	12 weeks	1. Change in SDI PRO score 2. Histologic measures of type 2 inflammation, endoscopically visualized anatomic measures, distensibility measures of esophagus 3. Adverse events	Yes
Dellon 2022 [22]	Australia, Canada, Europe, United States	A	81 (42 + 39)	33.9, 28.8	28/14, 21/18	300 mg weekly vs. placebo	24 weeks	1. Histologic remission 2. The absolute change from baseline in the DSQ score 3. Other secondary outcomes 4. Adverse events	Yes
		B	240 (80 + 81 + 79)	28.7, 27.8, 27.9	50/30, 45/36, 58/21	300 mg weekly vs. 300 mg biweekly vs. placebo	24 weeks		Yes
		A → C	40 + 37			300 mg weekly → 300 mg weekly vs. placebo → 300 mg weekly	28 weeks		No
		B → C	Ongoing						No
Chehade 2024 [27]	United States, Canada	A	102 (37 + 31 + 34)	6.8, 7.2, 7.2	28/9, 25/6, 25/9	HE-DUPI vs. LE-DUPI vs. placebo #	16 weeks	1. Histologic remission 2. Secondary histologic and clinical endpoints 3. Adverse events	Yes
		B	Ongoing, following part A				36 weeks		No
		C	Ongoing				108 weeks		No

Abbreviations: DSQ, Dysphagia Symptom Questionnaire; HE-DUPI, high-exposure dupilumab; LE-DUPI, low-exposure dupilumab; SDI, Straumann Dysphagia Instrument. # The trough level at a steady state of HE-DUPI is equal to 300 mg weekly administration in adults and that of LE-DUPI is equal to 300 mg biweekly administration, respectively.

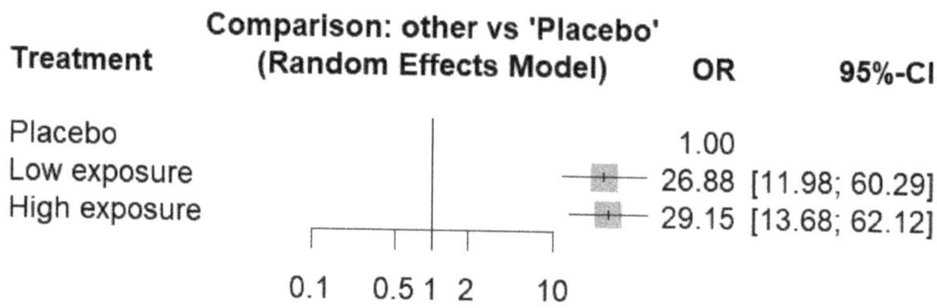

Figure 2. Forest plot of comparison of DUPI vs. placebo efficacy for histologic remission. OR, odds ratio; CI, confidence interval. The comparison presents the odds ratio for the incidence of histologic remission in low-exposure and high-exposure dupilumab groups versus placebo.

3.3. *Adverse Events Analysis*

Patients receiving DUPI treatment exhibited a non-significant increase in the incidence of all adverse events compared to those receiving a placebo (Figure 3). Regarding serious adverse events (SAEs), a non-significant increased risk was observed in the LE-DUPI group (Figure 4). However, a statistically significant increase in SAEs was reported in patients receiving HE-DUPI.

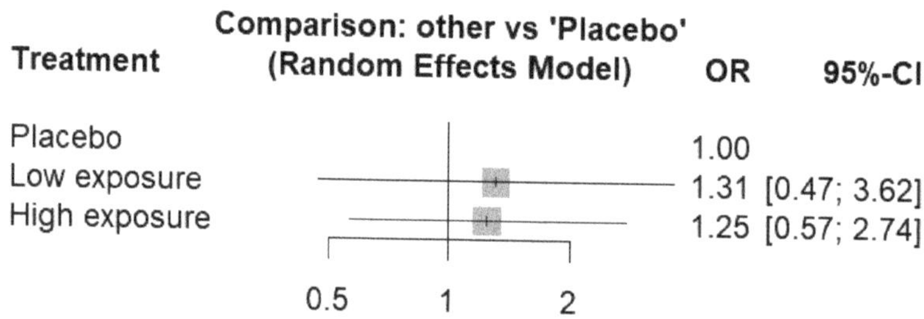

Figure 3. Forest plot of all adverse events in DUPI groups vs. placebo. OR, odds ratio; CI, confidence interval. The comparison presents the odds ratio for the incidence of all adverse events in the low-exposure and high-exposure dupilumab groups versus placebo.

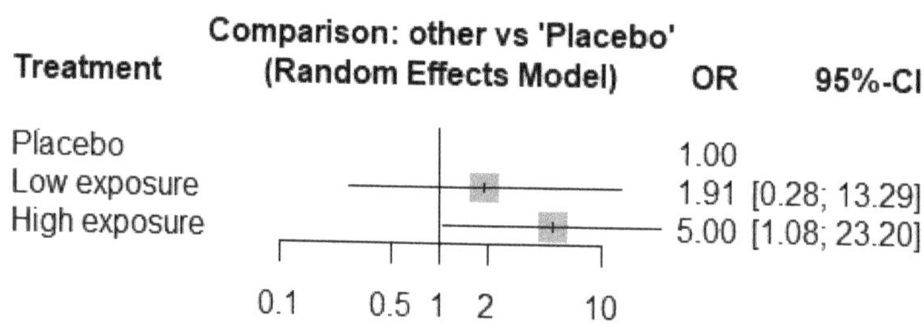

Figure 4. Forest plot of serious adverse events in DUPI groups vs. placebo. OR, odds ratio; CI, confidence interval. The comparison presents the odds ratio for the incidence of serious adverse events in low-exposure and high-exposure dupilumab groups versus placebo.

4. Discussion

The management of EoE remains challenging for a subset of patients, and the recent approval of DUPI represents a novel therapeutic approach. Our meta-analysis of available RCTs demonstrates significant improvement in histologic remission among patients treated with both HE-DUPI and LE-DUPI dosing regimens. Additionally, our analysis included studies focusing on young children, showing efficacy and safety outcomes comparable to those observed in adult populations receiving DUPI. Regarding safety profiles, while

HE-DUPI was associated with a higher incidence of SAEs, these were not attributed to the investigational product. Based on the current evidence, we propose that LE-DUPI may offer an optimal balance between efficacy and safety for the treatment of EoE.

Previous systematic reviews and meta-analyses have investigated the efficacy of DUPI in the treatment of EoE. Aziz et al. reviewed data from 287 patients across two RCTs and reported that DUPI demonstrated efficacy in both subjective and objective outcomes [23]. However, all the participants in their study were older than 12 years. In contrast, the present study includes 102 children younger than 12 years, thereby addressing the gap in the knowledge regarding the efficacy and safety of DUPI in the treatment of EoE in younger children. Additionally, Garg et al. conducted a systematic review and meta-analysis evaluating the real-world effectiveness of DUPI based on cohort studies [24]. While both RCTs and cohort studies are extensively utilized in clinical research, they differ significantly in study design, methodology, and application. RCTs are rigorously designed and carefully controlled to minimize confounding factors, thereby providing high-quality evidence on the efficacy and safety of investigational drugs [25]. The findings of the present study align with previous systematic reviews while supplementing critical data on the use of DUPI in children under 12 years of age.

DUPI, a human monoclonal antibody targeting the interleukin-4 receptor (IL-4R), inhibits downstream type 2 inflammatory cascades predominant in allergic diseases [17]. The strong association between EoE and atopic conditions, coupled with the elevated levels of IL-4, IL-13, and other inflammatory mediators observed in EoE patients, provides a robust theoretical framework for DUPI's efficacy [34–36]. The drug's mechanism of action, targeting the IL-4/IL-13 pathway, is particularly relevant to EoE pathophysiology, as these cytokines play crucial roles in tissue remodeling and eosinophil recruitment [37]. While dietary modifications and proton pump inhibitors remain first-line treatments and topical glucocorticoids such as budesonide and fluticasone are widely used, the introduction of DUPI expands the therapeutic armamentarium for clinicians [14,38]. Several cohort studies have explored the clinical efficacy of DUPI and demonstrated its promising effects in histologic improvement [24,39–41]. Improvements in clinical symptoms were also reported [24,40,42]. The present study, based on higher-level evidence from randomized controlled trials, reached the same conclusions as previous cohort studies.

The allergic etiology of EoE is further supported by its response to DUPI, an established treatment for other atopic conditions [36,43]. This therapeutic efficacy underscores the complex interplay between mucosal immunity, allergen exposure, and esophageal inflammation in EoE pathogenesis. The benefits of DUPI for EoE in adults and adolescents are relatively well established; however, its efficacy in children remains largely unclear [44]. A study by Chehade et al. provided compelling evidence supporting the histologic efficacy of DUPI in treating pediatric EoE [27]. Previous systematic reviews and meta-analyses examined the efficacy of DUPI in real-world cohort studies [24,41]. However, the efficacy of DUPI in young children was not addressed in these reviews. Our study strengthens the evidence of DUPI's efficacy specifically in the pediatric population, particularly young children. Further sensitivity analyses and subgroup analyses stratified by adults, adolescents, and young children yielded consistent results. DUPI has been used for several years to manage severe atopic dermatitis in children, with well-documented efficacy and safety profiles. Transient increases in eosinophil count have been observed in children undergoing DUPI treatment for allergic diseases; however, this elevation did not compromise clinical efficacy [45]. DUPI's application in the treatment of refractory EoE in children thus represents a reasonable therapeutic option for pediatricians [46,47].

The severity of EoE is primarily assessed using clinical symptoms, endoscopic findings, and histologic pathology [6,8]. Several scoring systems have been developed, and the correlation between clinical symptoms and pathological changes has been well established [48]. Our review focuses on children with EoE, where subjective symptom evaluation may be less reliable, particularly in younger children. Consequently, the primary outcome of our study emphasizes objective histologic remission. Additionally, the long-term efficacy of DUPI treatment remains largely uncertain, although previous studies have documented its 1-year efficacy in treating atopic dermatitis and EoE [20,32]. Future research investigating the long-term efficacy of DUPI is highly warranted.

Adverse events, particularly SAEs, are a critical consideration in clinical trials. Although the safety of DUPI has been well documented and no safety concerns were observed in a previous study [49], across the three trials analyzed, twenty-two participants experienced SAEs: fifteen in the HE-DUPI group, six in the LE-DUPI group, and one in the placebo group. The reported SAEs encompassed a diverse range of conditions, including procedural complications, infectious events, psychiatric manifestations, and systemic reactions. Notably, all the SAEs were deemed unrelated to the investigational product by the trial investigators. Non-serious adverse events occurred in approximately 75% of participants across all groups, with common manifestations including COVID-19, injection site reactions, upper respiratory tract infections, and various systemic symptoms. Our analysis revealed a non-significant increase in the overall number of AEs in both DUPI groups, but a significant increase in the number of SAEs in the HE-DUPI group. This safety profile informs our recommendation of LE-DUPI as the preferred regimen in patients with refractory EoE.

The strengths of our review lie in the inclusion of well-designed RCTs with robust methodological quality. Young children undergoing DUPI treatment were also included in our review. Additionally, we compared the histologic efficacy and adverse event profiles of different DUPI dosing regimens through a network meta-analysis. However, several limitations warrant consideration. Firstly, the absence of pharmacokinetic data on DUPI exposure in individual participants precludes a detailed analysis of dose–response relationships and potential correlations with adverse events. Secondly, while we focused on histologic remission as the primary outcome, the assessment of patient-reported outcomes and their correlation with histologic findings would provide a more comprehensive understanding of DUPI's clinical impact. Assessing subjective symptoms in young children remains challenging. Third, although the enrolled RCTs were of high quality and demonstrated a low risk of bias, several confounding factors may have influenced the clinical efficacy observed, such as differences in inclusion criteria, variations in disease severity, and prior treatment histories within the study populations. Finally, further studies are needed to explore the long-term efficacy of DUPI in treating EoE [50,51].

5. Conclusions

Eosinophilic esophagitis is a challenging condition with a clear immunological basis. Our meta-analysis demonstrates significant improvement in histologic remission with DUPI treatment. While HE-DUPI showed a higher incidence of SAEs, these were not attributed to the treatment itself. Based on the current evidence, we recommend LE-DUPI as a promising therapeutic option for patients with EoE who have shown inadequate response to conventional treatments. Further research is warranted to elucidate long-term efficacy, optimize dosing regimens, and identify patient subgroups most likely to benefit from this targeted biological therapy.

Supplementary Materials: The following supporting information can be downloaded at: https://www.mdpi.com/article/10.3390/life15020307/s1, Figure S1: Netgraph of enrolled studies; Figure S2: Forest plot of DUPI efficacy for histologic remission, Table S1: PICO of present systematic review. Table S2: RoB 2 bias risk assessment of enrolled trials.

Author Contributions: Conceptualization, S.-H.C., J.-J.C. and C.-Y.L.; methodology, C.-C.C., W.-T.L., L.Y.-M.L. and C.-Y.L.; software, W.-T.L. and C.-Y.L.; validation, C.-H.L., S.-L.W. and C.-Y.Y.; formal analysis, C.-Y.L.; investigation, S.-H.C., J.-J.C., C.-C.C. and W.-T.L.; data curation, Y.-L.T. and Y.-N.H.; writing—original draft preparation, S.-H.C. and C.-Y.L.; writing—review and editing, J.-J.C. and C.-C.C. All authors have read and agreed to the published version of the manuscript.

Funding: This research received no external funding.

Institutional Review Board Statement: Not applicable to studies not involving humans or animals.

Conflicts of Interest: The authors declare no conflicts of interest.

References

1. Liacouras, C.A.; Furuta, G.T.; Hirano, I.; Atkins, D.; Attwood, S.E.; Bonis, P.A.; Burks, A.W.; Chehade, M.; Collins, M.H.; Dellon, E.S.; et al. Eosinophilic esophagitis: Updated consensus recommendations for children and adults. *J. Allergy Clin. Immunol.* **2011**, *128*, 3–20.e26; quiz 21–22. [CrossRef] [PubMed]
2. Dellon, E.S.; Hirano, I. Epidemiology and natural history of eosinophilic esophagitis. *Gastroenterology* **2018**, *154*, 319–332.e3. [CrossRef]
3. Kapel, R.C.; Miller, J.K.; Torres, C.; Aksoy, S.; Lash, R.; Katzka, D.A. Eosinophilic esophagitis: A prevalent disease in the united states that affects all age groups. *Gastroenterology* **2008**, *134*, 1316–1321. [CrossRef] [PubMed]
4. Arias, Á.; Pérez-Martínez, I.; Tenías, J.M.; Lucendo, A.J. Systematic review with meta-analysis: The incidence and prevalence of eosinophilic oesophagitis in children and adults in population-based studies. *Aliment. Pharmacol. Ther.* **2016**, *43*, 3–15. [CrossRef] [PubMed]
5. Spergel, J.M.; Book, W.M.; Mays, E.; Song, L.; Shah, S.S.; Talley, N.J.; Bonis, P.A. Variation in prevalence, diagnostic criteria, and initial management options for eosinophilic gastrointestinal diseases in the united states. *J. Pediatr. Gastroenterol. Nutr.* **2011**, *52*, 300–306. [CrossRef]
6. Muir, A.; Falk, G.W. Eosinophilic esophagitis: A review. *JAMA* **2021**, *326*, 1310–1318. [CrossRef] [PubMed]
7. Furuta, G.T.; Katzka, D.A. Eosinophilic esophagitis. *N. Engl. J. Med.* **2015**, *373*, 1640–1648. [CrossRef] [PubMed]
8. Lucendo, A.J.; Molina-Infante, J.; Arias, Á.; von Arnim, U.; Bredenoord, A.J.; Bussmann, C.; Amil Dias, J.; Bove, M.; González-Cervera, J.; Larsson, H.; et al. Guidelines on eosinophilic esophagitis: Evidence-based statements and recommendations for diagnosis and management in children and adults. *United Eur. Gastroenterol. J.* **2017**, *5*, 335–358. [CrossRef] [PubMed]
9. Taft, T.H.; Kern, E.; Keefer, L.; Burstein, D.; Hirano, I. Qualitative assessment of patient-reported outcomes in adults with eosinophilic esophagitis. *J. Clin. Gastroenterol.* **2011**, *45*, 769–774. [CrossRef]
10. Simon, D.; Cianferoni, A.; Spergel, J.M.; Aceves, S.; Holbreich, M.; Venter, C.; Rothenberg, M.E.; Terreehorst, I.; Muraro, A.; Lucendo, A.J.; et al. Eosinophilic esophagitis is characterized by a non-ige-mediated food hypersensitivity. *Allergy* **2016**, *71*, 611–620. [CrossRef] [PubMed]
11. Spergel, J.M.; Brown-Whitehorn, T.F.; Beausoleil, J.L.; Franciosi, J.; Shuker, M.; Verma, R.; Liacouras, C.A. 14 years of eosinophilic esophagitis: Clinical features and prognosis. *J. Pediatr. Gastroenterol. Nutr.* **2009**, *48*, 30–36. [CrossRef] [PubMed]
12. Hirano, I.; Moy, N.; Heckman, M.G.; Thomas, C.S.; Gonsalves, N.; Achem, S.R. Endoscopic assessment of the oesophageal features of eosinophilic oesophagitis: Validation of a novel classification and grading system. *Gut* **2013**, *62*, 489–495. [CrossRef] [PubMed]
13. Kottyan, L.C.; Davis, B.P.; Sherrill, J.D.; Liu, K.; Rochman, M.; Kaufman, K.; Weirauch, M.T.; Vaughn, S.; Lazaro, S.; Rupert, A.M.; et al. Genome-wide association analysis of eosinophilic esophagitis provides insight into the tissue specificity of this allergic disease. *Nat. Genet.* **2014**, *46*, 895–900. [CrossRef]
14. Dellon, E.S.; Gonsalves, N.; Hirano, I.; Furuta, G.T.; Liacouras, C.A.; Katzka, D.A. ACG clinical guideline: Evidenced based approach to the diagnosis and management of esophageal eosinophilia and eosinophilic esophagitis (EOE). *Am. J. Gastroenterol.* **2013**, *108*, 679–692; quiz 693. [CrossRef] [PubMed]
15. Hahn, J.W.; Lee, K.; Shin, J.I.; Cho, S.H.; Turner, S.; Shin, J.U.; Yeniova, A.; Koyanagi, A.; Jacob, L.; Smith, L.; et al. Global incidence and prevalence of eosinophilic esophagitis, 1976–2022: A systematic review and meta-analysis. *Clin. Gastroenterol. Hepatol.* **2023**, *21*, 3270–3284.e7. [CrossRef]
16. Eluri, S.; Selitsky, S.R.; Perjar, I.; Hollyfield, J.; Betancourt, R.; Randall, C.; Rusin, S.; Woosley, J.T.; Shaheen, N.J.; Dellon, E.S. Clinical and molecular factors associated with histologic response to topical steroid treatment in patients with eosinophilic esophagitis. *Clin. Gastroenterol. Hepatol.* **2019**, *17*, 1081–1088.e2. [CrossRef] [PubMed]
17. Beck, L.A.; Thaçi, D.; Hamilton, J.D.; Graham, N.M.; Bieber, T.; Rocklin, R.; Ming, J.E.; Ren, H.; Kao, R.; Simpson, E.; et al. Dupilumab treatment in adults with moderate-to-severe atopic dermatitis. *N. Engl. J. Med.* **2014**, *371*, 130–139. [CrossRef]
18. Ledda, A.G.; Costanzo, G.; Sambugaro, G.; Caruso, C.; Bullita, M.; Di Martino, M.L.; Serra, P.; Firinu, D.; Del Giacco, S. Eosinophil cationic protein variation in patients with asthma and crswnp treated with dupilumab. *Life* **2023**, *13*, 1884. [CrossRef] [PubMed]

19. Marron, S.E.; Tomas-Aragones, L.; Moncin-Torres, C.A.; Gomez-Barrera, M.; Aranibar, F.J.G.-L.d. Patient reported outcome measure in atopic dermatitis patients treated with dupilumab: 52-weeks results. *Life* **2021**, *11*, 617. [CrossRef] [PubMed]
20. Blauvelt, A.; de Bruin-Weller, M.; Gooderham, M.; Cather, J.C.; Weisman, J.; Pariser, D.; Simpson, E.L.; Papp, K.A.; Hong, H.C.; Rubel, D.; et al. Long-term management of moderate-to-severe atopic dermatitis with dupilumab and concomitant topical corticosteroids (liberty ad chronos): A 1-year, randomised, double-blinded, placebo-controlled, phase 3 trial. *Lancet* **2017**, *389*, 2287–2303. [CrossRef] [PubMed]
21. U.S. Food and Drug Administration. FDA Approves First Treatment for Eosinophilic Esophagitis, a Chronic Immune Disorder. FDA News Release. Available online: https://www.prnewswire.com/news-releases/fda-approves-first-treatment-for-eosinophilic-esophagitis-a-chronic-immune-disorder-301552266.html (accessed on 30 June 2024).
22. Dellon, E.S.; Rothenberg, M.E.; Collins, M.H.; Hirano, I.; Chehade, M.; Bredenoord, A.J.; Lucendo, A.J.; Spergel, J.M.; Aceves, S.; Sun, X.; et al. Dupilumab in adults and adolescents with eosinophilic esophagitis. *N. Engl. J. Med.* **2022**, *387*, 2317–2330. [CrossRef] [PubMed]
23. Aziz, M.; Haghbin, H.; Gangwani, M.; Aziz, A.; Dahiya, D.S.; Ali, H.; Lee-Smith, W.; Goyal, H.; Kamal, F. Efficacy of dupilumab in eosinophilic esophagitis: A systematic review and meta-analysis of randomized controlled trials. *Am. J. Ther.* **2024**, *31*, e43–e45. [CrossRef]
24. Garg, A.; Moond, V.; Broder, A.; Mohan, B. S716 real-world effectiveness of dupilumab in eosinophilic esophagitis: A systematic review and meta-analysis. *Off. J. Am. Coll. Gastroenterol. ACG* **2024**, *119*, S495–S496. [CrossRef]
25. Hong, Y.D.; Jansen, J.P.; Guerino, J.; Berger, M.L.; Crown, W.; Goettsch, W.G.; Mullins, C.D.; Willke, R.J.; Orsini, L.S. Comparative effectiveness and safety of pharmaceuticals assessed in observational studies compared with randomized controlled trials. *BMC Med.* **2021**, *19*, 307. [CrossRef]
26. Hutton, B.; Salanti, G.; Caldwell, D.M.; Chaimani, A.; Schmid, C.H.; Cameron, C.; Ioannidis, J.P.; Straus, S.; Thorlund, K.; Jansen, J.P.; et al. The prisma extension statement for reporting of systematic reviews incorporating network meta-analyses of health care interventions: Checklist and explanations. *Ann. Intern. Med.* **2015**, *162*, 777–784. [CrossRef]
27. Chehade, M.; Dellon, E.S.; Spergel, J.M.; Collins, M.H.; Rothenberg, M.E.; Pesek, R.D.; Hirano, I.; Liu, R.; Laws, E.; Mortensen, E.; et al. Dupilumab for eosinophilic esophagitis in patients 1 to 11 years of age. *N. Engl. J. Med.* **2024**, *390*, 2239–2251. [CrossRef] [PubMed]
28. Sterne, J.A.C.; Savović, J.; Page, M.J.; Elbers, R.G.; Blencowe, N.S.; Boutron, I.; Cates, C.J.; Cheng, H.-Y.; Corbett, M.S.; Eldridge, S.M.; et al. Rob 2: A revised tool for assessing risk of bias in randomised trials. *BMJ* **2019**, *366*, l4898. [CrossRef] [PubMed]
29. Lu, G.; Ades, A.E. Combination of direct and indirect evidence in mixed treatment comparisons. *Stat. Med.* **2004**, *23*, 3105–3124. [CrossRef]
30. Chiu, N.C.; Chi, H.; Tu, Y.K.; Huang, Y.N.; Tai, Y.L.; Weng, S.L.; Chang, L.; Huang, D.T.; Huang, F.Y.; Lin, C.Y. To mix or not to mix? A rapid systematic review of heterologous prime-boost COVID-19 vaccination. *Expert. Rev. Vaccines* **2021**, *20*, 1211–1220. [CrossRef]
31. Hirano, I.; Dellon, E.S.; Hamilton, J.D.; Collins, M.H.; Peterson, K.; Chehade, M.; Schoepfer, A.M.; Safroneeva, E.; Rothenberg, M.E.; Falk, G.W.; et al. Efficacy of dupilumab in a phase 2 randomized trial of adults with active eosinophilic esophagitis. *Gastroenterology* **2020**, *158*, 111–122.e10. [CrossRef]
32. Rothenberg, M.E.; Dellon, E.S.; Collins, M.H.; Hirano, I.; Chehade, M.; Bredenoord, A.J.; Lucendo, A.J.; Spergel, J.M.; Sun, X.; Hamilton, J.D.; et al. Efficacy and safety of dupilumab up to 52 weeks in adults and adolescents with eosinophilic oesophagitis (liberty eoe treet study): A multicentre, double-blind, randomised, placebo-controlled, phase 3 trial. *Lancet Gastroenterol. Hepatol.* **2023**, *8*, 990–1004. [CrossRef] [PubMed]
33. Bredenoord, A.J.; Dellon, E.S.; Hirano, I.; Lucendo, A.J.; Schlag, C.; Sun, X.; Glotfelty, L.; Mannent, L.; Maloney, J.; Laws, E.; et al. Dupilumab demonstrated efficacy and was well tolerated regardless of prior use of swallowed topical corticosteroids in adolescent and adult patients with eosinophilic oesophagitis: A subgroup analysis of the phase 3 liberty eoe treet study. *Gut* **2024**, *73*, 398–406. [CrossRef]
34. Chehade, M.; Falk, G.W.; Aceves, S.; Lee, J.K.; Mehta, V.; Leung, J.; Shumel, B.; Jacob-Nara, J.A.; Deniz, Y.; Rowe, P.J.; et al. Examining the role of type 2 inflammation in eosinophilic esophagitis. *Gastro Hep Adv.* **2022**, *1*, 720–732. [CrossRef] [PubMed]
35. Syverson, E.P.; Rubinstein, E.; Lee, J.J.; McDonald, D.R.; Hait, E. The role of dupilumab in the treatment of eosinophilic esophagitis. *Immunotherapy* **2024**, *16*, 845–852. [CrossRef] [PubMed]
36. Lugović-Mihić, L.; Meštrović-Štefekov, J.; Potočnjak, I.; Cindrić, T.; Ilić, I.; Lovrić, I.; Skalicki, L.; Bešlić, I.; Pondeljak, N. Atopic dermatitis: Disease features, therapeutic options, and a multidisciplinary approach. *Life* **2023**, *13*, 1419. [CrossRef]
37. Gandhi, N.A.; Pirozzi, G.; Graham, N.M.H. Commonality of the il-4/il-13 pathway in atopic diseases. *Expert. Rev. Clin. Immunol.* **2017**, *13*, 425–437. [CrossRef] [PubMed]
38. Chan, J.; Flynn, D.M.; Gordon, M.; Parmar, R.; Moolenschot, K.; Jackman, L.; Gaynor, E.; Epstein, J.; Cordell, A.; Kannappan, H.; et al. Swallowed topical steroid therapy for eosinophilic oesophagitis in children: Practical, evidence-based guidance by the bspghan eosinophilic oesophagitis working group. *BMJ Paediatr. Open* **2024**, *8*, e002467. [CrossRef] [PubMed]

39. Becker, R.; Rigsby, M.; Suchi, M.; Lerner, D.G.; Chugh, A. Dupilumab in adolescent eosinophilic esophagitis: Experience with fibrostenosis and eosinophilic gastrointestinal disease with esophageal involvement. *J. Pediatr. Gastroenterol. Nutr.* **2024**, *78*, 1337–1341. [CrossRef] [PubMed]
40. Lee, C.J.; Dellon, E.S. Real-world efficacy of dupilumab in severe, treatment-refractory, and fibrostenotic patients with eosinophilic esophagitis. *Clin. Gastroenterol. Hepatol.* **2024**, *22*, 252–258. [CrossRef] [PubMed]
41. Russin, M.; Chen, J.; Rubenstein, J.H.; Chang, J.W. Real-world effectiveness and use of dupilumab in eosinophilic esophagitis. *Am. J. Gastroenterol.* **2024**. [CrossRef]
42. Spergel, J.M.; Chehade, M.; Dellon, E.S.; Bredenoord, A.J.; Sun, X.; Glotfelty, L.; Shabbir, A.; Tilton, S.T.; McCann, E. Dupilumab improves health-related quality of life and a range of symptoms in patients with eosinophilic esophagitis. *Am. J. Gastroenterol.* **2024**, *119*, 2398–2407. [CrossRef]
43. Aceves, S.S.; Dellon, E.S.; Greenhawt, M.; Hirano, I.; Liacouras, C.A.; Spergel, J.M. Clinical guidance for the use of dupilumab in eosinophilic esophagitis: A yardstick. *Ann. Allergy Asthma Immunol.* **2023**, *130*, 371–378. [CrossRef] [PubMed]
44. de Oliveira, F.D.; Costa, R.C.; de Santana Sato, E.D.B.; Khalil, S.M.; Meine, G.C. Efficacy and safety of monoclonal antibodies for the treatment of eosinophilic esophagitis: A systematic review and meta-analysis of randomized controlled trials. *Dig. Dis. Sci.* **2024**, *69*, 2530–2539. [CrossRef]
45. Wechsler, M.E.; Klion, A.D.; Paggiaro, P.; Nair, P.; Staumont-Salle, D.; Radwan, A.; Johnson, R.R.; Kapoor, U.; Khokhar, F.A.; Daizadeh, N.; et al. Effect of dupilumab on blood eosinophil counts in patients with asthma, chronic rhinosinusitis with nasal polyps, atopic dermatitis, or eosinophilic esophagitis. *J. Allergy Clin. Immunol. Pract.* **2022**, *10*, 2695–2709. [CrossRef]
46. Caminati, M.; Senna, G.; Maule, M.; Di Sabatino, A.; Rossi, C.M. Diagnosis, management and therapeutic options for eosinophilic esophagitis. *Curr. Opin. Allergy Clin. Immunol.* **2024**, *24*, 122–128. [CrossRef] [PubMed]
47. Chawla, K.; Alabbas, B.; Sheth, D.; Papademetriou, M. As easy as eoe: A novel and effective multidisciplinary approach to care of patients with eosinophilic esophagitis in the age of biologics. *Dig. Dis. Sci.* **2020**, *65*, 2196–2202. [CrossRef]
48. Dellon, E.S.; Khoury, P.; Muir, A.B.; Liacouras, C.A.; Safroneeva, E.; Atkins, D.; Collins, M.H.; Gonsalves, N.; Falk, G.W.; Spergel, J.M.; et al. A clinical severity index for eosinophilic esophagitis: Development, consensus, and future directions. *J. Allergy Clin. Immunol.* **2022**, *150*, 33–47. [CrossRef]
49. Sambugaro, G.; Brambilla, E.; Costanzo, G.; Bonato, V.; Ledda, A.G.; Del Giacco, S.; Scarpa, R.; Rattazzi, M.; Favero, E.; Cinetto, F.; et al. COVID-19 clinical features and outcome in italian patients treated with biological drugs targeting type 2 inflammation. *Life* **2024**, *14*, 378. [CrossRef]
50. González-Uribe, V.; Rodríguez-Bueno, C.P.A.; Mojica-González, Z.S.; Malagón-Liceaga, A.; Basile-Alvarez, M.R. Sustained clinical and histopathological remission in a patient with eosinophilic esophagitis and type-2 comorbidities at 18 months after discontinuation of dupilumab. *Clin. J. Gastroenterol.* **2024**, *17*, 803–808. [CrossRef]
51. Rothenberg, M.; Dellon, E.; Bredenoord, A.; Collins, M.; Hirano, I.; Chehade, M.; Lucendo, A.; Spergel, J.; Sun, X.; Hamilton, J.; et al. Dupilumab improves clinical and histologic aspects of disease in adult and adolescent patients with eosinophilic esophagitis at week 24: Results from part b of the 3-part liberty eoe treet study. *J. Allergy Clin. Immunol.* **2022**, *149*, AB312. [CrossRef]

life

MDPI

Article

The Role of the Subcostal Transversus Abdominis Plane Block in Facilitating Operating Room Extubation After Living Donor Liver Transplantation for Hepatocellular Carcinoma: A Propensity Score-Matching Analysis

Jaewon Huh and Min Suk Chae *

Department of Anesthesiology and Pain Medicine, Seoul St. Mary's Hospital, College of Medicine, The Catholic University of Korea, Seoul 06591, Republic of Korea
* Correspondence: shscms@catholic.ac.kr; Tel.: +82-2-2258-6150; Fax: +82-2-537-1951

Abstract: Background: Effective pain management is essential to early extubation and recovery in living donor liver transplantation (LDLT). The subcostal transversus abdominis plane (TAP) block has emerged as a potential strategy to address postoperative pain while reducing opioid consumption. This study evaluated the effectiveness of the TAP block in facilitating early extubation in the OR and examined its impact on re-intubation rates, postoperative fentanyl requirements, and pain intensity upon ICU admission to determine its role in perioperative pain management. **Methods:** This retrospective cohort study included adult patients who underwent LDLT for hepatocellular carcinoma within the Milan criteria. Propensity score matching was performed to compare outcomes between patients who received the subcostal TAP block and those who did not. The primary outcome was the rate of successful extubation in the operating room (OR). Secondary outcomes included re-intubation rates, postoperative fentanyl requirements, and peak numeric rating scale (NRS) pain scores upon ICU admission. **Results:** The subcostal TAP block was associated with a significantly higher rate of successful OR extubation compared with no TAP block. Multivariable analysis revealed that the TAP block independently increased the likelihood of successful extubation. Patients receiving the TAP block required less fentanyl for pain management and demonstrated lower peak NRS pain scores upon ICU admission. No complications related to the TAP block were observed, underscoring its safety in this high-risk population. **Conclusions:** The subcostal TAP block facilitates early OR extubation by effectively managing postoperative pain and reducing opioid requirements, promoting smoother recovery without increasing adverse events. These findings support its inclusion in multimodal analgesia protocols for optimizing perioperative outcomes in LDLT patients.

Keywords: subcostal TAP block; living donor liver transplantation; early extubation; operating room

1. Introduction

Advancements in perioperative care have markedly improved outcomes for liver transplantation (LT), yet challenges persist in achieving early postoperative rehabilitation. Managing pain effectively after surgery is crucial to speeding recovery and enhancing patient outcomes. However, pain control in LT patients is particularly complex due to impaired liver function and the frequent occurrence of renal dysfunction. Postoperative pain is a well-recognized issue in LT patients, with studies reporting moderate to severe pain in the early postoperative period, contributing to delayed recovery, prolonged ventilation, and increased ICU stay [1]. While opioids are often necessary for postoperative pain management, their use can lead to sedation, respiratory depression, nausea, and vomiting, which may delay recovery and increase the risk of complications [2,3]. Given these concerns, regional anesthesia techniques have gained attention as opioid-sparing strategies for postoperative pain control. Among them, the transversus abdominis plane (TAP) block has emerged as an effective option for managing pain after abdominal procedures, reducing opioid consumption and potentially enhancing recovery outcomes [4,5]. The subcostal TAP block, introduced by Hebbard et al., involves the administration of local anesthetics between the rectus abdominis and transversus abdominis muscles or, sometimes, in the posterior rectus sheath. This approach provides targeted analgesia to the T7 to T12 dermatomes [6–8]. The subcostal TAP block has been shown to be effective for upper-abdominal surgeries, such as open liver resections, and has demonstrated potential for use in LT [9,10]. A retrospective analysis of orthotopic LT patients revealed that the subcostal TAP block significantly reduced postoperative morphine requirements, highlighting its feasibility and clinical advantages [11]. Similarly, a prospective study by Assefi et al. demonstrated that the block reduced opioid consumption without compromising pain relief and reported no associated complications, reinforcing its safety and effectiveness [12].

Postoperative management for LT has traditionally relied on prolonged mechanical ventilation and sedation in the intensive care unit (ICU) [13]. However, findings from other surgical fields indicate that early tracheal extubation can significantly improve recovery and overall outcomes [14,15]. Additionally, ICU ventilator support constitutes a major contributor to the healthcare costs associated with LT, and successful early extubation has the potential to mitigate this financial burden [16]. Despite strong evidence supporting the safety and feasibility of early extubation after LT, many transplant centers remain reliant on routine postoperative mechanical ventilation in the ICU. This reliance often stems from concerns about the complexity of the procedure and potential risks, including cardiopulmonary complications, reoperation, failed extubation, and challenges in recovering from surgical stress [17]. Studies have identified effective pain control as a critical factor in achieving successful early extubation in the operating room (OR) after LT, emphasizing its feasibility and clinical benefits [2,12,17,18]. Similar observations in cardiac surgery have demonstrated the effectiveness of fascial plane blocks, such as the erector spinae plane block and the pecto-intercostal fascial block, as components of multimodal analgesia protocols. These techniques have been shown to improve patient comfort, shorten extubation times, and promote faster recovery and rehabilitation [19–21].

This study aimed to assess the effectiveness of the subcostal TAP block in promoting early extubation in the OR among patients undergoing living donor liver transplantation (LDLT). Additionally, it examined the block's impact on related clinical outcomes, such as the necessity for re-intubation, postoperative fentanyl requirements, and pain intensity at the time of ICU admission.

2. Patient and Methods

2.1. Ethical Consideration

This study was designed as a retrospective observational cohort and conducted in alignment with the ethical standards outlined in the Declaration of Helsinki. Approval for the research protocol was obtained from the Institutional Review Board and Ethics Committee (approval number KC21IRSI0576) on 17 September 2021. Given its retrospective nature, the requirement for obtaining informed consent from participants was waived. The results are reported following the recommendations provided by the Strengthening the Reporting of Observational Studies in Epidemiology (STROBE) guidelines.

2.2. Study Population

This study included adult patients aged 19 years or older who underwent elective LDLT at our hospital between September 2012 and September 2022. Eligible participants were those diagnosed with hepatocellular carcinoma (HCC) meeting the Milan criteria and deemed suitable for regional anesthesia, defined as having an international normalized ratio (INR) ≤ 2.0 and a platelet count $\geq 50 \times 10^9$/L [22,23]. Exclusion criteria encompassed pediatric patients (<19 years), individuals with other underlying liver disease etiologies (e.g., alcohol-induced, autoimmune, biliary pathology, acute hepatitis A, or drug-/toxin-related liver disease), and those with contraindications to regional anesthesia, such as active skin infections at the injection site or known hypersensitivity to local anesthetics. Patients on anticoagulant or antiplatelet therapy (e.g., aspirin and warfarin) within seven days prior to surgery were also excluded. Additional exclusions included cases involving deceased donor liver transplantation, ABO-incompatible LDLT, multi-organ transplants that included the liver, or re-transplantation. Patients with significant preoperative systemic comorbidities, such as uncontrolled cardiac, pulmonary, or renal conditions that contraindicated LDLT, were also omitted. Similarly, those requiring prolonged postoperative sedation (>24 h) or sedation reintroduction within 48 h, which could interfere with recovery assessments, were excluded. Finally, patients with incomplete or missing key data regarding recipient or donor graft characteristics were not included in this study.

During the study period, 677 patients underwent LDLT at our institution. After applying the inclusion and exclusion criteria, 388 patients were excluded, primarily due to non-HCC liver disease (190 patients), contraindications to regional anesthesia (123 patients), prolonged postoperative sedation requirements (70 patients), and incomplete or missing clinical data (5 patients), leaving 289 eligible patients for analysis.

To minimize potential confounding, propensity score (PS) matching was performed, yielding a final cohort of 186 matched patients. These patients were evenly divided into two groups based on the application of the subcostal TAP block, with 93 patients in the TAP block group and 93 in the no-TAP block group (Figure 1).

2.3. Surgical and Anesthetic Management

The recipient's surgical procedure and anesthetic management have been detailed in our prior studies [24,25]. In summary, the recipient surgery involved a J-shaped subcostal incision, followed by implantation of the donor liver. The piggyback technique was employed to optimize venous drainage without the need for complete caval clamping. To ensure proper hepatic venous outflow, reconstruction of the middle hepatic vein was performed as needed. After completing hepatic vessel and bile duct anastomoses, Doppler ultrasonography was used to confirm vascular patency and assess graft perfusion before closing the abdominal incision.

Anesthesia was managed by using a combination of desflurane, rocuronium, and remifentanil to achieve optimal muscle relaxation and maintain hemodynamic stability. Perioperative care was guided by invasive hemodynamic monitoring, including measurements of arterial blood pressure, central venous pressure, and cardiac output. Hemodynamic instability was managed with targeted fluid resuscitation and the careful use of vasopressors to maintain systemic perfusion pressures. Diuretics were administered as needed to address oliguria, fluid overload, or electrolyte imbalances, ensuring stable systemic hemodynamics.

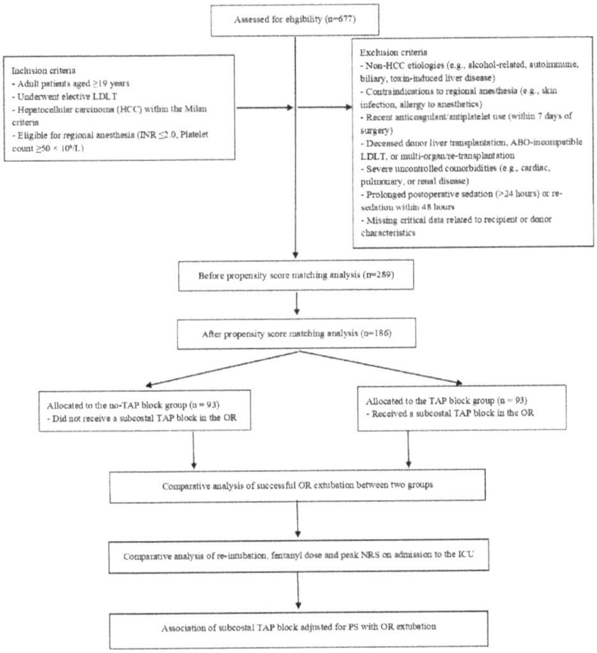

Figure 1. Study flow diagram.

To optimize postoperative analgesia while minimizing opioid use, a multimodal analgesia protocol was implemented. This included a combination of systemic analgesics and a subcostal TAP block, which was performed immediately before awakening at the conclusion of surgery. The subcostal TAP block was integrated into the analgesic strategy to provide targeted pain relief for the J-shaped subcostal incision, facilitating early extubation and reducing opioid requirements.

Postoperative analgesia was initiated at the time of surgical site closure, approximately 60 min before the planned extubation, using a combination of nefopam (1 mg/kg) and fentanyl (1 µg/kg) diluted in 100 mL of normal saline, provided there were no contraindications. Upon ICU admission, peak pain levels were assessed by using the numeric rating scale (NRS). Rescue analgesia with fentanyl (50 µg) was administered as needed, depending on the NRS score. For scores ≥ 5, additional fentanyl was provided every 15 min until the pain score fell below 5. All fentanyl doses were determined by the attending ICU physician, who was not involved in the study, and meticulously recorded by nursing staff.

2.4. Subcostal TAP Block

Since September 2012, the subcostal TAP block has been integrated into the perioperative management of LDLT patients as part of a multimodal analgesia strategy to enhance postoperative pain control and reduce opioid consumption. Introduced as an opioid-sparing technique, the TAP block aims to improve recovery outcomes while minimizing opioid-related adverse effects. It was selectively performed in LDLT patients deemed suitable for regional anesthesia, ensuring both safety and procedural efficacy, while those with significant coagulation abnormalities or contraindications to regional anesthesia were excluded.

In the OR, before awakening, a subcostal TAP block was performed by a single anesthesiologist with expertise in regional anesthesia to provide targeted pain relief for the J-shaped subcostal incision used in LDLT. The block was administered under real-time ultrasound guidance to ensure precision and reduce the risk of complications. With the patient in a supine position and the abdominal area aseptically prepared, a high-frequency linear ultrasound probe was placed along the subcostal margin on the surgical side, aligned parallel to the costal arch. The anatomical layers, including the external oblique, internal oblique, and transversus abdominis muscles, were clearly identified. An in-plane technique was used to advance a 21-gauge, 100 mm echogenic block needle under ultrasound guidance in a medial-to-lateral direction, targeting the fascial plane between the internal oblique and transversus abdominis muscles. Hydrodissection with 2–3 mL of normal saline was performed to confirm accurate needle placement within the fascial plane. Following confirmation, 20 mL of 0.25% ropivacaine was incrementally injected to ensure adequate spread and effective analgesic coverage of the incision site. The block was administered unilaterally on the side of the J-shaped incision and completed at the conclusion of surgery. Throughout the procedure, the patient was carefully monitored for signs of local anesthetic systemic toxicity (LAST) and other potential complications to ensure safety.

2.5. *OR Extubation Criteria*

In this study, decisions regarding extubation in the OR after LT were made by experienced anesthesiologists specializing in liver transplant anesthesia [24]. Extubation readiness was assessed based on a standardized set of criteria (Supplementary Table S1). Adequate oxygenation was defined as a peripheral oxygen saturation (SpO_2) of at least 95% with a fractional inspired oxygen concentration (FiO_2) of 0.5 or less. Ventilatory adequacy required a tidal volume greater than 5 mL/kg, a spontaneous respiratory rate below 25 breaths per minute, and end-tidal carbon dioxide ($ETCO_2$) levels within the normocarbic range of 30–40 mmHg. Hemodynamic stability was also essential, with minimal vasopressor support defined as a norepinephrine infusion rate of less than 0.1 µg/kg/min. Full reversal of neuromuscular blockade was confirmed through indicators such as a sustained head lift or a firm hand grasp. Neurological assessments ensured that patients could respond to simple verbal commands, had spontaneous eye opening, and retained protective reflexes like coughing and gagging. Metabolic stability requirements included a pH above 7.25, normal serum electrolyte levels, and evidence of euvolemia. A core body temperature of at least 35.5 °C was also required. Surgical considerations were reviewed, and extubation was performed only in the absence of significant bleeding or concerns about hepatic vascular patency. Routine consultation with the surgical team was not necessary unless specific complications arose. After extubation, all patients were transferred to the ICU for postoperative monitoring and care.

2.6. *Outcomes*

The primary outcome of this study was the rate of successful extubation in the OR immediately following LT. Successful extubation was defined as meeting all predefined extubation criteria without the need for postoperative mechanical ventilation before transfer to the ICU. Secondary outcomes included the rate of re-intubation within the first postoperative hour, the total fentanyl dose administered for pain management upon ICU admission, and the peak numeric rating scale (NRS) pain score recorded at the time of ICU admission. Re-intubation was noted if mechanical ventilation was required due to inadequate oxygenation, insufficient ventilation, hemodynamic instability, or other clinical concerns. Fentanyl dosage was documented to evaluate postoperative analgesic needs, and the peak NRS score served as an objective measure of immediate postoperative pain severity.

2.7. Clinical Variables for PS-Matching Analysis

For the PS-matching analysis, clinical variables were carefully chosen to ensure comparability between the subcostal TAP block group and the no-TAP block group. These variables included preoperative recipient characteristics, intraoperative parameters, and donor graft-related factors to address potential confounders and create balanced groups for analysis. Baseline demographic and clinical characteristics included sex, age, body mass index (BMI), and comorbidities such as hypertension and diabetes mellitus. Liver disease severity and complications were assessed by using the Model for End-Stage Liver Disease (MELD) score, history of varices, and the presence of ascites ($\geq$1 L). Preoperative cardiac function was evaluated through echocardiographic findings, including ejection fraction (%) and diastolic dysfunction ($\geq$grade II). Laboratory parameters considered included white blood cell count, hematocrit, aspartate aminotransferase (AST), alanine aminotransferase (ALT), serum sodium, potassium, albumin, ammonia, platelet count, and INR. Intraoperative factors included the total surgery duration and average vital signs, such as systolic and diastolic blood pressure and heart rate. Transfusion requirements were documented, including the number of packed red blood cell (PRBC) units and fresh frozen plasma (FFP) units administered. Donor graft-related variables included donor sex, age, and BMI, along with graft-specific factors such as the graft–recipient weight ratio (%), graft weight (g), fatty percentage (%), and total ischemic time (minutes). These variables were used in the PS-matching process to minimize baseline discrepancies between the groups, enabling a reliable comparison of perioperative outcomes associated with the subcostal TAP block.

2.8. Statistical Analysis

The Shapiro–Wilk test was used to evaluate the normality of continuous variables. Continuous data are reported as medians with interquartile ranges, while categorical data are presented as counts and percentages. To reduce confounding factors between the TAP block and no-TAP block groups, PS matching was applied. Propensity scores were calculated, and one-to-one matching was performed by using a greedy algorithm without replacement to achieve balance between the groups. Perioperative recipient and donor graft variables were analyzed by using the Mann–Whitney U test for continuous variables. For categorical variables, either the χ^2 test or Fisher's exact test was employed, depending on the data distribution and sample size. The effect of the subcostal TAP block on successful extubation in the OR was assessed through multivariable logistic regression analysis, adjusted for the PS. Results are presented as odds ratios with 95% confidence intervals, and a *p*-value of <0.05 was considered statistically significant. All statistical analyses were conducted by using SPSS for Windows (version 24.0; IBM Corp., Armonk, NY, USA) and Microsoft Excel.

3. Results

3.1. Demographic Variables

All patients had HCC within the Milan criteria and underwent elective LDLT. Among the 289 patients, 240 (83.0%) were male, with a mean age of 55.2 $\pm$ 7.5 years and a mean BMI of 24.6 $\pm$ 3.6 kg/m^2. Hypertension was observed in 68 patients (23.5%), and diabetes mellitus in 79 patients (27.3%). The mean MELD score was 11.6 $\pm$ 6.5 points. A history of varices was present in 49 patients (17.0%), and ascites was identified in 96 patients (33.2%). The mean PLT count was 150.9 $\pm$ 37.3 $\times$ 10^9/L, and the mean INR was 1.5 $\pm$ 0.5.

3.2. PS-Matching Analysis of Pre- and Intraoperative Recipient and Donor/Graft Variables According to Subcostal TAP Block

Before PS matching, several significant differences were observed between the no-TAP and TAP block groups (Table 1). Patients in the TAP block group had a lower median age (54.0 vs. 56.5 years, $p = 0.013$), higher MELD scores (13.6 vs. 6.7, $p < 0.001$), and lower hematocrit levels (30.1% vs. 34.3%, $p < 0.001$). Additionally, the TAP block group had higher ALT levels (median of 32.0 IU/L vs. 29.0 IU/L, $p = 0.002$) and lower albumin levels (median of 3.0 g/dL vs. 3.4 g/dL, $p < 0.001$). Comorbid hypertension was less prevalent in the TAP block group (16.6% vs. 30.6%, $p = 0.005$).

Table 1. Perioperative demographic variables in the no-TAP block and TAP block groups before and after propensity score matching.

	Before Propensity Score Matching				**After Propensity Score Matching**			
Group	**No-TAP Block**	**TAP Block**	***p*-Value**	**SD**	**No-TAP Block**	**TAP Block**	***p*-Value**	**SD**
n	**144**	**145**			**93**	**93**		
Preoperative recipient variables								
Sex (male)	122 (84.7%)	118 (81.4%)	0.449	0.086	80 (86.0%)	77 (82.8%)	0.544	0.083
Age (years)	56.5 (52.0–61.0)	54.0 (50.0–59.0)	0.013	−0.262	56.0 (52.0–60.0)	55.0 (51.0–60.0)	0.457	−0.091
BMI (kg/m^2)	24.2 (22.0–26.4)	24.4 (22.9–26.7)	0.195	0.146	24.1 (22.0–26.7)	24.2 (22.5–26.1)	0.727	0.044
Comorbidity								
Hypertension	44 (30.6%)	24 (16.6%)	0.005	−0.376	24 (25.8%)	19 (20.4%)	0.385	−0.144
Diabetes mellitus	38 (26.4%)	41 (28.3%)	0.719	0.042	24 (25.8%)	26 (28.0%)	0.741	0.048
MELD score (points)	6.7 (6.0–10.9)	13.6 (6.0–21.7)	<0.001	0.754	8.2 (6.0–11.9)	7.9 (6.0–15.0)	0.888	0.094
Complications								
Varix	16 (11.1%)	33 (22.8%)	0.008	0.277	12 (12.9%)	13 (14.0%)	0.83	0.026
Ascites (≥1 L)	42 (29.2%)	54 (37.2%)	0.145	0.166	31 (33.3%)	28 (30.1%)	0.636	−0.066
Echocardiography								
Ejection fraction (%)	64.0 (62.0–66.0)	65.0 (62.3–67.4)	0.096	0.149	64.0 (63.0–66.3)	65.0 (62.7–67.7)	0.249	0.123
Diastolic dysfunction (≥grade II)	22 (15.3%)	28 (19.3%)	0.365	0.102	16 (17.2%)	17 (18.3%)	0.848	0.027
Laboratory values								
White blood cell count ($\times 10^9$/L)	4.1 (2.8–5.2)	3.4 (2.6–5.4)	0.251	0.105	4.1 (2.5–5.2)	3.4 (2.5–4.9)	0.404	0.093
Hematocrit (%)	34.3 (28.7–39.2)	30.1 (25.8–36.1)	<0.001	−0.401	33.5 (27.5–37.7)	33.0 (27.1–37.9)	0.66	−0.040
Aspartate aminotransferase (IU/L)	34.5 (26.3–50.8)	50.0 (33.5–84.5)	<0.001	0.358	34.0 (26.0–51.0)	39.0 (29.0–61.5)	0.076	0.064
Alanine aminotransferase (IU/L)	29.0 (20.0–42.0)	32.0 (24.0–67.0)	0.002	0.323	28.0 (18.0–41.5)	31.0 (21.5–44.5)	0.126	0.048
Sodium (mEq/L)	141.0 (138.0–142.0)	139.0 (136.0–141.0)	<0.001	−0.305	141.0 (137.0–142.0)	140.0 (137.0–142.0)	0.549	−0.027

Table 1. *Cont.*

	Before Propensity Score Matching				After Propensity Score Matching			
Group	No-TAP Block	TAP Block	*p*-Value	SD	No-TAP Block	TAP Block	*p*-Value	SD
n	**144**	**145**			**93**	**93**		
Potassium (mEq/L)	4.0 (3.7–4.3)	4.0 (3.7–4.3)	0.601	−0.031	4.0 (3.8–4.3)	4.0 (3.8–4.3)	0.575	−0.040
Albumin (g/dL)	3.4 (2.8–3.9)	3.0 (2.6–3.6)	<0.001	−0.461	3.2 (2.8–3.8)	3.3 (2.7–3.7)	0.742	−0.056
Ammonia (μg/dL)	89.0 (62.5–134.8)	106.0 (71.0–166.0)	0.018	0.252	96.0 (68.5–143.0)	91.0 (65.0–133.0)	0.417	−0.060
Platelet count ($\times 10^9$/L)	151.0 (130.3–169.0)	147.0 (131.0–162.0)	0.28	−0.196	145.0 (126.5–161.0)	147.0 (128.0–162.0)	0.662	0.052
International normalized ratio	1.3 (1.1–1.4)	1.7 (1.2–2.2)	<0.001	0.832	1.3 (1.1–1.4)	1.2 (1.2–1.6)	0.24	0.098
Intraoperative recipient variables								
Operation time (min)	482.5 (435.0–540.0)	500.0 (460.0–595.0)	0.023	0.269	505.0 (442.5–545.0)	490.0 (457.5–572.5)	0.82	0.004
Average of vital signs								
Systolic blood pressure (mmHg)	106.3 (99.3–116.9)	108.3 (97.6–118.4)	0.91	0.016	104.0 (97.5–114.4)	107.5 (97.5–118.4)	0.257	0.153
Diastolic blood pressure (mmHg)	57.7 (53.1–63.7)	58.8 (52.8–64.9)	0.649	0.062	57.0 (52.0–63.8)	58.5 (52.0–64.4)	0.636	0.094
Heart rate (beats/min)	88.3 (80.1–97.9)	87.5 (78.5–100.6)	0.738	−0.022	88.5 (80.3–103.7)	87.3 (77.0–98.0)	0.252	−0.161
Blood transfusion								
Packed red blood cells (units)	5.0 (5.0–5.0)	5.0 (5.0–5.0)	0.746	0.049	5.0 (5.0–5.0)	5.0 (5.0–5.0)	0.444	0.088
Fresh frozen plasma (units)	5.0 (5.0–5.0)	5.0 (5.0–5.0)	0.099	0.284	5.0 (5.0–5.0)	5.0 (5.0–5.0)	0.798	0.094
Donor graft variables								
Sex (male)	87 (60.4%)	91 (62.8%)	0.682	−0.048	53 (57.0%)	57 (61.3%)	0.551	−0.089
Age (years)	35.2 (28.0–46.0)	31.0 (24.0–46.5)	0.023	−0.221	34.0 (27.0–41.5)	31.0 (24.5–48.0)	0.418	−0.052
BMI (kg/m^2)	20.2 (18.2–21.4)	20.2 (18.0–22.0)	0.771	0.008	20.2 (18.2–21.3)	20.2 (17.9–22.5)	0.729	0.062
Graft–recipient weight ratio (%)	1.2 (1.0–1.5)	1.1 (1.0–1.4)	0.075	−0.248	1.2 (1.0–1.4)	1.1 (1.0–1.4)	0.776	−0.061
Graft weight (g)	826.0 (692.5–926.0)	792.0 (669.0–900.0)	0.211	−0.119	800.0 (672.0–896.6)	802.0 (680.0–901.0)	0.977	−0.024
Fatty percentage (%)	4.9 (1.0–5.0)	5.0 (1.0–5.0)	0.156	0.176	4.9 (0.5–5.0)	5.0 (0.5–5.0)	0.485	0.153
Total ischemic time (min)	80.0 (63.5–113.8)	94.0 (67.0–119.5)	0.119	0.022	85.0 (65.5–117.0)	94.0 (66.0–125.5)	0.327	0.053

Abbreviations: TAP, transversus abdominis plane; BMI, body mass index; SD, standard deviation; MELD, model for end-stage liver disease. Values are expressed as numbers (percentages) and medians (interquartile ranges).

After PS matching, these variables were balanced between the no-TAP and TAP block groups. There were no significant differences in demographic characteristics, MELD scores (median of 7.9 vs. 8.2, $p = 0.888$), or laboratory parameters, such as hematocrit (33.0% vs. 33.5%, $p = 0.660$) and albumin levels (3.3 g/dL vs. 3.2 g/dL, $p = 0.742$). Furthermore, intraoperative variables, including operation time and transfusion requirements, showed no statistically significant differences between the two groups after matching.

3.3. OR Extubation and ICU Outcomes

In the PS-matched cohort of 186 patients (93 in each group), the rate of extubation in the OR was significantly higher in the TAP block group compared with the no-TAP block group (93.5% vs. 81.7%; $p = 0.014$). This finding, as shown in Table 2 and Figure 2, demonstrates a statistical association between the subcostal TAP block and successful OR extubation.

Table 2. Operating room extubation outcomes in propensity score-matched patients comparing no-TAP and TAP block groups.

Group	No-TAP Block	TAP Block	*p*-Value
n	**93**	**93**	
Extubation in the OR (%)	76 (81.7%)	87 (93.5%)	0.014
Re-intubation on admission to the ICU (%)	3 (3.2%)	1 (1.1%)	0.621
Fentanyl dose on admission to the ICU (μg)	150 (150–200)	50 (50–100)	<0.001
Peak NRS on admission to the ICU	8 (8–9)	6 (6–7)	<0.001

Abbreviations: TAP, transversus abdominis plane; OR, operating room; ICU, intensive care unit; NRS, numeric rating scale. Values are expressed as numbers (percentages) and medians (interquartile ranges).

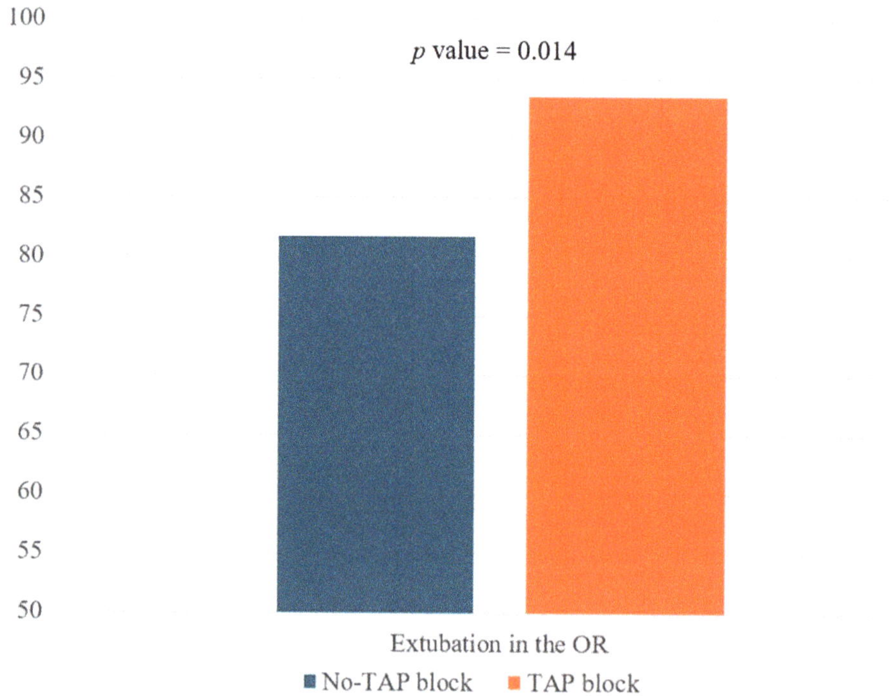

Figure 2. Operating room extubation rates in patients undergoing living donor liver transplantation, stratified by TAP block intervention. Patients in the TAP block group had a significantly higher rate of successful extubation in the operating room compared with the no-TAP block group (93.5% vs. 81.7%; $p = 0.014$). Abbreviations: TAP, transversus abdominis plane; OR, operating room.

The rate of re-intubation upon admission to the ICU was lower in the TAP block group (1.1% vs. 3.2%), although this difference was not statistically significant ($p = 0.621$).

Re-intubation in the no-TAP block group was primarily attributed to CO_2 retention caused by shallow tachypnea due to incisional pain, which disrupted deep and smooth breathing. In the TAP block group, a single case of re-intubation occurred, potentially due to incomplete analgesic coverage provided by the block. In all instances, re-intubation was resolved within one hour, with patients successfully weaned from ventilatory support and discharged from the ICU without further complications.

Patients in the TAP block group required significantly lower fentanyl doses upon ICU admission (median of 50 μg vs. 150 μg; $p < 0.001$) and reported lower peak visual analog scale (VAS) pain scores (median of 6 vs. 8; $p < 0.001$), reflecting improved postoperative pain management.

3.4. Association Between Subcostal TAP Block Adjusted for PS and OR Extubation

Multivariate analysis adjusted for PS demonstrated a significant association between the subcostal TAP block and successful OR extubation. The TAP block was independently associated with a higher likelihood of successful OR extubation, with an odds ratio of 3.243 (95% CI: 1.217–8.644; $p = 0.019$) (Table 3).

Table 3. Association of subcostal TAP block with facilitating operating room extubation in propensity score-matched patients.

	β	Odds Ratio	95% CI	*p*-Value
Subcostal TAP Block Adjusted for PS				
Successful extubation in the operating room	1.177	3.243	1.217–8.644	0.019

Abbreviations: TAP, transversus abdominis plane; PS, propensity score; CI, confidence interval.

3.5. Postoperative Subcostal TAP Block-Related Complications

In this study, no complications related to the subcostal TAP block were observed. Specifically, there were no incidences of local anesthetic systemic toxicity (LAST), which could result from inadvertent intravascular injection or excessive systemic absorption of the anesthetic agent. Similarly, no cases of hematoma formation at the injection site were reported, indicating that the procedure did not cause vascular injury.

Potential risks associated with regional anesthesia, such as infection at the injection site, were also absent in this cohort. Moreover, no mechanical complications, including inadvertent puncture of surrounding organs or structures, were documented. These results suggest that the subcostal TAP block was consistently performed without any observable adverse events, further supporting its safety as a perioperative analgesic technique.

4. Discussion

This study demonstrates that the subcostal TAP block is a feasible analgesic option in highly selected LDLT patients and is associated with certain perioperative benefits, including improved pain control and reduced opioid consumption. While these findings suggest a potential role for the TAP block in facilitating early extubation, the observational nature of this study and the inclusion of both preoperative and intraoperative selection criteria introduce the possibility of selection bias. Patients who received the TAP block had lower opioid requirements and improved pain scores upon ICU admission. Additionally, while the TAP block group showed a higher rate of successful extubation in the OR, these findings should be interpreted with caution due to the potential influence of confounding factors. The observed lower re-intubation rate in the TAP block group may reflect improved analgesia but could also be influenced by patient selection variables. Importantly, no TAP block-related complications were reported, supporting its safety and feasibility when performed under real-time ultrasound guidance.

Research in cardiac surgery has emphasized the role of fascial plane blocks in facilitating earlier tracheal extubation and reducing ICU stays. Revollo et al. found that patients who received fascial plane blocks, particularly the erector spinae plane block, had significantly shorter extubation times (reduced by 9.29 h; 95% CI: −11.98 to −6.60; $p = 0.022$) and shorter ICU stays by 1.1 days (95% CI: −1.43 to −0.79; $p < 0.0001$) compared with those managed with intravenous analgesia alone, with no complications reported [21]. Similarly, Wang et al. demonstrated that the pecto-intercostal fascial block (PIFB) reduced extubation times (9.4 ± 4.1 h vs. 12.1 ± 4.6 h; $p = 0.031$) and intraoperative opioid use (153.2 ± 48.3 μg vs. 199.4 ± 51.7 μg; $p = 0.002$). The PIFB group also experienced lower coughing pain scores (1.45 ± 1.43 vs. 3.00 ± 1.71; $p = 0.021$) without significant differences in resting pain scores or adverse events [20]. In our study, the subcostal TAP block demonstrated clear clinical benefits in promoting earlier extubation and improving postoperative outcomes in LDLT patients. The TAP block group had a significantly higher rate of successful extubation in the OR compared with the no-TAP block group (93.5% vs. 81.7%; $p = 0.014$). Multivariable analysis further revealed that the TAP block increased the odds of successful extubation in the OR by three times (odds ratio: 3.243; 95% CI: 1.217–8.644; $p = 0.019$). Beyond extubation, the TAP block significantly reduced fentanyl requirements upon ICU admission (median of 50 μg vs. 150 μg; $p < 0.001$) and lowered peak NRS pain scores (median of 6 vs. 8; $p < 0.001$), underscoring its efficacy in pain management. Importantly, no complications related to the TAP block were observed, demonstrating its safety and feasibility when performed under real-time ultrasound guidance [7,8,26]. The observed association between the TAP block and improved perioperative outcomes suggests that regional analgesia techniques may contribute to optimizing postoperative recovery in LDLT patients, particularly by reducing opioid consumption and facilitating early extubation. These effects could lead to better respiratory function, reduced postoperative sedation, and improved hemodynamic stability, all of which are critical in high-risk surgical populations. Furthermore, the findings underscore the importance of individualized pain management strategies in LDLT recipients. Given the variability in hepatic function and coagulation profiles among transplant patients, a targeted multimodal analgesia approach that includes regional techniques like the TAP block may help balance effective pain relief with safety considerations. Identifying optimal candidates for the TAP block through refined selection criteria may further enhance its utility while minimizing the risk of complications.

The concept of accelerated recovery following surgery, known as Enhanced Recovery After Surgery (ERAS), has gained significant attention in recent years. ERAS emphasizes standardized perioperative strategies aimed at optimizing healthcare resource use, minimizing complications, and enhancing patient outcomes [27]. A key aspect of this approach is the incorporation of multimodal analgesic techniques, including advanced regional anesthesia methods such as the pectoral plane block, serratus anterior plane block, and erector spinae plane (ESP) block. In line with ERAS principles, studies have shown that these interventions can reduce recovery times without increasing the risk of adverse events [28–30]. Effective pain management, early tracheal extubation, and the avoidance of prolonged mechanical ventilation are critical goals in perioperative care for LT. Adequate pain control not only improves patient comfort but also helps prevent complications related to impaired ventilation. Early extubation, a cornerstone of ERAS protocols, reduces risks associated with ventilator use and accelerates recovery. Avoiding prolonged mechanical ventilation further enhances outcomes by decreasing morbidity and healthcare costs [3,31]. This study aligns with the principles of ERAS, demonstrating the subcostal TAP block as a valuable component of a multimodal strategy to improve patient care in complex surgical procedures like LDLT. By providing effective pain relief, the TAP block minimizes opioid use, reducing associated risks and facilitating early extubation—a critical step toward rapid recovery. Specifically, the subcostal TAP block proved effective in managing pain from the J-shaped incision in LDLT, alleviating parietal pain-induced respiratory compromise. This enabled sufficient tidal volume without tachypnea, ensuring stable respiratory function and reducing the likelihood of prolonged mechanical ventilation. Further research should investigate the long-term benefits of the TAP block and refine protocols to enhance its application in liver transplantation.

The subcostal TAP block employed in this study is a regional anesthesia technique that targets the fascial plane between the transversus abdominis and internal oblique muscles. By delivering local anesthetic to this plane, the block interrupts nerve conduction in the anterior branches of the lower thoracic intercostal nerves (T7–T12) and, in some cases, the iliohypogastric and ilioinguinal nerves [7,8]. This technique is particularly effective for managing pain in dermatomes associated with upper-abdominal incisions, making it highly suitable for LT procedures involving J-shaped subcostal incisions. The block's primary effectiveness in LT lies in its ability to provide localized analgesia for parietal pain, which arises from the abdominal wall incision and prolonged retraction needed for liver exposure. Parietal pain significantly contributes to postoperative discomfort and respiratory challenges, such as limited diaphragmatic movement, shallow breathing, or tachypnea. By alleviating this pain, the subcostal TAP block helps maintain adequate tidal volume and stable respiratory function, reducing the need for extended ventilatory support and enabling earlier extubation [3,16,17,24,32]. For LT patients, who often have impaired liver function and coagulopathy, the TAP block offers a key safety advantage. Unlike neuraxial techniques such as epidural or paravertebral blocks, which carry a heightened risk of hematoma in anticoagulated individuals, the TAP block provides effective analgesia without breaching intrathecal or epidural spaces. Administering the block under real-time ultrasound guidance further minimizes the risk of vascular or visceral injury, ensuring precision and safety [11,12]. Additionally, the opioid-sparing benefits of the TAP block make it especially valuable in this patient population. Reduced opioid use is advantageous as excessive opioids can worsen hepatic encephalopathy, delay gastrointestinal recovery, and heighten the risk of respiratory depression [33,34]. These combined physiological and safety benefits establish the subcostal TAP block as a crucial element of the multimodal analgesic approach in LT, significantly improving postoperative outcomes while maintaining a robust safety profile.

This study has several limitations that should be acknowledged. First, its retrospective design introduces the potential for selection bias, as the administration of the TAP block was determined by both preoperative and intraoperative factors, which may have influenced the observed outcomes. Although propensity score matching was used to minimize confounding, residual biases cannot be entirely ruled out. Second, as a single-center study, the findings may not be fully generalizable to other institutions with different surgical approaches, perioperative protocols, or patient populations. Third, the evaluation of pain control and opioid consumption was limited to the immediate postoperative period, without assessing long-term outcomes such as chronic pain, opioid dependence, or overall quality of life, which could provide a more comprehensive understanding of the TAP block's impact. Fourth, while the TAP block was performed under ultrasound guidance, differences in operator experience and technique may have influenced its effectiveness and safety, though this aspect was not specifically analyzed. Lastly, this study focused exclusively on LDLT recipients with HCC within transplant eligibility criteria who were considered suitable candidates for regional anesthesia based on coagulation and platelet function assessments. These selection criteria may limit the generalizability of the findings, as the results may not directly apply to LDLT recipients with other liver diseases, patients undergoing deceased donor liver transplantation, or individuals with different perioperative risk profiles. Future research should aim to address these limitations through prospective, multicenter studies with larger cohorts. Additionally, randomized controlled trials with extended follow-up could further clarify the long-term benefits of the TAP block and help refine patient selection criteria for its use in liver transplantation.

5. Conclusions

This study demonstrates that the subcostal TAP block is a feasible analgesic technique in highly selected LDLT recipients and is associated with certain perioperative benefits, including improved pain control and reduced opioid requirements. While these findings suggest a potential role for the TAP block in facilitating early extubation and enhancing perioperative recovery, several limitations must be considered. The retrospective study design and selection criteria for TAP block administration introduce the possibility of selection bias, and despite propensity score matching, residual confounding factors cannot be entirely ruled out. Additionally, as a single-center study, the findings may not be fully generalizable to other institutions with different perioperative practices and patient populations. This study also focused on the immediate postoperative period, and long-term analgesic effects, functional recovery, and overall quality of life outcomes were not assessed. Given these limitations, our results should be interpreted with caution, and larger prospective, multicenter studies are needed to confirm its efficacy, refine patient selection criteria, and optimize clinical implementation. Nevertheless, the safety and feasibility of the TAP block, particularly when performed under ultrasound guidance, support its consideration as part of multimodal analgesia protocols in carefully selected LDLT patients. Future research should focus on optimizing dosing strategies, identifying patient subgroups that may derive the greatest benefit, and evaluating its potential role in broader liver transplant populations, including deceased donor liver transplantation and emergency surgical settings.

Supplementary Materials: The following supporting information can be downloaded at: https://www.mdpi.com/article/10.3390/life15020297/s1, Supplementary Table S1: Criteria for extubation in the operating room following living donor liver transplantation.

Author Contributions: Conceptualization, J.H. and M.S.C.; methodology, J.H. and M.S.C.; software, J.H. and M.S.C.; validation, J.H. and M.S.C.; formal analysis, J.H. and M.S.C.; investigation, J.H. and M.S.C.; resources, J.H. and M.S.C.; data curation, J.H. and M.S.C.; writing—original draft preparation, J.H. and M.S.C.; writing—review and editing, J.H. and M.S.C.; project administration, J.H. and M.S.C. All authors have read and agreed to the published version of the manuscript.

Funding: This research received no external funding.

Institutional Review Board Statement: This study was designed as a retrospective observational cohort and conducted in alignment with the ethical standards outlined in the Declaration of Helsinki. Approval for the research protocol was obtained from the Institutional Review Board and Ethics Committee (approval number KC21IRSI0576) on 17 September 2021. Given its retrospective nature, the requirement for obtaining informed consent from participants was waived. The results are reported following the recommendations provided by the Strengthening the Reporting of Observational Studies in Epidemiology (STROBE) guidelines.

Informed Consent Statement: As this study was conducted retrospectively, the requirement for informed consent was waived.

Data Availability Statement: Data are contained within the article.

Conflicts of Interest: The authors declare no conflict of interest.

References

1. Kutzler, H.L.; Gannon, R.; Nolan, W.; Meisterling, L.; Cech, M.; Gleason, D.; Uzl, J.; Rochon, C.; Maneckshana, B.; Serrano, O.K.; et al. Opioid avoidance in liver transplant recipients: Reduction in postoperative opioid use through a multidisciplinary multimodal approach. *Liver Transplant.* **2020**, *26*, 1254–1262. [CrossRef] [PubMed]
2. Brustia, R.; Monsel, A.; Skurzak, S.; Schiffer, E.; Carrier, F.M.; Patrono, D.; Kaba, A.; Detry, O.; Malbouisson, L.; Andraus, W.; et al. Guidelines for Perioperative Care for Liver Transplantation: Enhanced Recovery After Surgery (ERAS) Recommendations. *Transplantation* **2022**, *106*, 552–561. [CrossRef]
3. Day, R.W.; Aloia, T.A. Enhanced recovery in liver surgery. *J. Surg. Oncol.* **2019**, *119*, 660–666. [CrossRef] [PubMed]
4. McDonnell, J.G.; Curley, G.; Carney, J.; Benton, A.; Costello, J.; Maharaj, C.H.; Laffey, J.G. The analgesic efficacy of transversus abdominis plane block after cesarean delivery: A randomized controlled trial. *Anesth. Analg.* **2008**, *106*, 186–191. [CrossRef] [PubMed]
5. McDonnell, J.G.; O'Donnell, B.; Curley, G.; Heffernan, A.; Power, C.; Laffey, J.G. The analgesic efficacy of transversus abdominis plane block after abdominal surgery: A prospective randomized controlled trial. *Anesth. Analg.* **2007**, *104*, 193–197. [CrossRef] [PubMed]
6. Chen, Y.; Shi, K.; Xia, Y.; Zhang, X.; Papadimos, T.J.; Xu, X.; Wang, Q. Sensory Assessment and Regression Rate of Bilateral Oblique Subcostal Transversus Abdominis Plane Block in Volunteers. *Reg. Anesth. Pain Med.* **2018**, *43*, 174–179. [CrossRef] [PubMed]
7. Hebbard, P.D.; Barrington, M.J.; Vasey, C. Ultrasound-guided continuous oblique subcostal transversus abdominis plane blockade: Description of anatomy and clinical technique. *Reg. Anesth. Pain Med.* **2010**, *35*, 436–441. [CrossRef]
8. Hebbard, P.; Fujiwara, Y.; Shibata, Y.; Royse, C. Ultrasound-guided transversus abdominis plane (TAP) block. *Anaesth. Intensive Care* **2007**, *35*, 616–617. [PubMed]
9. Guo, J.G.; Li, H.L.; Pei, Q.Q.; Feng, Z.Y. The analgesic efficacy of subcostal transversus abdominis plane block with Mercedes incision. *BMC Anesthesiol.* **2018**, *18*, 36. [CrossRef] [PubMed]
10. Kıtlık, A.; Erdogan, M.A.; Ozgul, U.; Aydogan, M.S.; Ucar, M.; Toprak, H.I.; Colak, C.; Durmus, M. Ultrasound-guided transversus abdominis plane block for postoperative analgesia in living liver donors: A prospective, randomized, double-blinded clinical trial. *J. Clin. Anesth.* **2017**, *37*, 103–107. [CrossRef]
11. Milan, Z.B.; Duncan, B.; Rewari, V.; Kocarev, M.; Collin, R. Subcostal transversus abdominis plane block for postoperative analgesia in liver transplant recipients. *Transplant. Proc.* **2011**, *43*, 2687–2690. [CrossRef] [PubMed]
12. Assefi, M.; Trillaud, E.; Vezinet, C.; Duceau, B.; Baron, E.; Pons, S.; Clavieras, N.; Quemeneur, C.; Selves, A.; Scatton, O.; et al. Subcostal transversus abdominis plane block for postoperative analgesia in liver transplant recipients: A before-and-after study. *Reg. Anesth. Pain Med.* **2023**, *48*, 352–358. [CrossRef] [PubMed]
13. Stock, P.G.; Payne, W.D. Liver transplantation. *Crit. Care Clin.* **1990**, *6*, 911–926. [CrossRef] [PubMed]
14. Lanuti, M.; de Delva, P.E.; Maher, A.; Wright, C.D.; Gaissert, H.A.; Wain, J.C.; Donahue, D.M.; Mathisen, D.J. Feasibility and outcomes of an early extubation policy after esophagectomy. *Ann. Thorac. Surg.* **2006**, *82*, 2037–2041. [CrossRef] [PubMed]
15. Cohen, J.; Loewinger, J.; Hutin, K.; Sulkes, J.; Zelikovski, A.; Singer, P. The safety of immediate extubation after abdominal aortic surgery: A prospective, randomized trial. *Anesth. Analg.* **2001**, *93*, 1546–1549, table of contents. [CrossRef] [PubMed]
16. Mandell, M.S.; Lezotte, D.; Kam, I.; Zamudio, S. Reduced use of intensive care after liver transplantation: Influence of early extubation. *Liver Transpl.* **2002**, *8*, 676–681. [CrossRef] [PubMed]
17. Aniskevich, S.; Pai, S.L. Fast track anesthesia for liver transplantation: Review of the current practice. *World J. Hepatol.* **2015**, *7*, 2303–2308. [CrossRef]
18. Biancofiore, G.; Bindi, M.L.; Romanelli, A.M.; Boldrini, A.; Bisà, M.; Esposito, M.; Urbani, L.; Catalano, G.; Mosca, F.; Filipponi, F. Fast track in liver transplantation: 5 years' experience. *Eur. J. Anaesthesiol.* **2005**, *22*, 584–590. [CrossRef]
19. Çalişir, F.; Orak, Y.; Boran, Ö.F.; Ege, M.; Karabekiroğlu, M.E.; Biradli, H.; Doğaner, A. The effect of erector spinae plane block on postoperative extubation time and laboratory parameters in open heart surgery: A retrospective study. *Turk. J. Med. Sci.* **2024**, *54*, 121–127. [CrossRef] [PubMed]
20. Wang, L.; Jiang, L.; Xin, L.; Jiang, B.; Chen, Y.; Feng, Y. Effect of pecto-intercostal fascial block on extubation time in patients undergoing cardiac surgery: A randomized controlled trial. *Front. Surg.* **2023**, *10*, 1128691. [CrossRef] [PubMed]
21. Revollo, S.O.; Echevarria, G.C.; Fullerton, D.; Ramirez, I.; Farias, J.; Lagos, R.; Lacassie, H.J. Intraoperative Fascial Plane Blocks Facilitate Earlier Tracheal Extubation and Intensive Care Unit Discharge After Cardiac Surgery: A Retrospective Cohort Analysis. *J. Cardiothorac. Vasc. Anesth.* **2023**, *37*, 437–444. [CrossRef] [PubMed]
22. Harrop-Griffiths, W.; Cook, T.; Gill, H.; Hill, D.; Ingram, M.; Makris, M.; Malhotra, S.; Nicholls, B.; Popat, M.; Swales, H.; et al. Regional anaesthesia and patients with abnormalities of coagulation: The Association of Anaesthetists of Great Britain & Ireland The Obstetric Anaesthetists' Association Regional Anaesthesia UK. *Anaesthesia* **2013**, *68*, 966–972.

23. Mazzaferro, V.; Regalia, E.; Doci, R.; Andreola, S.; Pulvirenti, A.; Bozzetti, F.; Montalto, F.; Ammatuna, M.; Morabito, A.; Gennari, L. Liver transplantation for the treatment of small hepatocellular carcinomas in patients with cirrhosis. *N. Engl. J. Med.* **1996**, *334*, 693–699. [CrossRef]
24. Chae, M.S.; Kim, J.W.; Jung, J.Y.; Choi, H.J.; Chung, H.S.; Park, C.S.; Choi, J.H.; Hong, S.H. Analysis of pre- and intraoperative clinical for successful operating room extubation after living donor liver transplantation: A retrospective observational cohort study. *BMC Anesthesiol.* **2019**, *19*, 112. [CrossRef] [PubMed]
25. Chae, M.S.; Koo, J.M.; Park, C.S. Predictive Role of Intraoperative Serum Brain Natriuretic Peptide for Early Allograft Dysfunction in Living Donor Liver Transplantation. *Ann. Transplant.* **2016**, *21*, 538–549. [CrossRef] [PubMed]
26. Lee, T.H.; Barrington, M.J.; Tran, T.M.; Wong, D.; Hebbard, P.D. Comparison of extent of sensory block following posterior and subcostal approaches to ultrasound-guided transversus abdominis plane block. *Anaesth. Intensive Care* **2010**, *38*, 452–460. [CrossRef] [PubMed]
27. Ljungqvist, O.; Scott, M.; Fearon, K.C. Enhanced Recovery After Surgery: A Review. *JAMA Surg.* **2017**, *152*, 292–298. [CrossRef]
28. Chin, K.J.; El-Boghdadly, K. Mechanisms of action of the erector spinae plane (ESP) block: A narrative review. *Can. J. Anaesth.* **2021**, *68*, 387–408. [CrossRef] [PubMed]
29. Kumar, K.N.; Kalyane, R.N.; Singh, N.G.; Nagaraja, P.S.; Krishna, M.; Babu, B.; Varadaraju, R.; Sathish, N.; Manjunatha, N. Efficacy of bilateral pectoralis nerve block for ultrafast tracking and postoperative pain management in cardiac surgery. *Ann. Card. Anaesth.* **2018**, *21*, 333–338.
30. Blanco, R.; Parras, T.; McDonnell, J.G.; Prats-Galino, A. Serratus plane block: A novel ultrasound-guided thoracic wall nerve block. *Anaesthesia* **2013**, *68*, 1107–1113. [CrossRef] [PubMed]
31. Jin, B.; Gu, Y.; Xi, S.; Liu, X.; Wu, X.; Li, G. Application of enhanced recovery after surgery following liver transplantation. *World J. Surg. Oncol.* **2023**, *21*, 248. [CrossRef] [PubMed]
32. Brustia, R.; Slim, K.; Scatton, O. Enhanced recovery after liver surgery. *J. Visc. Surg.* **2019**, *156*, 127–137. [CrossRef] [PubMed]
33. Rubin, J.B.; Aby, E.S.; Barman, P.; Tincopa, M. Opioid use and risks in candidates and recipients of liver transplant. *Liver Transpl.* **2024**, *31*, 231–241. [CrossRef] [PubMed]
34. Sussman, J.; Calderon, E.; Ubl, D.S.; Croome, K.P.; Taner, C.B.; Heimbach, J.K.; Moss, A.; Habermann, E.B.; Mathur, A.K. Variation in opioid prescribing patterns after abdominal transplant surgery. *Clin. Transplant.* **2021**, *35*, e14439. [CrossRef] [PubMed]

life

MDPI

Article

Epidemiology of Biliary Acute Pancreatitis—A Seven-Year Experience of a Large Tertiary Center

Andrei Vicențiu Edu [1,2], Mihai Radu Pahomeanu [1,2,*], Alexandru Olăreanu [1], Dana Gabriela Corbu [1], Andreea Ramona Treteanu [1], Alexandru Constantinescu [1,2], Vasile Șandru [1,3], Narcis Octavian Zărnescu [1,4] and Lucian Negreanu [1,2]

[1] Faculty of Medicine, Carol Davila University of Medicine and Pharmacy Bucharest, 050474 Bucharest, Romania; danacorbu1@gmail.com (D.G.C.); andreea-ramona.treteanu0720@stud.umfcd.ro (A.R.T.)
[2] Internal Medicine & Gastroenterology Department, University Emergency Hospital of Bucharest, 050098 Bucharest, Romania
[3] Gastroenterology Department, Emergency Clinical Hospital of Bucharest, 014461 Bucharest, Romania
[4] Abdominal Surgery Department, University Emergency Hospital of Bucharest, 050098 Bucharest, Romania
* Correspondence: mihairadu.pahomeanu@gmail.com; Tel.: +40-724039210

Abstract: (1) Introduction: One of the most common causes of acute pancreatitis is cholelithiasis, which is considered to be associated with female sex, older age, and recurrence. Our aim was to define a group of patients with B-AP to facilitate their diagnosis and management, while more judiciously using medical resources. (2) Materials and Methods: This retrospective, large cohort study, which was conducted by extracting data from the BUC-API registry, consisted of 1855 cases between 1 June 2015 and 1 April 2022. Each admission of the same patient was considered a separate case if it did not have signs of chronic pancreatitis. Severity and morphology were stratified according to the Revised Atlanta Classification. (3) Results: A total of 732 cases of B-AP were analyzed, with 92.5% occurring at the first attack. The median age was 65 years, with 61.9% of the patients being female. The majority (82.2%) were surgical cases, and the length of stay (LoS) was 7 days. There were 10.2% severe cases, with a mortality rate of 4%. (4) Discussion: We found positive associations between sex, age, recurrence, and morphology and biliary etiology. Compared with the general population, female sex and age over 65 years correlate better with a biliary etiology. In most scenarios, patients suffer from first attacks, with a lower probability of developing local complications. There was a tendency for biliary pancreatitis patients to be admitted to surgical wards.

Keywords: epidemiology; acute pancreatitis; biliary pancreatitis; gastroenterology; severity; length of stay; pancreatitis

1. Introduction

Acute pancreatitis represents one of the most common causes of gastrointestinal hospitalization. Being a disease characterized by the localized destruction and inflammation of the pancreas or a systemic inflammatory response. AP remains one of the most common gastroenterological conditions worldwide, with data from the Global Burden of Disease Study revealing a global incidence for pancreatitis of 2.75 million incident cases in 2021, representing an 8.5% increase compared to 2010 [1]. The incidence varies across countries and regions, ranging from a low incidence of 15.0 cases/100,000 in Denmark [2], 29.2 cases/100,000 in Romania to 83.7 cases/100,000 in Sweden [3]. Eastern Europe, in particular, shows high disability-adjusted life years, age-standardized incidence rates, and age-standardized mortality rates regarding AP [1].

The most common causes of AP are cholelithiasis, alcoholism, and hypertriglyceridemia. While alcoholism is more often encountered in Eastern Europe, the biliary etiology prevails in almost every other region [4] and seems to be twice as prevalent as the latter [5]. Furthermore, acute biliary pancreatitis is often more severe compared with alcoholic pancreatitis with a higher risk of complications [6]. While mild AP typically resolves on its own and has a positive prognosis, severe cases have high mortality rates ranging from 20% to 40% [7]. Aside from its intrinsic mortality, AP is a significant risk factor for pancreatic neoplasia, a condition that is diagnosed late in evolution and has a very low 5-year survival rate [8,9].

There is a high degree of heterogeneity in the management of B-AP, with multiple guidelines and no clear consensus in this area [10]. Several recent meta-analyses have shown that early cholecystectomy might lower the rates of complications and recurrence and could shorten the length of stay (LoS) [11,12]. Although there is a clear association between biliary pancreatitis and female sex, older age, and recurrence [13,14], there seems to be no difference among etiological groups regarding the outcome of AP [15].

The aim of this study was to define the group of patients with B-AP by clinical and demographic criteria, especially to determine whether there are any associations between age and biliary etiology. The following associations were investigated: B-AP with sex, severity, cost, recurrence, ward of care, LoS, intensive care unit (ICU) admission, and LoS-ICU.

2. Materials and Methods

This was a retrospective cohort study that used data from the BUC-API registry. This registry is a single-center repository that includes 2042 consecutive cases of various pancreatic pathologies (acute pancreatitis, recurrent acute pancreatitis, and acute-on-chronic pancreatitis).

The registry was developed with the approval of the ethics committee of the University Emergency Hospital of Bucharest (protocol code 68629/19, date of approval: 18 October 2024). All patients provided informed consent for the use of their data for medical research prior to admission to the hospital. The study followed the ethical guidelines stated in the 1975 Declaration of Helsinki and those from the STROBE guidelines.

For this particular study, any admission for the same patient was considered a separate case. The electronic health records of the University Emergency Hospital of Bucharest were used to identify cases. ICD-10 specific codes for pancreas-related diseases (K85, B26.3 and B25.2) were used to refine the search among all discharges from the hospital that occurred between 1 June 2015 and 1 April 2022.

Initially, there were 2520 extracted cases from EHRs, those cases were assessed by trained medical staff, and then, 426 were excluded, because they were duplicates, together with other 52 cases that were miscoded, because they did not fulfill 2 out of 3 diagnostic criteria for AP [16]. From the remaining 2042 cases, after thorough inspection, another 187 cases that were in fact acute-on-chronic pancreatitis were excluded from the study, as they fulfilled both evidence-based medicine imaging diagnostic criteria of chronic pancreatitis [17] (atrophy, fibrosis, dilated ducts, calcifications, and fibrosis) and those of AP [16]. The final number of cases included in the analysis was 1572, after excluding idiopathic AP cases in order to simplify the statistical analysis and the conclusions of this study. (See cases flowchart in Figure 1).

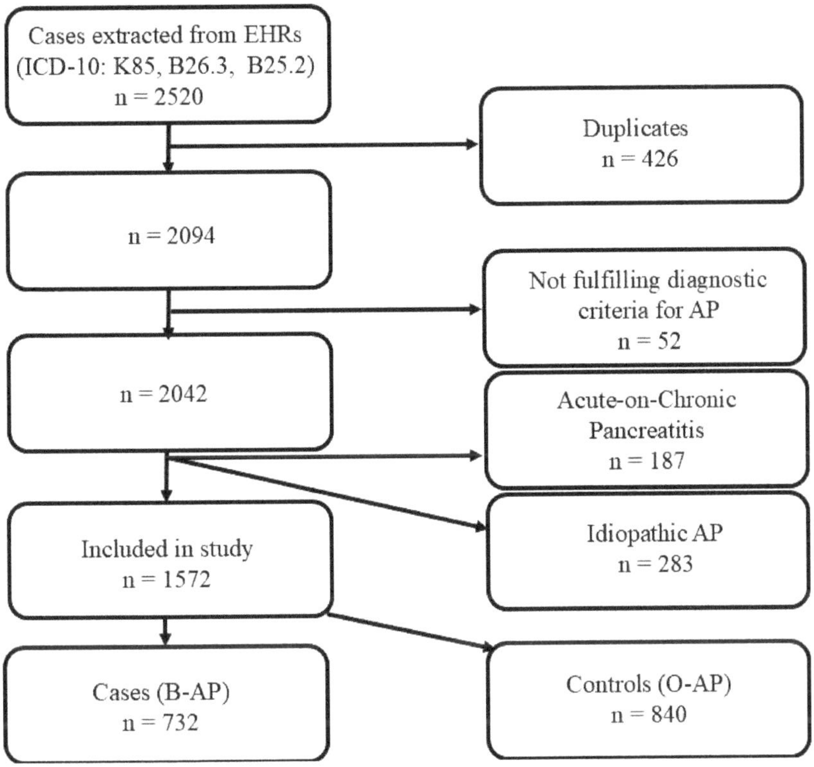

Figure 1. Cases flowchart.

In order to establish the etiology, the criteria stated by Besselink et al. [16] were used. Any patient who had at least one of the following criteria for biliary–etiological AP was included: ALT > 150 U/L within the first 48 h from admission and imaging (ultrasound or CT) evidence of biliary pathology that might influence pancreatic secretion and/or known gallstone disease without another evident etiology was considered as part of the B-AP group. To simplify the statistical analysis, all other known etiology cases were merged into a single group that was compared with the biliary cases.

Any case of AP without signs of chronic pancreatitis that was previously admitted to the hospital within the time frame of the BUC-API registry and/or was known with previous episodes of AP was considered a recurrent case. Severity and morphology (local complications) were stratified according to the Revised Atlanta Classification [18].

The decision to be admitted to a particular ward was made by a multidisciplinary council in the ER comprising representatives of emergency medicine, a gastroenterologist, a surgeon, and a radiologist.

For this study, the data were organized using Microsoft 365 © (Microsoft Inc., Redmond, WA, USA) and Google Docs © (Alphabet Inc., Mountain View, CA, USA). To observe the general characteristics of the cohort, frequency tests were employed. To examine the correlation between two categorical variables, we employed the Pearson chi-square test and Phi Cramer's V test, receiver operating curve and its derivatives, and multinomial logistic regression. The Mann–Whitney U-test was used to examine the correlation among continuous and categorical variables. SPSS Statistics version 29.0.0.0 © (IBM Inc., Armonk, NY, USA) was used for all the statistical analyses and charts from this study.

Zotero 6 © (Corporation for Digital Scholarship, Vienna, VA, USA) for Windows and Zotero Connector for Google Chrome were used to manage the references and bibliography.

3. Results

3.1. Population Characteristics

In the GP population of the AP cases, the first attack prevails (82.8%), which is the same as that in the B-AP cases (92.5%). The median age was 57.0 years in the GP group but was greater in the B-AP group (65.0 years). In the GP group, there was a minority of females; whereas, in the B-AP subgroup, they represented the majority (40.8% vs. 61.9%). With respect to the ward of care, in the GP, there were a minority of surgical cases; whereas, in the B-AP cohort, they were the most common (49.3% vs. 82.2%).

The morphology of the GP group was predominantly interstitial edema (38.5%), similar to that of the B-AP (37.4%), but there were fewer data available in the B-AP group (30.3% vs. 32.4%) and more cases of normal pancreas at discharge than in the GP group (14.8% vs. 20.2%). Both the GP and B-AP healed outcomes at discharge were highly prevalent (83.0% vs. 83.7%), and there were similar mortality rates between the two aforementioned pathologies (5.8% and 4.0%, respectively).

An identical median LoS between the GP and B-AP patients (7.0 days) was observed. Most of the GP cases had biliary (39.5%), alcoholic (33.9%), or idiopathic (15.2%) etiologies. There were 12.9% severe cases in the GP group and a mildly lower rate of 10.2% in the B-AP group. A slightly lower ICU admittance rate in the B-AP group than in the GP group (8,7% vs. 9.6%) was found. The rates of rurality were similar for both GPs (27.3%) and B-APs (27.6%) (Tables 1 and 2).

Table 1. Population characteristics.

AP Cases		*n* = 1855
	Recurrence	
First known attack		1536 (82.8%)
Recurrent AP		319 (17.2%)
	Age (years)	
Median		57 (IQR = 26.0)
Mean		56.9 (SD = 17.1)
	Length of stay (LoS)	
Median		7.0 (IQR = 6.0)
Mean		8.8 (SD = 7.8)
	Daily cost of hospitalization (EUR)	
Median		185.3 (IQR = 87.0)
Mean		433.2 (SD = 3446.7)
	Etiology	
Biliary		732 (39.5%)
All other known causes		840 (45.3%)
Idiopathic		283 (15.2%)
	Gender	
Male		1098 (59.2%)
Female		757 (40.8%)
	Severity	
Mild		954 (51.4%)
Moderately severe		677 (36.5%)
Severe		224 (12.1%)
	Morphology	
Interstitial		715 (38.5%)
Normal pancreas		274 (14.8%)
Fluid collections		179 (11.4%)
Necrosis		65 (4.1%)
No data		562 (30.3%)

Table 1. *Cont.*

AP Cases	n = 1855
Outcome	
Healed/ameliorated	1540 (83.0%)
Discharged at will	116 (6.3%)
Deceased	108 (5.8%)
Transferred	79 (4.3%)
Stationary	12 (0.6%)
ICU	
No	1676 (90.4%)
Yes	179 (9.6%)
Ward of care	
Gastroenterology	941 (50.7%)
Surgery	914 (49.3%)
Rurality	
Urban	1332 (71.8%)
Rural	507 (27.3%)
No data	16 (0.9%)

Table 2. Comparison of elements between the two etiological groups. All statistically significant p-values are marked with *.

	B-AP (n = 732)	O-AP (n = 840)	p-Value
Severity			
Mild	394 (53.8%)	421 (50.1%)	0.25
Moderately severe	263 (35.9%)	316 (37.6%)	
Severe	75 (10.2%)	103 (12.3%)	
ICU			
No	668 (91.3%)	769 (91.5%)	0.84
Yes	64 (8.7%)	71 (8.5%)	
Ward of care			
Gastroenterology	130 (17.8%)	656 (78.1%)	<0.01 *
Surgery	602 (82.2%)	184 (21.9%)	
Gender			
Male	279 (38.1%)	675 (80.4%)	<0.01 *
Female	453 (61.9%)	165 (19.6%)	
Outcome			
Healed/ameliorated	613 (83.7%)	705 (83.9%)	<0.01 *
Stationary	6 (0.8%)	5 (0.6%)	
Transfer	57 (7.8%)	16 (1.9%)	
Discharge at will	27 (3.7%)	73 (8.7%)	
Deceased	29 (4.0%)	41 (4.9%)	
Recurrence			
First attack	677 (92.5%)	612 (72.9%)	<0.01 *
Recurrence	55 (7.5%)	228 (27.1%)	
Morphology			
Interstitial	274 (37.4%)	349 (41.5%)	<0.01 *
Fluid collections	49 (6.7%)	130 (15.5%)	
Necrosis	24 (3.3%)	41 (4.9%)	
Normal pancreas	148 (20.2%)	94 (11.2%)	
No data	237 (32.4%)	226 (26.9%)	
Rurality			
Urban	526 (71.9%)	588 (70.0%)	0.43
Rural	202 (27.6%)	241 (28.7%)	
No data	4 (0.5%)	11 (1.3%)	
Age (years)			
Mean	61.8 (SD = 18.4)	52.3 (SD = 14.1)	<0.01 *
Median	65.0 (IQR = 27.0)	51.0 (IQR = 20.7)	
Length of stay (days)			
Mean	8.4 (SD = 5.7)	9.0 (SD = 8.4)	0.34
Median	7.0 (IQR = 6.0)	7.0 (IQR = 5.0)	
ICU Length of stay (days)			
Mean	5.0 (SD = 4.7)	5.4 (SD = 5.9)	0.54
Median	2.5 (IQR = 5.0)	4.0 (IQR = 4.0)	

3.2. Age

Mann–Whitney U-tests were used to determine whether there were any differences in etiology or age. The results indicated that B-AP patients were significantly older than O-AP patients were, U = 202,354.5, Z = −11.7, $p < 0.01$. The median age was 65.0 years (IQR = 17.0) in the B-AP and 51.0 years (IQR = 20.7) in the OAP (Table 2, Figure 2).

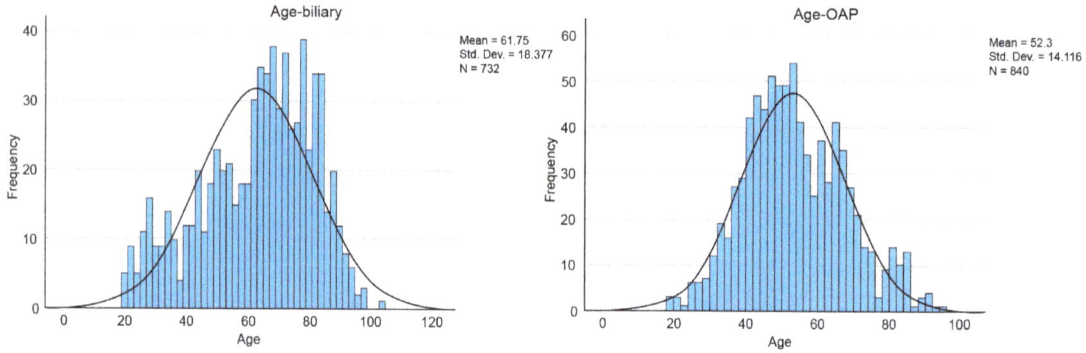

Figure 2. Age distribution amongst the two groups.

A receiver operating characteristic (ROC) curve analysis yielded an AUC of 0.67 (95% CI [0.64, 0.70]), suggesting moderate statistical discriminatory ability in regard to age as a predictor of B-AP. The optimal cut-off for the model was determined using Youden's index (J). As such a J = 0.31, with a sensitivity of 59.7% and a specificity of 71.5% at a threshold of 60.50 years (Figure 3).

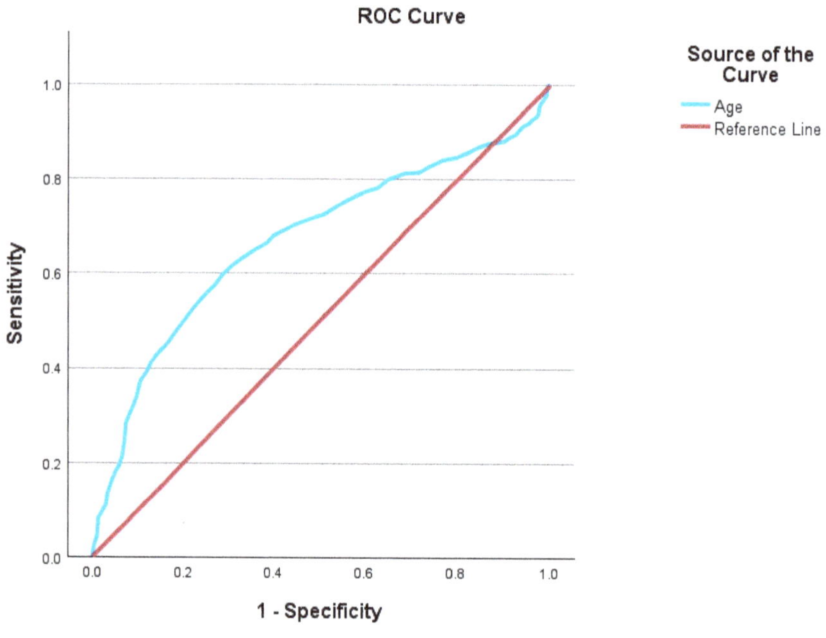

Figure 3. ROC for age.

3.3. Gender

To compare the distributions of sex in the two etiology groups, a chi-square test of independence was run. The aforementioned test revealed a significant difference between the two variables (X2(1) = 292.6, $p < 0.01$). A Cramer V of 0.43 implies that there is a medium–strong magnification association. As a post hoc test, we obtained an adjusted standardized residual (ASR) of +17.1 with respect to women with B-AP, which means that there is an important difference from the expected frequencies, with women being more prone to developing B-AP (Table 2).

3.4. Recurrence

The chi-square test revealed that the number of previous attacks of AP without chronicization differed significantly (X2(1) = 102.1, $p < 0.01$). Cramer's V of 0.26 suggests a medium-strength association. When ASR was used as a post hoc test, the first attack of B-AP differed in frequency from the expected ASR of +10.1 (Table 2).

3.5. Outcome

To check for any distinction between outcomes at discharge and etiology, a chi-square test of independence was used. There were statistically significant differences (X2(4) = 45.6, $p < 0.01$). Cramer's V (V = 0.17) suggests a medium-strength association. In post hoc testing, differences in the expected frequency with respect to transfer (ASR = +5.5 in the B-AP group) and discharge-at-will (ASR = −4.1 in the B-AP group) were obtained, implying that B-APs are more likely to be transferred to another unit and less likely to be discharged at will (Table 2).

3.6. Morphology

A chi-square test of independence revealed a statistically significant difference (X2(4) = 55.3, $p < 0.01$) between morphology and etiology. Cramer's V (V = 0.18) indicates a medium-strength association. Determining the ASR via post hoc tests revealed differences in the expected frequency of the B-AP group: normal pancreas (ASR = +4.9), local fluid complications (ASR = −5.5), and no data (ASR = +2.4) (Table 2).

3.7. Ward of Care

There was a noticeable difference between the ward of care and etiology using a chi-square test of independence (X2(1) = 569.6, $p < 0.01$). Cramer's V (V = 0.60) also revealed a strong association. By calculating the post hoc ASR, we observed a meaningful difference in the expected frequency with respect to B-APs and surgical wards (ASR = +23.9) (Table 2).

3.8. Multinomial Logistic Regression for the Model

A multinomial logistic regression analysis was performed to observe the relationship between etiology and the following predictor variables: age, sex, recurrence, and ward of care. The model was statistically significant, indicating that it was able to differentiate among the etiologies based on the predictor variables X^2 (4) = 708.9, $p < 0.01$. For B-AP compared with O-AP, all the variables were significant predictors. Each year increase in age was associated with a 3% increase in the likelihood of suffering from B-AP (Exp(B) = 1.03, $p < 0.01$, 95% CI [1.03, 1.04]). Sex was a significant predictor, as males were 82% less likely to suffer from B-AP (Exp(B) = 0.18, $p < 0.01$, 95% CI [0.14, 0.24]). The recurrence was an important predictor, as those suffering from their first attack of AP were 110% more likely to suffer from B-AP (Exp(B) = 2.10, $p < 0.01$, 95% CI [1.38, 3.21]). The ward of care was also a predictor, as those that were cared for in surgical wards were 14 times more likely to suffer from B-AP (Exp(B) = 15.14, $p < 0.01$, 95% CI [11.35, 20.19]).

3.9. Other Aims

No statistically meaningful differences between etiology and the following outcomes were observed: severity (X2(2) = 2.7, p = 0.26), ICU admission rate (X2(1) = 0.4, p = 0.84) or LoS-ICU (U = 2136.0, Z = −0.6, p = 0.54), rurality (X2(3) = 2.8, p = 0.43), or LoS (U = 298,934.0, Z = −0.9, p = 0.34) (Table 2).

4. Discussion

The findings suggest a correlation between sex and etiology, as it appears that female sex is correlated with B-AP with respect to O-AP. This finding is in accordance with another study [19] that reported a greater female predilection for B-AP than for alcoholic AP. We do not find this surprising, as it is well established [20] that estrogen heightens the risk for developing cholesterol gallstones by augmenting the cholesterol saturation of bile secretion.

B-AP was more common in patients over 60 years of age. This contradicts the data from Cho et al. [21], as they were not able to find any significant differences regarding age. However, in other cohorts [13,19], a similar association between older age and B-AP was found. This heterogeneity can be explained by the different numbers of patients included (153 in Cho et al.) and greater than 700 patients in the other groups.

B-APs are associated with a greater probability of a normal pancreas during imaging investigations; whereas, O-APs are more likely to develop with fluid collections (APFCs and pseudocysts). This finding correlates with the findings of Du et al. [22], who reported a lower probability of developing local complications in B-AP patients, and with the findings of another paper [21], who reported significant differences with regard to pseudocyst development, which is more often found in alcoholic AP than in B-AP. While there are few reports in the literature regarding local complications stratified by etiology, our results may facilitate a timely and definitive solution involving cholecystectomy and/or ERCP in B-AP patients, as ERCP remains a method of choice in common bile duct lithiasis [23].

The study data showed that B-AP is more commonly seen as a first attack of AP. In the literature [24,25], there seems to be a large consensus that B-AP is associated with a single episode; whereas, other etiologies (mainly alcoholic) may be linked with recurrence. This effect is most likely caused by the instrumentation of the biliary tract in the B-AP with a definitive solution, as stressed by other peer researchers [26,27].

With respect to the ward of care, any previous analysis regarding the correlation between the type of ward and etiology were hard to find, as we observed a tendency for biliary cases to be admitted to surgical wards instead of gastroenterological wards. Nevertheless. Several studies that address this problem are suggesting that admission directly to surgical wards could lower the recurrence rate, shorten LoS, and lower costs [28]. Another retrospective study [29] revealed that patients with B-AP who were cared for by surgeons had a lower count of consulting services, laboratory tests, and antibiotics. As such, it is considered that admittance to surgical wards might translate to better care for B-AP patients and a more rapid, definitive solution, which will probably also translate to a lower cost of care.

In a previous study [30] on the same population but focusing on alcohol-induced AP, the other most prevalent etiology, it was found that the epidemiology of those patients differs a lot from those with B-AP. The first ones are more probable to be middle-aged male patients with recurrent AP. As such, there could be a better stratification of the etiology based also on demographic and historical factors in addition to medical ones.

Exploring the outcome, we find that there is a significantly greater probability for B-AP to be transferred; whereas, for O-AP, there is a greater probability of discharge-at-will. As we could not find any data on this topic stratified by transfer and/or discharge, it should be considered that both of these outcomes might be influenced by the fact that this study is unicentric. More multicenter studies on this topic are required, as this might be a local effect and not a disease-related effect. No statistically relevant differences with respect to mortality could be found.

Although not part of the aim of the study, we cannot end this paper without reminding that a large part of B-AP patients can suffer a second attack of AP after the instrumentalization of the common bile duct with ERCP for choledochal lithiasis extraction. The post-ERCP pancreatitis in this particular indication was very well described by previous studies in the literature [31].

In this study, it was a lack of any significant differences regarding severity, rurality, LoS, ICU admission, or ICU-LoS. It was difficult to determine whether this lack of difference might be caused by limitations in the study design, such as its retrospective design, the unicentricity of the study, missing data from EHRs, and/or any potential confounding variables that could not be accounted for. Although rare, it is possible that this study may have missed some AP cases related to biliary heterotopia of the pancreatic tissue [32], as we have not accounted for them. Other limitations of this study can arise from the fact that we have not checked for any surgical or endoscopical interventions required in order to solve the biliary pathology.

As strong points of this study, the large number of cases analyzed and the lack of selection bias stand out, as all cases were consecutive admissions with clear inclusion and exclusion criteria and long durations.

5. Conclusions

The ROC and multinomial logistic regression showed us a possible reliable future model for predicting biliary etiology based solely on demographic factors. This should include in the analysis: age, sex, recurrence, and ward of care. Based on our study, the typical sketch of a biliary acute pancreatitis patient should be female in her sixties at her first attack of AP admitted to a surgical ward. Other factors that might contribute to the predictive model are pancreatic morphology and outcome at discharge.

Author Contributions: A.V.E. drafted the original manuscript with the exception of Results section and Patients and Methodology section, as well as providing the funding acquisition. M.R.P. drafted the Results section and Methodology section and performed all statistical tests. A.O., D.G.C. and A.R.T. were in charge of data curation. A.C., V.Ș. and N.O.Z. reviewed and edited the manuscript. L.N. supervised the project and contributed to reviewing and editing the final version of the manuscript. All authors have read and agreed to the published version of the manuscript.

Funding: This research received no external funding.

Institutional Review Board Statement: The study was conducted in accordance with the Declaration of Helsinki and approved by the Ethics Committee of University Emergency Hospital of Bucharest (protocol code 68629/19, date of approval: 18 October 2024).

Informed Consent Statement: Informed consent was obtained from all subjects involved in the study prior to hospitalization.

Data Availability Statement: Data available upon reasonable request from the corresponding author.

Acknowledgments: The publication of this paper was supported by the University of Medicine and Pharmacy Carol Davila through the institutional program Publish not Perish. Author would like to thank the following for their decisive contribution to the BUC-API registry: Andreea Irina Ghiță, Irina Ștefania Diaconu, Tudor Mitu, Hosein Nayyerani, Anamaria Simona Odorog, Damiana Ojog, Diana Nițu, Dalia Ioana Constantinescu, Miruna Untea, Matei Mitrache, Arina Gheorghe, Miruna Olteanu, and Daniela Gabriela Grigore.

Conflicts of Interest: The authors declare no conflicts of interest.

References

1. Li, T.; Qin, C.; Zhao, B.; Li, Z.; Zhao, Y.; Lin, C.; Wang, W. Global and Regional Burden of Pancreatitis: Epidemiological Trends, Risk Factors, and Projections to 2050 from the Global Burden of Disease Study 2021. *BMC Gastroenterol.* **2024**, *24*, 398. [CrossRef] [PubMed]
2. Nøjgaard, C. Prognosis of Acute and Chronic Pancreatitis—A 30-Year Follow-Up of a Danish Cohort. *Dan. Med. Bull.* **2010**, *57*, B4228.
3. Ekbom, A.; McLaughlin, J.K.; Karlsson, B.-M.; Nyrén, O.; Gridley, G.; Adami, H.-O.; Fraumeni, J.F., Jr. Pancreatitis and Pancreatic Cancer: A Population-Based Study. *JNCI J. Natl. Cancer Inst.* **1994**, *86*, 625–627. [CrossRef] [PubMed]
4. Gimenez, T.R.; Calvo, A.G.; Vicent, J.G. Etiology of Acute Pancreatitis. *Cent. Eur. J. Med.* **2014**, *9*, 530–542. [CrossRef]
5. Zilio, M.B.; Eyff, T.F.; Azeredo-Da-Silva, A.L.F.; Bersch, V.P.; Osvaldt, A.B. A Systematic Review and Meta-Analysis of the Aetiology of Acute Pancreatitis. *HPB* **2019**, *21*, 259–267. [CrossRef] [PubMed]
6. Kamal, A.; Akshintala, V.S.; Kamal, M.M.; El Zein, M.; Besharati, S.; Kumbhari, V.; Ngamruengphong, S.; Shin, E.J.; Singh, V.K.; Kalloo, A.N.; et al. Does Etiology of Pancreatitis Matter? Differences in Outcomes Among Patients With Post–Endoscopic Retrograde Cholangiopancreatography, Acute Biliary, and Alcoholic Pancreatitis. *Pancreas* **2019**, *48*, 574. [CrossRef] [PubMed]
7. Hu, J.-X.; Zhao, C.-F.; Wang, S.-L.; Tu, X.-Y.; Huang, W.-B.; Chen, J.-N.; Xie, Y.; Chen, C.-R. Acute Pancreatitis: A Review of Diagnosis, Severity Prediction and Prognosis Assessment from Imaging Technology, Scoring System and Artificial Intelligence. *World J. Gastroenterol.* **2023**, *29*, 5268–5291. [CrossRef] [PubMed]
8. Carrière, C.; Young, A.L.; Gunn, J.R.; Longnecker, D.S.; Korc, M. Acute Pancreatitis Markedly Accelerates Pancreatic Cancer Progression in Mice Expressing Oncogenic Kras. *Biochem. Biophys. Res. Commun.* **2009**, *382*, 561–565. [CrossRef] [PubMed]
9. Munigala, S.; Almaskeen, S.; Subramaniam, D.S.; Bandi, S.; Bowe, B.; Xian, H.; Sheth, S.G.; Burroughs, T.E.; Agarwal, B. Acute Pancreatitis Recurrences Augment Long-Term Pancreatic Cancer Risk. *Off. J. Am. Coll. Gastroenterol. ACG* **2023**, *118*, 727. [CrossRef] [PubMed]
10. Loveday, B.P.T.; Srinivasa, S.; Vather, R.; Mittal, A.; Petrov, M.S.; Phillips, A.R.J.; Windsor, J.A. High Quantity and Variable Quality of Guidelines for Acute Pancreatitis: A Systematic Review. *Off. J. Am. Coll. Gastroenterol. ACG* **2010**, *105*, 1466. [CrossRef]
11. Yang, D.-J.; Lu, H.-M.; Guo, Q.; Lu, S.; Zhang, L.; Hu, W.-M. Timing of Laparoscopic Cholecystectomy After Mild Biliary Pancreatitis: A Systematic Review and Meta-Analysis. *J. Laparoendosc. Adv. Surg. Tech.* **2018**, *28*, 379–388. [CrossRef]
12. Prasanth, J.; Prasad, M.; Mahapatra, S.J.; Krishna, A.; Prakash, O.; Garg, P.K.; Bansal, V.K. Early Versus Delayed Cholecystectomy for Acute Biliary Pancreatitis: A Systematic Review and Meta-Analysis. *World J. Surg.* **2022**, *46*, 1359–1375. [CrossRef] [PubMed]
13. Pu, W.; Luo, G.; Chen, T.; Jing, L.; Hu, Q.; Li, X.; Xia, H.; Deng, M.; Lü, M.; Chen, X. A 5-Year Retrospective Cohort Study: Epidemiology, Etiology, Severity, and Outcomes of Acute Pancreatitis. *Pancreas* **2020**, *49*, 1161–1167. [CrossRef] [PubMed]
14. Ragnarsson, T.; Andersson, R.; Ansari, D.; Persson, U.; Andersson, B. Acute Biliary Pancreatitis: Focus on Recurrence Rate and Costs When Current Guidelines Are Not Complied. *Scand. J. Gastroenterol.* **2017**, *52*, 264–269. [CrossRef] [PubMed]
15. Gullo, L.; Migliori, M.; Oláh, A.; Farkas, G.; Levy, P.; Arvanitakis, C.; Lankisch, P.; Beger, H. Acute Pancreatitis in Five European Countries: Etiology and Mortality. *Pancreas* **2002**, *24*, 223. [CrossRef]
16. Deviere, J. IAP/APA Evidence-Based Guidelines for the Management of Acute Pancreatitis. *Pancreatology* **2013**, *13*, e1–e15. [CrossRef]
17. Conwell, D.L.; Lee, L.S.; Yadav, D.; Longnecker, D.S.; Miller, F.H.; Mortele, K.J.; Levy, M.J.; Kwon, R.; Lieb, J.G.; Stevens, T.; et al. American Pancreatic Association Practice Guidelines in Chronic Pancreatitis: Evidence-Based Report on Diagnostic Guidelines. *Pancreas* **2014**, *43*, 1143. [CrossRef] [PubMed]
18. Banks, P.A.; Bollen, T.L.; Dervenis, C.; Gooszen, H.G.; Johnson, C.D.; Sarr, M.G.; Tsiotos, G.G.; Vege, S.S. Classification of Acute Pancreatitis—2012: Revision of the Atlanta Classification and Definitions by International Consensus. *Gut* **2013**, *62*, 102–111. [CrossRef]
19. Samanta, J.; Dhaka, N.; Gupta, P.; Singh, A.K.; Yadav, T.D.; Gupta, V.; Sinha, S.K.; Kochhar, R. Comparative Study of the Outcome between Alcohol and Gallstone Pancreatitis in a High-Volume Tertiary Care Center. *JGH Open* **2019**, *3*, 338–343. [CrossRef] [PubMed]
20. Wang, H.H.; Liu, M.; Clegg, D.J.; Portincasa, P.; Wang, D.Q.-H. New Insights into the Molecular Mechanisms Underlying Effects of Estrogen on Cholesterol Gallstone Formation. *Biochim. Biophys. Acta BBA-Mol. Cell Biol. Lipids* **2009**, *1791*, 1037–1047. [CrossRef] [PubMed]
21. Cho, J.H.; Kim, T.N.; Kim, S.B. Comparison of Clinical Course and Outcome of Acute Pancreatitis According to the Two Main Etiologies: Alcohol and Gallstone. *BMC Gastroenterol.* **2015**, *15*, 87. [CrossRef]
22. Du, J.; Zhang, J.; Zhang, X.; Jiang, R.; Fu, Q.; Yang, G.; Fan, H.; Tang, M.; Chen, T.; Li, X.; et al. Computed Tomography Characteristics of Acute Pancreatitis Based on Different Etiologies at Different Onset Times: A Retrospective Cross-Sectional Study. *Quant. Imaging Med. Surg.* **2022**, *12*, 4448–4461. [CrossRef] [PubMed]
23. Coman, I.S.; Radu, E.-V.; Sandru, V.; Cristinel Barsan, I.; Dumitru Badiu, C.; Constantinescu, G.; Titus Grigorean, V. Retained Common Bile Duct Lithiasis at a Pacient with Periampullary Duodenal Diverticulum. *Chirurgia* **2016**, *111*, 517. [CrossRef]

24. Cho, J.H.; Jeong, Y.H.; Kim, K.H.; Kim, T.N. Risk Factors of Recurrent Pancreatitis after First Acute Pancreatitis Attack: A Retrospective Cohort Study. *Scand. J. Gastroenterol.* **2020**, *55*, 90–94. [CrossRef]
25. Song, K.; Guo, C.; Li, C.; Ding, N. Risk Factors of Recurrence of Acute Pancreatitis: A Retrospective Research. *Turk. J. Gastroenterol.* **2021**, *32*, 971. [CrossRef] [PubMed]
26. Hwang, S.S.; Li, B.H.; Haigh, P.I. Gallstone Pancreatitis Without Cholecystectomy. *JAMA Surg.* **2013**, *148*, 867–872. [CrossRef] [PubMed]
27. García de la Filia Molina, I.; García García de Paredes, A.; Martínez Ortega, A.; Marcos Carrasco, N.; Rodríguez De Santiago, E.; Sánchez Aldehuelo, R.; Foruny Olcina, J.R.; González Martin, J.Á.; López Duran, S.; Vázquez Sequeiros, E.; et al. Biliary Sphincterotomy Reduces the Risk of Acute Gallstone Pancreatitis Recurrence in Non-Candidates for Cholecystectomy. *Dig. Liver Dis.* **2019**, *51*, 1567–1573. [CrossRef] [PubMed]
28. Kulvatunyou, N.; Watt, J.; Friese, R.S.; Gries, L.; Green, D.J.; Joseph, B.; O'Keeffe, T.; Tang, A.L.; Vercruysse, G.; Rhee, P. Management of Acute Mild Gallstone Pancreatitis under Acute Care Surgery: Should Patients Be Admitted to the Surgery or Medicine Service? *Am. J. Surg.* **2014**, *208*, 981–987. [CrossRef] [PubMed]
29. Judkins, S.E.; Moore, E.E.; Witt, J.E.; Barnett, C.C.; Biffl, W.L.; Burlew, C.C.; Johnson, J.L. Surgeons Provide Definitive Care to Patients with Gallstone Pancreatitis. *Am. J. Surg.* **2011**, *202*, 673–678. [CrossRef]
30. Gűnșahin, D.; Edu, A.V.; Pahomeanu, M.R.; Mitu, T.Ș.; Ghiță, A.I.; Odorog, A.S.; Preda, C.M.; Negreanu, L. Alcoholic Acute Pancreatitis, a Retrospective Study about Clinical Risk Factors and Outcomes—A Seven-Year Experience of a Large Tertiary Center. *Biomedicines* **2024**, *12*, 1299. [CrossRef]
31. Boicean, A.; Birlutiu, V.; Ichim, C.; Todor, S.B.; Hasegan, A.; Bacila, C.; Solomon, A.; Cristian, A.; Dura, H. Predictors of Post-ERCP Pancreatitis (P.E.P.) in Choledochal Lithiasis Extraction. *J. Pers. Med.* **2023**, *13*, 1356. [CrossRef]
32. Şerboiu, C.S.; Aliuș, C.; Dumitru, A.; Țăpoi, D.; Costache, M.; Nica, A.E.; Alexandra-Ana, M.; Antoniac, I.; Grădinaru, S. Gallbladder Pancreatic Heterotopia—The Importance of Diagnostic Imaging in Managing Intraoperative Findings. *Medicina* **2023**, *59*, 1407. [CrossRef] [PubMed]

life

MDPI

Article

Laparoscopic and Open Distal Pancreatectomy—An Initial Single-Institution Experience with a Propensity Score Matching Analysis

Irena Plahuta [1,2], Žan Šarenac [2], Medeja Golob [2], Špela Turk [1], Bojan Ilijevec [1], Tomislav Magdalenić [1], Stojan Potrč [1,2] and Arpad Ivanecz [1,2,*]

[1] Clinical Department of Abdominal and General Surgery, University Medical Centre Maribor, Ljubljanska Ulica 5, 2000 Maribor, Slovenia; irena.plahuta@ukc-mb.si (I.P.)
[2] Department of Surgery, Faculty of Medicine, University of Maribor, Taborska Ulica 8, 2000 Maribor, Slovenia
* Correspondence: arpad.ivanecz@ukc-mb.si

Abstract: Laparoscopic distal pancreatectomy is a minimally invasive approach for the surgical treatment of neoplasms in the distal pancreas. This study aimed to compare this approach to the open procedure. A retrospective analysis of a prospectively maintained database of 400 pancreatectomies was performed. The laparoscopic distal pancreatectomy group (LDP) was compared to the open distal pancreatectomy group (ODP). A propensity score matching analysis (PSM) was performed. From 2016 to 2023, 108 distal pancreatectomies were carried out, 19 (17.6%) laparoscopically and 89 (82.4%) openly. The conversion rate was 13.6%. The severe morbidity rates were 28.1% in the ODP group, 47.4% in the LDP group, and 15.8% in the ODP-PSM group. The difference between the latter two was statistically significant ($p = 0.034$) due to the high rate of Clavien–Dindo grade 3a complications (42.1% versus 10.5%, $p = 0.042$) in the LDP group. The 90-day mortality rates were 3.3% in the ODP group and 5.3% in the other two groups. The LDP group had a shorter duration of intravenous narcotic analgesia (5 versus 7 days, $p = 0.041$). There was no difference in the R0 resection or postoperative pancreatic fistula rates. Our attention should be drawn to preventing postoperative complications because the oncological outcomes are already comparable with those of the open procedure, and postoperative pain management is promising.

Keywords: laparoscopic distal pancreatectomy; splenectomy; postoperative pancreatic fistula; intravenous narcotic analgesia; morbidity; mortality; resection rate

1. Introduction

The first successful laparoscopic distal pancreatectomy was reported by Alfred Cuschieri thirty years ago [1]. However, the pancreas was long considered unsuitable for minimal access surgical approaches. Obstacles to the wide implementation of laparoscopic distal pancreatectomy include the difficult exposure of the pancreas in the retroperitoneum, the intimate proximity of major vascular structures, the complex technical nature and high complication profile of these operations, concern over adherence to oncological principles, and challenges in training surgeons to perform these low-volume, complex operations [2].

Minimally invasive surgery is a standard for many gastrointestinal surgical procedures, but pancreatic surgery is considered unique and highly specific. The expertise gained in minimally invasive procedures applied in other gastrointestinal areas does not necessarily provide a sufficient guarantee of good outcomes for pancreatic surgery [3].

The initial reports of technical feasibility and safety evaluations were followed through a large multicenter retrospective cohort study (DIPLOMA) and prospective multicenter (LEOPARD) and single-center (LAPOP) randomized control trials comparing laparoscopic with open distal pancreatectomy [4–7]. These reports confirmed the feasibility and safety of laparoscopic distal pancreatectomy, which is routine in many medical centers worldwide.

There is growing international interest in moving the field forward in an organized manner. A dedicated session for minimally invasive distal pancreatectomy was held at the first international conference on minimally invasive pancreatic resection in conjunction with the annual meeting of the International Hepato-Pancreato-Biliary Association in 2016 [2–4]. The first evidence-based guidelines on minimally invasive pancreatic resection were presented in 2019 [8]. The first internationally validated European guidelines on minimally invasive pancreatic surgery achieved consensus in Brescia, Italy, in 2022, and outcome benchmarks have also been established [9–11].

The present single tertiary center research has aimed to demonstrate that the laparoscopic approach is not inferior to the open procedure in the entire patient population with neoplasms in the distal pancreas.

2. Materials and Methods

A retrospective review of a prospectively maintained database of all consecutive patients who underwent pancreatic resection at a single tertiary referral center was performed. The first laparoscopic distal pancreatectomy was undertaken in April 2016, and data were collected until December 2023.

The patients' demographics, preoperative clinical characteristics, intraoperative details, histopathological data, and postoperative outcomes were retrieved from the database.

The approach was mainly the surgeons' preference, but the selection criteria for the laparoscopic one were applied as proposed, as follows: at the beginning, patients with small, presumably benign tumors in the pancreatic tail were selected. With growing experience, patients with malignant, bigger, and more proximal tumors were selected. Caution is still present when the tumor is large, presumably malignant, locally advanced, near the neck of the pancreas, or close to the celiac trunk and its branches [12].

The surgical technique was applied as follows: for laparoscopic distal pancreatectomy, after general anesthesia, the patient was kept supine and was positioned in a 30–45 right lateral decubitus. The surgeon stood on the patient's right, while the first assistant and the scrub nurse stood on the patient's left. Pneumoperitoneum was achieved using an optical trocar (Covidien, Medtronic plc, Minneapolis, MN, USA), and three other ports were placed. A 10-mm 30° telescope (Olympus, Tokyo, Japan) was used for visualization. The gastrocolic ligament was dissected to access the pancreas. Laparoscopic ultrasonography (Esaote, Genoa, Italy) was used to determine the tumor and its relationship to the splenic vessels.

After mobilization of the distal pancreas from the retroperitoneum, the splenic artery and vein were clipped. The pancreas was divided at the neck using an Endo GIA™ 60 mm Articulating Extra Thick Reinforced Reload with Tri-Staple™ 2.0 Technology instrument (Covidien, Medtronic plc, Minneapolis, MN, USA). Then, the splenic ligaments were cut.

The specimen was removed using an endo-bag through the Pfannenstiel incision. Passive drainage was placed at the pancreatic bed through the laparoscopic port site.

An open distal pancreatectomy was performed through a left subcostal incision. The steps of the operation were similar to those of a laparoscopic approach, and the same kind of stapler was used. The splenic artery and vein were separately ligated with a 2-0 polyglactin 910 suture. A drain was placed next to the remnant pancreas and brought out through a separate stab incision. The abdominal wall was closed in layers, and the skin was stapled [13,14].

Only pure laparoscopic distal pancreatectomy with splenectomy was carried out, and no hand-assisted or hybrid procedures were performed. There were no multi-visceral or vascular resections. The operative time was defined as the interval from the incision to the skin suturing. The conversion into an open approach was defined as the requirement for laparotomy at any time of the procedure, except for the extraction of the resected specimen.

Diagnoses were based on the final histopathological reports. The histological surgical margins for malignant lesions were defined as microscopically positive (<1 mm, R1) or negative. R0 resection was defined as complete tumor removal with a clear microscopic margin [15,16].

Postoperative morbidity was graded according to the Clavien–Dindo classification and based on the most severe complication. Grades 1 and 2 indicate minor complications that required medical therapies for treatment. Severe complications encompassed grades $\geq$ 3a, as follows: Grades 3a and 3b necessitate interventional radiological or surgical procedures, grades 4a and 4b involved organ support, and grade 5 signified mortality [17].

A postoperative pancreatic fistula, post-pancreatectomy hemorrhage, and delayed gastric emptying were based on the criteria established by the International Study Group of Pancreatic Surgery [18–20]. Reoperation was defined as any surgical procedure performed before discharge from the hospital or in the first 30 postoperative days [14].

The Numeric Pain Rating Scale [21] was used [21] to assess postoperative pain. It consists of a 0–10 scale, with 0 meaning "no pain" and 10 meaning "the worst pain imaginable" [22].

The length of hospital stay was calculated as the interval from the day of surgery to the day of discharge. Patients were discharged when they tolerated oral fluids and a solid diet without intravenous fluid supplementation requirements, their pain was controlled with oral analgesics, and they were mobile enough to take care of themselves [23,24].

Patients consented before the surgery that their anonymous data could be used for research. Therefore, their records were anonymized and deidentified before analysis. The Institutional Ethics Committee approved the research (UKC-MB-KME-41/24). All methods were performed following the relevant guidelines and regulations.

The patients who underwent distal pancreatectomy were divided into two groups and compared according to the type of approach, as follows: laparoscopic distal pancreatectomy (LDP) and open distal pancreatectomy (ODP) groups. Then, a propensity score matching analysis (PSM) was performed, and the groups were compared again.

All consecutive patients with benign or malignant lesions in the body or tail of the pancreas who underwent laparoscopic distal pancreatectomy were eligible for inclusion in this study. There were no exclusion criteria.

The primary endpoints were intraoperative outcomes (operative time and transfusion required). The secondary endpoints were postoperative outcomes (morbidity, severe morbidity, mortality, pancreas-specific morbidity (postoperative pancreatic fistula, post-pancreatectomy hemorrhage, and delayed gastric emptying), reoperation, intensive care unit admission, high-dependency unit stay, time to oral food intake and stool passing, intravenous narcotics requirement, length of hospital stay, readmission, and incisional hernias).

Oncological outcomes (R0 resection and number of harvested lymph nodes) were analyzed in a subset of patients with pancreatic malignant neoplasms.

IBM SPSS for Windows Version 29.0.0.0 (IBM Corporation, Armonk, NY, USA) was used for statistical computations. Percentages are reported to one decimal place. A p value < 0.05 was considered statistically significant.

The categorical variables are displayed as numbers with percentages. The differences between categorical variables were tested using Fisher's Exact test. When more than two categories were present, the Fisher–Freeman–Halton test was used. Continuous variables were expressed as median (interquartile range) and analyzed with the Mann–Whitney test since the distribution analysis showed a non-normal data distribution.

PSM was used to minimize selection bias [25,26]. The patients were matched using relevant variables to equate the complexity of surgical cases. A matched group of patients (ODP-PSM group) was created with a 1:1 ratio without replacement. Standardized mean difference (SMD) was used to assess the balance of the clinical backgrounds between the two groups. An SMD < 0.2 indicated very small differences between the means (optimal balance regarding a variable was generally achieved), an SMD between 0.2 and 0.8 indicated medium differences (a fairly sufficient balance regarding a variable was generally achieved), and an SMD > 0.8 indicated considerable differences (poor balance regarding a variable was generally achieved) [14].

After PSM, the statistical analysis of continuous variables was performed with the Wilcoxon signed-ranks test, and the analysis of categorical variables was performed with the Related-samples Cochran's Q test and with Related-samples marginal homogeneity test when more than two categories were present [25,27,28].

3. Results

Figure 1 shows the study flowchart. Our institution performed 400 pancreatic resections from January 2016 to December 2023, including 108 distal pancreatectomies with splenectomies.

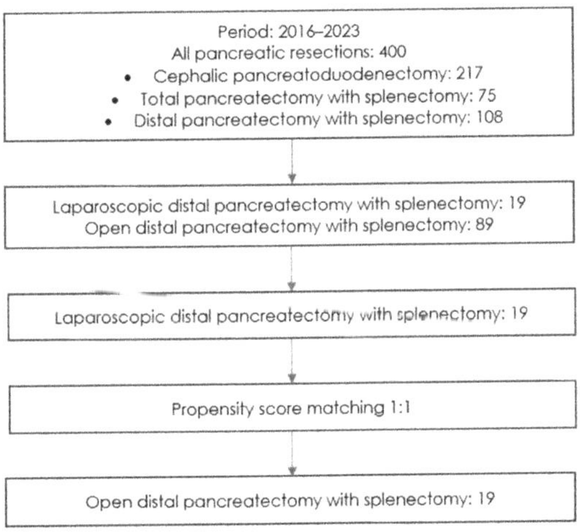

Figure 1. The study flowchart of pancreatectomies from 2016 to 2023.

Our dedicated hepato-pancreato-biliary team consisted of five surgeons who performed open pancreatic resections. Three of them, who were also experienced laparoscopic liver and gastric surgeons, were deployed into the laparoscopic distal pancreatectomy program [29–31]. The chronology of the distal pancreatectomy is given in Figure 2.

From the laparoscopic group, 3 (13.6%) cases required conversion to an open procedure, while 19 (86.4%) cases were completed as planned.

The characteristics of LDP versus ODP before and after PSM analysis are summarized in Tables 1–3. Table 1 shows the preoperative characteristics of patients and their tumors.

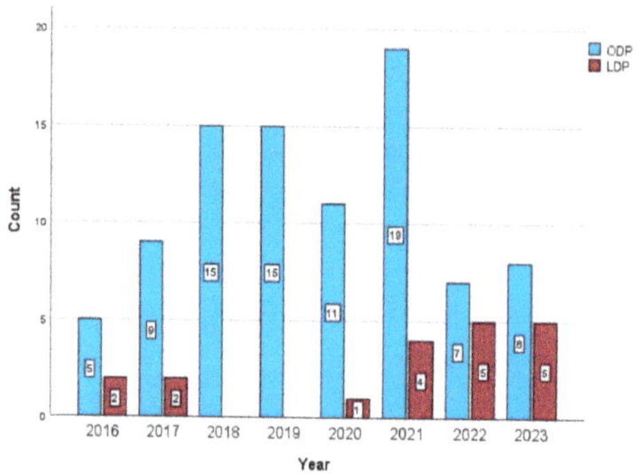

Figure 2. The chronology of distal pancreatectomies at our institution. LDP = laparoscopic distal pancreatectomy; ODP = open distal pancreatectomy.

Table 1. Preoperative characteristics of 108 patients and their tumors before and after a propensity score matching analysis of LDP versus ODP.

Variable	Overall Analysis				Propensity Score Matched Patients		
	All Patients 108 (%)	LDP (n = 19, 17.6%)	ODP (n = 89, 82.4%)	p Value	LDP (n = 19, 100%)	ODP-PSM (n = 19, 100%)	p Value
Male sex	50 (46.3)	8 (42.1)	42 (47.2)	0.802 [a]	8 (42.1)	7 (36.8)	0.705 [b]
Age (years)	66 (19)	69 (14)	64 (19)	0.085 [c]	69 (14)	66 (13)	0.090 [d]
Body mass index (kg/m^2)	27.3 (8.2)	26.7 (8.9)	27.3 (8)	0.623 [c]	26.7 (8.9)	27.6 (7.4)	0.717 [d]
ASA score III	27 (25.0)	5 (26.3)	22 (24.7)	1.000 [a]	5 (26.3)	5 (26.3)	0.480 [b]
Comorbidities present	75 (69.4)	14 (73.7)	61 (68.5)	0.787 [a]	14 (73.7)	14 (73.7)	1.000 [b]
Number of comorbidities	2 (2)	2 (2)	2 (3)	0.663 [c]	2 (2)	2 (4)	0.931 [d]
Previous abdominal surgery	42 (38.9)	11 (57.9)	31 (34.8)	0.073 [a]	11 (57.9)	9 (47.4)	0.480 [b]
C-reactive protein > 5 mg/L	28 (25.9)	4 (21.1)	24 (27.0)	0.775 [a]	4 (21.1)	5 (26.3)	0.705 [b]
Carcinoembryonic antigen > 5 µg/L	17 (15.7)	1 (5.3)	16 (18.0)	0.297 [a]	1 (5.3)	4 (21.1)	0.180 [b]
Carbohydrate antigen 19-9 > 37 kU/L	42 (38.9)	7 (36.8)	35 (39.3)	1.000 [a]	7 (36.8)	7 (36.8)	1.000 [b]
Malignant tumors	69 (63.9)	13 (68.4)	56 (62.9)	0.794 [a]	13 (68.4)	11(57.9)	0.414 [b]
Tumor size (mm)	35 (27)	29 (26)	35 (25)	0.124 [c]	29 (26)	35 (25)	0.121 [d]
Tumor in the neck/body	57 (52.8)	7 (36.8)	50 (56.2)	0.138 [a]	7 (36.8)	5 (26.3)	0.480 [b]

[a] Categorical variable reported as n (%), Fisher's Exact test and [b] the Related-samples Cochran's Q test; [c] continuous variable, non-normal distribution, reported as median (interquartile range), Mann-Whitney test and [d] Wilcoxon signed-ranks test. ASA = American Society of Anesthesiologists; LDP = laparoscopic distal pancreatectomy; ODP = open distal pancreatectomy; PSM = propensity score matching.

For the PSM, the method was closest to the neighborhood method, with a caliper width of 0.20. The relevant variables were patient-related (sex, age, body mass index, American Society of Anesthesiologists (ASA) score, previous abdominal surgery, and C-reactive protein) and tumor-related (malignancy, tumor size, and tumor site). A matched group of patients was created with a 1:1 ratio (13, 21). The standardized mean difference (SMD) was 0.21. Table 2 shows the outcomes of surgery.

Table 2. Outcomes of 108 patients: intraoperative outcomes, recovery, morbidity, and mortality before and after a propensity score matching analysis of LDP versus ODP.

Outcome	Overall Analysis				Propensity Score Matched Patients		
	All Patients *n* (%)	**LDP (*n* = 19, 17.6%)**	**ODP (*n* = 89, 82.4%)**	***p* Value**	**LDP (*n* = 19, 100%)**	**ODP-PSM (*n* = 19, 100%)**	***p* Value**
Operative time (min)	190 (80)	202 (110)	185 (90)	0.084 [c]	202 (110)	190 (140)	0.602 [d]
Blood loss (mL)	209 (241)	134 (64)	226 (279)	0.073 [c]	134 (64)	245 (330)	0.121 [d]
Intraoperative blood transfusion	6 (5.6)	1 (5.3)	5 (5.6)	1.000 [a]	1 (5.3)	1 (5.3)	1.000 [b]
No complications	22 (20.4)	1 (5.3)	21 (23.6)		1 (5.3)	6 (31.6)	
Clavien–Dindo 1	25 (23.1)	7 (36.8)	18 (20.2)		7 (36.8)	4 (21.1)	
Clavien–Dindo 2	27 (25.0)	2 (10.5)	25 (28.1)		2 (10.5)	6 (31.6)	
Clavien–Dindo 3a	21 (19.4)	8 (42.1)	13 (14.6)	0.018 [e]	8 (42.1)	2 (10.5)	0.042 [f]
Clavien–Dindo 3b	8 (7.4)	0 (0.0)	8 (9.0)		0 (0.0)	0 (0.0)	
Clavien–Dindo 4b	1 (0.9)	0 (0.0)	1 (1.1)		0 (0.0)	0 (0.0)	
Clavien–Dindo 5	4 (3.7)	1 (5.3)	3 (3.3)		1 (5.3)	1 (5.3)	
Severe morbidity (Clavien–Dindo $\geq$ 3a)	34 (30.6)	9 (47.4)	25 (28.1)	0.111 [a]	9 (47.4)	3 (15.8)	0.034 [b]
30-day mortality	1 (0.9)	0 (0.0)	1 (1.1)	1.000 [a]	0 (0.0)	1 (5.3)	0.317 [b]
90-day mortality	4 (3.7)	1 (5.3)	3 (3.3)	0.444 [a]	1 (5.3)	1 (5.3)	1.000 [b]
Post-pancreatectomy hemorrhage (all three grades)	3 (2.8)	0 (0.0)	3 (3.4)	1.000 [a]	0 (0.0)	1 (5.3)	0.317 [b]
Delayed gastric emptying	2 (1.9)	1 (5.3)	1 (1.1)	0.322 [a]	1 (5.3)	1 (5.3)	1.000 [b]
Postoperative pancreatic fistula type B	32 (29.6)	7 (36.8)	25 (28.1)	0.580 [a]	7 (36.8)	5 (26.3)	0.527 [b]
Postoperative pancreatic fistula type C	8 (7.4)	0 (0.0)	8 (9.0)	0.346 [a]	0 (0.0)	1 (5.3)	0.317 [b]
Reoperation	11 (10.2)	1 (5.3)	10 (11.2)	0.685 [a]	1 (5.3)	0 (0.0)	0.317 [b]
Readmission	23 (21.3)	3 (15.8)	20 (22.5)	0.759 [a]	3 (15.8)	1 (5.3)	0.317 [b]
Hospital stay (days)	11 (7)	9 (7)	11 (8)	0.074 [c]	9 (7)	12 (11)	0.538 [d]
Intensive care unit admission	7 (6.5)	1 (5.3)	6 (6.7)	1.000 [a]	1 (5.3)	1 (5.3)	1.000 [b]
High-dependency unit stay (days)	5 (2)	5 (3)	5 (2)	0.849 [c]	5 (3)	5 (2)	0.451 [d]
Time to oral food intake (days)	4 (2)	4 (2)	4 (2)	0.878 [c]	4 (2)	4 (3)	0.647 [d]
Time to stool passing (days)	4 (1)	3 (1)	4 (1)	0.866 [c]	3 (1)	3 (2)	0.523 [d]
Intravenous narcotics requirement (days)	6 (3)	5 (4)	6 (3)	0.214 [c]	5 (4)	7 (2)	0.041 [d]
Incisional hernia	14 (13.0)	2 (10.5)	12 (13.5)	1.000 [a]	2 (10.5)	3 (15.8)	0.655 [b]

[a] Categorical variable reported as *n* (%), Fisher's Exact test and [b] the Related-samples Cochran's Q test; [c] continuous variable, non-normal distribution, reported as median (interquartile range), Mann-Whitney test, and [d] Wilcoxon signed-ranks test; [e] categorical variable with more than two groups, reported as *n* (%), Fisher–Freeman–Halton test and [f] Related-samples marginal homogeneity test. LDP = laparoscopic distal pancreatectomy; ODP = open distal pancreatectomy; PSM = propensity score matching.

Table 3. An overview of severe complications.

	ODP Without ODP-PSM Group	LDP Group	ODP-PSM Group
Clavien–Dindo 3a (intervention without general anesthesia)			
Thoracic drainage		1	
Postoperative pancreatic fistula drainage	11	6	2
Subphrenic abscess drainage	2	1	
Gastric bleeding–endoscopic hemostasis			1
Clavien–Dindo 3b (intervention under general anesthesia)			
Subtotal colectomy due to toxic megacolon	1		
Reduction in internal hernia	1		
Drainage of the abscess	3		1
Duodenum-preserving pancreatectomy	2		
Hemostasis of bleeding from lienal artery	2		
Partial omentectomy due to necrosis	1		
Lymphorrhea–sutures of cisterna chyli	1		
Colostomy due to the colocutaneous fistula		1	
Clavien–Dindo 4b (multiorgan dysfunction)			
Septic shock due to portal vein thrombosis	1		
Clavien–Dindo 5 (death)			
Pulmonary embolism			1
Acute myocardial infarction	1		
Septic shock	1		
Coronavirus disease 2019 pneumonia		1	

LDP = laparoscopic distal pancreatectomy; ODP = open distal pancreatectomy; PSM = propensity score matching.

The difference between the LDP and ODP groups was significant when comparing the overall complications; moreover, the difference was due to complications of Clavien–Dindo grade 3a. These also contributed to the significant difference between the LDP and ODP-PSM groups regarding severe complications. Table 3 provides their basic overview, but percentages are not given because one patient can have more than one complication. The time-trend analysis of complications of Clavien–Dindo grades $\geq$ 3a among groups is given in Figure 3. The 90-day mortality rate was 3.7%. The causes of death are given in Table 3.

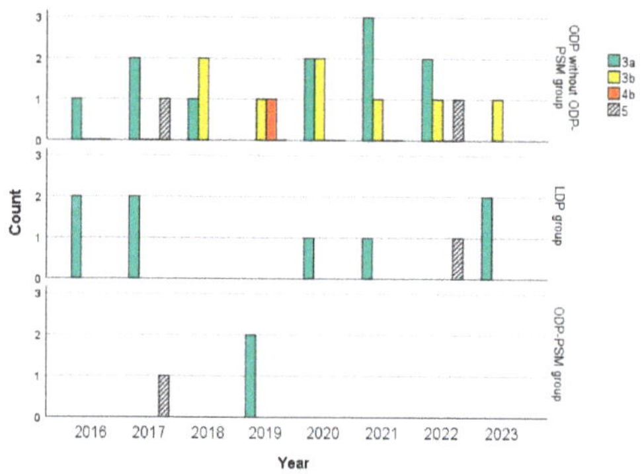

Figure 3. The time-trend analysis of complications of Clavien–Dindo grades $\geq$ 3a among groups (concordant with Table 2). LDP = laparoscopic distal pancreatectomy; ODP = open distal pancreatectomy; PSM = propensity score matching.

The oncological results are given in Table 4.

Table 4. Histopathological reports of 69 (63.9%) patients with malignant tumors before and after a propensity score matching analysis of LDP versus ODP.

Outcome	Overall Analysis				Propensity Score Matched Patients		
	All Patients $n = 69$	LDP ($n = 13$, 68.4%)	ODP ($n = 56$, 62.9%)	p Value	LDP ($n = 13$, 68.4%)	ODP-PSM ($n = 11$, (57.9%)	p Value
Diagnosis							
Pancreatic ductal adenocarcinoma	39 (56.5)	5 (38.5)	34 (60.7)	0.191 [e]	5 (38.5)	6 (54.5)	0.564 [f]
Nonfunctioning pancreatic neuroendocrine neoplasms	27 (39.1)	8 (61.5)	19 (33.9)		8 (61.5)	4 (36.4)	
Other	3 (4.3)	0 (0.0)	3 (5.4)		0 (0.0)	1 (9.1)	
Number of harvested lymph nodes	14 (12)	14 (9)	15 (16)	0.685 [c]	14 (9)	15 (22)	0.284 [d]
Resection margin (mm)	3 (8)	4 (11)	3 (9)	0.786 [c]	4 (11)	6 (15)	0.929 [d]
R0 resection	57 (82.6)	11 (84.6)	46 (82.1)	1.000 [a]	11 (84.6)	10 (90.9)	1.000 [b]

[a] Categorical variable reported as n (%), Fisher's Exact test, and [b] the Related-samples Cochran's Q test; [c] continuous variable, non-normal distribution, reported as median (interquartile range), Mann-Whitney test, and [d] Wilcoxon signed-ranks test; [e] categorical variable with more than two groups, reported as n (%), Fisher–Freeman–Halton test, and [f] Related-samples marginal homogeneity test. LDP = laparoscopic distal pancreatectomy; ODP = open distal pancreatectomy.

4. Discussion

This research has shown some significant differences between the LDP and ODP groups. The first was a statistically significant difference in the overall postoperative complication rate (p = 0.018). It was due to complications of Clavien–Dindo grade 3a, which was 42.1% in the LDP group and 14.6% in the ODP group. The rate in the ODP-PSM group was 10.5%, and the difference was significant (p = 0.042). This grade of complications also contributed to the significant difference (p = 0.034) between the LDP (42.1%) and ODP-PSM groups (14.6%) in terms of severe complications. The next difference was a shorter duration of intravenous narcotic analgesia (5 vs. 7 days, p = 0.041) in the LDP group, which became significant after PSM.

The present study was designed to provide a comprehensive picture of the current laparoscopic distal pancreatectomy in a single tertiary referral center, where the first procedure was performed in 2016. Along with many studies that dealt mainly with pancreatic ductal adenocarcinoma or nonfunctioning pancreatic neuroendocrine neoplasms, our cohort comprises patients with all kinds of diseases that can arise in the distal pancreas [5,14,32–35].

The clinical characteristics of patients in the LDP and ODP groups did not differ (Table 1), as also reported by Casadei et al., where the differences among the groups became insignificant after PSM [14]. Along with proficiency with open pancreatic resections, the equable selection of patients in both groups could be assigned to the surgeons' broad experience from laparoscopic liver and gastric surgery [29,36,37]. However, our rate of conversions into the open approach was 13.6%. It was close to the median value of 12.3% in the study by Giani et al., while the benchmark is 2.5% [11] (Table 5). This could be explained by an unfinished learning curve that demands the completion of 25 laparoscopic distal pancreatectomies to gain individual expertise [30,38].

Table 5. Range, median, and benchmark values in minimally invasive distal pancreatectomy with splenectomy at a glance (adopted from Giani et al. [11]).

Outcome	Range	Median Value	Benchmark
Duration of operation (min)	132.5–361.5	232.5	160
Conversion (%)	0–54.5	12.3	2.5
Intraoperative blood transfusion (%)	0–10.8	2.6	0.5
Overall morbidity (%)	25.6–100	58.0	30.4
Severe morbidity (%)	4.4–54.7	17.4	8.4
Postoperative pancreatic fistula (%)	6.3–47.4	21.9	8.3
Reoperations (%)	0–20.0	5.4	1.8
Duration of hospital stay (days)	5–13	8	5
Readmissions (%)	0–40	13.0	4.1
90–days mortality	0–17.6	0	0

Nevertheless, these three patients were included in the ODP group because the intention-to-treat principle, essential in randomized controlled trials, is more difficult to apply to a retrospective clinical study comparing the outcomes of surgical approaches [39]. One patient had a percutaneous drainage of a postoperative pancreatic fistula (Clavien-Dindo grade 3a) and none of them was not included in the ODP-PSM group.

The primary endpoints were the duration of the operation and the transfusion requirement. Our study showed no differences between the LDP and ODP groups for both outcomes. The median duration of the laparoscopic operation was 202 min, the median in the study by Giani et al. was 232.5 min, and the benchmark was 160 min. The benchmark for intraoperative transfusion application was 0.5% [11]. Our intraoperative blood transfusion rate was 5.3%, without any significant difference with the ODP group (Table 2). This could be explained by a quarter of ASA score III patients and their median age of 69. These patients are prone to bleeding due to tissue fragility [40]. However, more attention should be given to the preoperative anemia correction [41].

This research showed that a shorter duration of intravenous narcotic analgesia (5 vs. 7 days, $p = 0.041$) in the LDP group became significant after PSM (Table 2). Less pain is, apart from the cosmetic effect, the desired consequence of reduced trauma of the abdominal wall [14]. For the assessment of postoperative pain, the Numeric Pain Rating Scale was used [21]. It contained a 0–10 scale, with 0 meaning "no pain" and 10 meaning "the worst pain imaginable" [22]. The intravenous narcotic, namely piritramide, was administered when the patients estimated their pain ≥ 6.

It is proposed that narcotic analgesia can contribute to the occurrence of postoperative pancreatic fistula after distal pancreatectomy due to the spasm of the sphincter of Oddi, which increases pressure within the pancreatic duct stump [42,43]. However, pancreas-specific morbidity was insignificant between the groups (Table 2). For postoperative pancreatic fistula type B, our rates in the ODP group were 28.1%, 36.8% in the LDP group, and 26.3% in the ODP-PSM group. Postoperative pancreatic fistula type C was observed only in open distal pancreatectomies. The benchmark for fistula type B/C was set at 8.3% [11].

In 2021, our institution unified the surgical technique, where one type of stapler is used in open and laparoscopic distal pancreatectomies. The staplers are proven useful when the pancreatic thickness is <12 mm [44–46]. Recently, has been suggested that a pre-firing pancreatic compression for at least 10 min might reduce the risk of clinically relevant postoperative pancreatic fistula development, especially when a pancreatic gland tissue is thick [47,48].

Among the secondary endpoints, our overall morbidity rate was 76.4% in the ODP group, 94.7% in the LDP group, and 68.4% in the ODP-PSM group. Both comparisons were statistically significant (Table 2). This skyrocketing rate in the LDP group was due to the complications of Clavien–Dindo grade 3a (42.1%), which signified percutaneous drainages of fluid collections in the thorax or abdomen (Table 3). They also contributed to the statistical significance of the severe morbidity rates (Clavien–Dindo $\geq$ 3a) in this group (47.4%). However, this rate was insignificant compared to the ODP group (28.1%) but showed significance when compared to the ODP-PSM group (10.5%; $p = 0.034$). The benchmark was 8.4% [11]. The proposed risk factors for severe morbidity were ASA grade > II, multi-visceral resections, and robotic resections [11]. However, one-quarter of our patients were ASA grade III, but there were no multi-visceral or robotic resections. As can be observed in Figures 2 and 3, the count of LDP had a growing trend, and the count of its severe complications had a decreasing one. Of note, leaving the drain in place for sufficient time could diminish the rate of complications of Clavien–Dindo grade 3a, since the rates of postoperative pancreatic fistula type B were insignificant among the groups.

Mortality rates, reoperations, and readmissions did not differ between the LDP and ODP groups (Table 2). The 90-day mortality rate of 3.7% in the whole cohort was caused by medical complications in three patients (Table 3). One patient died of irreversible septic shock following a toxic megacolon due to a postoperative pancreatic fistula. Perioperative mortality close to zero has always been a desired benchmark (Table 5) [11]. On the other hand, the rate of reoperations was 0 in the LDP group and 9% in the ODP group. The reasons for reoperations are given in Table 3.

The duration of a high-dependence unit or hospital stay depends on many factors, including the availability of personnel, facilities, and social and cultural factors, which differ between wards and lands [49]. Nevertheless, there was no difference in these variables among our groups; moreover, the LDP group (nine days) was close to the median of the duration of the hospital stay in this study (eight days). Furthermore, a readmission rate is proposed as a more unified outcome, and the time to functional recovery may become a replacement outcome for the duration of a hospital stay [11]. The readmission rates were indifferent among the groups; furthermore, the LDP group had a rate of 15.8%, while the median was 13%, and the benchmark was 4.1%. There was no difference between the groups in the functional recovery of patients, which included four days to oral food intake and three days to stool passing in both groups after PSM. Therefore, a benchmark of five days of hospital stay is obtainable (Tables 2 and 5).

Furthermore, the oncological outcomes were analyzed in a subset of patients with pancreatic malignant neoplasms. As shown in Table 4, there were no differences between the LDP and ODP groups. After PSM, the rate of R0 resections was 84.6% in the LDP group and 90.9% in the matched group. In 2014, the International Study Group on Pancreatic Surgery set guidelines for lymphadenectomy in pancreatic ductal adenocarcinoma. For tumors of the pancreatic body and tail, removal of stations 10, 11, and 18 was set as the standard, also because of adequate nodal staging [50]. The first and second echelons were recently established in pancreatoduodenectomy [16]. Several research studies have confirmed the importance of those stations for distal pancreatectomy, adding that the optimal extent of lymphadenectomy should be estimated based on the tumor location [51–53]. The analysis by Zhun Hong Wong et al. showed no significant difference between laparoscopic, robotic, and open distal pancreatectomies for harvested lymph nodes, resection margins, and tumor recurrence; however, the patients' survival rate was better in laparoscopic and robotic groups when compared to the open resection group [33].

Moreover, Partelli et al. published a study on nonfunctioning pancreatic neuroendocrine neoplasms, in which the rate of severe postoperative morbidity was lower and the duration of hospital stay was shorter in the laparoscopic group. Despite the significantly lower number of harvested lymph nodes in the laparoscopic group (13 versus 10, $p = 0.0036$), similar disease-free and overall survival rates were reported for both groups [35].

The present study has several limitations. First, the number of patients in the LDP group is relatively low, which can lead to the loss of statistical power. Second, given the retrospective nature of this study, selection bias may have been present. Although propensity score matching was performed to overcome potential bias and make the two groups similar, it is less effective than a prospective randomized trial. Another important issue is the failure to meet many of the international benchmarks. Therefore, a future clinical direction will be to increase the volume of LDP in order to overcome the challenges of the learning curve. Future research aims to compare the long-term survival rates of patients with malignant tumors in the distal pancreas.

To conclude, our attention should be drawn to preventing postoperative complications, because the oncological outcomes are already comparable with those of the open procedure, and postoperative pain management is promising. Much will have to be done to achieve the benchmark values.

Author Contributions: Conceptualization: I.P. and A.I.; methodology: I.P., A.I. and Š.T.; software: I.P.; validation: A.I.; formal analysis: I.P. and B.I.; investigation: Ž.Š., M.G. and T.M.; resources: Ž.Š., M.G. and T.M.; data curation: S.P., B.I. and I.P.; writing—original draft preparation: I.P. and A.I.; writing—review and editing: I.P., Š.T., A.I. and S.P.; visualization: I.P.; supervision: S.P.; project administration: A.I.; funding acquisition: Š.T., T.M., A.I. and I.P. All authors have read and agreed to the published version of the manuscript.

Funding: The University Medical Centre Maribor funded the article procession charge, IRP-2023/02-10.

Institutional Review Board Statement: This study was conducted according to the guidelines of the Declaration of Helsinki and approved by the Institutional Ethics Committee of the University Medical Centre Maribor (UKC-MB-KME-41/24, 25 September 2024).

Informed Consent Statement: Informed consent was obtained from all subjects involved in this study.

Data Availability Statement: Due to the patients' privacy, the data presented in this study are available upon request from the corresponding author.

Conflicts of Interest: The authors declare no conflicts of interest. The sponsor had no role in the design, execution, interpretation, or writing of this study.

References

1. Cuschieri, A. Laparoscopic surgery of the pancreas. *J. R. Coll. Surg. Edinb.* **1994**, *39*, 178–184.
2. Vollmer, C.M.; Asbun, H.J.; Barkun, J.; Besselink, M.G.; Boggi, U.; Conlon, K.C.; Han, H.S.; Hansen, P.D.; Kendrick, M.L.; Montagnini, A.L.; et al. Proceedings of the first international state-of-the-art conference on minimally-invasive pancreatic resection (MIPR). *HPB* **2017**, *19*, 171–177. [CrossRef]
3. Bassi, C.; Andrianello, S. Identifying key outcome metrics in pancreatic surgery, and how to optimally achieve them. *HPB* **2017**, *19*, 178–181. [CrossRef]
4. Røsok, B.I.; de Rooij, T.; van Hilst, J.; Diener, M.K.; Allen, P.J.; Vollmer, C.M.; Kooby, D.A.; Shrikhande, S.V. Minimally invasive distal pancreatectomy. *HPB* **2017**, *19*, 205–214. [CrossRef]
5. van Hilst, J.; de Rooij, T.; Klompmaker, S.; Rawashdeh, M.; Aleotti, F.; Al-Sarireh, B.; Alseidi, A.; Ateeb, Z.; Balzano, G.; Berrevoet, F.; et al. Minimally Invasive versus Open Distal Pancreatectomy for Ductal Adenocarcinoma (DIPLOMA): A Pan-European Propensity Score Matched Study. *Ann. Surg.* **2019**, *269*, 10–17. [CrossRef]
6. de Rooij, T.; van Hilst, J.; van Santvoort, H.; Boerma, D.; van den Boezem, P.; Daams, F.; van Dam, R.; Dejong, C.; van Duyn, E.; Dijkgraaf, M.; et al. Minimally Invasive Versus Open Distal Pancreatectomy (LEOPARD): A Multicenter Patient-blinded Randomized Controlled Trial. *Ann. Surg.* **2019**, *269*, 2–9. [CrossRef]

7. Björnsson, B.; Larsson, A.L.; Hjalmarsson, C.; Gasslander, T.; Sandström, P. Comparison of the duration of hospital stay after laparoscopic or open distal pancreatectomy: Randomized controlled trial. *Br. J. Surg.* **2020**, *107*, 1281–1288. [CrossRef]
8. Asbun, H.J.; Moekotte, A.L.; Vissers, F.L.; Kunzler, F.; Cipriani, F.; Alseidi, A.; D'Angelica, M.I.; Balduzzi, A.; Bassi, C.; Björnsson, B.; et al. The Miami International Evidence-based Guidelines on Minimally Invasive Pancreas Resection. *Ann. Surg.* **2020**, *271*, 1–14. [CrossRef]
9. Abu Hilal, M.; van Ramshorst, T.M.E.; Boggi, U.; Dokmak, S.; Edwin, B.; Keck, T.; Khatkov, I.; Ahmad, J.; Al Saati, H.; Alseidi, A.; et al. The Brescia Internationally Validated European Guidelines on Minimally Invasive Pancreatic Surgery (EGUMIPS). *Ann. Surg.* **2024**, *279*, 45–57. [CrossRef]
10. van Ramshorst, T.M.E.; van Hilst, J.; Boggi, U.; Dokmak, S.; Edwin, B.; Keck, T.; Khatkov, I.; Balduzzi, A.; Pulvirenti, A.; Ahmad, J.; et al. Standardizing definitions and terminology of left-sided pancreatic resections through an international Delphi consensus. *Br. J. Surg.* **2024**, *111*, znae039. [CrossRef]
11. Giani, A.; van Ramshorst, T.; Mazzola, M.; Bassi, C.; Esposito, A.; de Pastena, M.; Edwin, B.; Sahakyan, M.; Kleive, D.; Jah, A.; et al. Benchmarking of minimally invasive distal pancreatectomy with splenectomy: European multicentre study. *Br. J. Surg.* **2022**, *109*, 1124–1130. [CrossRef]
12. Liang, S.; Hameed, U.; Jayaraman, S. Laparoscopic pancreatectomy: Indications and outcomes. *World J. Gastroenterol.* **2014**, *20*, 14246–14254. [CrossRef]
13. Casadei, R.; Ricci, C.; D'Ambra, M.; Marrano, N.; Alagna, V.; Rega, D.; Monari, F.; Minni, F. Laparoscopic versus open distal pancreatectomy in pancreatic tumours: A case-control study. *Updates Surg.* **2010**, *62*, 171–174. [CrossRef]
14. Casadei, R.; Ingaldi, C.; Ricci, C.; Alberici, L.; De Raffele, E.; Vaccaro, M.C.; Minni, F. Laparoscopic versus open distal pancreatectomy: A single centre propensity score matching analysis. *Updates Surg.* **2021**, *73*, 1747–1755. [CrossRef]
15. Kwon, J.; Lee, S.R.; Park, S.Y.; Lee, J.H.; Song, K.B.; Hwang, D.W.; Shin, J.H.; Kim, S.C. Effect of resection margin status on recurrence pattern and survival in distal pancreatectomy for left-sided pancreatic ductal adenocarcinoma. *J. Hepatobiliary Pancreat. Sci.* **2023**, *30*, 633–643. [CrossRef]
16. Malleo, G.; Maggino, L.; Casciani, F.; Lionetto, G.; Nobile, S.; Lazzarin, G.; Paiella, S.; Esposito, A.; Capelli, P.; Luchini, C.; et al. Importance of Nodal Metastases Location in Pancreatoduodenectomy for Pancreatic Ductal Adenocarcinoma: Results from a Prospective, Lymphadenectomy Protocol. *Ann. Surg. Oncol.* **2022**, *29*, 3477–3488. [CrossRef]
17. Clavien, P.A.; Barkun, J.; de Oliveira, M.L.; Vauthey, J.N.; Dindo, D.; Schulick, R.D.; de Santibanes, E.; Pekolj, J.; Slankamenac, K.; Bassi, C.; et al. The Clavien-Dindo classification of surgical complications: Five-year experience. *Ann. Surg.* **2009**, *250*, 187–196. [CrossRef]
18. Bassi, C.; Marchegiani, G.; Dervenis, C.; Sarr, M.; Abu Hilal, M.; Adham, M.; Allen, P.; Andersson, R.; Asbun, H.J.; Besselink, M.G.; et al. The 2016 update of the International Study Group (ISGPS) definition and grading of postoperative pancreatic fistula: 11 Years After. *Surgery* **2017**, *161*, 584–591. [CrossRef]
19. Wente, M.N.; Veit, J.A.; Bassi, C.; Dervenis, C.; Fingerhut, A.; Gouma, D.J.; Izbicki, J.R.; Neoptolemos, J.P.; Padbury, R.T.; Sarr, M.G.; et al. Postpancreatectomy hemorrhage (PPH): An International Study Group of Pancreatic Surgery (ISGPS) definition. *Surgery* **2007**, *142*, 20–25. [CrossRef]
20. Wente, M.N.; Bassi, C.; Dervenis, C.; Fingerhut, A.; Gouma, D.J.; Izbicki, J.R.; Neoptolemos, J.P.; Padbury, R.T.; Sarr, M.G.; Traverso, L.W.; et al. Delayed gastric emptying (DGE) after pancreatic surgery: A suggested definition by the International Study Group of Pancreatic Surgery (ISGPS). *Surgery* **2007**, *142*, 761–768. [CrossRef]
21. Breivik, H.; Borchgrevink, P.C.; Allen, S.M.; Rosseland, L.A.; Romundstad, L.; Hals, E.K.; Kvarstein, G.; Stubhaug, A. Assessment of pain. *Br. J. Anaesth.* **2008**, *101*, 17–24. [CrossRef] [PubMed]
22. Nugent, S.M.; Lovejoy, T.I.; Shull, S.; Dobscha, S.K.; Morasco, B.J. Associations of Pain Numeric Rating Scale Scores Collected during Usual Care with Research Administered Patient Reported Pain Outcomes. *Pain. Med.* **2021**, *22*, 2235–2241. [CrossRef] [PubMed]
23. Wang, Y.; Li, J.; Weng, Y.; Deng, X.; Jin, J.; Peng, C. A new enhanced recovery after surgery pathway for left-sided pancreatic cancer patients after distal pancreatectomy. *Transl. Cancer Res.* **2019**, *8*, 2613–2620. [CrossRef] [PubMed]
24. Lassen, K.; Coolsen, M.M.; Slim, K.; Carli, F.; de Aguilar-Nascimento, J.E.; Schäfer, M.; Parks, R.W.; Fearon, K.C.; Lobo, D.N.; Demartines, N.; et al. Guidelines for perioperative care for pancreaticoduodenectomy: Enhanced Recovery After Surgery (ERAS®) Society recommendations. *Clin. Nutr.* **2012**, *31*, 817–830. [CrossRef]
25. Austin, P.C. An Introduction to Propensity Score Methods for Reducing the Effects of Confounding in Observational Studies. *Multivar. Behav. Res.* **2011**, *46*, 399–424. [CrossRef]
26. Yao, X.I.; Wang, X.; Speicher, P.J.; Hwang, E.S.; Cheng, P.; Harpole, D.H.; Berry, M.F.; Schrag, D.; Pang, H.H. Reporting and Guidelines in Propensity Score Analysis: A Systematic Review of Cancer and Cancer Surgical Studies. *J. Natl. Cancer Inst.* **2017**, *109*, djw323. [CrossRef]
27. Donner, A.; Li, K.Y. The relationship between chi-square statistics from matched and unmatched analyses. *J. Clin. Epidemiol.* **1990**, *43*, 827–831. [CrossRef]

28. Dunnigan, K. Tests of marginal homogeneity and special cases. *Pharm. Stat.* **2013**, *12*, 213–216. [CrossRef]
29. Jagric, T. East meets West: The initial results of laparoscopic gastric cancer resections with Eastern principles in a single Western centre—A propensity score-matched study. *Langenbecks Arch. Surg.* **2021**, *406*, 2699–2708. [CrossRef]
30. Ivanecz, A.; Plahuta, I.; Mencinger, M.; Perus, I.; Magdalenic, T.; Turk, S.; Potrc, S. The learning curve of laparoscopic liver resection utilising a difficulty score. *Radiol. Oncol.* **2021**, *56*, 111–118. [CrossRef]
31. Potrc, S.; Ivanecz, A.; Pivec, V.; Marolt, U.; Rudolf, S.; Iljevec, B.; Jagric, T. Impact Factors for Perioperative Morbidity and Mortality and Repercussion of Perioperative Morbidity and Long-term Survival in Pancreatic Head Resection. *Radiol. Oncol.* **2018**, *52*, 54–64. [CrossRef] [PubMed]
32. Gavriilidis, P.; Roberts, K.J.; Sutcliffe, R.P. Comparison of robotic vs laparoscopic vs open distal pancreatectomy. A systematic review and network meta-analysis. *HPB* **2019**, *21*, 1268–1276. [CrossRef] [PubMed]
33. Zhun Hong Wong, N.; Wei Ting Yap, D.; Lei Ng, S.; Yu Ning Ng, J.; James, J.J.; Wei Chieh Kow, A. Oncological outcomes in minimally invasive vs. open distal pancreatectomy: A systematic review and network meta-analysis. *Front. Surg.* **2024**, *11*, 1369169. [CrossRef] [PubMed]
34. Korrel, M.; Vissers, F.L.; van Hilst, J.; de Rooij, T.; Dijkgraaf, M.G.; Festen, S.; Groot Koerkamp, B.; Busch, O.R.; Luyer, M.D.; Sandström, P.; et al. Minimally invasive versus open distal pancreatectomy: An individual patient data meta-analysis of two randomized controlled trials. *HPB* **2021**, *23*, 323–330. [CrossRef] [PubMed]
35. Partelli, S.; Andreasi, V.; Rancoita, P.M.V.; Perez-Sanchez, E.; Muffatti, F.; Balzano, G.; Crippa, S.; Di Serio, C.; Falconi, M. Outcomes after distal pancreatectomy for neuroendocrine neoplasms: A retrospective comparison between minimally invasive and open approach using propensity score weighting. *Surg. Endosc.* **2021**, *35*, 165–173. [CrossRef]
36. Ivanecz, A.; Plahuta, I.; Magdalenic, T.; Mencinger, M.; Perus, I.; Potrc, S.; Krebs, B. The external validation of a difficulty scoring system for predicting the risk of intraoperative complications during laparoscopic liver resection. *BMC Surg.* **2019**, *19*, 179. [CrossRef]
37. Ivanecz, A.; Plahuta, I.; Magdalenic, T.; Ilijevec, B.; Mencinger, M.; Perus, I.; Potrc, S. Evaluation of the Iwate Model for Predicting the Difficulty of Laparoscopic Liver Resection: Does Tumor Size Matter? *J. Gastrointest. Surg.* **2021**, *25*, 1451–1460. [CrossRef]
38. Chan, K.S.; Wang, Z.K.; Syn, N.; Goh, B.K.P. Learning curve of laparoscopic and robotic pancreas resections: A systematic review. *Surgery* **2021**, *170*, 194–206. [CrossRef]
39. McCoy, C.E. Understanding the Intention-to-treat Principle in Randomized Controlled Trials. *West. J. Emerg. Med.* **2017**, *18*, 1075–1078. [CrossRef]
40. Lu, Q.; Lu, J.W.; Wu, Z.; Liu, X.M.; Li, J.H.; Dong, J.; Yin, G.Z.; Lv, Y.; Zhang, X.F. Perioperative outcome of elderly versus younger patients undergoing major hepatic or pancreatic surgery. *Clin. Interv. Aging* **2018**, *13*, 133–141. [CrossRef]
41. Pecorelli, N.; Guarneri, G.; Quattromani, R.; Arru, G.G.; Gozzini, L.; Lee, Y.H.; Vallorani, A.; Turi, S.; Partelli, S.; Crippa, S.; et al. The impact of preoperative anemia on pancreatic resection outcomes. *HPB* **2022**, *24*, 717–726. [CrossRef] [PubMed]
42. Kowalsky, S.J.; Zenati, M.S.; Dhir, M.; Schaefer, E.G.; Dopsovic, A.; Lee, K.K.; Hogg, M.E.; Zeh, H.J.; Vollmer, C.M.; Zureikat, A.H. Postoperative narcotic use is associated with development of clinically relevant pancreatic fistulas after distal pancreatectomy. *Surgery* **2018**, *163*, 747–752. [CrossRef] [PubMed]
43. Boyev, A.; Prakash, L.R.; Chiang, Y.J.; Childers, C.P.; Jain, A.J.; Newhook, T.E.; Bruno, M.L.; Arvide, E.M.; Dewhurst, W.L.; Kim, M.P.; et al. Postoperative Opioid Use Is Associated with Increased Rates of Grade B/C Pancreatic Fistula After Distal Pancreatectomy. *J. Gastrointest. Surg.* **2023**, *27*, 2135–2144. [CrossRef] [PubMed]
44. Kang, M.K.; Kim, H.; Byun, Y.; Han, Y.; Choi, Y.J.; Kang, J.S.; Kwon, W.; Han, I.W.; Shin, S.H.; Choi, D.W.; et al. Optimal stapler cartridge selection to reduce post-operative pancreatic fistula according to the pancreatic characteristics in stapler closure distal pancreatectomy. *HPB* **2021**, *23*, 633–640. [CrossRef]
45. Murata, Y.; Maeda, K.; Ito, T.; Gyoten, K.; Hayasaki, A.; Iizawa, Y.; Fujii, T.; Tanemura, A.; Kuriyama, N.; Kishiwada, M.; et al. Efficacy of Reinforced Stapler Versus Hand-sewn Closure of the Pancreatic Stump During Pure Laparoscopic Distal Pancreatectomy to Reduce Pancreatic Fistula. *Surg. Laparosc. Endosc. Percutan Tech.* **2023**, *33*, 99–107. [CrossRef]
46. Xia, N.; Li, J.; Huang, X.; Tian, B.; Xiong, J. Reinforced stapling does not reduce postoperative pancreatic fistula in distal pancreatectomy: A systematic review and meta-analysis. *Updates Surg.* **2023**, *75*, 2063–2074. [CrossRef]
47. Quero, G.; Laterza, V.; Schena, C.A.; Massimiani, G.; Lucinato, C.; Fiorillo, C.; Mezza, T.; Taglioni, F.; Menghi, R.; Di Cesare, L.; et al. Prolonged pre-firing pancreatic compression with linear staplers in distal pancreatectomy: A valuable technique for post-operative pancreatic fistula prevention. *Langenbecks Arch. Surg.* **2024**, *409*, 184. [CrossRef]
48. Kjeseth, T.; Yaqub, S.; Edwin, B.; Kleive, D.; Sahakyan, M.A. Peri-firing compression in prevention of pancreatic fistula after distal pancreatectomy: A systematic review and a cohort study. *Scand. J. Surg.* **2024**, *113*, 73–79. [CrossRef]
49. Barresi, V.; Reggiani Bonetti, L.; Ieni, A.; Caruso, R.A.; Tuccari, G. Histological grading in colorectal cancer: New insights and perspectives. *Histol. Histopathol.* **2015**, *30*, 1059–1067. [CrossRef]

50. Tol, J.A.; Gouma, D.J.; Bassi, C.; Dervenis, C.; Montorsi, M.; Adham, M.; Andrén-Sandberg, A.; Asbun, H.J.; Bockhorn, M.; Büchler, M.W.; et al. Definition of a standard lymphadenectomy in surgery for pancreatic ductal adenocarcinoma: A consensus statement by the International Study Group on Pancreatic Surgery (ISGPS). *Surgery* **2014**, *156*, 591–600. [CrossRef]
51. Seo, S.; Uemura, K.; Sumiyoshi, T.; Kondo, N.; Okada, K.; Otsuka, H.; Murakami, Y.; Takahashi, S. Optimal lymph-node dissection for pancreatic tail cancer. *Surg. Today* **2022**, *52*, 1307–1312. [CrossRef] [PubMed]
52. Ishida, H.; Ogura, T.; Takahashi, A.; Miyamoto, R.; Matsudaira, S.; Amikura, K.; Tanabe, M.; Kawashima, Y. Optimal Region of Lymph Node Dissection in Distal Pancreatectomy for Left-Sided Pancreatic Cancer Based on Tumor Location. *Ann. Surg. Oncol.* **2022**, *29*, 2414–2424. [CrossRef] [PubMed]
53. Imamura, T.; Yamamoto, Y.; Sugiura, T.; Okamura, Y.; Ito, T.; Ashida, R.; Ohgi, K.; Uesaka, K. Reconsidering the Optimal Regional Lymph Node Station According to Tumor Location for Pancreatic Cancer. *Ann. Surg. Oncol.* **2021**, *28*, 1602–1611. [CrossRef] [PubMed]

life

MDPI

Review

Inflammatory Bowel Diseases and Nephropathies: Exploring the Gut–Kidney Axis

Roberto de Sire [1,2,*], Alessia La Mantia [1], Livio Bonacci [1], Anna Testa [1], Alessia Dalila Guarino [1], Antonio Rispo [1], Olga Maria Nardone [1] and Fabiana Castiglione [1]

[1] IBD Unit, Department of Clinical Medicine and Surgery, University Federico II, 80126 Naples, Italy; alessialamantia7@gmail.com (A.L.M.); liviobonacci@gmail.com (L.B.); annatesta82@virgilio.it (A.T.); ale.tizi@hotmail.it (A.D.G.); antonio.rispo2@unina.it (A.R.); olga.nardone@libero.it (O.M.N.); fabcasti@unina.it (F.C.)

[2] Endoscopy Unit, Department of Gastroenterology, IRCCS Humanitas Research Hospital, 20089 Rozzano, Italy

* Correspondence: roberto.desire@libero.it

Abstract: Inflammatory bowel disease (IBD) can extend beyond the gastrointestinal tract, affecting extraintestinal organs and significantly increasing morbidity and mortality. Despite early studies revealing kidney involvement in nearly a quarter of patients with IBD, renal manifestations have been notably overlooked. Among these manifestations, nephrolithiasis, obstructive uropathy, and fistula formation between the bowel and urinary tract are the most reported occurrences. Additionally, renal parenchymal involvement in IBD, including glomerulonephritis (GN), tubulointerstitial nephritis, and amyloidosis, has been documented. GN is particularly noteworthy, as a significant proportion of patients progress to end-stage kidney disease (ESKD). Although GN has long been recognized as a potential extraintestinal manifestation (EIM) of IBD, it has often been dismissed as an anecdotal association. Recently, several studies highlighted the clinical correlation between GN and IBD, suggesting a pathogenic interplay involving gut inflammation, dysbiosis, and intrinsic glomerular processes. Thus, our objective is to elucidate the basis of IBD-related nephropathies, with a specific focus on IgA nephropathy (IgAN) and the gut–kidney axis.

Keywords: inflammatory bowel disease; IBD; nephropathies; IgAN; gut microbiota; gut-kidney axis

1. Introduction

Inflammatory bowel disease (IBD) can extend to other organs, significantly impacting health outcomes [1]. Extraintestinal manifestations (EIMs) are characterized as inflammatory conditions occurring in every system of the body and can broadly be classified as classical (inflammatory process occurring at distant sites), associations (associations with other immune-mediated disorders), and complications (complications of systemic inflammation); moreover, some manifestations occur as a side effect of IBD therapy [2,3]. These manifestations either result from the spread of immune responses from the intestine, which may occur independently even if they are influenced by IBD, or share similar environmental or genetic factors [4–7].

The renal manifestations associated with IBD have been relatively understudied despite early findings indicating kidney involvement in nearly a quarter of IBD patients. Initial research identified nephrolithiasis, obstructive uropathy, and fistula formation between the bowel and urinary tract as common occurrences [8,9]. Moreover, renal parenchymal involvement in IBD, including glomerulonephritis (GN), tubulointerstitial nephritis, and amyloidosis, has been documented. However, due to the absence of systematic analyses, the true prevalence remains unclear [10,11].

In recent years, the introduction of more potent medications for IBD treatment has heightened concerns about potential nephrotoxic effects, emphasizing the significance of this area of study [12]. Renal parenchymal involvement can affect various compartments, including the glomerular, tubular, or interstitial regions. GN is particularly noteworthy due to its significant implications, as approximately 20–30% of patients may progress to end-stage kidney disease (ESKD) if left untreated [13]. While GN has been acknowledged as a potential EIM of IBD for some time, it was frequently viewed as an anecdotal association [14]. Nevertheless, in recent years, several studies have emphasized the clinical correlation between GN and IBD, suggesting a pathogenic interplay involving gut inflammation, dysbiosis, and intrinsic glomerular processes [15–17].

Several studies have highlighted notable disparities in the gut microbiota (GM) composition between individuals with IBD and healthy controls [18,19]. Notably, patients with Crohn's Disease (CD) often exhibit a decrease in the Firmicutes phylum, specifically *Faecalibacterium prausnitzii*, in their stool samples, while members of the Proteobacteria phylum, such as Enterobacteriaceae (including *Escherichia coli*), are frequently elevated compared to healthy controls [20–22]. This imbalance results in gut dysbiosis, characterized by a shift in the equilibrium between beneficial and potentially harmful microorganisms. An imbalance in microbial communities can disrupt the GM, potentially leading to intestinal dysbiosis by compromising the integrity of the intestinal barrier [23].

Furthermore, there are reports indicating that viable bacteria, primarily from the Proteobacteria phylum—particularly species such as *Escherichia coli*—can migrate from the gut to extraintestinal sites, including the kidneys. This bacterial translocation is often associated with bacterial dysbiosis, overgrowth, and weakened host immune defenses [24–26]. The pathological relationship between GM and kidney diseases is referred to as the gut–kidney axis, and it appears to play a role in various clinical manifestations, including IgA nephropathy (IgAN) [27,28].

In this narrative review, our objective is to elucidate the basis of IBD-related nephropathies, with a specific focus on IgAN and the gut–kidney axis.

2. The Gut–Kidney Axis

The connection between GM and chronic kidney disease (CKD) is termed the "gut–kidney axis" [29,30]. It is widely recognized that the intestinal microbiome, consisting of diverse microorganisms like bacteria, viruses, protozoa, and fungi, profoundly influences the host's homeostasis during both health and disease [31,32]. Gut microbes and their metabolites play vital roles in maintaining gut epithelial integrity, providing energy, defending against pathogens, and modulating the immune system. Consequently, changes in microbial composition, known as dysbiosis, are thought to initiate the progression of several diseases, including CKD [33,34].

Emerging evidence indicates that GM contributes to CKD pathogenesis, interacting with systemic metabolic and inflammatory pathways [35,36]. Indeed, certain bacteria within the GM are responsible for synthesizing uremic toxins, which are implicated in CKD progression. Three bacterial families, namely Clostridiaceae, Enterobacteriaceae, and Verrucomicrobiaceae, harbor the tryptophanase gene responsible for indole production. Additionally, five families—Cellulomonadaceae, Dermabacteraceae, Micrococcaceae, Polyangiaceae, and Xanthomonadaceae—possess the uricase gene, while two families—Clostriadiaceae and Enterobacteriaceae—are capable of deaminating tyrosine into p-cresol [37]. These bacterial families are predominant in patients with ESKD. The high abundance of bacterial families possessing urease, uricase, and indole- and p-cresol-forming enzymes may hasten CKD progression by influencing the synthesis of uremic toxins [38]. Imbalances in the GM can lead to the heightened production of potentially harmful metabolites like indoxyl sulfate and p-cresyl sulfate, alongside increased permeability, and harm to the intestinal barrier. This damage to the barrier allows for greater exposure to uremic toxins and endotoxins [39]. The buildup of uremic toxins in the system exacerbates oxidative stress and inflammation, thereby fostering the onset of CKD [40].

In a recent systematic review, Stanford et al. highlighted that individuals with CKD demonstrate a decreased presence of the Prevotellaceae family and Roseburia genus, alongside an increase in potential pathobionts from the Enterobacteriaceae and Streptococcaceae families, as well as the *Enterococcus* genus, in comparison to healthy controls [41]. Additionally, considering kidney stones' role in CKD development and progression, they also explored the correlation between GM and nephrolithiasis, reporting that this condition is associated with a significant reduction in *Bifidobacterium* and *Faecalibacterium* taxa, while *Bacteroides* was more prevalent [41].

Ren et al. investigated variations in microbial structure across different stages of CKD [42]. Their analysis, using linear discriminant analysis (LDA), revealed that Tenericutes and Mollicutes were elevated in CKD stages 1–2, Parasutterella was enriched in CKD stages 3–4, and Akkermansia, Blautia, and Verrucomicrobia were increased in CKD stage 5 [42]. Additionally, adults undergoing hemodialysis or peritoneal dialysis exhibited higher levels of Alphaproteobacteria, Streptococcaceae, and Streptococcus compared to controls [41].

Figure 1 shows the key players in the gut–kidney axis.

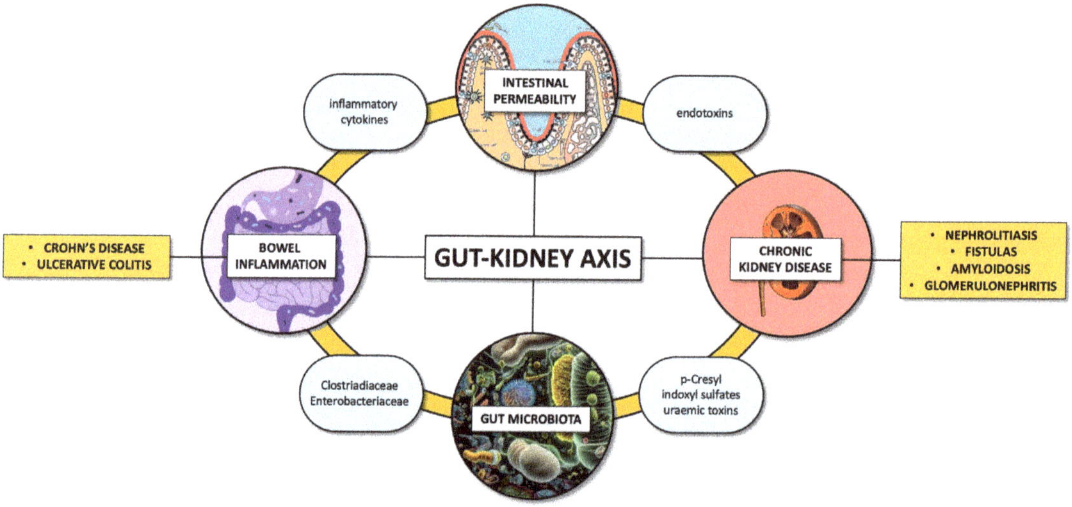

Figure 1. The gut–kidney axis: the link between IBD and CKD.

3. Renal Involvement in IBD

Single or multiple EIMs may manifest before or after the onset of intestinal symptoms or the formal diagnosis of IBD. These manifestations include systemic inflammatory, autoimmunity susceptibility, and metabolic and nutritional dysregulation. The appearance of EIMs in patients with IBD is reported with variable frequency (from 4 to 49%) based on variability in the definition of EIMs, the heterogeneity of sites affected by inflammation, and the potential simultaneous involvement of multiple sites [5]. While almost any organ can be impacted, the joints, skin, eyes, liver, and biliary tract are most frequently mentioned as sites of EIMs.

Surprisingly, kidney involvement, reported in early studies in nearly 25% of IBD patients, has received considerably less attention [8]. The most prevalent occurrences included nephrolithiasis, obstructive uropathy, the development of fistulas connecting the bowel and urinary tract, and renal parenchymal involvement in forms such as glomerulonephritis, tubulointerstitial nephritis, and amyloidoisis. Furthermore, the spread of advanced drugs for treating IBD, some associated with nephrotoxicity, may impact the incidence of renal involvement. Approximately 30–50% of patients with ulcerative colitis and around 15% of those with Crohn's disease are treated with 5-aminosalicylate (5-ASA), while anti-Tumor Necrosis Factor α (TNF-α) is prescribed to roughly 20–40% of IBD patients, especially those with moderate to severe disease. Both treatments have been associated with the development of progressive renal impairment.

3.1. Nephrolitiasis

Numerous studies demonstrate a heightened risk of nephrolithiasis in individuals with IBD compared to the general population [43]. The primary mechanisms leading to the formation of uric acid and calcium oxalate stones, two predominant types in IBD patients, involve diarrhea, malabsorption-related low urine volume and pH, and increased intestinal oxalate absorption-related hyperoxaluria. Additional mechanisms may contribute to the formation of oxalate stones. The bacterium *Oxalobacter formigenes* plays a role in degrading dietary oxalate, and its depletion in the gut can result in the increased absorption of oxalate. Administering *Oxalobacter* orally has been shown to reduce urinary oxalate concentration [44]. Low levels of antilithogenic substances such as magnesium and citrate in the urine also contribute to the formation of kidney stones in individuals with IBD [45]. Ideally, magnesium and citrate replacements should focus on normalizing urinary levels rather than serum levels [45]. Preventive measures include adopting a diet low in oxalate and fat, along with pyridoxine supplementation [46]. Oral cholestyramine, while increasing oxalate excretion, concurrently decreases citrate excretion [47]. The toxic effects of oxalate on renal epithelial and tubular cells can lead to oxalate nephropathy, characterized by persistent hyperoxaluria, and, in conjunction with stone formation, represents a significant but rare contributor to the development of CKD.

3.2. Fistulas

Crohn's disease (CD), affecting the entire thickness of the intestinal wall, increases the susceptibility to bowel perforation and the development of fistulas [48–50]. The adhesion of inflamed intestinal segments to the bladder wall can lead to erosion and the development of colo- and entero-vesical fistulas in 2% to 4% of individuals with CD [51]. The appearance of fistulas may be preceded by subacute small bowel obstruction, especially in the presence of coexisting intestinal strictures [52]. Entero-vesical fistulas often coincide with the development of intrapelvic abscesses. Clinical symptoms of entero-vesical fistulas may include air bubbles in urine (pneumaturia), urinary tract infections, and the presence of stool in urine (fecaluria) [53]. Diagnosing this condition is often difficult, necessitating a high level of clinical suspicion. Cases might present with non-specific symptoms like fever and abdominal discomfort, lacking typical signs. Early and collaborative consultations involving specialists—such as a gastroenterologist, surgeon, radiologist, and pathologist—are essential to devise an effective, personalized treatment strategy. Intestinal Ultrasound (IUS) has emerged as a valuable, non-invasive tool in detecting colo vesical fistulas, with the addition of an oral contrast potentially improving diagnostic accuracy [54]. Contrast enhanced CT scans, widely used in clinical settings, offer a rapid and sensitive method for identifying fistulas, though they expose patients to radiation, an important consideration for young IBD patients who require frequent imaging over time [55]. Alternatively, MRI provides a precise visualization of fistula tracts without radiation exposure, offering a superior soft tissue contrast to CT while maintaining high sensitivity and specificity. Comprehensive imaging, often using multiple modalities, is usually necessary, and management typically integrates both medical and surgical approaches.

3.3. Amyloidosis

Serum amyloid protein (SAA) amyloidosis, also known as secondary amyloidosis, is an uncommon complication of IBD. It is caused by an extracellular deposition of insoluble amyloid fibrils derived from circulating acute-phase reactant serum amyloid A protein, with renal involvement recognized as the most frequently fatal manifestation of IBD-associated amyloidosis [56]. SAA amyloidosis typically emerges relatively late in the natural course of IBD due to prolonged and chronic uncontrolled inflammation, and its renal involvement typically presents with a nephrotic syndrome [4]. With a diagnostic gold standard represented by the kidney biopsy, SAA amyloidosis is associated with a faster progression to an ESKD, leading to increased rates of infection, severe sepsis, and multi-organ system involvement, and thus to reduced patient survival [57]. For these reasons, patients with IBD should be routinely screened for proteinuria with urinary dipsticks and serial measurement of SAA concentration. However, in about 15% of cases, neither proteinuria nor elevated serum creatinine is found [56]. Since SAA amyloidosis is strictly related to prolonged and uncontrolled inflammation, treatment should be targeted to the underlying IBD activity to reduce the new deposition of SAA.

3.4. Glomerulonephritis

Glomerulonephritis is another uncommon complication of IBD. Although infrequent reports have brought into question whether there is a causal link, the onset of glomerulonephritis often coincides with an acute exacerbation of intestinal inflammation, with renal function improving through treatment of the underlying IBD. Various types of glomerulonephritis associated with IBD have been documented, encompassing IgAN, crescentic glomerulonephritis, focal segmental glomerulosclerosis, membranous glomerulonephritis, minimal change disease, membranoproliferative glomerulonephritis, and mesangiocapillary glomerulonephritis [58]. In a histopathological examination reviewing kidney biopsy results from 83 IBD patients (45 with CD; 38 with UC), IgAN emerged as the most prevalent diagnosis [58].

3.5. Nephrotoxicity

3.5.1. 5-ASA

The occurrence of nephrotoxicity linked to 5-ASA in IBD patients is uncommon and presents in an idiosyncratic manner, irrespective of the dosage, posing a challenge in establishing a definitive causal relationship explaining the numerous contradictory series reported in the literature. A genome-wide association study has established an association between human leukocyte antigen (HLA), particularly HLA-DRB1*03:01, and nephrotoxicity induced by 5-ASA [59]. Nephrotoxicity induced by 5-ASA typically occurs after a median treatment duration of three years, is more prevalent in males, and can manifest at any age. The most frequent histological observation is chronic tubulointerstitial nephritis. While uncommon, it is advisable to conduct an annual monitoring of renal function to identify nephrotoxicity associated with 5-ASA [12].

3.5.2. Immunosuppressants

Tacrolimus and ciclosporin, both calcineurin inhibitors, are widely utilized in medical practice, particularly to prevent rejection incidents following solid-organ transplants [60]. Ciclosporin, in addition, has a recognized application in managing acute severe UC. However, its use is limited by its high toxicity profile, particularly nephrotoxicity, which affects its overall safety [12,61]. The nephrotoxic effects associated with ciclosporin are believed to stem from vasoconstriction of the kidney's afferent arterioles, resulting in a reduced renal blood flow and lowered glomerular filtration rates [62]. Over time, this vasoconstriction may lead to chronic kidney damage, manifesting as interstitial fibrosis and a structural disruption of the arterioles [63].

3.5.3. Biologic Drugs

TNF-α inhibitors, such as infliximab, adalimumab, certolizumab pegol, and golimumab, are increasingly being used in the treatment of Crohn's Disease (CD) and Ulcerative Colitis (UC). There have been cases of infliximab-induced focal segmental glomerulosclerosis, which led to severe nephrotic syndrome in a UC patient [64]. The rise in novel therapeutic options for inflammatory bowel disease (IBD) has highlighted concerns regarding their toxicity and safety profiles. Vedolizumab (VDZ), a humanized monoclonal antibody targeting the $\alpha4\beta7$ integrin, is prescribed for moderate to severe cases of UC and CD. A case report associated VDZ with acute tubulointerstitial nephritis; however, renal function was fully restored with glucocorticoid treatment, and the re-administration of VDZ was well-tolerated [65]. Ustekinumab (USK), an anti-IL-23 biologic, is another treatment option for moderate to severe UC and CD. While there has been an isolated case linking it to nephrotic syndrome secondary to focal segmental glomerulosclerosis [66], recent real-world studies confirm its safety and efficacy as a long-term treatment, with no renal complications reported [67]. Tofacitinib (TOFA), the first oral Janus kinase (JAK) inhibitor approved for UC treatment, has previously been linked to an increase in serum creatinine, though its clinical impact remains unclear [68]. Other JAK inhibitors, like upadacitinib (UPA) and filgotinib (FILGO), show no nephrotoxic effects [69]; however, pharmacokinetic studies indicate that FILGO concentration increases in patients with an estimated glomerular filtration rate (eGFR) below 60 mL/min/1.73 m^2, prompting recommendations of dosage adjustments in such cases [70].

3.6. Dietary Factors

In patients with both IBD and CKD, dietary factors, such as oxalates, vitamin C, and caffeine, play a crucial role in disease management, influencing both gut and kidney health through a complex interplay of absorption, metabolism, and excretion.

The altered intestinal environment seen in IBD patients often leads to increased intestinal permeability and malabsorption, particularly of fats and bile acids. This malabsorption contributes to hyperoxaluria, where excess oxalate—derived from dietary sources or produced endogenously—accumulates in the body, significantly increasing the risk of calcium oxalate kidney stones [71]. In CKD, the role of oxalates becomes even more problematic. In CKD, gut dysbiosis can contribute to alterations in the metabolism of dietary components like oxalates. In this context, reduced *Oxalobacter formigenes* levels may impair oxalate degradation, potentially exacerbating calcium oxalate stone formation and renal damage [72].

Moreover, high doses of vitamin C—commonly used for its antioxidant properties—can exacerbate this condition because it metabolizes into oxalate, contributing further to the risk of oxalate nephropathy, particularly in CKD patients [73]. Therefore, while vitamin C is generally beneficial, excessive supplementation needs to be carefully monitored in these populations.

Caffeine consumption, often overlooked, also presents risks for both IBD and CKD patients. Caffeine has diuretic effects that can lead to dehydration, which increases urine concentration and enhances the risk of stone formation. Furthermore, caffeine increases calcium excretion in the urine, further compounding the risk of calcium oxalate stone formation in susceptible individuals [74]. While moderate caffeine intake is generally considered safe, in patients with IBD and CKD, particularly those prone to nephrolithiasis, careful regulation of caffeine consumption is advised.

Overall, managing the dietary intake of oxalates, vitamin C, and caffeine is essential in reducing the risk of complications such as kidney stones and further renal impairment in patients with comorbid IBD and CKD. Proper dietary interventions, including the restriction of high-oxalate foods and the cautious use of vitamin C supplements, alongside moderation of caffeine intake, are important strategies to minimize these risks and improve overall patient outcomes.

4. IgAN and IBD: Causation or Correlation?

IgAN is the most common primary glomerulonephritis, and it is characterized by a highly variable clinical presentation, ranging from microscopic haematuria to rapidly progressive glomerulonephritis and ESKD requiring chronic haemodialysis or kidney transplantation. The widely accepted pathogenesis of IgAN is the "multiple-hit hypothesis". Gut dysbiosis can compromise the integrity of the intestinal mucosal barrier, leading to the release of galactose-deficient IgA1 (Gd-IgA1) into the bloodstream [75]. Upon binding with specific antibodies, the IgA1 deposits in renal tissues, contributing to the development of IgAN [75]. In this process, gut dysbiosis plays a role as a potential "trigger point", being associated with increased gut permeability and aberrant immune responses, which may exacerbate kidney damage [75].

A recent study using metagenomic sequencing explored the characteristics and functional pathways of GM in patients with IgAN [76]. The findings revealed significant differences between IgAN patients and healthy controls. In the IgAN group, *E. coli* was notably more abundant compared to the control group ($p < 0.05$). Among patients with abnormal renal function, distinct microorganisms such as Enterococcaceae, *Moraxella*, and *Acinetobacter* were identified [76]. The study also demonstrated that the functional pathways of the gut microbiota that differed between IgAN patients and controls were primarily associated with bile acid metabolism [76].

Gleeson et al. explored how the GM, particularly *A. muciniphila* (a mucin-degrading bacterium), contributes to IgAN [77]. In humans and mice, *A. muciniphila* deglycosylated human IgA1, enabling it to travel from the gut to kidney glomeruli via circulation, causing autoimmune kidney disease [77]. Mice with human IgA1 and Fc α receptor I developed IgA nephropathy when colonized by *A. muciniphila*. In humans, the protective correlation between α-defensin 6 and *A. muciniphila* was lost in IgA nephropathy patients. Additionally, *A. muciniphila*-modified IgA1 was recognized by autoantibodies in patient sera, highlighting its role in disease pathogenesis [77].

A kidney biopsy series established the association between IgAN and IBD [78]. Therefore, there is a need to precisely understand the pathophysiological mechanisms underlying the various phenotypical manifestations to improve clinical and therapeutic management. More recently, some studies have shed light on the possible role of the gut–kidney axis in IgAN pathogenesis, with particular attention being paid to IBD. Patients with IBD showed IgAN as the most frequent abnormal finding upon kidney biopsy (24%), with a significantly higher prevalence compared to patients without IBD (8%, $p < 0.001$), which may reflect a common pathogenic mechanism between IgAN and IBD. This was also supported by a Swedish population-based cohort study, which demonstrated that patients with IgAN have a higher risk of developing IBD and that IgAN in IBD patients is more likely to progress to ESKD than in patients with isolated IgAN [79].

IgAN is considered as an immune-mediated disease influenced by a combination of genetic and environmental factors. The typical pathological feature is the development of immune complexes of galactose-deficient IgA1 (Gd-IgA1) which cannot be cleared from the circulation and thus deposit in the glomerular mesangium, potentially activating the complement system and triggering inflammation [80]. The development of immune complexes is found to be a heritable trait [81] and genome-wide association study (GWAS) data sets have identified multiple susceptibility loci for IgAN along with several risk alleles associated with intestinal epithelial barrier maintenance and mucosal immunity [82–84]. Some of the loci involved in IgAN, such as CARD9 or HORMAD2, are shared with IBD [85,86], and have also been associated with immune-mediated diseases, such as Systemic Lupus Erythematosus (SLE) [87].

Two specific single-nucleotide polymorphisms (SNPs), namely rs4151657 and rs549182, have been linked to IgAN [88]. The SNP rs4151657 is found within the intron of the complement factor B (CFB) gene, which is crucial for initiating the alternative complement pathway, thought to be a primary mechanism in IgAN development. Studies suggest that CFB is locally elevated in colonic biopsies from patients with IBD [89–91]. Additionally, these patients exhibit signs of complementary activation within the intestinal mucosa and increased circulating complement factors. This finding supports the idea that alternative pathway activation in IBD, coupled with the release of complement components and inflammatory mediators into the bloodstream, may contribute to IgAN. Abnormalities in IgA, such as irregular glycosylation, self-aggregation, receptor shedding, or the formation of immune complexes (ICs) with dietary antigens, are known to trigger inflammatory conditions impacting both the intestines and kidneys. Furthermore, LIGHT, an essential molecule for the activation of T cells that migrate to the gut, may provoke intense gut inflammation and IgA deposits in the kidneys, potentially contributing to IBD, IgAN, and even celiac disease [92,93].

On the other hand, the SNP rs549182 is mapped to the NOTCH4 gene and was found to be correlated to the process of glomerulosclerosis, which occurs in IgAN [94]. Since it is involved in cell proliferation, inflammation, and innate immunity, the Notch receptor family and signaling pathways are also involved in the development of IBD. Moreover, in patients with IgAN, advanced glomerulosclerosis and tubulointerstitial changes were found to be more severe in patients with IBD than in patients without IBD [95], leading to the hypothesis that IBD can promote inflammation in IgAN. In fact, patients with IBD are more exposed to nephrotoxicity due to the risk of dehydration, which can activate the renin–angiotensin–aldosterone system involved in glomerular ischemia and interstitial fibrosis, and due to the systemic inflammation characterized by the production of IL-23 and TNF-α, which could contribute to the exacerbation of tubulointerstitial lesions in IgAN. Additionally, it has been reported that CD16+ macrophages may contribute to intestinal fibrosis [96], as well as abnormal B cell activation [97], which can also play a role in interstitial inflammation in CKD, including IgAN [98]. Recently, it was found that IBD and IgAN share some changes in SDEGs, miRNAs and SIRGs, which are involved in the T cell receptor (TCR) pathway, related to humoral immunity, leading to the activation and differentiation of CD4+ T cells. Moreover, it was found that these SDEGs and SIRGs were related to the differentiation of Th17 cells, which cause autoimmunity and inflammation, promote the immune response, and activate various inflammatory pathways through the IL-17 signaling pathway. Therefore, infections and other factors can up-regulate the expression of Th17 cells and Th17-related cytokines in mucosal immunity, inducing or aggravating IgAN and IBD. This may represent not only a common pathogenetic mechanism but also a potential therapeutic target [99]. Moreover, SDEGs and SIRGs are both associated with the regulation of inflammatory mediators of transient receptor potential (TRP) channels. These channels are distributed throughout the gastrointestinal tract and play a role in intestinal inflammation. TRP channels are expressed in immune cells and contribute to the immune response by activating macrophages and CD4+T cells. Several studies have implicated them in the immune pathogenesis of IBD [100,101]. Therefore, the modulation of TRP channels, either through inhibition or activation, could be a therapeutic strategy for intestinal inflammation [99]. Additionally, since inhibiting TRP channel-related genes, such as TRPC5, could protect podocytes in the kidney and prevent kidney failure, TRP channels may also emerge as promising targets for the prevention and treatment of both IgAN and IBD [102].

Table 1 shows the main studies that explored the relationship between IBD and IgAN [16,17,101,103,104].

Table 1. Main studies that explored the relationship between IBD and IgAN.

Author, Year	Study Design	Study Population	Intervention	Outcomes	Key Findings
Xiao et al., 2022 [103]	Mendelian randomization (MR) study	The summary statistics of exposures included IBD (N = 31,665 cases and 33,977 controls), UC (N = 6,968 cases and 20,464 controls), and CD (N = 5956 cases and 14,927 controls). For IgAN, the GWAS summary statistics included 977 subjects with IgAN and 4980 disease-free controls	In this two-sample MR study, significant and independent single-nucleotide polymorphisms (SNPs) were chosen as IVs to clarify the causal association at the genetic level using the GWAS data	Clarify if IBD, UC, and CD have a potential causal effect on IgAN and whether a reverse causal effect exists	The results of this two-sample MR analysis suggested that IBD, UC, and CD were causally associated with the risk of IgAN, while there was no sufficient evidence for the causal effect of IgAN on IBD, UC, or CD

Table 1. *Cont.*

Author, Year	Study Design	Study Population	Intervention	Outcomes	Key Findings
Qing et al., 2022 [101]	Case-control study	45UC patients (adults), 47CD patients (adults) and 47 healthy controls (adults). 12IgAN patients and 8 healthy controls	The differential expression analysis and weighted gene co-expression network analysis (WGCNA) were conducted on gene expression data of IgAN, UC and CD, which were obtained from the Gene Expression Omnibus (GEO)	Focusing on the genetic effects and abnormal immunity in IgAN and IBD	This work revealed that the differentiation of Th17 cells may mediate the abnormal humoral immunity in IgAN and IBD patients and identified novel gene candidates that could be used as biomarkers or potential therapeutic targets
Nurmi et al., 2021 [104]	Retrospective study	629 patients with newly diagnosed IgAN during the years 1976–2012	Data on diagnosis of IBD and celiac disease were retrospectively collected from medical records. Further, to detect unrecognized celiac disease, IgA-class tissue transglutaminase antibodies (tTGA) were measured from serum samples taken at the time of kidney biopsy during years 1980–2012 (defined as screen-detected celiac disease autoimmunity)	Studying the prevalence of IBD and celiac disease in IgAN patients over time	The prevalence of IBD increased over time in IgAN patients, which exceeds the prevalence of 0.6% in the Finnish general population
Lian et al., 2023 [16]	Mendelian randomization (MR) study	They selected a group of single-nucleotide polymorphisms (SNPs) specific to IBD as instrumental variables from a published genome-wide association study (GWAS) with 86,640 individuals of European ancestry	Summary statistics for multiple kidney diseases were obtained from the publicly available GWAS. Genetic data from one GWAS involving 210 extensive T-cell traits were used to estimate the mediating effect on specific kidney disease	Examining the causal association between genetically predicted IBD and the risk of multiple kidney diseases. Evaluating which type of kidney disease primarily reflects this causal relationship	This study provides genetic evidence supporting a positive causal association between IBD, including its subclassification as ulcerative colitis and Crohn's disease, and the risk of IgAN. However, no causal association was found between IBD and other types of kidney diseases

Table 1. *Cont.*

Author, Year	Study Design	Study Population	Intervention	Outcomes	Key Findings
Joher et al., 2021 [17]	Retrospective multicentre study	24 patients with biopsy-proven IgAN occurring in a context of CD or UC	These patients were compared with 134 patients with primary biopsy-proven IgAN and 19 patients with IBD-associated IgAN identified through a systematic literature review	Assessing the clinical significance of the association between IgAN and IBD by reviewing clinical, histological and therapeutic data and outcomes for patients with IgAN occurring in a context of CD or UC	IBD-associated IgAN has frequent inflammatory lesions at onset and variable long-term outcomes. Interestingly, the IgAN diagnosis was not associated with IBD flare. TNF-α blockade had no impact on the presentation and course of IBD-IgAN

5. Conclusions

Renal involvement in IBD is often underestimated, despite its affecting nearly a quarter of patients. Emerging research highlights the gut–kidney axis as an influential factor in nephropathy development, particularly through its impact on systemic inflammation and metabolite homeostasis. Dysbiosis-induced systemic inflammation may exacerbate renal involvement in IBD, although the causality of this remains under investigation. Notably, IgAN stands out as an immune-mediated condition influenced by both genetic and environmental factors. Studies indicate that patients with IgAN have a higher risk of developing IBD, and when IgAN co-occurs with IBD, there is an increased likelihood of progression to ESKD, suggesting a pathogenic link between these conditions through the gut–kidney axis. Among IBD treatments, certain drugs, such as 5-ASA and anti-TNF-α agents, may increase the risk of renal complications, whereas other biologics and small molecules show minimal nephrotoxic effects. Thus, the careful selection and monitoring of therapies are essential to mitigate potential renal risks in IBD patients. Future research should focus on understanding the detailed mechanisms of the gut–kidney axis and developing targeted therapies to improve the outcomes of patients with IBD and nephropathies.

Author Contributions: Conceptualization, R.d.S. and F.C.; writing—original draft preparation, R.d.S., A.L.M. and L.B.; writing—review and editing, R.d.S. and A.T.; visualization, A.D.G., A.R. and O.M.N.; supervision, F.C. All authors have read and agreed to the published version of the manuscript.

Funding: This research received no external funding.

Institutional Review Board Statement: Not applicable.

Informed Consent Statement: Not applicable.

Data Availability Statement: Not applicable.

Conflicts of Interest: The authors declare no conflicts of interest.

References

1. Hedin, C.R.H.; Vavricka, S.R.; Stagg, A.J.; Schoepfer, A.; Raine, T.; Puig, L.; Pleyer, U.; Navarini, A.; van der Meulen-de Jong, A.E.; Maul, J.; et al. The Pathogenesis of Extraintestinal Manifestations: Implications for IBD Research, Diagnosis, and Therapy. *J. Crohn's Colitis* **2019**, *13*, 541–554. [CrossRef] [PubMed]
2. van Sommeren, S.; Janse, M.; Karjalainen, J.; Fehrmann, R.; Franke, L.; Fu, J.; Weersma, R.K. Extraintestinal Manifestations and Complications in Inflammatory Bowel Disease: From Shared Genetics to Shared Biological Pathways. *Inflamm. Bowel Dis.* **2014**, *20*, 987–994. [CrossRef]
3. Gordon, H.; Burisch, J.; Ellul, P.; Karmiris, K.; Katsanos, K.; Allocca, M.; Bamias, G.; Acosta, M.B.-D.; Braithwaite, T.; Greuter, T.; et al. ECCO Guidelines on Extraintestinal Manifestations in Inflammatory Bowel Disease. *J. Crohns Colitis* **2024**, *18*, 1–37. [CrossRef] [PubMed]

4. Kumar, S.; Pollok, R.; Goldsmith, D. Renal and Urological Disorders Associated with Inflammatory Bowel Disease. *Inflamm. Bowel Dis.* **2023**, *29*, 1306–1316. [CrossRef]
5. Rogler, G.; Singh, A.; Kavanaugh, A.; Rubin, D.T. Extraintestinal Manifestations of Inflammatory Bowel Disease: Current Concepts, Treatment, and Implications for Disease Management. *Gastroenterology* **2021**, *161*, 1118–1132. [CrossRef]
6. Rothfuss, K.S.; Stange, E.F.; Herrlinger, K.R. Extraintestinal Manifestations and Complications in Inflammatory Bowel Diseases. *World J. Gastroenterol.* **2006**, *12*, 4819–4831. [CrossRef]
7. Adams, D.H.; Eksteen, B. Aberrant Homing of Mucosal T Cells and Extraintestinal Manifestations of Inflammatory Bowel Disease. *Nat. Rev. Immunol.* **2006**, *6*, 244–251. [CrossRef] [PubMed]
8. Shield, D.E.; Lytton, B.; Weiss, R.M.; Schiff, M., Jr. Urologic Complications of Inflammatory Bowel Disease. *J. Urol.* **1976**, *115*, 701–706. [CrossRef]
9. Greenstein, A.J.; Janowitz, H.D.; Sachar, D.B. The Extra-intestinal Complications of Crohn's Disease and Ulcerative Colitis: A Study of 700 Patients. *Medicine* **1976**, *55*, 401–412. [CrossRef]
10. Angeletti, A.; Arrigo, S.; Madeo, A.; Molteni, M.; Vietti, E.; Arcuri, L.; Coccia, M.C.; Gandullia, P.; Ghiggeri, G.M. Different Renal Manifestations Associated with Very Early Onset Pediatric Inflammatory Bowel Disease: Case Report and Review of Literature. *BMC Nephrol.* **2021**, *22*, 146. [CrossRef]
11. Corica, D.; Romano, C. Renal Involvement in Inflammatory Bowel Diseases. *J. Crohns Colitis* **2016**, *10*, 226–235. [CrossRef] [PubMed]
12. Lamb, C.A.; Kennedy, N.A.; Raine, T.; Hendy, P.A.; Smith, P.J.; Limdi, J.K.; Hayee, B.H.; Lomer, M.C.E.; Parkes, G.C.; Selinger, C.; et al. British Society of Gastroenterology Consensus Guidelines on the Management of Inflammatory Bowel Disease in Adults. *Gut* **2019**, *68* (Suppl. S3), s1–s106. [CrossRef] [PubMed]
13. Heaf, J.G.; Sørensen, S.S.; Hansen, A. Increased Incidence and Improved Prognosis of Glomerulonephritis: A National 30-Year Study. *Clin. Kidney J.* **2020**, *14*, 1594–1602. [CrossRef]
14. Doumas, S.A.; Tsironis, C.; Bolaji, A.A.; Garantziotis, P.; Frangou, E. Glomerulonephritis and Inflammatory Bowel Disease: A Tale of Gut-Kidney Axis Dysfunction. *Autoimmun. Rev.* **2023**, *22*, 103327. [CrossRef]
15. Yan, Q.; Zhao, Z.; Liu, D.; Li, J.; Pan, S.; Duan, J.; Liu, Z. Novel Immune Cross-talk between Inflammatory Bowel Disease and IgA Nephropathy. *Ren Fail.* **2024**, *46*, 2337288. [CrossRef]
16. Lian, X.; Wang, Y.; Wang, S.; Peng, X.; Wang, Y.; Huang, Y.; Chen, W. Does Inflammatory Bowel Disease Promote Kidney Diseases: A Mendelian Randomization Study with Populations of European Ancestry. *BMC Med. Genom.* **2023**, *16*, 225. [CrossRef]
17. Joher, N.; Gosset, C.; Guerrot, D.; Pillebout, E.; Hummel, A.; Boffa, J.J.; Faguer, S.; Rabant, M.; Higgins, S.; Moktefi, A.; et al. Immunoglobulin A Nephropathy in Association with Inflammatory Bowel Diseases: Results from a National Study and Systematic Literature Review. *Nephrol. Dial. Transplant.* **2022**, *37*, 531–539. [CrossRef] [PubMed]
18. De Sire, R.; Talocco, C.; Petito, V. Microbiota and Inflammatory Bowel Disease: An Update. *Recenti Prog. Med.* **2018**, *109*, 570–573. [CrossRef]
19. Nardone, O.M.; de Sire, R.; Petito, V.; Testa, A.; Villani, G.; Scaldaferri, F.; Castiglione, F. Inflammatory Bowel Diseases and Sarcopenia: The Role of Inflammation and Gut Microbiota in the Development of Muscle Failure. *Front. Immunol.* **2021**, *12*, 694217. [CrossRef]
20. Sokol, H.; Pigneur, B.; Watterlot, L.; Lakhdari, O.; Bermúdez-Humarán, L.G.; Gratadoux, J.J.; Blugeon, S.; Bridonneau, C.; Furet, J.P.; Corthier, G.; et al. Faecalibacterium prausnitzii is an Anti-inflammatory Commensal Bacterium Identified by Gut Microbiota Analysis of Crohn Disease Patients. *Proc. Natl. Acad. Sci. USA* **2008**, *105*, 16731–16736. [CrossRef]
21. Qiu, X.; Zhang, M.; Yang, X.; Hong, N.; Yu, C. Faecalibacterium prausnitzii Upregulates Regulatory T Cells and Anti-inflammatory Cytokines in Treating TNBS-induced Colitis. *J. Crohns Colitis* **2013**, *7*, e558–e568. [CrossRef] [PubMed]
22. Martín, R.; Chain, F.; Miquel, S.; Lu, J. The Commensal Bacterium Faecalibacterium prausnitzii is Protective in DNBS-induced Chronic Moderate and Severe Colitis Models. *Inflamm. Bowel Dis.* **2014**, *20*, 417–430. [CrossRef]
23. Graziani, C.; Gasbarrini, A.; Scaldaferri, F.; Talocco, C.; Sire, R.; Petito, V.; Lopetuso, L.R.; Gervasoni, J.; Persichilli, S.; Franceschi, F.; et al. Intestinal Permeability in Physiological and Pathological Conditions: Major Determinants and Assessment Modalities. *Eur. Rev. Med. Pharmacol. Sci.* **2019**, *23*, 795–810. [CrossRef]
24. Mielcarek, C.; Romond, P.C.; Romond, M.B.; Bezirtzoglou, E. Modulation of Bacterial Translocation in Mice Mediated through Lactose and Human Milk Oligosaccharides. *Anaerobe* **2011**, *17*, 361–366. [CrossRef] [PubMed]
25. Berg, R.D. Bacterial Translocation from the Gastrointestinal Tract. *Adv. Exp. Med. Biol.* **1999**, *473*, 11–30. [CrossRef] [PubMed]
26. Gebbers, J.O.; Laissue, J.A. Bacterial Translocation in the Normal Human Appendix Parallels the Development of the Local Immune System. *Ann. N. Y. Acad. Sci.* **2004**, *1029*, 337–343. [CrossRef]
27. Stavropoulou, E.; Kantartzi, K.; Tsigalou, C.; Konstantinidis, T.; Romanidou, G.; Voidarou, C.; Bezirtzoglou, E. Focus on the Gut-Kidney Axis in Health and Disease. *Front. Med.* **2021**, *7*, 620102. [CrossRef]
28. Tan, D.S.Y.; Akelew, Y.; Snelson, M.; Nguyen, J.; O'Sullivan, K.M. Unravelling the Link between the Gut Microbiome and Autoimmune Kidney Diseases: A Potential New Therapeutic Approach. *Int. J. Mol. Sci.* **2024**, *25*, 4817. [CrossRef]
29. Cabała, S.; Ożgo, M.; Herosimczyk, A. The Kidney-Gut Axis as a Novel Target for Nutritional Intervention to Counteract Chronic Kidney Disease Progression. *Metabolites* **2024**, *14*, 78. [CrossRef]
30. Mafra, D.; Borges, N.; Alvarenga, L.; Esgalhado, M.; Cardozo, L.; Lindholm, B.; Stenvinkel, P. Dietary Components That May Influence the Disturbed Gut Microbiota in Chronic Kidney Disease. *Nutrients* **2019**, *11*, 496. [CrossRef]

31. Thursby, E.; Juge, N. Introduction to the Human Gut Microbiota. *Biochem. J.* **2017**, *474*, 1823–1836. [CrossRef] [PubMed]
32. Lin, L.; Zhang, J. Role of Intestinal Microbiota and Metabolites on Gut Homeostasis and Human Diseases. *BMC Immunol.* **2017**, *18*, 2. [CrossRef]
33. Huang, H.W.; Chen, M.J. Exploring the Preventive and Therapeutic Mechanisms of Probiotics in Chronic Kidney Disease through the Gut-Kidney Axis. *J. Agric. Food Chem.* **2024**, *72*, 8347–8364. [CrossRef]
34. Cosola, C.; Rocchetti, M.T.; Sabatino, A.; Fiaccadori, E.; Di Iorio, B.R.; Gesualdo, L. Microbiota Issue in CKD: How Promising Are Gut-targeted Approaches? *J. Nephrol.* **2019**, *32*, 27–37. [CrossRef] [PubMed]
35. Magliocca, G.; Mone, P.; Di Iorio, B.R.; Heidland, A.; Marzocco, S. Short-Chain Fatty Acids in Chronic Kidney Disease: Focus on Inflammation and Oxidative Stress Regulation. *Int. J. Mol. Sci.* **2022**, *23*, 5354. [CrossRef]
36. Lambert, K.; Rinninella, E.; Biruete, A.; Sumida, K.; Stanford, J.; Raoul, P.; Mele, M.C.; Wang, A.Y.; Mafra, D. Targeting the Gut Microbiota in Kidney Disease: The Future in Renal Nutrition and Metabolism. *J. Ren. Nutr.* **2023**, *33* (Suppl. S6), S30–S39. [CrossRef]
37. Wong, J.; Piceno, Y.M.; DeSantis, T.Z.; Pahl, M.; Andersen, G.L.; Vaziri, N.D. Expansion of Urease- and Uricase-Containing, Indole- and p-Cresol-Forming Intestinal Microbiota in ESRD. *Am. J. Nephrol.* **2014**, *39*, 230–237. [CrossRef] [PubMed]
38. Lin, X.; Liang, W.; Li, L.; Xiong, Q.; He, S.; Zhao, J.; Guo, X.; Xiang, S.; Zhang, P.; Wang, H.; et al. The Accumulation of Gut Microbiome-derived Indoxyl Sulfate and p-Cresyl Sulfate in Patients with End-Stage Renal Disease. *J. Ren. Nutr.* **2022**, *32*, 578–586. [CrossRef]
39. Liu, W.C.; Tomino, Y.; Lu, K.C. Impacts of Indoxyl Sulfate and p-Cresol Sulfate on Chronic Kidney Disease and Mitigating Effects of AST-120. *Toxins* **2018**, *10*, 367. [CrossRef]
40. Rysz, J.; Franczyk, B.; Ławiński, J.; Olszewski, R.; Ciałkowska-Rysz, A.; Gluba-Brzózka, A. The Impact of CKD on Uremic Toxins and Gut Microbiota. *Toxins* **2021**, *13*, 252. [CrossRef]
41. Stanford, J.; Charlton, K.; Stefoska-Needham, A.; Ibrahim, R.; Lambert, K. The Gut Microbiota Profile of Adults with Kidney Disease and Kidney Stones: A Systematic Review of the Literature. *BMC Nephrol.* **2020**, *21*, 215. [CrossRef] [PubMed]
42. Ren, Z.; Fan, Y.; Li, A.; Shen, Q.; Wu, J.; Ren, L.; Lu, H.; Ding, S.; Ren, H.; Liu, C.; et al. Alterations of the Human Gut Microbiome in Chronic Kidney Disease. *Adv. Sci.* **2020**, *7*, 2001936. [CrossRef] [PubMed]
43. Parks, J.H.; Worcester, E.M.; O'Connor, R.C.; Coe, F.L. Urine Stone Risk Factors in Nephrolithiasis Patients with and without Bowel Disease. *Kidney Int.* **2003**, *63*, 255–265. [CrossRef]
44. Parmar, M.S. Kidney Stones. *BMJ* **2004**, *328*, 1420–1424. [CrossRef] [PubMed]
45. McConnell, N.; Campbell, S.; Gillanders, I.; Rolton, H.; Danesh, B. Risk Factors for Developing Renal Stones in Inflammatory Bowel Disease. *BJU Int.* **2002**, *89*, 835–841. [CrossRef]
46. Nazzal, L.; Puri, S.; Goldfarb, D.S. Enteric Hyperoxaluria: An Important Cause of End-stage Kidney Disease. *Nephrol. Dial. Transplant.* **2016**, *31*, 375–382. [CrossRef]
47. Nordenvall, B.; Backman, L.; Burman, P.; Larsson, L.; Tiselius, H.G. Low-oxalate, Low-fat Dietary Regimen in Hyperoxaluria Following Jejunoileal Bypass. *Acta Chir. Scand.* **1983**, *149*, 89–91.
48. Rispo, A. David Against Goliath: Direct Comparison of Handheld Bowel Sonography and Magnetic Resonance Enterography for Diagnosis of Crohn's Disease. *Inflamm. Bowel Dis.* **2023**, *29*, 563–569. [CrossRef]
49. Levy, C.; Tremaine, W.J. Management of Internal Fistulas in Crohn's Disease. *Inflamm. Bowel Dis.* **2002**, *8*, 106–111. [CrossRef]
50. Castiglione, F. Exploring the Concept of Deep Remission in Crohn's Disease: Correlation between Transmural Healing and Biomarkers. *Therap. Adv. Gastroenterol.* **2022**, *15*, 17562848221110643. [CrossRef]
51. Taxonera, C.; Barreiro-de-Acosta, M.; Bastida, G.; Martinez-Gonzalez, J.; Merino, O.; García-Sánchez, V.; Gisbert, J.P.; Marín-Jiménez, I.; López-Serrano, P. Outcomes of Medical and Surgical Therapy for Entero-urinary Fistulas in Crohn's Disease. *J. Crohns Colitis* **2016**, *10*, 657–662. [CrossRef] [PubMed]
52. Keady, C.; Hechtl, D.; Joyce, M. When the Bowel Meets the Bladder: Optimal Management of Colorectal Pathology with Urological Involvement. *World J. Gastrointest. Surg.* **2020**, *12*, 208–225. [CrossRef] [PubMed]
53. Gruner, J.S.; Sehon, J.K.; Johnson, L.W. Diagnosis and Management of Enterovesical Fistulas in Patients with Crohn's Disease. *Am. Surg.* **2002**, *68*, 714–719. [CrossRef]
54. Maconi, G.; Sampietro, G.M.; Parente, F.; Pompili, G.; Russo, A.; Cristaldi, M.; Arborio, G.; Ardizzone, S.; Matacena, G.; Taschieri, A.M.; et al. Contrast Radiology, Computed Tomography, and Ultrasonography in Detecting Internal Fistulas and Intra-abdominal Abscesses in Crohn's Disease: A Prospective Comparative Study. *Am. J. Gastroenterol.* **2003**, *98*, 1545–1555. [CrossRef]
55. Rao, N.; Kumar, S.; Taylor, S.; Plumb, A. Diagnostic Pathways in Crohn's Disease. *Clin. Radiol.* **2019**, *74*, 578–591. [CrossRef]
56. Tosca Cuquerella, J.; Bosca-Watts, M.M.; Anton Ausejo, R.; Tejedor Alonso, S.; Mora De Miguel, F.; Minguez Perez, M. Amyloidosis in Inflammatory Bowel Disease: A Systematic Review of Epidemiology, Clinical Features, and Treatment. *J. Crohns Colitis* **2016**, *10*, 1245–1253. [CrossRef]
57. Sharma, P.; Aguilar, R.; Siddiqui, O.A.; Nader, M.A. Secondary Systemic Amyloidosis in Inflammatory Bowel Disease: A Nation-wide Analysis. *Ann. Gastroenterol.* **2017**, *30*, 504–511. [CrossRef] [PubMed]
58. Ambruzs, J.M.; Larsen, C.P. Renal Manifestations of Inflammatory Bowel Disease. *Rheum. Dis. Clin. N. Am.* **2018**, *44*, 699–714. [CrossRef] [PubMed]

59. Heap, G.A.; So, K.; Weedon, M.; Edney, N.; Bewshea, C.; Singh, A.; Annese, V.; Beckly, J.; Buurman, D.; Chaudhary, R. Clinical Features and HLA Association of 5-Aminosalicylate (5-ASA)-Induced Nephrotoxicity in Inflammatory Bowel Disease. *J. Crohns Colitis* **2016**, *10*, 149–158. [CrossRef]
60. Naesens, M.; Kuypers, D.R.; Sarwal, M. Calcineurin Inhibitor Nephrotoxicity. *Clin. J. Am. Soc. Nephrol.* **2009**, *4*, 481–508. [CrossRef]
61. Van Assche, G.; D'Haens, G.; Noman, M.; Vermeire, S.; Hiele, M.; Asnong, K.; Arts, J.; D'Hoore, A.; Penninckx, F.; Rutgeerts, P. Randomized, Double-Blind Comparison of 4 mg/kg versus 2 mg/kg Intravenous Cyclosporine in Severe Ulcerative Colitis. *Gastroenterology* **2003**, *125*, 1025–1031. [CrossRef] [PubMed]
62. Ciarcia, R.; Damiano, S.; Florio, A.; Spagnuolo, M.; Zacchia, E.; Squillacioti, C.; Mirabella, N.; Florio, S.; Pagnini, U.; Garofano, T.; et al. The Protective Effect of Apocynin on Cyclosporine A-induced Hypertension and Nephrotoxicity in Rats. *J. Cell. Biochem.* **2015**, *116*, 1848–1856. [CrossRef] [PubMed]
63. Burdmann, E.A.; Andoh, T.F.; Yu, L.; Bennett, W.M. Cyclosporine Nephrotoxicity. *Semin. Nephrol.* **2003**, *23*, 465–476. [CrossRef] [PubMed]
64. Dumitrescu, G.; Dahan, K.; Treton, X.; Corcos, O.; Bouhnik, Y.; Stefanescu, C. Nephrotic Syndrome after Infliximab Treatment in a Patient with Ulcerative Colitis. *J. Gastrointestin. Liver Dis.* **2015**, *24*, 249–251. [CrossRef]
65. Bailly, E.; Von Tokarski, F.; Beau-Salinas, F.; Picon, L.; Miquelestorena-Standley, E.; Rousseau, G.; Jonville-Bera, A.P.; Halimi, J.M. Interstitial Nephritis Secondary to Vedolizumab Treatment in Crohn Disease and Safe Rechallenge Using Steroids: A Case Report. *Am. J. Kidney Dis.* **2018**, *71*, 142–145. [CrossRef]
66. Pérez Fernández, M.; Piteiro Bermejo, A.B.; Peña Esparragoza, J.K.; Blasco Martínez, A.; Aracil Moreno, I.; Mancha Ramos, J.; Moreno Barrio, F. Nephrotic Syndrome in Relation to Treatment with Ustekinumab. *Nefrologia* **2019**, *39*, 100–102. [CrossRef]
67. Chaparro, M.; Baston-Rey, I.; Fernández-Salgado, E.; González García, J.; Ramos, L.; Diz-Lois Palomares, M.T.; Argüelles-Arias, F.; Flores, E.I.; Cabello, M.; Iturria, S.R.; et al. Long-Term Real-World Effectiveness and Safety of Ustekinumab in Crohn's Disease Patients: The SUSTAIN Study. *Inflamm. Bowel Dis.* **2022**, *28*, 1725–1736. [CrossRef]
68. Kremer, J.M.; Kivitz, A.J.; Simon-Campos, J.A.; Nasonov, E.L.; Tony, H.P.; Lee, S.K.; Vlahos, B.; Hammond, C.; Bukowski, J.; Li, H.; et al. Evaluation of the Effect of Tofacitinib on Measured Glomerular Filtration Rate in Patients with Active Rheumatoid Arthritis: Results from a Randomized Controlled Trial. *Arthritis Res. Ther.* **2015**, *17*, 95. [CrossRef]
69. Mohamed, M.F.; Trueman, S.; Feng, T.; Anderson, J.; Marbury, T.C.; Othman, A.A. Characterization of the Effect of Renal Impairment on Upadacitinib Pharmacokinetics. *J. Clin. Pharmacol.* **2019**, *59*, 856–862. [CrossRef]
70. D'Amico, F.; Magro, F.; Peyrin-Biroulet, L.; Danese, S. Positioning Filgotinib in the Treatment Algorithm of Moderate to Severe Ulcerative Colitis. *J. Crohns Colitis* **2022**, *16*, 835–844. [CrossRef]
71. Torricelli, F.C.; Reichard, C.; Monga, M. Urolithiasis in Complicated Inflammatory Bowel Disease: A Comprehensive Analysis of Urine Profile and Stone Composition. *Int. Urol. Nephrol.* **2021**, *53*, 205–209. [CrossRef] [PubMed]
72. Fernandez-Prado, R.; Esteras, R.; Perez-Gomez, M.V.; Gracia-Iguacel, C.; Gonzalez-Parra, E.; Sanz, A.B.; Ortiz, A.; Sanchez-Niño, M.D. Nutrients Turned into Toxins: Microbiota Modulation of Nutrient Properties in Chronic Kidney Disease. *Nutrients* **2017**, *9*, 489. [CrossRef] [PubMed]
73. Kędzierska-Kapuza, K.; Szczuko, U.; Stolińska, H.; Bakaloudi, D.R.; Wierzba, W.; Szczuko, M. Demand for Water-Soluble Vitamins in a Group of Patients with CKD versus Interventions and Supplementation—A Systematic Review. *Nutrients* **2023**, *15*, 860. [CrossRef] [PubMed]
74. Kikut, J.; Konecka, N.; Ziętek, M.; Kulpa, D.; Szczuko, M. Diet Supporting Therapy for Inflammatory Bowel Diseases. *Eur. J. Nutr.* **2021**, *60*, 2275–2291. [CrossRef] [PubMed]
75. Zhi, W.; Li, A.; Wang, Q.; Yuan, X.; Qing, J.; Zhang, C.; Wang, Y.; Li, Y. Safety and Efficacy of Fecal Microbiota Transplantation as an Adjunctive Treatment for IgA Nephropathy: An Exploratory Clinical Trial. *Sci. Rep.* **2024**, *14*, 22935. [CrossRef]
76. Deng, Y.; Nong, Z.; Wei, M.; Xu, Y.; Luo, Y.; Li, X.; Zhao, R.; Yang, Z.; Pan, L. Characteristics and Function of the Gut Microbiota in Patients with IgA Nephropathy Investigated Using Metagenomic Sequencing Technology. *Ren. Fail.* **2024**, *46*, 2393754. [CrossRef]
77. Gleeson, P.J.; Benech, N.; Chemouny, J.; Metallinou, E.; Berthelot, L.; da Silva, J.; Bex-Coudrat, J.; Boedec, E.; Canesi, F.; Boumaix, C.; et al. The Gut Microbiota Post-Translationally Modifies IgA1 in Autoimmune Glomerulonephritis. *Sci. Transl. Med.* **2024**, *16*, eadl6149. [CrossRef]
78. Ambruzs, J.M.; Walker, P.D.; Larsen, C.P. The Histopathologic Spectrum of Kidney Biopsies in Patients with Inflammatory Bowel Disease. *Clin. J. Am. Soc. Nephrol.* **2014**, *9*, 265–270. [CrossRef]
79. Rehnberg, J.; Symreng, A.; Ludvigsson, J.F.; Emilsson, L. Inflammatory Bowel Disease Is More Common in Patients with IgA Nephropathy and Predicts Progression of ESKD: A Swedish Population-Based Cohort Study. *J. Am. Soc. Nephrol.* **2021**, *32*, 411–423. [CrossRef]
80. Pattrapornpisut, P.; Avila-Casado, C.; Reich, H.N. IgA Nephropathy: Core Curriculum 2021. *Am. J. Kidney Dis.* **2021**, *78*, 429–441. [CrossRef]
81. Kiryluk, K.; Moldoveanu, Z.; Sanders, J.T.; Eison, T.M.; Suzuki, H.; Julian, B.A.; Novak, J.; Gharavi, A.G.; Wyatt, R.J. Aberrant Glycosylation of IgA1 is Inherited in Both Pediatric IgA Nephropathy and Henoch-Schönlein Purpura Nephritis. *Kidney Int.* **2011**, *80*, 79–87. [CrossRef] [PubMed]

82. Yu, X.Q.; Li, M.; Zhang, H.; Low, H.Q.; Wei, X.; Wang, J.Q.; Sun, L.D.; Sim, K.S.; Li, Y.; Foo, J.N.; et al. A Genome-wide Association Study in Han Chinese Identifies Multiple Susceptibility Loci for IgA Nephropathy. *Nat. Genet.* **2011**, *44*, 178–182. [CrossRef] [PubMed]
83. Kiryluk, K.; Li, Y.; Scolari, F.; Sanna-Cherchi, S.; Choi, M.; Verbitsky, M.; Fasel, D.; Lata, S.; Prakash, S.; Shapiro, S.; et al. Discovery of New Risk Loci for IgA Nephropathy Implicates Genes Involved in Immunity Against Intestinal Pathogens. *Nat. Genet.* **2014**, *46*, 1187–1196. [CrossRef] [PubMed]
84. Li, M.; Wang, L.; Shi, D.C.; Foo, J.N.; Zhong, Z.; Khor, C.C.; Lazzani, C.; Chitterio, L.; Salvi, E.; Yin, P.-R.; et al. Genome-Wide Meta-Analysis Identifies Three Novel Susceptibility Loci and Reveals Ethnic Heterogeneity of Genetic Susceptibility for IgA Nephropathy. *J. Am. Soc. Nephrol.* **2020**, *31*, 2949–2963. [CrossRef]
85. Liu, J.Z.; Van Sommeren, S.; Huang, H.; Ng, S.C.; Alberts, R.; Takahashi, A.; Ripke, S.; Lee, J.C.; Jostins, L.; Shah, T.; et al. International Multiple Sclerosis Genetics Consortium; International IBD Genetics Consortium. Association Analyses Identify 38 Susceptibility Loci for Inflammatory Bowel Disease and Highlight Shared Genetic Risk Across Populations. *Nat. Genet.* **2015**, *47*, 979–986. [CrossRef]
86. Jostins, L.; Ripke, S.; Weersma, R.K.; Duerr, R.H.; McGovern, D.P.; Hui, K.Y.; Lee, J.C.; Schumm, L.P.; Sharma, Y.; Anderson, A.C.; et al. Host-microbe Interactions Have Shaped the Genetic Architecture of Inflammatory Bowel Disease. *Nature* **2012**, *491*, 119–124. [CrossRef] [PubMed]
87. De Jager, P.L.; Graham, R.; Farwell, L.; Sawcer, S.; Richardson, A.; Behrens, T.W.; Compston, A.; Hafler, D.A.; Kere, J.; Vyse, T.J.; et al. The Role of Inflammatory Bowel Disease Susceptibility Loci in Multiple Sclerosis and Systemic Lupus Erythematosus. *Genes Immun.* **2006**, *7*, 327–334. [CrossRef]
88. Shi, D.; Zhong, Z.; Wang, M.; Cai, L.; Fu, D.; Peng, Y.; Guo, L.; Mao, H.; Yu, X.; Li, M. Identification of Susceptibility Locus Shared by IgA Nephropathy and Inflammatory Bowel Disease in a Chinese Han Population. *J. Hum. Genet.* **2020**, *65*, 241–249. [CrossRef]
89. Ostvik, A.E.; Granlund, A.V.; Gustafsson, B.I.; Torp, S.H.; Espevik, T.; Mollnes, T.E.; Damås, J.K.; Sandvik, A.K. Mucosal Toll-like Receptor 3-dependent Synthesis of Complement Factor B and Systemic Complement Activation in Inflammatory Bowel Disease. *Inflamm. Bowel Dis.* **2014**, *20*, 995–1003. [CrossRef]
90. Halstensen, T.S.; Mollnes, T.E.; Garred, P.; Fausa, O.; Brandtzaeg, P. Epithelial Deposition of Immunoglobulin G1 and Activated Complement (C3b and Terminal Complement Complex) in Ulcerative Colitis. *Gastroenterology* **1990**, *98*, 1264–1271. [CrossRef]
91. Zimmermann-Nielsen, E.; Grønbaek, H.; Dahlerup, J.F.; Baatrup, G.; Thorlacius-Ussing, O. Complement Activation Capacity in Plasma Before and During High-Dose Prednisolone Treatment and Tapering in Exacerbations of Crohn's Disease and Ulcerative Colitis. *BMC Gastroenterol.* **2005**, *5*, 31. [CrossRef] [PubMed]
92. Wang, J.; Anders, R.A.; Wu, Q.; Peng, D.; Cho, J.H.; Sun, Y.; Karaliukas, R.; Kang, H.S.; Turner, J.R.; Fu, Y.X. Dysregulated LIGHT Expression on T Cells Mediates Intestinal Inflammation and Contributes to IgA Nephropathy. *J. Clin. Investig.* **2004**, *113*, 826–835. [CrossRef] [PubMed]
93. Papista, C.; Berthelot, L.; Monteiro, R.C. Dysfunctions of the IgA System: A Common Link Between Intestinal and Renal Diseases. *Cell. Mol. Immunol.* **2011**, *8*, 126–134. [CrossRef] [PubMed]
94. Murea, M.; Park, J.K.; Sharma, S.; Kato, H.; Gruenwald, A.; Niranjan, T.; Si, H.; Thomas, D.B.; Pullman, J.M.; Melamed, M.L.; et al. Expression of Notch Pathway Proteins Correlates with Albuminuria, Glomerulosclerosis, and Renal Function. *Kidney Int.* **2010**, *78*, 514–522. [CrossRef] [PubMed]
95. Akiyama, M.; Shimomura, K.; Yoshimoto, H.; Sako, M.; Kodama, M.; Abe, K.; Gunji, M.; Kang, D.; Takaki, T.; Wada, Y.; et al. Crohn's Disease May Promote Inflammation in IgA Nephropathy: A Case-Control Study of Patients Undergoing Kidney Biopsy. *Virchows Arch.* **2022**, *481*, 553–563. [CrossRef]
96. Salvador, P.; Macías-Ceja, D.C.; Gisbert-Ferrándiz, L.; Hernández, C.; Bernardo, D.; Alós, R.; Navarro-Vicente, F.; Esplugues, J.V.; Ortiz-Masiá, D.; Barrachina, M.D.; et al. CD16+ Macrophages Mediate Fibrosis in Inflammatory Bowel Disease. *J. Crohns Colitis* **2018**, *12*, 589–599. [CrossRef]
97. Sieber, G.; Herrmann, F.; Zeitz, M.; Teichmann, H.; Rühl, H. Abnormalities of B-Cell Activation and Immunoregulation in Patients with Crohn's Disease. *Gut* **1984**, *25*, 1255–1261. [CrossRef]
98. Heller, F.; Lindenmeyer, M.T.; Cohen, C.D.; Brandt, U.; Draganovici, D.; Fischereder, M.; Kretzler, M.; Anders, H.-J.; Sitter, T.; Mosberger, I.; et al. The Contribution of B Cells to Renal Interstitial Inflammation. *Am. J. Pathol.* **2007**, *170*, 457–468. [CrossRef]
99. Du, Y.; Chen, J.; Shen, L.; Wang, B. TRP channels in inflammatory bowel disease: Potential therapeutic targets. *Biochem. Pharmacol.* **2022**, *203*, 115195. [CrossRef]
100. Chen, Y.; Mu, J.; Zhu, M.; Mukherjee, A.; Zhang, H. Transient Receptor Potential Channels and Inflammatory Bowel Disease. *Front. Immunol.* **2020**, *11*, 180. [CrossRef]
101. Qing, J.; Li, C.; Hu, X.; Song, W.; Tirichen, H.; Yaigoub, H.; Li, Y. Differentiation of T Helper 17 Cells May Mediate the Abnormal Humoral Immunity in IgA Nephropathy and Inflammatory Bowel Disease Based on Shared Genetic Effects. *Front. Immunol.* **2022**, *13*, 916934. [CrossRef] [PubMed]
102. Zhou, Y.; Castonguay, P.; Sidhom, E.H.; Clark, A.R.; Dvela-Levitt, M.; Kim, S.; Sieber, J.; Wieder, N.; Jung, J.Y.; Andreeva, S.; et al. A Small-Molecule Inhibitor of TRPC5 Ion Channels Suppresses Progressive Kidney Disease in Animal Models. *Science* **2017**, *358*, 1332–1336. [CrossRef] [PubMed]

103. Xiao, M.; Ran, Y.; Shao, J.; Lei, Z.; Chen, Y.; Li, Y. Causal Association between Inflammatory Bowel Disease and IgA Nephropathy: A Bidirectional Two-Sample Mendelian Randomization Study. *Front. Genet.* **2022**, *13*, 1002928. [CrossRef] [PubMed]
104. Nurmi, R.; Pohjonen, J.; Metso, M.; Pörsti, I.; Niemelä, O.; Huhtala, H.; Mustonen, J.; Kaukinen, K.; Mäkelä, S. Prevalence of Inflammatory Bowel Disease and Celiac Disease in Patients with IgA Nephropathy over Time. *Nephron* **2021**, *145*, 78–84. [CrossRef] [PubMed]

life

MDPI

Article

Fruit and Vegetable Consumption and Inflammatory Bowel Disease: A Case-Control Study

Anas M. Almofarreh [1], Haytham A. Sheerah [2,*], Ahmed Arafa [3,4], Fairuz A. Algori [5], Ghonem R. Almutairi [6], Kafi A. Alenzi [7], Madiha M. Al-Alsehemi [8], Banan H. Mekwar [9], Osama Alzeer [10] and Haneen N. Molla [10]

1 Assistant Deputyship for Health Investment Development, Ministry of Health, Riyadh 11451, Saudi Arabia; aalmofarreh@moh.gov.sa
2 Office of the Vice Minister of Health, Ministry of Health, Riyadh 11451, Saudi Arabia
3 Department of Preventive Cardiology, National Cerebral and Cardiovascular Center, Suita 564-8565, Japan; ahmed011172@med.bsu.edu.eg
4 Department of Public Health and Community Medicine, Faculty of Medicine, Beni-Suef University, Beni-Suef 62521, Egypt
5 Assistant Deputyship for Preventive Health, Ministry of Health, Riyadh 11451, Saudi Arabia
6 General Administration for Health Facilities Licensing, Ministry of Health, Riyadh 11451, Saudi Arabia; gralmotari@moh.gov.sa
7 Assistant Deputyship for Medical Assistance Services, Ministry of Health, Riyadh 11451, Saudi Arabia
8 Department of Legislation and Regulations, General Directorate of Nursing and Midwifery Affairs, Ministry of Health, Riyadh 11451, Saudi Arabia
9 Deputyship for Therapeutic Services, Ministry of Health, Riyadh 11451, Saudi Arabia; bmekwar@moh.gov.sa
10 Department of Clinical Nutrition, King Khalid University Hospital, King Saud University Medical City, Riyadh 12372, Saudi Arabia
* Correspondence: hasheerah@moh.gov.sa

Abstract: Background: Inflammatory bowel diseases (IBD), including ulcerative colitis (UC) and Crohn's disease (CD), are chronic conditions with complex etiologies that may involve dietary factors. This study investigates the association between fruit and vegetable consumption and the risk of UC and CD, focusing on gender-specific differences. Methods: A hospital-based case–control study, comprising 158 UC patients (93 men and 65 women), 245 CD patients (167 men and 78 women), and 395 controls without IBD (256 men and 139 women), was conducted in Riyadh, Saudi Arabia. Fruit and vegetable consumption data were gathered through a self-administered questionnaire distributed before diagnosis. Logistic regression analysis was applied to estimate the odds ratios (ORs) and 95% confidence intervals (95% CIs) for UC and CD among the participants reporting the daily consumption of fruits and vegetables. Results: Among men, daily vegetable consumption was associated with higher odds of UC in the age-adjusted model [OR (95% CI): 1.78 (1.02, 3.10)], but this association became non-significant after further adjustment for body mass index, smoking, anemia, and elevated liver enzymes [OR (95% CI): 1.70 (0.91, 3.18)]. No significant associations were observed between vegetable consumption and CD. In contrast, the women who consumed vegetables every day had a non-significant inverse association with UC and a significant inverse association with CD in both the age-adjusted and multivariable-adjusted models [ORs (95% CIs): 0.44 (0.23, 0.87) and 0.41 (0.20, 0.84), respectively]. Fruit consumption was neither associated with UC nor CD in either sex. Conclusions: Daily vegetable consumption was significantly associated with decreased odds of CD among women, but not men, highlighting potential sex-specific dietary influences on IBD risk.

Keywords: Crohn's disease; diet; food; observational study; ulcerative colitis; vegetables

1. Introduction

Inflammatory bowel disease (IBD) refers to a group of chronic, relapsing inflammatory conditions of the gastrointestinal tract, primarily including ulcerative colitis (UC) and Crohn's disease (CD). Both conditions are characterized by chronic inflammation, which may affect various parts of the digestive tract, leading to symptoms such as abdominal pain, diarrhea, and fatigue. Despite extensive research, the exact etiology of IBD remains unclear, but it is believed to result from a complex interaction between genetic, environmental, and immune factors [1].

The burden of IBD is substantial, affecting millions of individuals worldwide, with rising incidence rates, particularly in newly industrialized regions [2,3]. Between 1990 and 2019, the age-standardized prevalence rate of IBD increased in 13 out of the 21 Global Burden of Disease (GBD) regions, and by 2019, there were approximately 4.9 million IBD patients worldwide [2]. In countries with historically low IBD prevalence, including those in the Arab region, an increase in cases has been observed over recent decades, likely driven by urbanization and the Westernization of diets. A meta-analysis of 16 studies investigating Arab populations put UC and CD incidences at 2.33 and 1.46 per 100,000 person–years, respectively [4]. In Saudi Arabia, where the rapid shift toward a Western lifestyle has been pronounced, IBD represents an emerging public health challenge [5], but limited data exist on its risk factors within the local population.

Diet has long been suggested as a key modifiable factor in the development and progression of IBD. Emerging evidence has highlighted the potential role of fruits and vegetables in influencing IBD risk [6,7], given their rich content of fiber, antioxidants, vitamins, and anti-inflammatory properties [8]. However, a few studies have investigated the association between fruit and vegetable consumption and IBD risk and even reached inconsistent conclusions. In a population-based case–control study involving 256 UC patients, 186 CD patients, and 940 controls from eight Asian countries and Australia, fruit and vegetable consumption was not associated with UC and CD [9]. In a prospective cohort study using data from the US Nurses' Health Study II (103 UC and 70 CD incident cases), women who reported a high-school diet, involving greater amounts of fruits, vegetables, and fish, had a lower risk of CD, but not UC [10]. In a case–control study, including 51 UC patients, 81 CD patients, and 104 controls from Australia, the daily consumption of fruits was negatively associated with UC but not CD, while the daily consumption of vegetables was neither associated with UC nor CD [11]. In another case–control study involving 144 UC patients, 123 CD patients, and 267 controls from Denmark, the daily consumption of fruits and vegetables was associated with lower odds of UC and CD [12].

In addition, there is a significant gap in the knowledge about the association between dietary factors and IBD among Arab populations. Most studies have been conducted in Western countries, and it is unclear whether these findings apply to populations in different sociocultural contexts, such as Saudi Arabia. In addition, although sex-based differences in IBD pathogenesis, risk factors, disease course, and response to therapy have been documented [13], previous studies did not highlight the sex-specified associations between dietary factors and IBD.

In this context, this study aims to investigate the association between fruit and vegetable consumption and the risk of UC and CD among men and women in Saudi Arabia.

2. Methods

2.1. Study Population

The sample size calculation for this study has been detailed elsewhere [14]. The study population was drawn from individuals, aged ≥18 years, diagnosed at a private polyclinic in Riyadh, Saudi Arabia between January 2009 and December 2017. This case–control study included 171 patients with UC, 251 with CD, and 400 individuals with other gastrointestinal conditions, who acted as the control group. Eligibility for the UC and CD groups required a recent diagnosis, while the control participants needed to be free from IBD, malignancy, polyposis, and diverticulosis. The participants lacking fruit and vegetable consumption data were excluded, resulting in a final sample of 158 UC patients, 245 CD patients, and 395 controls for the statistical analysis.

2.2. Diagnosis of Ulcerative Colitis and Crohn's Disease

As outlined in previous studies [14–16], the participants presenting with symptoms indicative of IBD, including abdominal pain, diarrhea, bloating, loss of appetite, unexplained weight loss, or bloody stool, underwent laboratory testing. These tests included urine and stool analyses for inflammatory biomarkers, as well as blood tests to measure the complete blood count, C-reactive protein, the erythrocyte sedimentation rates, bilirubin, alanine aminotransferase, creatinine, and the alkaline phosphatase levels. The participants with both clinical symptoms and laboratory results consistent with IBD were further evaluated through gastrointestinal endoscopy. A histopathological examination of the biopsy samples was then performed to confirm the diagnosis.

2.3. Assessment of Fruit and Vegetable Consumption

Data on fruit and vegetable consumption were gathered through a self-administered questionnaire distributed before ascertaining the IBD diagnosis. To evaluate their typical weekly consumption, the participants were asked, "How often do you eat fruits?" and "How often do you eat vegetables?" The response options for both questions were "once per month or less", "once per week", "twice per week", "every day", "do not remember" and "NA". For statistical analysis, the responses "once per month or less", "once per week", and "twice per week" were combined into a single category labeled "infrequent consumption". The participants who selected "do not remember" or "NA" were excluded from the analysis. The illiterate participants received assistance from data collectors.

2.4. Statistical Analysis

Logistic regression was used to compute the odds ratios (ORs) and 95% confidence intervals (CIs) for the UC and CD of frequent versus infrequent fruit and vegetable consumption. The results were adjusted for age only in Model I and were further adjusted for body mass index (BMI), smoking, anemia, and elevated liver enzymes in Model II. Since sex interacted with the association between fruit and vegetable consumption and IBD (p-values for sex interactions were <0.10), all the analyses were stratified by sex. Age and BMI, on the other hand, showed no interaction (p-values for age and BMI interactions were >0.20). The Statistical Package for Social Science (SPSS) 2013 (IBM SPSS Statistics for Windows, Version 22.0, IBM Corporation, Armonk, NY, USA) was used for data analysis.

3. Results

Among the 516 men in the study, 93 were diagnosed with UC, 167 with CD, and 256 served as controls. The men with UC were significantly older than those in the CD and control groups; 47.3% of the UC patients were aged ≥40 years, compared to 25.2% of the CD patients and 34.0% of the controls. The proportion of individuals with a BMI ≥ 25 kg/m^2 was lower among the UC and CD patients compared to the controls, with 39.0% in UC, 27.5% in CD, and 57.4% in the control group. Additionally, the control group had a higher proportion of current smokers (32.0%) than the UC (18.3%) and CD (26.9%) groups. While the proportion of daily fruit consumption did not significantly differ across the groups—11.8% in UC, 15.0% in CD, and 14.1% in the controls—the UC patients reported more daily vegetable consumption (73.1%) compared to the CD patients (55.1%) and the controls (59.8%). The prevalence of anemia also varied significantly, with 11.7% in the controls, 47.3% in the UC patients, and 18.0% in the CD patients (Table 1).

Among the 282 women, 65 were diagnosed with UC, 78 with CD, and 139 served as controls. The women with CD were significantly younger than those with UC and the controls; 42.3% of the CD patients were <30 years old, compared to 21.5% of the UC patients and 18.0% of the controls. The proportion of women with a BMI ≥ 25 kg/m^2 was lower in the CD group compared to the UC and control groups: 35.9% in CD, 60.3% in UC, and 63.3% in the controls. While the proportion of daily fruit consumption did not significantly vary across the groups, 13.8% in UC, 11.5% in CD, and 12.9% in the controls, the UC and CD patients reported less daily vegetable consumption (66.2% and 50.0%, respectively) compared to the controls (79.1%). Anemia was less common in the control group (22.3%) compared to the UC (38.5%) and CD (30.8%) groups (Table 1).

Table 1. Comparison between cases and controls in the case–control study.

Characteristics		Ulcerative Colitis	Crohn's Disease	Control
Men (n = 516)				
Number of participants		93	167	256
Age, years, %	<30	19.4	29.3	18.4
	30–39	33.3	45.5	47.6
	≥40	47.3	25.2	34.0
Body mass index, kg/m^2, %	<18.5	7.5	17.4	9.4
	18.5–24.9	53.8	55.1	33.2
	25.0–29.9	21.5	16.8	27.7
	≥30	17.2	10.7	29.7
Fruit consumption, %	Daily	11.8	15.0	14.1
	Infrequent	88.2	85.0	85.9
Vegetable consumption, %	Daily	73.1	55.1	59.8
	Infrequent	26.9	44.9	40.2
Current smoking, %		18.3	26.9	32.0
Anemia, %		47.3	18.0	11.7
Elevated liver enzymes, %		4.3	6.6	9.8
Women (n = 282)				
Number of participants		65	78	139
Age, years, %	<30	21.5	42.3	18.0
	30–39	36.9	41.0	33.1
	≥40	41.6	16.7	48.9
Body mass index, kg/m^2, %	<18.5	9.8	20.5	9.4
	18.5–24.9	29.9	43.6	27.3
	25.0–29.9	27.5	26.9	28.8
	≥30	32.8	9.0	34.5
Fruit consumption, %	Daily	13.8	11.5	12.9
	Infrequent	86.2	88.5	87.1
Vegetable consumption, %	Daily	66.2	50.0	79.1
	Infrequent	33.8	50.0	20.9
Current smoking, %		1.5	1.3	0.0
Anemia, %		38.5	30.8	22.3
Elevated liver enzymes, %		7.7	7.7	4.3

In the age-adjusted and multivariable-adjusted regression models, daily fruit consumption was not associated with UC or CD in either sex (Table 2). Among men, daily vegetable consumption was associated with increased odds of UC in the age-adjusted model [OR (95% CI): 1.78 (1.02, 3.10)]; however, this association lost statistical significance after further adjustments [OR (95% CI): 1.70 (0.91, 3.18)]. No significant associations were found between vegetable consumption and CD (Table 3). In women, daily vegetable consumption was inversely associated with UC in the age-adjusted model, despite not reaching statistical significance [OR (95% CI): 0.50 (0.23, 1.07)], and the association remained similar in the multivariable-adjusted model [OR (95% CI): 0.48 (0.22, 1.06)]. Daily vegetable consumption was significantly associated with lower odds of CD in both the age-adjusted and multivariable-adjusted models [ORs (95% CIs): 0.44 (0.23, 0.87) and 0.41 (0.20, 0.84), respectively] (Table 3).

Table 2. Association between daily fruit consumption and inflammatory bowel disease.

	Model I	Model II
Men		
Control	1 (Reference)	1 (Reference)
Ulcerative colitis	0.72 (0.34, 1.50)	0.99 (0.45, 2.22)
Crohn's disease	1.28 (0.72, 2.27)	1.30 (0.71, 2.39)
Women		
Control	1 (Reference)	1 (Reference)
Ulcerative colitis	1.15 (0.48, 2.76)	1.23 (0.50, 3.02)
Crohn's disease	1.31 (0.52, 3.32)	1.27 (0.48, 3.33)

Table 3. Association between daily vegetable consumption and inflammatory bowel disease.

	Model I	Model II
Men		
Control	1 (Reference)	1 (Reference)
Ulcerative colitis	1.78 (1.02, 3.10)	1.70 (0.91, 3.18)
Crohn's disease	1.01 (0.66, 1.54)	1.02 (0.66, 1.60)
Women		
Control	1 (Reference)	1 (Reference)
Ulcerative colitis	0.50 (0.23, 1.07)	0.48 (0.22, 1.06)
Crohn's disease	0.44 (0.23, 0.87)	0.41 (0.20, 0.84)

4. Discussion

In this case–control study, we investigated the association between fruit and vegetable consumption and the risk of developing UC and CD, in a population from Riyadh, Saudi Arabia. Our findings suggest that the women, but not men, who reported higher vegetable consumption showed a reduced risk of IBD, particularly UC. No significant association was observed between fruit consumption and IBD risk in either sex. These results highlight the potential protective role of vegetables in reducing IBD risk but indicate that fruit consumption might not have the same effect in this population. They also highlight the sex-based differences in the dietary factors related to IBD.

The observed protective effect of vegetables may be explained by their rich fiber content, antioxidants, vitamins, and anti-inflammatory compounds. Vegetables, particularly leafy greens, are high in insoluble fiber, which promotes gut health by improving bowel regularity, enhancing microbial diversity, and producing short-chain fatty acids (SCFAs), such as butyrate. SCFAs have anti-inflammatory effects and play a crucial role in maintaining the intestinal barrier function, which is often compromised in IBD [8,17,18]. Additionally, the antioxidants found in vegetables, including vitamins A, C, and E, help neutralize oxidative stress, a key contributor to the chronic inflammation observed in IBD [19,20]. In contrast, the lack of a significant association between fruit consumption and IBD risk could be attributed to fruits' fermentable sugars, such as fructose, which can lead to gastrointestinal symptoms, particularly in individuals with gut inflammation [21]. These sugars may disrupt gut microbiota balance, potentially counteracting any protective effects from fiber or antioxidants.

The sex-based differences in the nutritional factors related to IBD are not well-documented [13]; however, the differences in our study could be attributed to the dietary behaviors across the sexes. Women often consume more vegetables than men [22,23]. This higher intake could lead to a more obvious protective effect in women, while men might not consume enough vegetables to experience the same benefit.

Of note, a meta-analysis of observational studies showed that fruit consumption (measured as g/day in three studies) was negatively associated with UC and CD [ORs (95% CIs): 0.69 (0.55, 0.86) and 0.47 (0.38, 0.58), respectively]. Similarly, fruit consumption (measured as g/day) was negatively associated with UC and CD [ORs (95% CIs): 0.56 (0.48, 0.66) and 0.52 (0.46, 0.59), respectively] [24]. When the meta-analysis investigated the associations with additional servings of fruits and vegetables, fruit and vegetable consumption was negatively associated with CD. In contrast, the association with UC did not reach statistical significance. It is also worth mentioning that all the sub-analyses of this meta-analysis showed moderate to high heterogeneity across the studies [24].

Beyond their role in IBD development, the impact of fruit and vegetable consumption on IBD activation has shown mixed results. One study found that consuming both leafy and non-leafy vegetables, as well as fruits, exacerbated the IBD symptoms [25]. In contrast, a more recent study reported that fruit and vegetable intake reduced the prevalence of active IBD by 44% and helped prevent remission [26].

From the perspective of preventive medicine, our findings have important clinical and public health implications since they reinforce the role of a vegetable-rich diet in maintaining gut health and preventing inflammatory conditions like IBD. Clinicians and public health professionals should encourage higher vegetable consumption as part of the dietary guidelines aimed at reducing IBD risk, especially in regions like Saudi Arabia, where the incidence of IBD is rising. Since vegetables appear to offer protective effects against inflammation in the gut, integrating them into daily diets may serve as a cost-effective, preventive measure. On a clinical level, dietary interventions focusing on increasing vegetable intake could be considered as part of a holistic management approach for patients at high risk of IBD or those in the early stages of the disease.

This study presents several strengths, such as investigating an understudied population and utilizing standardized diagnostic methods for UC and CD. However, several limitations should be acknowledged. First, the data were collected from a single polyclinic in Riyadh. Since this is a private institution, the patients likely represent a higher socioeconomic group. This may limit the generalizability of our results. Second, recruitment occurred over an extended period, during which dietary habits and trends related to fruit and vegetable consumption may have shifted. Third, the food frequency questions were neither validated nor pre-tested. Fourth, a limitation of this questionnaire is that it assessed fruit and vegetable consumption in aggregate rather than individually, without specifying the types of fruits and vegetables consumed. In addition, the study did not account for the specific components of the fruits and vegetables (e.g., fiber, antioxidants, and vitamins), which could have varying effects on IBD risk. This approach may overlook variations in nutrient content and the health benefits associated with different fruits and vegetables. Fifth, due to the limited number of cases in each fruit and vegetable consumption frequency group, we combined the non-daily consumers into one group. This precluded the analysis of a potential dose–response relationship. Finally, we did not adjust our results for important confounders, such as total caloric intake. Seventh, our control group comprised patients with other gastrointestinal conditions. This may have led to an underestimation of the association between fruit and vegetable consumption and IBD due to overlapping dietary patterns.

5. Conclusions

This study found a negative association between daily vegetable consumption and the risk of CD among women but not men, suggesting that a higher intake of vegetables may have a protective effect against CD in Arab women. In addition, daily vegetable consumption showed a tendency of a protective effect against UC risk in women but not men. These findings highlight the importance of considering gender-specific dietary patterns in the prevention of IBD. On the other hand, no similar associations were observed with fruit consumption, indicating that the protective dietary factors against IBD may be more specific to vegetable intake. Further research, especially with larger cohorts, diverse populations, and prospective cohort designs, is needed to confirm these associations and to explore the underlying mechanisms.

Author Contributions: Conceptualization, A.M.A. and H.A.S.; Methodology, A.M.A. and H.A.S.; Software, A.M.A. and H.A.S.; Validation, A.M.A. and H.A.S.; Formal analysis, A.M.A. and H.A.S.; Investigation, A.M.A. and H.A.S.; Resources, A.M.A. and H.A.S.; Data curation, A.M.A. and H.A.S.; Writing—original draft, A.M.A. and H.A.S.; Writing—review & editing, H.A.S., A.A., F.A.A., G.R.A., K.A.A., M.M.A.-A., B.H.M., O.A. and H.N.M.; Visualization, A.M.A. and H.A.S.; Supervision, H.A.S. All authors have read and agreed to the published version of the manuscript.

Funding: This research received no external funding.

Institutional Review Board Statement: King Fahd Medical City's (KFMC) institutional review board (IRB) approved the study protocol on 18 October 2018. IRB log Number: 18-543E. IRB Registration Number with KACST, KSA: H-01-R012. IRB Registration Number with OHRP/NIH, USA: IRB00010471. Approval Number Federal Wide Assurance NIH, USA: FWA00018774.

Informed Consent Statement: Informed consent was obtained from all the participants. This study was conducted according to the Declaration of Helsinki. IRB registration number: H-01-R-012.

Data Availability Statement: Upon reasonable request, data will be provided by the corresponding author after consulting the IRB of KFMC.

Acknowledgments: We thank all the participants and staff.

Conflicts of Interest: All authors declare no conflicts of interest.

References

1. Wehkamp, J.; Götz, M.; Herrlinger, K.; Steurer, W.; Stange, E.F. Inflammatory bowel disease. *Dtsch. Arztebl. Int.* **2016**, *113*, 72–82. [PubMed]
2. Wang, R.; Li, Z.; Liu, S.; Zhang, D. Global, regional and national burden of inflammatory bowel disease in 204 countries and territories from 1990 to 2019: A systematic analysis based on the Global Burden of Disease Study 2019. *BMJ Open* **2023**, *13*, e065186. [CrossRef] [PubMed]
3. Li, C.J.; Wang, Y.K.; Zhang, S.M.; Ren, M.D.; He, S.X. Global burden of inflammatory bowel disease 1990–2019: A systematic examination of the disease burden and twenty-year forecast. *World J. Gastroenterol.* **2023**, *29*, 5751–5767. [CrossRef]
4. Mosli, M.; Alawadhi, S.; Hasan, F.; Abou Rached, A.; Sanai, F.; Danese, S. Incidence, prevalence, and clinical epidemiology of inflammatory bowel disease in the Arab world: A systematic review and meta-analysis. *Inflamm. Intest. Dis.* **2021**, *6*, 123–131. [CrossRef]
5. Al Fadda, M.; Peedikayil, M.C.; Kagevi, I.; Al Kahtani, K.; Mousa, A.A.; Al Ashgar, H.I.; Al Sohaibani, F.; Al Quaiz, M.; Abdulla, M.; Khan, M.Q.; et al. Inflammatory bowel disease in Saudi Arabia: A hospital-based clinical study of 312 patients. *Ann. Saudi Med.* **2012**, *32*, 276–282. [CrossRef]
6. Spooren, C.E.; Pierik, M.J.; Zeegers, M.P.; Feskens, E.J.; Masclee, A.A.; Jonkers, D.M. Review article: The association of diet with onset and relapse in patients with inflammatory bowel disease. *Aliment. Pharmacol. Ther.* **2013**, *38*, 1172–1187. [CrossRef] [PubMed]
7. de Castro, M.M.; Pascoal, L.B.; Steigleder, K.M.; Siqueira, B.P.; Corona, L.P.; Ayrizono, M.L.S.; Milanski, M.; Leal, R.F. Role of diet and nutrition in inflammatory bowel disease. *World J. Exp. Med.* **2021**, *11*, 1–16. [CrossRef]
8. Khalili, H.; Chan, S.S.M.; Lochhead, P.; Ananthakrishnan, A.N.; Hart, A.R.; Chan, A.T. The role of diet in the aetiopathogenesis of inflammatory bowel disease. *Nat. Rev. Gastroenterol. Hepatol.* **2018**, *15*, 525–535. [CrossRef] [PubMed]
9. Ng, S.C.; Tang, W.; Leong, R.W.; Chen, M.; Ko, Y.; Studd, C.; Niewiadomski, O.; Bell, S.; Kamm, M.A.; de Silva, H.J.; et al. Environmental risk factors in inflammatory bowel disease: A population-based case-control study in Asia-Pacific. *Gut* **2015**, *64*, 1063–1071. [CrossRef]

10. Ananthakrishnan, A.N.; Khalili, H.; Song, M.; Higuchi, L.M.; Richter, J.M.; Nimptsch, K.; Wu, K.; Chan, A.T. High school diet and risk of Crohn's disease and ulcerative colitis. *Inflamm. Bowel Dis.* **2015**, *21*, 2311–2319.
11. Niewiadomski, O.; Studd, C.; Wilson, J.; Williams, J.; Hair, C.; Knight, R.; Prewett, E.; Dabkowski, P.; Alexander, S.; Allen, B.; et al. Influence of food and lifestyle on the risk of developing inflammatory bowel disease. *Intern. Med. J.* **2016**, *46*, 669–676. [CrossRef] [PubMed]
12. Hansen, T.S.; Jess, T.; Vind, I.; Elkjaer, M.; Nielsen, M.F.; Gamborg, M.; Munkholm, P. Environmental factors in inflammatory bowel disease: A case-control study based on a Danish inception cohort. *J. Crohns Colitis* **2011**, *5*, 577–584. [CrossRef] [PubMed]
13. Rustgi, S.D.; Kayal, M.; Shah, S.C. Sex-based differences in inflammatory bowel diseases: A review. *Therap. Adv. Gastroenterol.* **2020**, *13*, 1756284820915043. [CrossRef]
14. Almofarreh, A.M.; Sheerah, H.A.; Arafa, A.; Al Mubarak, A.S.; Ali, A.M.; Al-Otaibi, N.M.; Alzahrani, M.A.; Aljubayl, A.R.; Aleid, M.A.; Alhamed, S.S. Dairy consumption and inflammatory bowel disease among Arab adults: A case-control study and meta-analysis. *Nutrients* **2024**, *16*, 2747. [CrossRef]
15. Almofarreh, A.; Sheerah, H.A.; Arafa, A.; Ahamed, S.S.; Alzeer, O.; Al-Hunaishi, W.; Mhimed, M.M.; Al-Hazmi, A.; Lim, S.H. Beverage consumption and ulcerative colitis: A case-control study from Saudi Arabia. *Int. J. Environ. Res. Public Health* **2022**, *19*, 2287. [CrossRef]
16. Almofarreh, A.; Sheerah, H.A.; Arafa, A.; Alzeer, O.; Alohali, E.; Cao, J.; Liu, K.; Almuzaini, Y.; Almishary, M. Association between coffee, tea, and soft drinks consumption and Crohn's disease in Arab populations: A case-control study. *Clin. Nutr. Open Sci.* **2024**, *55*, 116–122. [CrossRef]
17. Di Rosa, C.; Altomare, A.; Imperia, E.; Spiezia, C.; Khazrai, Y.M.; Guarino, M.P.L. The Role of Dietary Fibers in the Management of IBD Symptoms. *Nutrients* **2022**, *14*, 4775. [CrossRef]
18. Parada Venegas, D.; De la Fuente, M.K.; Landskron, G.; González, M.J.; Quera, R.; Dijkstra, G.; Harmsen, H.J.M.; Faber, K.N.; Hermoso, M.A. Short chain fatty acids (SCFAs)-mediated gut epithelial and immune regulation and its relevance for inflammatory bowel diseases. *Front. Immunol.* **2019**, *10*, 277.
19. Jarmakiewicz-Czaja, S.; Ferenc, K.; Filip, R. Antioxidants as protection against reactive oxidative stress in inflammatory bowel disease. *Metabolites* **2023**, *13*, 573. [CrossRef]
20. Chen, J.; Ruan, X.; Yuan, S.; Deng, M.; Zhang, H.; Sun, J.; Yu, L.; Satsangi, J.; Larsson, S.C.; Therdoratou, E.; et al. Antioxidants, minerals and vitamins in relation to Crohn's disease and ulcerative colitis: A Mendelian randomization study. *Aliment. Pharmacol. Ther.* **2023**, *57*, 399–408. [CrossRef]
21. Ma, X.; Nan, F.; Liang, H.; Shu, P.; Fan, X.; Song, X.; Hou, Y.; Zhang, D. Excessive intake of sugar: An accomplice of inflammation. *Front. Immunol.* **2022**, *13*, 988481. [CrossRef] [PubMed]
22. Martin, S. Surprise! Women eat healthier than men. *CMAJ* **2002**, *167*, 913. [PubMed]
23. Feraco, A.; Armani, A.; Amoah, I.; Guseva, E.; Camajani, E.; Gorini, S.; Strollo, R.; Padua, E.; Caprio, M.; Lombardo, M. Assessing gender differences in food preferences and physical activity: A population-based survey. *Front. Nutr.* **2024**, *11*, 1348456. [CrossRef] [PubMed]
24. Milajerdi, A.; Ebrahimi-Daryani, N.; Dieleman, L.A.; Larijani, B.; Esmaillzadeh, A. Association of dietary fiber, fruit, and vegetable consumption with risk of inflammatory bowel disease: A systematic review and meta-analysis. *Adv. Nutr.* **2021**, *12*, 735–743. [CrossRef]
25. Cohen, A.B.; Lee, D.; Long, M.D.; Kappelman, M.D.; Martin, C.F.; Sandler, R.S.; Lewis, J.D. Dietary patterns and self-reported associations of diet with symptoms of inflammatory bowel disease. *Dig. Dis. Sci.* **2013**, *58*, 1322–1328. [CrossRef]
26. Sauer, P.; Luft, V.C.; Dall'Alba, V. Patients with inflammatory bowel disease who regularly consume fruits and vegetables present lower prevalence of disease activation: A cross-sectional study. *Clin. Nutr. ESPEN* **2024**, *61*, 420–426. [CrossRef]

life

MDPI

Article

Phase Angle (PhA) Is an Easy and Complementary Tool for Assessing Nutritional Status in Ulcerative Colitis (UC) Patients: A Cross-Sectional Study

Viridiana Montsserrat Mendoza-Martínez [1], Roberto Baños-Vázquez [1], Guillermo Melendez-Mier [2], Javier Ivanovychs Carrillo-Rojas [3], Martha Alison Santoyo-Chávez [1], Sarahi Ontiveros-López [3], Annel Gómez-Coello [4], Galileo Escobedo [1], Jorge Luis de León-Rendón [5] and Nallely Bueno-Hernández [1,3,*]

1 Proteomics and Metabolomics Laboratory, Research Directorate, General Hospital of Mexico "Dr. Eduardo Liceaga", Mexico City 06720, Mexico; viiriidiios@gmail.com (V.M.M.-M.); robertobanos25@hotmail.com (R.B.-V.); santoyoalison@gmail.com (M.A.S.-C.); gescobedog@msn.com (G.E.)
2 Faculty of Public Health and Nutrition (FASPyN), Autonomous University of Nuevo León, Monterrey 66455, Mexico; melendez651@gmail.com
3 Specialty Hospital of the National Medical Center "La Raza", Mexico City 02990, Mexico; ivancarrillorojas@gmail.com (J.I.C.-R.); ontiveros.sarahi@hotmail.com (S.O.-L.)
4 Phoniatrics Department, National Institute of Rehabilitation "Luis Guillermo Ibarra Ibarra", Mexico City 14389, Mexico; annelgomezc@gmail.com
5 Inflammatory Bowel Disease Clinic of the Gastroenterology Service of the General Hospital of Mexico "Dr. Eduardo Liceaga", Mexico City 06720, Mexico; dr.jorgedeleon@hotmail.com
* Correspondence: nallely_bh5@yahoo.com.mx

Abstract: Background: Accumulating evidence has proposed phase angle (PhA) as a marker for assessing cellular integrity and nutritional status in ulcerative colitis (UC) patients; the aim of the study was to evaluate the efficacy of PhA in assessing nutritional status in patients with UC, investigating its potential as a biomarker of disease activity. Methods: We conducted a cross-sectional study in patients with UC and healthy controls. We determined PhA by electrical bioimpedance and categorized participants through bioelectrical impedance analysis. They were classified as normal PhA > 6.1° and low PhA < 6.1° in men and normal PhA > 5.6° and low PhA < 5.6° in women. Results: PhA was significantly lower in UC patients than in controls (5.8 ± 0.8 vs. 6.6 ± 0.7°; $p < 0.001$). Among UC patients, participants with low PhA showed a decrease in lean, dry mass (LDM) ($p < 0.001$), total body water ($p = 0.008$), and intracellular water ($p = 0.005$), accompanied by an increase in extracellular water ($p = 0.001$) compared to UC patients with normal PhA. Conclusions: PhA significantly decreases in UC patients compared to healthy controls and is even more reduced when UC is active. A cut-off point of <6.1 for men and <5.6 for women could be suitable for nutritional diagnosis in patients with UC, but it still needs to be validated.

Keywords: phase angle; nutritional status; inflammatory bowel disease; ulcerative colitis; bioelectrical impedance

1. Introduction

Inflammatory bowel disease (IBD) is a chronic inflammatory condition, including both Crohn's disease (CD) and ulcerative colitis (UC). UC is marked by symptoms such as bloody diarrhea stemming from persistent inflammation that begins in the rectum and may spread throughout the colon. In addition to gastrointestinal symptoms, UC often involves extraintestinal manifestations like joint pain, skin and eye complications, anemia, and, notably, malnutrition [1]. Given these complications, nutritional assessment in UC patients is essential. Malnutrition is common due to both the disease's impact on nutrient absorption and the body's increased metabolic demands during inflammation. Nutritional evaluation can help identify deficiencies early, allowing for targeted interventions that may improve patient outcomes and quality of life [2].

In UC patients, malnutrition occurs in up to 70% of patients with active disease and up to 38% of patients in remission and is associated with a high number of hospitalizations, frequency of relapses, need for surgery, and postoperative complications [3,4]. These complications are attributed to several factors, including digestive discomfort, pharmacological treatment, abdominal pain, reduced oral intake, inflammatory status, and disease severity. However, there is currently no consensus on the diagnosis of malnutrition in UC patients [5]. The criteria from the Global Leadership Initiative on Malnutrition (GLIM) for the diagnosis of malnutrition in UC are based on the patient's body mass index (BMI) [6].

However, assessing nutritional status based only on BMI may be inappropriate in UC. In this sense, the European Society for Clinical Nutrition and Metabolism (ESPEN) guidelines, developed to provide evidence-based recommendations for managing clinical nutrition and metabolism in IBD, acknowledge that BMI does not allow the accurate identification of patients with obesity, which often complicates the disease [5], because even patients with increased adiposity may have lower lean mass despite having an average BMI [7].

This information underlines the need to find other markers to provide information about the UC patient's nutritional status. In fact, there are alternative methods to assess a person's nutritional status, such as bioelectrical impedance analysis (BIA) and Phase Angle (PhA). In particular, PhA is a bioelectrical impedance parameter that provides insight into cell membrane integrity and cellular health. It reflects the body's ability to retain electrical charges across cell membranes, which is closely related to cell function and overall nutritional status. In patients with IBD, a lower PhA often indicates compromised cell membrane integrity, potentially due to inflammation, malnutrition, or both [8]. Signori-Urbano et al. found an inverse correlation between the inflammatory markers C-reactive protein (CRP) and erythrocyte sedimentation rate (ESR) and PhA in UC patients [9], suggesting that PhA may help monitor nutritional status in UC patients, serving as a simple, non-invasive tool that can offer valuable information on a patient's nutritional status and disease progression.

Thus, our primary goal was to evaluate the efficacy of PhA for assessing nutritional status in UC patients while also examining a possible relationship with disease activity.

2. Materials and Methods

2.1. Trial Design

We conducted a multicenter, cross-sectional study according to the STROBE (Observational Studies in Epidemiology) guidelines [10] (Figure 1), enrolling patients between 2020 and 2023 in the General Hospital of Mexico Dr. Eduardo Liceaga (HGMEL) and La Raza Medical Center (RMC). All participants had clinical, anthropometric, and biochemical evaluations.

2.2. Ethical Considerations

All participants signed a letter of informed consent and gave their authorization for the publication of the data obtained. The principles of Article 17 of the General Health Law regarding research and the ethical guidelines of the Declaration of Helsinki were followed. The ethical committees of both hospitals approved this project under the numbers DI 19/501/03/098 (HGMEL) and R-2023-3501-079 (RMC), and all participants signed a consent form. We collected data from the protocol registry on ClinicalTrials.gov with the number NCT04143633.

2.3. Eligibility Criteria for Participants

We enrolled patients of both sexes above 18 years with an intestinal biopsy-proven diagnosis of UC. We assessed disease activity by True Love and Witts, asking patients about medication use based on their current prescriptions. We excluded from the study participants with surgical, radiologic, methotrexate, or chemotherapy treatment, dementia, visible edema, pregnancy, amputations, and pacemakers. Besides UC patients, we enrolled a healthy control group with no history of high blood glucose, hypertension, or dyslipidemia. We also excluded participants who consumed alcohol or tobacco due to the possible exacerbation of gastrointestinal symptoms. To ensure accurate measurements, participants were required to be fasting, with no prior fluid intake, and were prohibited from intense exercise and alcohol consumption for one day before the assessment.

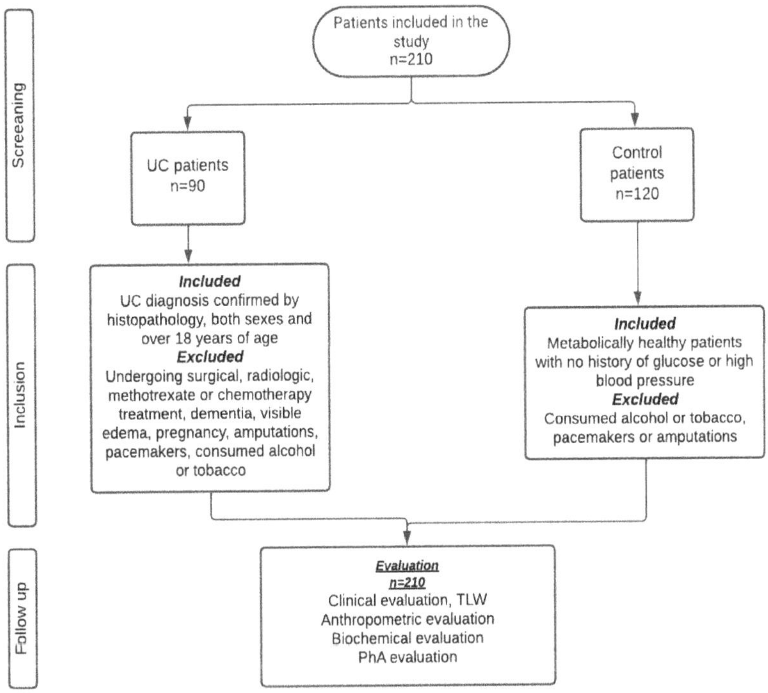

Figure 1. The flowchart illustrates the selection process of the study participants according to the STROBE criteria.

2.4. Outcomes

In the subjects of this research, the aim was to evaluate for the first time the effectiveness of PhA for the assessment of nutritional status by clinical, anthropometric, and biochemical evaluation in UC patients. It also aimed to investigate a possible association with disease activity, whether active or in remission, and to quantify ESR and CRP levels.

2.5. Clinical, Anthropometric, and Biochemical Evaluation of Volunteers

We collected and registered all study participants' demographic, anthropometric, clinical, and laboratory parameters, such as ESR, CRP, cholesterol, triglycerides, lymphocytes, and platelets. We performed BIA analysis and anthropometric assessments by standardized nutritionists using the RJL Quantum IV system (RJL Systems Inc. Clinton Township, MI, USA) to measure body composition and estimate fat mass (FM), lean dry mass (LDM), total body water (TBW), extracellular water (ECW), intracellular water (ICW), and skeletal muscle mass (SMM). The formula for Mexican adults [11] was used to calculate SMM: SMM (kg) = $[(Ht2|R \times 0.401) + (gender \times 3.825) + (age \times -0.071)] + 5.102$ [12].

We used Reactance(Xc)/Resistance(R)*($180/\pi$) to estimate PhA [13]. Weight (Weighing Machine, MS 50 SECA; Hamburg, Germany) and height (scale, MD 213 SECA; Hamburg, Germany) were measured, and body mass index (BMI) was calculated using the formula

BMI = weight (kg)/height (m)^2. The body circumferences, including waist circumference, were measured by placing a tape (Lufkin tape measure 6 mm × 2 m diameter pocket tape) between the iliac crest and the lumbar rib. We measured hip circumference by placing the tape at the predominant point of the buttocks, following the National Institute of Public Health recommendations [14]. To ensure accurate measurements, participants were required to be fasting, with no prior fluid intake, and were prohibited from intense exercise and alcohol consumption one day before the assessment. Biochemical parameters were extracted from the patient's electronic medical records, including results from standard blood tests relevant to the study.

2.6. Sample Size

We estimated the sample size using the GPower v.3.1 9.2 program, assuming an effect size of 0.4, an alpha error of 0.05, and a power of 80%. This resulted in a sample size of 90 participants per group. We included an additional 10% of patients to account for possible losses. We decided to increase the number of participants to 120 in the control group to improve the study's statistical power and detect genuine associations in both groups.

2.7. Statistical Analysis

We categorized UC patients according to the PhA value. For women, a PhA < 5.5° was classified as a "low PhA patient group with PhA < 6.1°" and a PhA > 5.6° as a "normal PhA patient group". For men, the cutoff was maintained at 6.1°, consistent with PhA > 6.1°, following Peng et al.'s 2022 guidelines. We used the PhA cutoff value proposed by the GLIM criteria as the gold standard [15]. After assessing the normality of data by the Kolmogorov–Smirnov test, we performed the Mann–Whitney U and t-test to compare data between UC patients and healthy controls. We performed bivariate associations by the Pearson correlation coefficient (r) for body composition variables with PhA in UC patients, defining null correlation values as ranging from 0.00 to 0.09, weak correlations from 0.10 to 0.29, moderate correlations from 0.30 to 0.49, and strong correlations from 0.50 to 1.0, according to the guidelines of Hernández Lalinde J.D. et al. [16]. We used the statistical package IBM-SPSS version 23 (IBM, Armonk, NY, USA) for the analysis, considering a p-value < 0.05 as significant.

3. Results

Two hundred and ten patients met the inclusion criteria and agreed to participate in the study. There were ninety UC patients and one hundred and twenty healthy controls; the average age of participants in both groups was 30 ± 12 years, and they were predominantly women (62%) (Table 1).

3.1. Differences Between UC Patients and Controls

Concerning disease activity, we found that up to 35% of UC patients were in remission, and 65% had active disease. While 100% of UC patients took mesalazine, almost 8% of them also took steroids. UC patients had higher platelet count (307.1 ± 144.2 vs. 249.4 ± 48.8 K/μL, $p < 0.001$) and lower resistance (629.1 ± 99.1 vs. 692.7 ± 110.7, $p < 0.001$), reactance (64.4 ± 9.9 vs. 80 ± 10.7, $p < 0.001$), weight (61.6 ± 11.9 vs. 65.4 ± 12.8 kg, $p = 0.043$), LDM (11.1 ± 3.1 vs. 17.2 ± 4.3 kg, $p < 0.001$), and SMM (18.2 ± 5.3 vs. 21.4 ± 4.9 kg, $p < 0.001$) compared to controls. In addition, PhA was significantly lower in UC patients than in controls (5.9 ± 0.9 vs. 6.6 ± 0.7°, $p < 0.001$). We found no differences in BMI between UC patients and controls (24.2 ± 3.9 vs. 24.1 ± 3.4 kg/m^2, $p = 0.534$) (Table 1). Of the patients with UC, 52.2% had a low PhA. Among these, 49% were women and 51% were men. In contrast, in the control group, eight patients had a low PhA, with five being women and three being men.

Table 1. Demographic, biochemical, and body composition parameters in the study population.

	Total Population (n = 210)	UC Patients (n = 90)	Control (n = 120)	p-Value
Age, years (mean ± SD)	30 ± 12	39 ± 12	23 ± 3	<0.001 *
Gender, n (%)				
Men	90 (38)	43 (36)	47 (39)	0.134
Women	120 (62)	47 (64)	73 (61)	
Weight, kg (mean ± SD)	64 ± 12.4	62 ± 11.9	65.4 ± 12.8	0.043 *
Waist, cm (mean ± SD)	81.1 ± 9.9	82.5 ± 10.4	80.3 ± 9.5	0.085
Hip, cm (mean ± SD)	97.9 ± 8.1	97.4 ± 7.1	98.2 ± 7.4	0.596
BMI, kg/m^2 (mean ± SD)	24.2 ± 3.6	24.2 ± 3.9	24.1 ± 3.4	0.534
Cholesterol, mg/dL (mean ± SD)	168.1 ± 37.1	172.1 ± 45.1	165.4 ± 29.5	0.224
Triglycerides, mg/dL (mean ± SD)	110.8 ± 75.9	118.9 ± 75.6	104.8 ± 75.1	0.186
Lymphocytes, count (mean ± SD)	2038.1 ± 662.7	2150.8 ± 856.8	1963.5 ± 465.6	0.065
Platelets K/µL (mean ± SD)	273.5 ± 103.8	307.1 ± 144.2	249.4 ± 48.8	<0.001 *
Resistance, ohms (mean ± SD)	665.5 ± 110.2	629.1 ± 99.1	692.7 ± 110.7	<0.001 *
Reactance, ohms (mean ± SD)	73.3 ± 12.9	64.4 ± 9.9	80 ± 10.7	<0.001 *
Fat, kg (mean ± SD)	20.3 ± 7.3	21.8 ± 8.1	23.6 ± 6.8	0.326
LDM, kg (mean ± SD)	14.1 ± 3.5	11.1 ± 3.1	17.2 ± 4.3	<0.001 *
SMM, kg (mean ± SD)	20.1 ± 5.3	18.2 ± 5.3	21.4 ± 4.9	<0.001 *
TBW L (mean ± SD)	28.4 ± 6.8	29.1 ± 7.1	30.1 ± 6.7	0.412
ICW, L (mean ± SD)	15.5 ± 4.4	15.6 ± 4.5	57.1 ± 3.1	0.729
ECW, L (mean ± SD)	13 ± 2.7	13.2 ± 2.8	42.9 ± 3.1	0.235
PhA, degrees (mean ± SD)	6.3 ± 0.9	5.9 ± 0.9	6.6 ± 0.7	<0.001 *

BMI: Body Mass Index, UC: Ulcerative Colitis. SD: Standard Deviation, TBW: Total Body Water, ICW: Intracellular Water, ECW: Extracellular Water, L: liters, mg: milligrams, dL: deciliter, PhA: Phase Angle, K/µL: thousand per microliter, LDM: lean dry mass SD: Standard Deviation, t-test for independent samples. * Significant p-value < 0.05.

3.2. Phase Angle and Disease Activity

When comparing patients with active disease to those in remission, we observed notable differences in CRP levels (11.7 ± 18.3 vs. 4.1 ± 3.7 mg/L, $p = 0.044$) (Table 2). However, we found no significant differences in other biochemical parameters. Furthermore, we found no differences in BMI (24.4 ± 4.2 vs. 24.2 ± 3.4 kg/m^2, $p = 0.696$) or PhA (5.9 ± 1 vs. 5.9 ± 0.9°, $p = 0.853$) when comparing UC patients with active disease to UC patients in remission. Conversely, there were significant differences in PhA when comparing UC patients with healthy controls (5.9 ± 0.9 vs. 6.6 ± 0.7°, $p < 0.001$) (Table 1).

Comparing patients with low PhA and those with normal PhA values, we found a decrease in LDM (10.1 ± 2.7 vs. 13.1 ± 2.4 kg, $p < 0.001$ in patients with active disease; 8.9 ± 2.2 vs. 12.1 ± 3.6 kg, $p = 0.008$ in patients in remission), SMM (14.9 ± 3.6 vs. 21.7 ± 5.8 kg, $p < 0.001$ in patients with active disease; 15.7 ± 3.3 vs. 20.7 ± 3.5 kg, $p < 0.001$ in patients in remission), and ICW (13.1 ± 3.3 vs. 17.6 ± 5.2 L, $p < 0.001$ in patients with active disease; 15.1 ± 4.1 vs. 17.3 ± 3.3 L, $p = 0.103$ in patients in remission). Only patients with active disease and low PhA exhibited a decrease in weight (57.7 ± 13.4 vs. 65.2 ± 12 kg, $p = 0.030$), TBW (25.7 ± 5.6 vs. 31.8 ± 8.2 L, $p = 0.002$), and ECW (12.3 ± 2.6 vs. 14.1 ± 3.1 L, $p < 0.001$) compared to patients with normal PhA. Conversely, patients with active disease and low PhA showed a significant increase in ESR (22.7 ± 14.4 vs. 15.1 ± 13.7 mm/h, $p = 0.050$) and CRP (17.8 ± 23.9 vs. 5.6 ± 6.2 mg/L, $p = 0.013$) compared to patients with normal PhA (Table 3).

In the study, the distribution of PhA among UC patients and controls revealed distinct patterns. Among UC patients with active disease, 52.5% had a low PhA, while 47.5% had a normal PhA. In contrast, among UC patients in remission, 51.6% had a low PhA, and 48.4% had a normal PhA (Table 3).

Table 2. Metabolic parameters in UC patients according to disease activity.

	Active Disease (n = 58)	Remission (n = 32)	*p*-Value
Weight, kg (mean ± SD)	61.4 ± 13.4	62.7 ± 9.2	0.308
Waist, cm (mean ± SD)	97.8 ± 8.5	82.5 ± 11.5	0.671
Hip, cm (mean ± SD)	97.3 ± 9.7	97.8 ± 8.5	0.664
BMI, kg/m^2 (mean ± SD)	24.5 ± 4.2	24.1 ± 3.3	0.593
PhA, degrees (mean ± SD)	5.8 ± 0.9	5.9 ± 0.9	0.646
FMI, kg/m^2 (mean ± SD)	9.1 ± 4.1	8.7 ± 3.4	0.768
FMSMM kg/m^2 (mean ± SD)	7.1 ± 1.5	6.9 ± 1.2	0.636
ESR, mm/h (mean ± SD)	19.1 ± 14.5	18.1 ± 12.8	0.989
CRP, mg/L (mean ± SD)	11.7 ± 18.3	4.1 ± 3.7	0.044 *
Cholesterol, mg/dL (mean ± SD)	171.3 ± 42.4	173.5 ± 50.6	0.652
Triglycerides, mg/dL (mean ± SD)	124.9 ± 86.3	107.7 ± 48.8	0.394
Lymphocytes, count(mean ± SD)	2163.7 ± 871.7	2126.5 ± 842.5	0.933
Platelets K/μL (mean ± SD)	320.6 ± 167.5	281.2 ± 80.5	0.635
Fat, kg (mean ± SD)	21.6 ± 8.3	22.7 ± 7.8	0.409
LDM, kg (mean ± SD)	11.6 ± 3	10.3 ± 3.4	0.072
SMM, kg (mean ± SD)	18.3 ± 5.9	18.1 ± 4.3	0.799
TBW L (mean ± SD)	28.8 ± 7.6	29.6 ± 5.9	0.268
ICW, L (mean ± SD)	13.2 ± 3.1	13.4 ± 2.5	0.188
ECW, L (mean ± SD)	13.2 ± 3.1	13.4 ± 2.5	0.254

BMI: Body Mass Index, UC: Ulcerative Colitis, ESR: Erythrocyte Sedimentation Rate, PhA: Phase Angle, CRP: C-Reactive Protein, TBW: Total Body Water, ICW: Intracellular Water, ECW: Extracellular Water, L: liters, mg: milligrams, dL: deciliter, cm: centimeters, SD: Standard Deviation, * Significant *p*-value < 0.05. The statistical analyzes were done with *t*-test & Mann–Whitney U test.

Table 3. Differences between UC patients experiencing active disease or remission are categorized by low and normal PhA.

	Active Disease			Remission		
	Low PhA (n = 37)	Normal PhA (n = 21)	*p*-Value	Low PhA (n = 19)	Normal PhA (n = 13)	*p*-Value
Age, years (mean ± SD)	37 ± 11	37 ± 9	0.876	49 ± 13	40 ± 15	0.134
Weight, kg (mean ± SD)	57.9 ± 13.1	68.5 ± 11.2	0.004 *	61.8 ± 10.2	64.1 ± 7.8	0.529
Waist, cm (mean ± SD)	81.4 ± 11.6	84.7 ± 10.7	0.304	82.9 ± 9.1	82.1 ± 0.5	0.816
Hip, cm (mean ± SD)	95.9 ± 10.7	100.1 ± 7.1	0.127	98.1 ± 9.8	97.4 ± 6.8	0.814
WC: Waist-to-Hip Ratio (mean ± SD)						
Women	0.86 ± 0.06	0.87 ± 0.08	0.805	0.83 ± 0.06	0.84 ± 0.12	0.906
Men	0.82 ± 0.09	0.81 ± 0.08	0.863	0.86 ± 0.09	0.84 ± 0.06	0.680
Total Cholesterol, mg/dL (mean ± SD)	167.3 ± 42.2	179.7 ± 43.7	0.310	177.1 ± 54.4	168.5 ± 46.5	0.658
Triglycerides, mg/dL (mean ± SD)	114.7 ± 47.3	146.1 ± 131.6	0.208	105.1 ± 51.3	111.6 ± 47.1	0.729
Lymphocytes count (mean ± SD)	2206.1 ± 876.8	2115.4 ± 896.7	0.721	2129.9 ± 999.4	2121.7 ± 595	0.980
Platelets K/μL (mean ± SD)	326.9 ± 167.8	318.3 ± 170.9	0.859	276.1 ± 93.5	288.8 ± 60.6	0.688
ESR, mm/h (mean ± SD)	23.1 ± 13.4	12.4 ± 14.1	0.008 **	17.9 ± 13.4	18.3 ± 12.4	0.939
CRP, mg/L (mean ± SD)	15.6 ± 21.8	5.4 ± 6.2	0.015 *	3.1 ± 2.1	5.5 ± 5.2	0.119
Resistance, ohms (mean ± SD)	681.4 ± 100.3	587.5 ± 91.5	0.001	643.1 ± 97.8	590.7 ± 59.3	0.084
Reactance, ohms (mean ± SD)	61.7 ± 9.3	67.6 ± 9	0.001	58.9 ± 8.2	69.6 ± 10.6	0.004 *
Fat, kg (mean ± SD)	22.3 ± 9.1	20.2 ± 6.7	0.356	24.7 ± 7.5	19.9 ± 7.6	0.104
LDM, kg (mean ± SD)	10.2 ± 2.5	14.1 ± 2.1	<0.001 **	8.7 ± 2.3	12.5 ± 3.6	0.002 **
SMM, kg (mean ± SD)	15.3 ± 3.4	23.9 ± 5.4	<0.001 **	15.6 ± 3.1	28.3 ± 6.6	<0.001 **
TBW L (mean ± SD)	25.8 ± 5.5	34.2 ± 8.1	<0.001 **	28.3 ± 6.6	31.4 ± 4.3	0.166
ICW, L (mean ± SD)	13.2 ± 3.3	19.2 ± 5.1	<0.001 **	14.9 ± 3.9	17.9 ± 3.1	0.041 **
ECW, L (mean ± SD)	12.3 ± 2.5	14.9 ± 3.1	0.001 **	13.3 ± 2.9	13.5 ± 1.8	0.839

ICC: Waist-to-Hip Ratio, BMI: Body Mass Index, UC: Ulcerative Colitis, ESR: Erythrocyte Sedimentation Rate, CRP: C-reactive protein, LDM: Lean Dry Mass, TBW: Total Body Water, ICW: Intracellular Water, ECW: Extracellular Water, SMM: Skeletal Muscles Mass, L: liters, mg: milligrams, dL: deciliter, cm: centimeters, PhA: Phase Angle. PhA low: <6.1°, PhA normal: >6.1° SD: Standard Deviation, * Significant *p*-value < 0.05 with independent samples *t*-test & ** Significant *p*-value < 0.05 with Mann–Whitney U test.

3.3. Correlations of Phase Angle with Body Composition Markers

We found a significant correlation between TBW (r = 0.509; $p < 0.001$), ICW ($r = 0.585$; $p < 0.001$), ECW (r = 0.366; $p < 0.001$), SMM (r = 0.803; $p < 0.001$), and LDM (r = 0.656; $p < 0.001$) with PhA in UC patients. Similar results were observed in the control group: TBW (r = 0.493; $p < 0.001$), ICW (r = 0.558; $p = 0.001$), ECW (r = 0.342; $p < 0.001$), SMM (r = 0.704; $p < 0.001$), and LDM (r = 0.617; $p < 0.001$) (Figure 2).

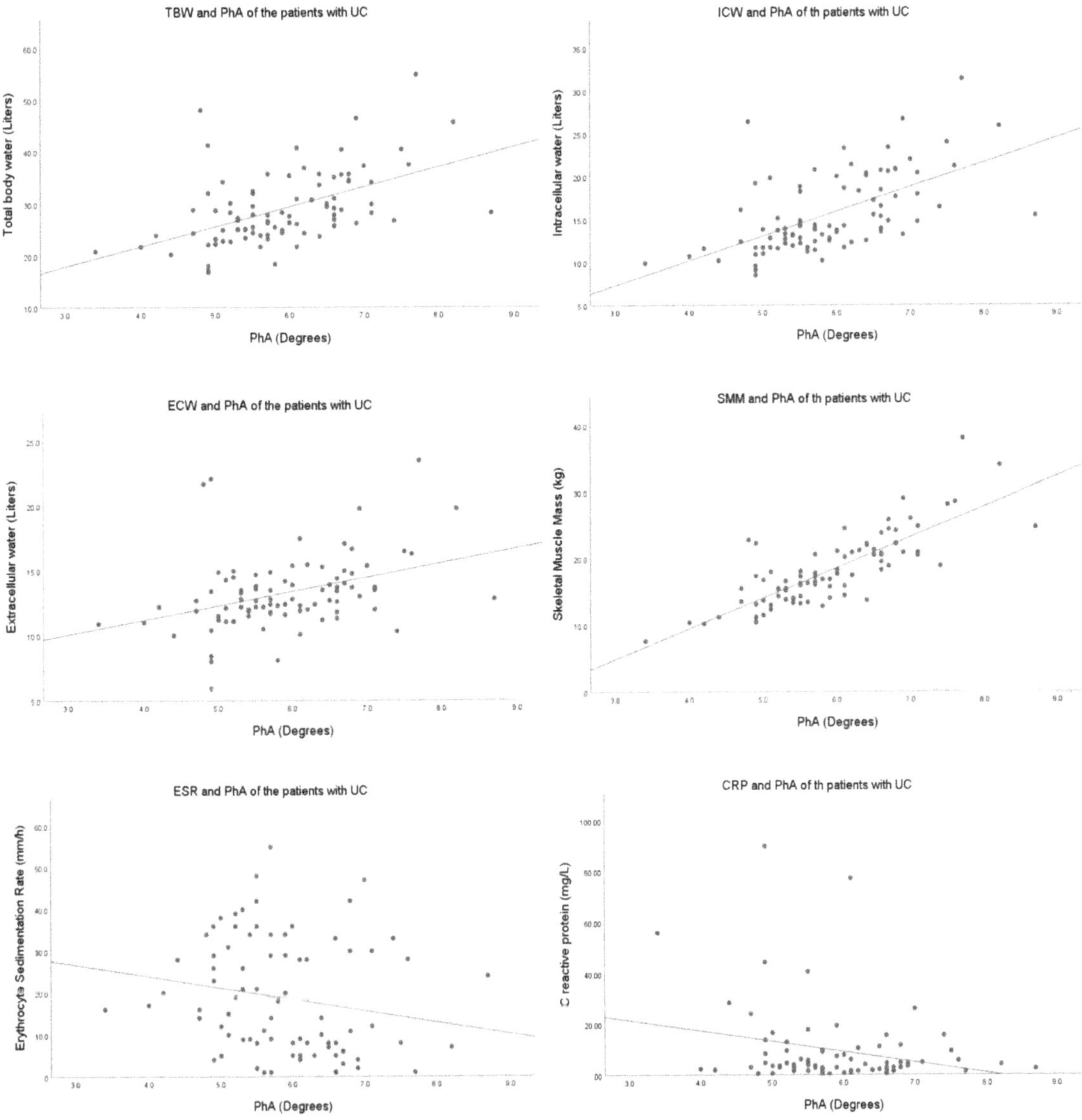

Figure 2. Correlations between PhA, body composition and biochemical parameters in UC patients. TBW: total body water, ICW: intracellular water, ECW: extracellular water, CRP: C-reactive protein, ESR: erythrocyte sedimentation rate, PhA: phase angle, UC: ulcerative colitis.

4. Discussion

PhA is considered a marker of cellular integrity and is directly related to prognosis and mortality in numerous diseases [16]. Furthermore, it serves as a predictor of malnutrition, which is defined by The World Health Organization (WHO) as a deficiency, excess, or imbalance in a person's intake of energy and/or nutrients [17]. However, there are few studies examining PhA in patients with IBD, primarily focused on CD. Peng et al. studied 169 CD patients, finding that PhA = 6.01° in men and 5.2° in women is associated with malnutrition. We found similar PhA values in UC patients, which suggests that low PhA may be a marker of the disease (Figure 3) [15].

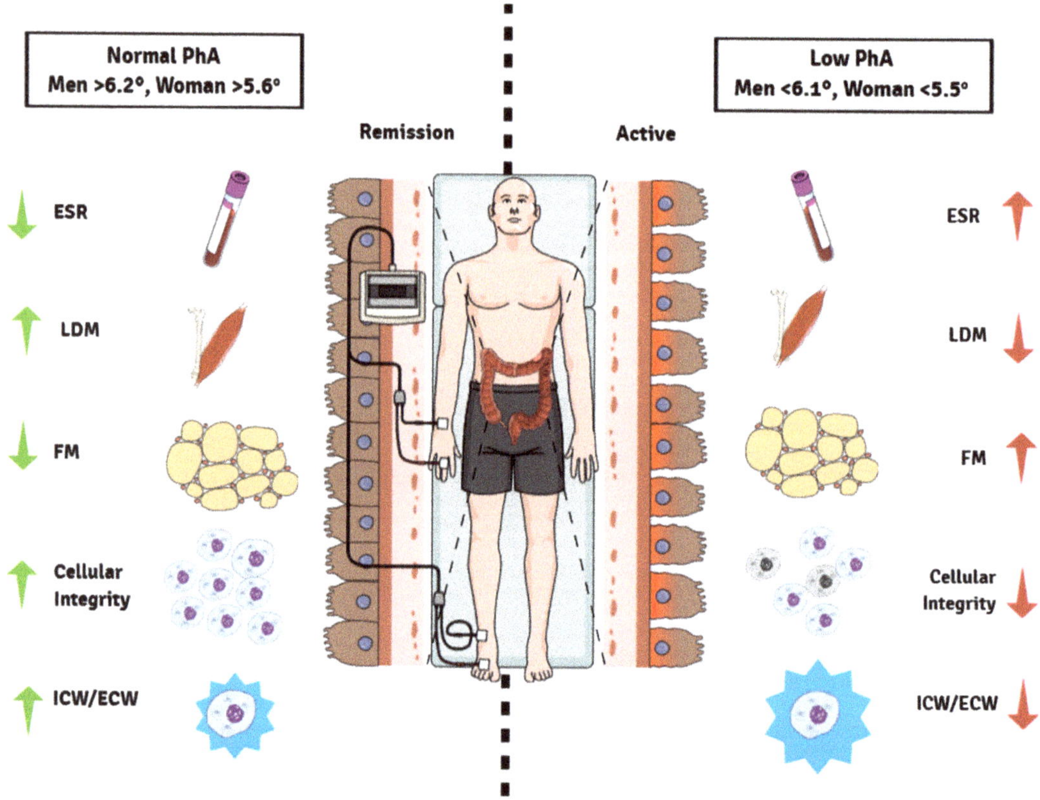

Figure 3. Proposal of the main metabolic changes in UC patients with low PhA. The metabolic alterations in UC patients with low PhA are associated with disease activity, increased ESR, decreased lean, dry mass, increased fat, and increased fluid retention. ESR: erythrocyte sedimentation rate, PhA: phase angle, TBW: total body water, ICW: intracellular water, ECW: extracellular water, UC: ulcerative colitis. Red arrows indicate that changes are detrimental. Green arrows indicate that changes are beneficial.

The findings in CD are possible because the disease is transmural, leading to increased cell death and decreased nutrient absorption, thus magnifying malnutrition compared to that observed in UC patients. However, this phenomenon could also occur in UC patients due to medication use, disease activity, and poor nutrient absorption. The same research team mentioned that patients with PhA < 6.1° in men and <5.5 in women have a higher risk of malnutrition as a manifestation of the inflammatory process (Figure 3). So far, this finding aligns with the study by Coffi et al. (2020), which also reported that lower PhA values were indicative of poorer nutritional status and higher levels of inflammation in IBD patients [18]. Otherwise, these data are consistent with those reported by Więch et al., where they showed that IBD children and adolescents with low PhA (<5°) display poor nutritional and functional status compared to healthy subjects [19]. In addition, low PhA is associated with reduced exercise capacity and physical activity in IBD patients. Normando C. et al. showed that low PhA correlates with decreased daily activities, especially in the elderly (Figure 3) [20]. In UC, the behavior is similar, as patients reduce their physical activity for fear of losing weight and muscle mass, which could also explain the decrease in PhA in our study population.

In addition, Cioffi et al. pointed out that inflammation and malnutrition negatively affect the electrical properties of tissue, leading to decreased PhA in UC patients compared to healthy individuals [21,22]. This phenomenon occurs because acute inflammation is the body's response to damage under transitory conditions; however, when inflammation becomes chronic, as in IBD patients, tissue damage and physiological imbalance occur due to the abnormal production of proinflammatory cytokines [22]. Inflammation related to disease activity leads to low PhA. In our population of UC patients, lower PhA was more evident in patients with active disease than in patients in remission, and this reduction was more significant in women. Thus, active disease and female sex can be considered factors related to malnourishment in UC; nevertheless, we need to conduct further studies before making solid conclusions [15].

Urbano et al. showed that PhA negatively correlates with CRP and ESR in UC patients, a finding also observed herein. Chronic inflammation contributes to metabolic abnormalities, changes in body composition, and chronic diseases such as sarcopenia, diabetes, and metabolic syndrome [9,21]. In our study, UC patients with low PhA (<6.1°) had lower weight, LDM, water, and ICW, accompanied by higher FM, compared to patients with normal PhA and regardless of disease activity [23]. However, inflammation and disease activity can affect fluid levels and influence PhA. According to the study by Bongiolo et al., PhA may reflect muscle mass loss independently of the disease activity. In our study, patients with UC who had low PhA (<6.1°) had lower weight, lower LDM, less water, especially ICW, and a higher amount of FM regardless of disease activity compared to patients with regular PhA (Figure 3) [23]. Based on the study of Bongiolo et al., PhA can reflect muscle mass depletion independently of active disease [24]. Many known risk factors for IBD trigger the loss of muscle and fat reserves, altering cellular fluid distribution. This change in body composition is associated with the prognosis, severity, and stage of UC [25]. We want to note that none of our patients had low BMI, which strengthens the argument for using other parameters, such as PhA, to monitor nutritional status in UC. The applicability of these data is helpful for physicians and nutritionists, as they can make a more objective assessment based on the activity of the disease and not only on the BMI. Interestingly, 40% of patients in our study population were overweight. However, the analysis of body composition and PhA revealed that patients could be at risk of malnutrition or sarcopenia [20]. In our study, patients with low PhA and active disease had higher CHF, an index related to cardiovascular risk. Although CHF levels do not determine risk, chronic inflammation leads to several cardiovascular and metabolic events, as well as sarcopenia, malnutrition, and poor nutrient absorption, especially in women compared to men [25–28].

In this study, we found changes related to the amount of ICW and ECW in UC patients compared to controls. This phenomenon may occur because low PhA is associated with altered distribution of ECW, hemoglobin, hematocrit, and muscle mass [26], as well as an imbalance of TBW and ECW in patients with cancer [29].

Several studies have shown that patients with IBD have lower levels of LDM, an indicator of the amount of minerals, visceral proteins, and muscles, particularly in pediatric patients [30]. Herein, we observed that UC patients display a significant decrease in LDM compared to controls. Since LDM also decreased in UC patients with active disease, we speculate that the amount of muscle and visceral proteins may decrease as disease severity and inflammation increase. A study conducted by Dhillon RJ et al. reported a decrease in muscle mass associated with the release of inflammatory mediators, such as tumor necrosis factor-alpha (TNF-α) and interleukin-6 (IL-6) [22,24,31]. Moreover, Bellido et al. emphasized that standardizing test protocols will facilitate the diagnosis and assessment of the risk associated with reduced PhA and aid in evaluating responses to therapeutic interventions [32]. Our results align with previous reports, showing that inflammatory markers such as ESR and CRP increase according to disease activity and PhA [33].

Regardless of disease activity, PhA may represent an alternative method to assess nutritional status in UC patients during active disease or remission to avoid malnourishment. Moreover, considering PhA may help improve the subjective results using non-specific measurements such as BMI or waist circumference. These traditional measures cannot accurately identify individuals with overt malnutrition who require short-term dietary support. Data from this study are relevant and may contribute to implementing personalized nutritional therapy that could lead to a better disease prognosis in UC. In parallel, a long-term follow-up of the patients could improve the study, which may also allow us to increase the sample size to recalculate parameters that did not reach significance but showed a trend. Additionally, we did not measure the amount of skeletal muscle and only registered LDM, a measurement that can be affected by the patient's bone mineral density. This study may open new research avenues focused on detecting and preventing malnutrition in UC patients. Future longitudinal studies on PhA in UC patients should include a diverse cohort and standardized measurement protocols to ensure consistency. Increasing the sample size will help minimize random variation. Regular, long-term follow-up is needed to correlate PhA changes with clinical outcomes like disease activity and quality of life. Appropriate statistical methods should be used to analyze trends and control for confounding variables. These steps will enhance the understanding of PhA's prognostic value in UC management.

5. Conclusions

We found that PhA significantly decreases in UC patients, particularly those with active disease. These findings suggest that PhA may help detect inflammatory activity and monitor changes in body composition in UC patients.

PhA appears to work as a complementary tool to assess nutritional status in UC patients when considering PhA $< 6.1^{\circ}$ to identify individuals with high inflammatory response and low LDM levels.

PhA exhibits correlations with inflammatory parameters that persist even after disease remission, which aligns with previous reports. It is worth noting that our results did not find significant differences in patients' BMI, confirming that this parameter is not strong enough to detect UC-related malnutrition. This finding reveals how relevant it may be to incorporate PhA in assessing nutritional status in UC patients. We still need to conduct prospective studies to evaluate the cutoff for different disease stages and validate it in this population.

Author Contributions: The authors' responsibilities were as follows: Conceptualization, V.M.M.-M. and N.B.-H.; methodology, R.B.-V.; software, G.M.-M.; validation, S.O.-L. and A.G.-C.; formal analysis, J.I.C.-R.; investigation, M.A.S.-C.; resources, G.E.; data curation, J.L.d.L.-R.; writing—original draft preparation, V.M.M.-M. and N.B.-H.; writing—review and editing, G.M.-M.; visualization, G.M.-M.; supervision, G.E.; project administration, V.M.M.-M.; funding acquisition, G.M.-M. and N.B.-H. All authors have read and agreed to the published version of the manuscript.

Funding: This research did not receive support from public institutions, commercial sectors, or non-profit organizations.

Institutional Review Board Statement: The study was conducted in accordance with the Declaration of Helsinki and approved by the Institutional Review Board and Ethics Committee of General Hospital of Mexico and La Raza Medical Center (protocol code DI 19/501/03/098; 1 February 2020 and R-2023-3501-079; 20 January 2023).

Informed Consent Statement: Informed consent was obtained from all subjects involved in the study.

Data Availability Statement: The data supporting the findings of this study are available on the link: "C:\Users\nalle\Dropbox\HospitalGeneral\1PROTOCOLOS\AF-CUCI\Basede datos\Base de datos CUCI y controles.sav".

Conflicts of Interest: The authors declare no conflict of interest.

References

1. Zhang, Y.Z.; Li, Y.Y. Inflammatory bowel disease: Pathogenesis. *World J. Gastroenterol.* **2014**, *20*, 91–99. [CrossRef] [PubMed]
2. Gompertz, M.; Sedano, R. Manifestaciones clínicas y endoscópicas en enfermedad inflamatoria intestinal. *Rev. Médica Clínica Las Condes* **2019**, *30*, 273–282. [CrossRef]
3. Li, S.; Ney, M.; Eslamparast, T.; Vandermeer, B.; Ismond, K.P.; Kroeker, K.; Halloran, B.; Raman, M.; Tandon, P. Systematic review of nutrition screening and assessment in inflammatory bowel disease. *World J. Gastroenterol.* **2019**, *25*, 3823–3837. [CrossRef] [PubMed]
4. Nishikawa, H.; Nakamura, S.; Miyazaki, T.; Kakimoto, K.; Fukunishi, S.; Asai, A.; Nishiguchi, S.; Higuchi, K. Inflammatory Bowel Disease and Sarcopenia: Its Mechanism and Clinical Importance. *J. Clin. Med.* **2021**, *10*, 4214. [CrossRef]
5. Bischoff, S.C.; Bager, P.; Escher, J.; Forbes, A.; Hébuterne, X.; Hvas, C.L.; Joly, F.; Klek, S.; Krznaric, Z.; Ockenga, J.; et al. ESPEN guideline on Clinical Nutrition in inflammatory bowel disease. *Clin. Nutr.* **2023**, *42*, 352–379. [CrossRef]
6. Fiorindi, C.; Luceri, C.; Dragoni, G.; Piemonte, G.; Scaringi, S.; Staderini, F.; Nannoni, A.; Ficari, F.; Giudici, F. GLIM Criteria for Malnutrition in Surgical IBD Patients: A Pilot Study. *Nutrients* **2020**, *12*, 2222. [CrossRef]
7. Forbes, A.; Escher, J.; Hébuterne, X.; Kłęk, S.; Krznaric, Z.; Schneider, S.; Shamir, R.; Stardelova, K.; Wierdsma, N.; Wiskin, A.E.; et al. ESPEN guideline: Clinical nutrition in inflammatory bowel disease. *Clin. Nutr.* **2017**, *36*, 321–347. [CrossRef]
8. Llames, L.; Baldomero, V.; Iglesias, M.L.; Rodota, L.P. Values of the phase angle by bioelectrical impedance; nutritional status and prognostic value. *Nutr. Hosp.* **2013**, *28*, 286–295.
9. Urbano, A.P.S.; Sassaki, L.Y.; Dorna, M.S.; Presti, P.T.; Carvalhaes, M.; Martini, L.A.; Ferreira, A.L.A. Associations among body composition, inflammatory profile and disease extent in ulcerative colitis patients. *Rev. Assoc. Med. Bras. (1992)* **2018**, *64*, 133–139. [CrossRef]
10. Vandenbroucke, J.P.; Von Elm, E.; Altman, D.G.; Gotzsche, P.C.; Mulrow, C.D.; Pocock, S.J.; Poole, C. Strengthening the reporting of observational studies in epidemiology (STROBE): Explanation and elaboration. *Gac. Sanit.* **2009**, *23*, 158. [CrossRef]
11. Macias, N.; Aleman-Mateo, H.; Esparza-Romero, J.; Valencia, M.E. Body fat measurement by bioelectrical impedance and air displacement plethysmography: A cross-validation study to design bioelectrical impedance equations in Mexican adults. *Nutr. J.* **2007**, *6*, 18. [CrossRef] [PubMed]
12. Janssen, I.; Heymsfield, S.B.; Baumgartner, R.N.; Ross, R. Estimation of skeletal muscle mass by bioelectrical impedance analysis. *J. Appl. Physiol. (1985)* **2000**, *89*, 465–471. [CrossRef] [PubMed]
13. Siddiqui, N.I.; Khan, S.A.; Shoeb, M.; Bose, S. Anthropometric Predictors of Bio-Impedance Analysis (BIA) Phase Angle in Healthy Adults. *J. Clin. Diagn. Res.* **2016**, *10*, CC01–CC04. [CrossRef] [PubMed]
14. Rojas, M.C.; Vargas, R.V. La medición de la talla y el peso. In *guía para el personal de la salud del primer nivel de atención*; Instituto Nacional de Salud: Lima, Peru, 2004.
15. Peng, Z.; Xu, D.; Li, Y.; Peng, Y.; Liu, X. Phase Angle as a Comprehensive Tool for Nutritional Monitoring and Management in Patients with Crohn's Disease. *Nutrients* **2022**, *14*, 2260. [CrossRef]
16. Lalinde, J.D.H.; Castro, F.E.; Rodríguez, J.E.; Rangel, J.G.C.; Sierra, C.A.T.; Torrado, M.K.A.; Bermúdez Pirela, V.J. Sobre el uso adecuado del coeficiente de correlación de Pearson: Definición, propiedades y suposiciones. *Arch. Venez. De Farmacol. Ter.* **2018**, *37*, 587–595.
17. Sellen, D. Physical status: The use and interpretation of anthropometry. Report of a WHO Expert Committee. *World Health Organ Tech. Rep. Ser.* **1995**, *854*, 1–452.
18. Cioffi, I.; Marra, M.; Imperatore, N.; Pagano, M.C.; Santarpia, L.; Alfonsi, L.; Testa, A.; Sammarco, R.; Contaldo, F.; Castiglione, F.; et al. Assessment of bioelectrical phase angle as a predictor of nutritional status in patients with Crohn's disease: A cross sectional study. *Clin. Nutr.* **2020**, *39*, 1564–1571. [CrossRef]
19. Wiech, P.; Dabrowski, M.; Bazalinski, D.; Salacinska, I.; Korczowski, B.; Binkowska-Bury, M. Bioelectrical Impedance Phase Angle as an Indicator of Malnutrition in Hospitalized Children with Diagnosed Inflammatory Bowel Diseases—A Case Control Study. *Nutrients* **2018**, *10*, 499. [CrossRef]
20. Norman, K.; Stobäus, N.; Fau-Pirlich, M.; Pirlich, M.; Fau-Bosy-Westphal, A.; Bosy-Westphal, A. Bioelectrical phase angle and impedance vector analysis—Clinical relevance and applicability of impedance parameters. *Clin. Nutr.* **2012**, *31*, 854–861. [CrossRef]
21. Mentella, M.C.; Scaldaferri, F.; Pizzoferrato, M.; Gasbarrini, A.; Miggiano, G.A.D. The Association of Disease Activity, BMI and Phase Angle with Vitamin D Deficiency in Patients with IBD. *Nutrients* **2019**, *11*, 2583. [CrossRef]
22. da Silva, B.R.; Orsso, C.E.; Gonzalez, M.C.; Sicchieri, J.M.F.; Mialich, M.S.; Jordao, A.A.; Prado, C.M. Phase angle and cellular health: Inflammation and oxidative damage. *Rev. Endocr. Metab. Disord.* **2023**, *24*, 543–562. [CrossRef] [PubMed]
23. Jablonska, B.; Mrowiec, S. Nutritional Status and Its Detection in Patients with Inflammatory Bowel Diseases. *Nutrients* **2023**, *15*, 1991. [CrossRef] [PubMed]

24. Bongiolo, A.M.; Machado, M.J.; Lazarotto, B.A.; Rupp, M.L.C.; Dal-Pizzol, F.; Pires, M.M.S. Phase Angle as a Predictor of Muscle Mass in Patients with Inflammatory Bowel Disease. *Arq. Gastroenterol.* **2024**, *61*, e23095. [CrossRef] [PubMed]
25. Casirati, A.; Crotti, S.; Raffaele, A.; Caccialanza, R.; Cereda, E. The use of phase angle in patients with digestive and liver diseases. *Rev. Endocr. Metab. Disord.* **2023**, *24*, 503–524. [CrossRef]
26. Ryan, E.; McNicholas, D.; Creavin, B.; Kelly, M.E.; Walsh, T.; Beddy, D. Sarcopenia and Inflammatory Bowel Disease: A Systematic Review. *Inflamm. Bowel Dis.* **2019**, *25*, 67–73. [CrossRef]
27. Nunez, P.; Garcia Mateo, S.; Quera, R.; Gomollon, F. Inflammatory bowel disease and the risk of cardiovascular diseases. *Gastroenterol. Hepatol.* **2021**, *44*, 236–242.
28. Cao, Q.; Yu, S.; Xiong, W.; Li, Y.; Li, H.; Li, J.; Li, F. Waist-hip ratio as a predictor of myocardial infarction risk: A systematic review and meta-analysis. *Medicine* **2018**, *97*, e11639. [CrossRef]
29. Katsura, N.; Yamashita, M.; Ishihara, T. Extracellular water to total body water ratio may mediate the association between phase angle and mortality in patients with cancer cachexia: A single-center, retrospective study. *Clin. Nutr. ESPEN* **2021**, *46*, 193–199. [CrossRef]
30. Thangarajah, D.; Hyde, M.J.; Konteti, V.K.; Santhakumaran, S.; Frost, G.; Fell, J.M. Systematic review: Body composition in children with inflammatory bowel disease. *Aliment. Pharmacol. Ther.* **2015**, *42*, 142–157. [CrossRef]
31. Dhillon, R.J.; Hasni, S. Pathogenesis and Management of Sarcopenia. *Clin. Geriatr. Med.* **2017**, *33*, 17–26. [CrossRef]
32. Bellido, D.; García-García, C.; Talluri, A.; Lukaski, H.C.; García-Almeida, J.M. Future lines of research on phase angle: Strengths and limitations. *Rev. Endocr. Metab. Disord.* **2023**, *24*, 563–583. [CrossRef]
33. Sands, B.E. Biomarkers of Inflammation in Inflammatory Bowel Disease. *Gastroenterology* **2015**, *149*, 1275–1285.e2. [CrossRef]

life

MDPI

Review

Management of a Rare Case of Superior Mesenteric Artery Aneurysm Associated with a Pancreatic Cyst Complicated by Acute Rupture: A Case Report and Review of Literature

Petru Razvan Dragulescu [1], Roxana Carmen Geana (Anghel) [1,*], Mircea Robu [1,2,*], Reza Nayyerani [1,2], Cristian Dumitrescu [1], Anca Dragan [3], Catalin Vasilescu [2], Vlad Anton Iliescu [1,2] and Ovidiu Stiru [1,2]

1 Department of Cardiac Surgery, Prof. Dr. C.C. Iliescu Emergency Institute for Cardiovascular Diseases, 022322 Bucharest, Romania; razvan.dragulescu@ymail.com (P.R.D.); reza.nayyerani@drd.umfcd.ro (R.N.); dumitrescu.cristian@aol.com (C.D.); vladanton.iliescu@gmail.com (V.A.I.); ovidiu.stiru@umfcd.ro (O.S.)

2 Faculty of Medicine, Carol Davila University of Medicine and Pharmacy, 050474 Bucharest, Romania; cartalin.vasilescu@umfcd.ro

3 1st Department of Cardiovascular Anaesthesiology and Intensive Care, Prof. Dr. C.C. Iliescu Emergency Institute for Cardiovascular Diseases, 022328 Bucharest, Romania; anca.dragan1978.14@gmail.com

* Correspondence: geana.roxana22@gmail.com (R.C.G.); mircea.robu@drd.umfcd.ro (M.R.)

Abstract: Superior mesenteric artery aneurysms are a rare pathology, and rupture due to a pancreatic cyst in the context of alcohol-induced pancreatitis is an even rarer condition. The first line of treatment is usually an endovascular approach. We present the case of a 51-year-old male with alcohol-induced pancreatitis, diagnosed with a superior mesenteric artery aneurysm with active bleeding in close contact with a large pancreatic cyst. A covered stent was used to treat this condition. The patient developed hemorrhagic shock 12 h after the procedure and an urgent laparotomy was performed. A second rupture of the arterial wall at the distal end of the stent was observed and in order to obtain distal perfusion, first, an infrarenal aorta to superior mesenteric artery bypass distal to the rupture was performed in order to exclude the aneurysm. Secondly, a bypass originating from the distal end of the first bypass to the distal end of the superior mesenteric artery was performed. The patient had an uneventful recovery and was discharged after 10 days. We reviewed the literature regarding the incidence and the therapeutic management of superior mesenteric artery aneurysm complicated by pancreatic cyst. An advanced search on PubMed from 2004 to 2024 returned 194 results and after applying the inclusion–exclusion criteria, 11 publications were selected. Although the endovascular approach is usually the first line of treatment with obvious advantages for the patient, a patient-tailored approach should be made in such cases and surgery could be the first option, when considering that the mechanism of aneurysm rupture is due to erosion of the arterial wall by the pancreatic enzymes. Surgery has the advantage of cyst drainage and aneurysm exclusion and in our case proved lifesaving.

Keywords: superior mesenteric artery; rupture arterial aneurysms; chronic pancreatitis; pancreatic cyst

1. Introduction

Superior mesenteric artery (SMA) pseudoaneurysms, though rare, present significant clinical challenges due to their potential for life-threatening complications such as rupture and hemorrhage [1–4]. These pseudoaneurysms are often associated with underlying conditions, particularly pancreatitis, which can erode the arterial wall through the release of pancreatic enzymes. Understanding the pathophysiology of SMA pseudoaneurysms is crucial, as timely diagnosis and intervention can markedly improve patient outcomes [4–8].

Current diagnostic techniques, especially advanced imaging modalities like computed tomography (CT) and CT angiography, have revolutionized the management of SMA pseudoaneurysms. These methods allow for precise visualization of vascular anatomy and the identification of aneurysms, facilitating early intervention. In particular, CT angiography offers a non-invasive means to evaluate the presence and extent of aneurysms, guiding the choice between endovascular and surgical treatment strategies [9–11].

From a therapeutic perspective, endovascular approaches have gained prominence as first-line treatments due to their minimally invasive nature and reduced recovery times. Techniques such as covered stent placement allow for immediate exclusion of the aneurysm while preserving blood flow to the distal vascular bed. However, the anatomical complexity often seen in patients with pancreatic pathology can complicate these interventions, necessitating a thorough understanding of the vascular anatomy and the potential for anatomical variations [9].

Despite advancements in treatment modalities, the management of SMA pseudoaneurysms remains challenging. The risk of rupture, especially in the context of pancreatitis, underscores the importance of personalized medicine approaches tailored to individual patient circumstances. This includes considering the patient's overall health, the extent of vascular involvement, and the presence of comorbid conditions [10,11].

Therefore, we performed a literature review regarding the incidence of SMA aneurysm in association with pancreatic cyst and its therapeutic management. This review aims to comprehensively explore the current state of knowledge regarding SMA pseudoaneurysms, emphasizing the interplay between advanced imaging techniques and therapeutic strategies, while highlighting the critical role of personalized medicine in optimizing patient outcomes.

2. Case Report

A 51-year-old male patient was admitted to the emergency department for severe epigastric pain, nausea, and vomiting with a 2-day onset. His medical history was consistent with alcohol-induced chronic pancreatitis with several episodes of acute decompensation. Physical examination revealed diffuse abdominal tenderness with slight muscular defense. On palpation, an epigastric mass was objectified, and abdominal auscultation revealed normoactive intestinal sounds. The patient denied any transit modifications, fever, or shivers. On admission, the patient had a BMI of 22.5 kg/m^2 and was hemodynamically stable with a blood pressure of 140/65 mmHg, heart rate of 83 bpm, normal sinus rhythm, and peripheral oxygen saturation of 97% in atmospheric air. Laboratory blood tests revealed elevated pancreatic enzymes: Amylase 91 U/L, Lipase 32 U/L (10 days prior to admission, they were 288 and 147 on a routine check-up). Also, the patient was anemic (Hb 9.5 g/dL), had a GGT of 134 U/L, and had an inflammatory syndrome (fibrinogen 465 mg/dL, and C Reactive Protein 102 mg/L).

The computer tomography (CT) scan revealed an SMA aneurysm with a small bleeding observed into a large size pancreatic cyst of 92 mm × 110 mm in the cephalic region (Figures 1 and 2). Another pancreatic cyst of 70 mm × 90 mm in the caudal region and also a right accessory hepatic artery (RAHA) proximally to the aneurysm were found.

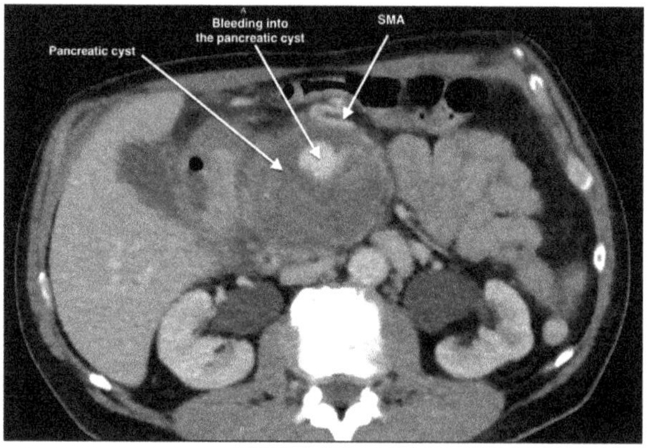

Figure 1. Preoperative CTA aspect of the ruptured SMAA-coronal view describing the course of the SMA and its rupture into the pancreatic cyst.

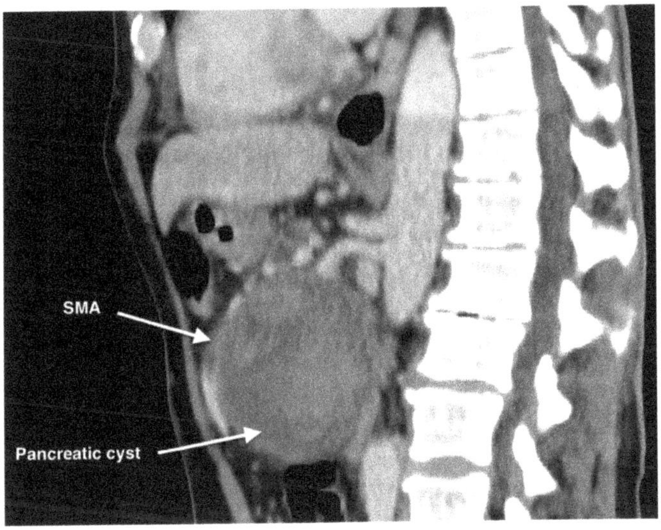

Figure 2. Preoperative CTA aspect of the ruptured SMAA and the pancreatic cyst-sagittal view describing the course of the SMA along the pancreatic cyst.

Angiography was performed (Figure 3) and the decision to implant a double-covered stent (Ivascular 5 × 37 mm) in the SMA was made. The endovascular approach was without any periprocedural complications and with a favorable result (Figure 4).

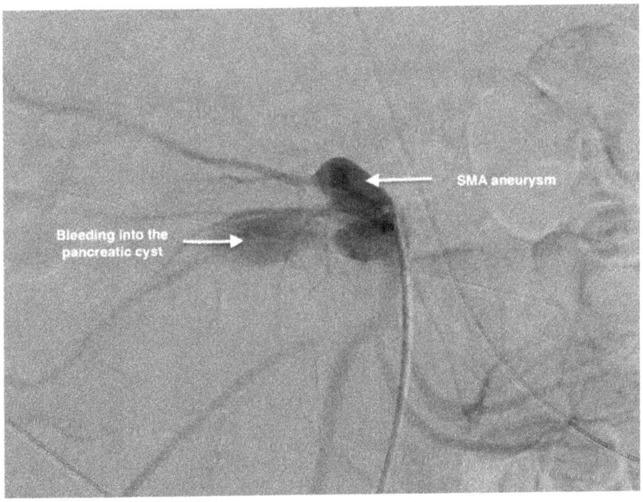

Figure 3. Preoperative arteriography of the superior mesenteric artery and its branches showing the bleeding of the SMAA into the pancreatic cyst.

After twelve hours from the endovascular procedure, the patient became severely hypotensive, with a blood pressure of 78/60 mmHg. Blood tests revealed a hemoglobin level of 4 g/dL and the patient was immediately transferred to the operating room for urgent exploratory laparotomy.

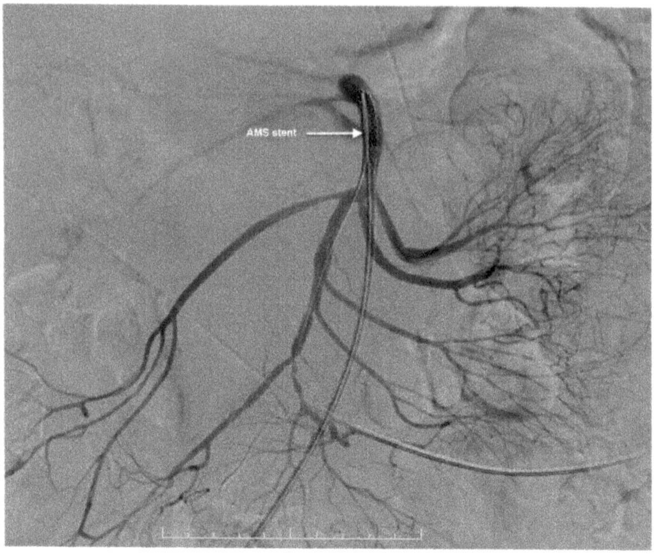

Figure 4. Preoperative arteriography aspect of the SMA after the endovascular treatment of the SMAA showing the Ivascular double-covered stent's position in the superior mesenteric artery.

Surgical Technique

After rapid induction of general anesthesia, a median laparotomy was done. We suspected that the cause of the hemorrhagic shock was the rupture of the SMA aneurism. In order to access the origin of the SMA, the Cattell-Braasch maneuver was performed for right-sided medial visceral rotation. The retroperitoneum was incised and the SMA course was identified. A pancreatic cyst was found in direct contact with the wall of the SMA aneurysm. Proximal and distal isolation of the SMA was performed with vessel loops. The splenic artery with the origin from SMA was isolated and clamped. Prior to arterial clamping, 100 IU per kilogram of unfractionated heparin was administered. After clamping of the SMA near the aorta, the cyst was incised and a mix of old and fresh blood was found. Visceral protection was achieved via the delivery of 1000 mL of cold (4C) Custodiol solution into the distal SMA, using a 14Fr Foley catheter. The stent was identified and the initial arterial wall rupture was also identified at the medial portion of the stent. At the distal end of the stent, we identified a second rupture in a friable area of the wall. This second rupture was not seen in the initial angiography study and we presumed that it was caused by the continuing erosion of the pancreatic enzymes. After stent removal and aneurysm exclusion by proximal and distal ligation, an end-to-side anastomosis with a 6 mm ePTFE graft with a 6.0 Polypropylene suture was performed distal to the ruptured artery wall. The proximal end of the graft was implanted with the same technique in the infrarenal aorta. Intraoperative epivascular Doppler of the distal SMA revealed a low distal flow with good perfusion of a hepatic accessory artery that originated from the SMA aneurysm. In order to address this distal visceral hypoperfusion, another interposition with a 6 mm ePTFE graft was performed from the distal end of the original bypass to the distal end of the SMA. Epivascular Doppler ultrasound of the distal SMA was within normal limits (Figures 5 and 6). The pancreatic cyst was drained and a drain tube was placed in the proximal area. The surgery was concluded in the usual manner.

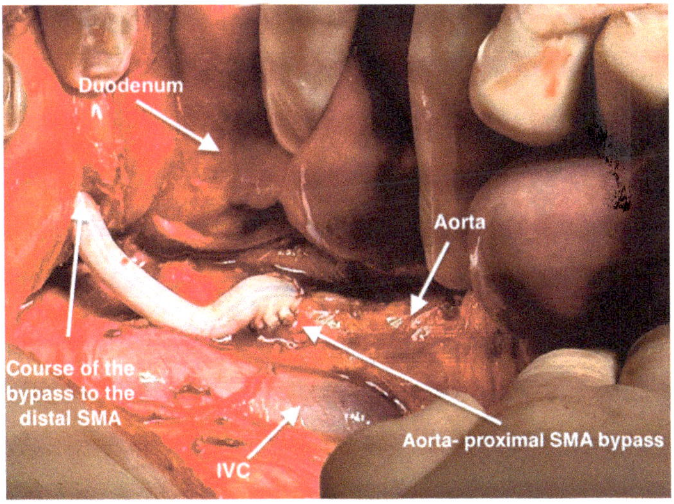

Figure 5. Medial visceral rotation in order to expose retroperitoneal structures. Intraoperative view of the bypass from the aorta to the proximal portion of the superior mesenteric artery. IVC-inferior vena cava.

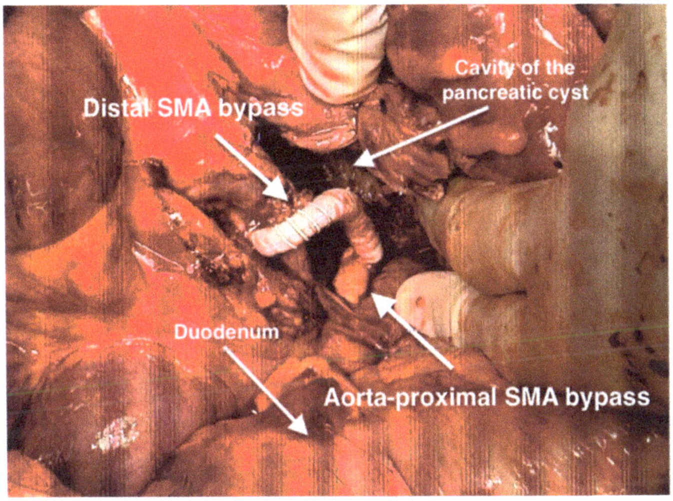

Figure 6. Intraoperative aspect of the bypass from the proximal segment of the SMA to the distal segment of the SMA. The cavity of the drained pancreatic cyst is visible.

The patient was transferred to the intensive care unit (ICU) and had a favorable postoperative evolution. He was extubated at 8 h postoperatively and was hemodynamically stable without the need for vasopressors. Intravenous anticoagulation started 3 h from surgery. Serum lactate and pancreatic enzymes were checked every 3 h in the first 24 h, with no detected elevation. Maximum lipase level was 30 U/L and maximum amylase level was 40 U/L. Serum lactate had a peak of 2.2 mmol/L. Oral anticoagulation intake was started on postoperative day four with a target INR between two and three. On the eighth postoperative day, the drains were removed at a drainage of 50 mL/24 h and after normal intestinal transit.

Postoperatively contrast enhanced CT evaluation showed patent SMA bypasses with good distal perfusion of the SMA and its branches (Figure 7). The patient was discharged 10 days postoperatively and remains asymptomatic.

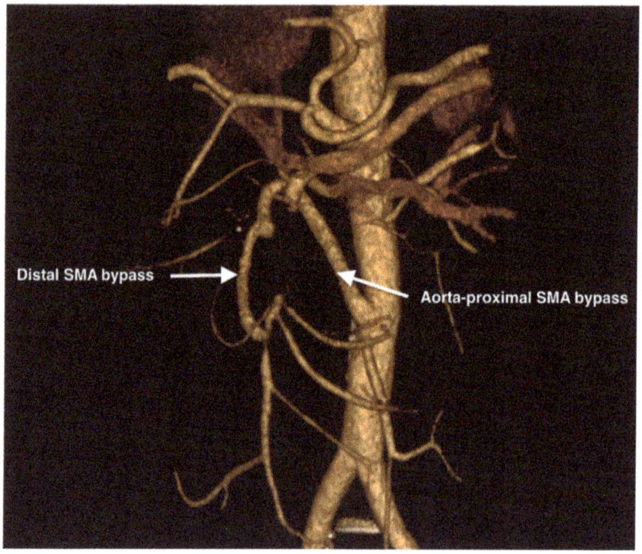

Figure 7. Postoperative 3D reconstruction of the computed angiography of the aorta and the SMA showing the patency of the bypass.

3. Discussion

Visceral artery aneurysm is a rare condition. Despite a low incidence, it is associated with a high mortality rate upon rupture, estimated at 25–75% [1,5]. The incidence of this condition rose in recent years mostly due to imaging techniques and the aging population [3,4,11]. Regarding SMA aneurysms, the prevalence is unclear and it is estimated between 0.5 and 2 per 10,000 [12,13].

The definition of visceral aneurysms includes both true aneurysms and pseudoaneurysms, but their etiologies and natural evolution are very different. It appears that SMA aneurysms tend to affect predominantly men, with the average age of presentation of 50 years [5,11,14,15]. Infection is the most common etiology of SMAAs. Mycotic aneurysms sum up for almost 60%. Pseudoaneurysms of the SMA are rare, trauma, or inflammation in the context of pancreatitis being the most frequent cases [14,16,17].

Superior mesenteric artery pseudoaneurysm in patients with pancreatitis is a rare vascular complication of pancreatitis. Various mechanisms have been proposed to explain the formation of pseudoaneurysms, with the two most widely accepted theories being: the presence of a pseudocyst that erodes and weakens the wall of a nearby artery, leading to the development of a pseudoaneurysm, and the activation of proteolytic enzymes within the pancreatic tissue, which results in the auto-digestion of pancreatic and adjacent structures. When a pseudoaneurysm ruptures, it results in uncontrolled hemorrhage into the abdominal cavity, which can rapidly lead to hypovolemic shock and death if not promptly managed. The risk of rupture is heightened by the ongoing enzymatic activity and the inflammatory environment created by pancreatitis [8,15,18,19].

Other possible etiologies of SMA aneurysms are connective tissue diseases such as the Marfan syndrome. Patients with the Marfan syndrome usually present with aortic root dilatation associated with aortic insufficiency, but the aneurysmal development may occur at any level of the aorta including the SMA. These patients usually have a multi-stage treatment approach because the pathological alterations of the arterial wall continue to develop. Because of this fact, subsequent surgeries at other sites besides the thoracic aorta are needed for a significant number of patients [20].

In our case, the etiology of the SMA pseudoaneurysm is most likely due to alcohol-induced pancreatitis considering the patient's past medical history, with multiple decompensation episodes. The mechanism implicated in the rupture of the SMA pseudoaneurysm that led to the hemorrhagic shock could be the weakening of the arterial wall by the pancreatic enzymes released from the level of the cyst. Also, mechanical stress could contribute to rupture of the SMA aneurysm when considering the close proximity of the cyst to the wall of the SMA.

The clinical presentation of a ruptured SMA pseudoaneurysm can be dramatic and nonspecific, often complicating early diagnosis. Patients typically present with sudden, severe abdominal pain, which may radiate to the back. Symptoms of hemorrhagic shock are common. Additionally, patients may exhibit signs of gastrointestinal bleeding, such as hematemesis or melena, if the rupture communicates with the gastrointestinal tract.

Given the overlap in symptoms with other abdominal emergencies, a high index of suspicion is necessary, especially in patients with a history of pancreatitis or known pancreatic pseudocysts.

One of the major differential diagnoses that must be taken into consideration are the abdominal complications of acute aortic dissection, such as bowel malperfusion caused by superior mesenteric artery dissection. In such cases, the patient's treatment approach must be individualized based on multiple considerations like the entire aortic anatomy and the static or dynamic nature of the intimal flap obstruction, and it may consist of classic surgical treatment combined with percutaneous endovascular techniques in order to achieve a full blood flow restoration [21].

Accurate and rapid diagnosis of a ruptured SMA pseudoaneurysm is crucial for effective management with imaging studies playing a main role in this regard.

Computed tomography (CT) or computed tomography angiography (CTA) is recommended as the first-line choice for diagnosis and treatment planning due to its advantages in depicting the relationship between aneurysms and associated blood vessels, enabling 3D vascular reconstruction, and supplying essential data for determining the appropriate surgical approach. Computed tomography angiography is also considered essential in evaluating the entire aorta in order to diagnose the special cases of superior mesenteric artery aneurisms that occur in connective tissue disorders such as the Marfan syndrome.

Review of Literature

We conducted a review of the literature on PubMed database from 2004 to 2024. The main objective of the research was to identify the incidence and therapeutic management of superior mesenteric artery aneursysm associated with pancreatic cyst. We conducted an advanced search on PubMed using the syntax: (superior mesenteric artery aneurysm) AND ((pancreatic cyst) OR (pseudopancreactic cyst) OR (pancreatic cyst rupture) OR (pancreatitis)), which returned 194 results, and after applying the inclusion and exclusion criteria, we selected 11 articles. The inclusion criteria consisted of the following: relevant manuscript for the search topic; full manuscript published in recognized journals; and manuscripts that included the management of this association of these pathologies. The exclusion criteria were represented by the following: publications that were not relevant to the topic; and letters, covers, correction or comments to published manuscripts.

The reported rupture rate for superior mesenteric artery aneurysms is approximately 38%. However, the exact rupture rates for less common superior mesenteric artery aneurysms remain unclear [22].

Visceral artery pseudoaneurysms always require treatment, regardless of their size or symptoms. Table 1 highlights the main studies dealing with the management of SMA aneurysms. Conservative management is not advised due to the high rupture rate and up to 90% mortality in untreated cases. The primary goal of treatment is to exclude the aneurysm sac. As stated in the Society of Vascular Surgery guidelines, once diagnosed, a SMAA should be treated as soon as possible [23].

Table 1. Main studies regarding the management of SMA aneurysm. SMAA: superior mesenteric artery aneurysm; NS: not specified; NA: not available.

Authors	Year	Country	Number of Patients	Mean Age (Years)	SMAA	Pancreatic Cyst	Treatment	Follow-Up (Months)	Mortality
Pulli et al. [12]	2008	Italy	55	59.3	2	1	Surgery	120	50%
Wang et al. [17]	2020	China	18	49.1	18	2	Surgery 9 pts Endovascular 3 pts Conservative 3 pts	47	0%
Zyromski et al. [16]	2007	USA	35	59.3	3	3	Surgery	NS	NS
Guo et al. [24]	2016	China	8	55.3	8	1	Endovascular	NS	NS
Arias et al. [7]	2020	Spain	1	NS	1	1	Endovascular	NS	NS
Saftoiu et al. [11]	2004	Romania	1	66	1	1	Surgery	NA	100%
Bouassida et al. [18]	2012	Tunisia	1	50	0	1	Surgery	NA	100%
Kaszczewski et al. [2]	2023	Poland	1	41	1	0	Endovascular	12	0%
Pitcher et al. [4]	2022	USA	131	60	41	1	Surgery 36 Endovascular 8	43.6	NS
Okubo et al. [10]	2023	Japan	1	92	1	0	Endovascular	21	0%
Saltzberg et al. [13]	2005	USA	65	64.9	3	0	Endovascular 18 (27.7%) Surgery 9 (13.9%)	14.9	NS

The main treatments for superior mesenteric artery aneurysm include open surgery, endovascular surgery, and conservative management.

Classical open surgical treatments include simple aneurysm resection or resection combined with revascularization. The choice of surgical method depends on the aneurysm's location, whether it is ruptured, and its relationship with the branching vessels. The challenges of open surgery lie in the complex anatomy of the superior mesenteric artery aneurysm and the difficulty of achieving a good surgical field.

With advances in interventional techniques, endovascular surgery has become a common approach for treating superior mesenteric artery aneurysms in recent years. This includes procedures such as covered stent grafts, multi-layer bare stent implantation, and coil or embolic material embolization. However, the limitations of endovascular treatment originate primarily from the complex anatomy of the superior mesenteric artery, which leads to an increased risk of covering critical branches at the main trunk of the superior mesenteric artery and also poses a real challenge in maneuvering the guide wire and catheter to the lesion site on distal branches [24,25].

The endovascular treatment is deemed safer, especially in patients with multiple comorbidities, but it should not be used when an infectious etiology is suspected. The location of the SMA aneurysm is of the utmost importance, because it may be difficult to place a stent near the origin owing to the lack of an adequate landing zone. Large aneurysms may not be suitable to the use of a covered stent owing to instability in a large lumen. The stent should extend at least 1 cm proximally and distally to achieve a complete seal.

Coil embolization is also an option to treat SMAA, but it carries the risk of incomplete coiling, leading to aneurysm progression. Bare stent-assisted coiling is deemed safer and does not bear the risk of side branch obstruction. Stent-assisted coiling requires longer procedure times and higher doses of radiation. Covered stent implantation is safe when anatomy is favorable, and there is no risk of side branch occlusion. All the necessary measurements can be determined from the preoperative CT angiogram and should be compared with the diagnostic angiogram obtained before the endovascular procedure [22,26]. Table 1 summarizes the main studies regarding the management of SMA aneurysms.

From the selected studies, 45.4% [5] were published in the last five years, showing that the incidence of the association of these pathologies is increasing. This may be due to the development of imagistic evaluation, which leads to an earlier and more accurate diagnosis.

Regarding the management of the patients included in the selected studies, 36.3% [4] of the publications described the surgical approach, 36.3% [4] used endovascular interventions, and 27.2% [3] combined the surgical and endovascular treatments. The studies that used endovascular procedures, alone or combined with surgery, were more recently published. The treatment strategy in this association of pathologies is guided by the patient's status. In our case, the patient became hemodynamically unstable; he was in a hemorrhaging shock, with hemoglobin levels of 4 g/dL, and we decided on an emergent surgical approach. In some situations, the endovascular treatment can stabilize the hemodynamic status of the patient. In those cases, endoscopic transpapillary drainage or endoscopic ultrasound drainage can be considered as a treatment option for the pancreatic pseudocyst.

The management of a ruptured SMA pseudoaneurysm requires a multidisciplinary approach and often involves both immediate resuscitative measures and definitive surgical or endovascular intervention. In our case, we initially opted for an interventional approach with a covered stent, considering that the patient was stable and only a small quantity of contrast agent was observed extravasated from the aneurysm. However, this strategy proved to be insufficient with the patient entering into hypovolemic shock, suggesting that a classical exploratory laparotomy is needed. Intraoperatively, we have found a second rupture at the distal end of the stent, which was not initially seen in preoperative studies, demonstrating the rapidly evolutive nature of this condition. If the initial rupture was with high probability caused by the erosion of the pancreatic enzymes from the cyst into the wall of the SAM, the question arises as to whether the placement of the stent could have contributed to the further weakening of the SMA wall. The location of the second rupture, at the distal end of the stent, could suggest this. Considering this, we could say that surgical management from the beginning could have been a more suitable approach when dealing with a ruptured SMAA caused by a pancreatic cyst.

In our case, the etiology of the SMA pseudoaneurysm was likely alcohol-induced pancreatitis, resulting in recurrent episodes and eventual formation of the aneurysm. The clinical presentation can be ambiguous, with symptoms of severe abdominal pain and signs of hemorrhagic shock complicating diagnosis. A high index of suspicion is vital, particularly in patients with known pancreatitis or pancreatic cysts.

This case highlights the need for personalized treatment strategies. While the initial approach in our patient involved endovascular stenting, the subsequent rapid deterioration necessitated surgical intervention, emphasizing the dynamic nature of SMA pseudoaneurysms. Given the potential for complications, a surgical approach may sometimes be more appropriate from the outset, particularly in cases with significant anatomical concerns.

In the presented case, both major indications for open surgical treatment were met, firstly because the patient was hemodynamically unstable, in hypovolemic shock, and secondly because our patient had previously received endovascular treatment for the SMAA.

The prognosis for patients with a ruptured SMA pseudoaneurysm is uncertain, with outcomes heavily dependent on the timing of diagnosis and intervention.

4. Conclusions

A ruptured superior mesenteric artery pseudoaneurysm associated with pancreatitis represents a rare and life-threatening medical and also surgical emergency. Early recognition, prompt imaging, and fast intervention are critical in order to improve patient outcomes. A patient-tailored management should be considered and in the particular case of an SMA aneurysm in close contact with a pancreatic cyst, a surgical approach as the initial treatment could be a safer option.

From the review of the literature, we concluded that advances in imaging and endovascular techniques have enhanced the diagnostic and therapeutic capabilities for this condition, but the high morbidity and mortality rates underline the need for ongoing active follow-up and multidisciplinary collaboration in managing complex pancreatic and vascular pathologies. Further studies with long-term follow-up are necessary in order to evaluate the best therapeutic strategies.

Author Contributions: Conceptualization, O.S., M.R., R.C.G., P.R.D. and V.A.I.; methodology, M.R., O.S., A.D. and C.D.; software M.R., A.D. and C.V.; validation, M.R., V.A.I., R.C.G. and R.N.; formal analysis, M.R., O.S., R.N. and V.A.I.; investigation, M.R., A.D., R.C.G., C.V. and O.S.; resources, M.R., P.R.D. and C.D.; data curation, M.R., A.D., C.V., C.D. and V.A.I.; writing—original draft preparation, M.R., R.C.G., C.D. and A.D.; writing—review and editing O.S., R.N. and C.D.; visualization, M.R., O.S., C.V. and V.A.I.; supervision, O.S. and V.A.I.; project administration, R.C.G., P.R.D. and V.A.I.; funding acquisition, O.S. All authors have read and agreed to the published version of the manuscript.

Funding: The publication of this paper was supported by the University of Medicine and Pharmacy Carol Davila through the institutional program Publish not Perish.

Institutional Review Board Statement: This study was conducted in accordance with the Declaration of Helsinki and approved by the Romanian National Ethics Committee of Emergency Institute for Cardiovascular Disease "Prof. Dr. C.C. Iliescu". (Approval Code: 167; Approval Date: 24 January 2022).

Informed Consent Statement: Informed consent was obtained from the patient.

Data Availability Statement: Data available on request.

Conflicts of Interest: The authors declare no conflicts of interest.

References

1. Erben, Y.; Brownstein, A.J.; Rajaee, S.; Li, Y.; Rizzo, J.A.; Mojibian, H.; Ziganshin, B.A.; Elefteriades, J.A. Natural history and management of splanchnic artery aneurysms in a single tertiary referral center. *J. Vasc. Surg.* **2018**, *68*, 1079–1087. [CrossRef] [PubMed]
2. Kaszczewski, P.; Kozubek, H.; Ostrowski, T.; Maciąg, R.; Chudziński, W.; Skórski, M.; Gałązka, Z. Rapid Formation and Hybrid Treatment of a Large Superior Mesenteric Artery Aneurysm. *Am. J. Case Rep.* **2023**, *24*, e939558. [CrossRef] [PubMed] [PubMed Central]
3. Corey, M.R.; Ergul, E.A.; Cambria, R.P.; English, S.J.; Patel, V.I.; Lancaster, R.T.; Kwolek, C.J.; Conrad, M.F. The natural history of splanchnic artery aneurysms and outcomes after operative intervention. *J. Vasc. Surg.* **2016**, *63*, 949–957. [CrossRef] [PubMed]
4. Pitcher, G.S.; Cirillo-Penn, N.C.; Mendes, B.C.; Shuja, F.; DeMartino, R.R.; Kalra, M.; Bower, T.C.; Harmsen, W.S.; Colglazier, J.J. Aneurysms of the superior mesenteric artery and its branches. *J. Vasc. Surg.* **2022**, *76*, 149–157. [CrossRef] [PubMed]
5. Piasek, E.; Sojka, M.; Kuczyńska, M.; Światłowski, Ł.; Drelich-Zbroja, A.; Furmaga, O.; Jargiełło, T. Visceral artery aneurysms—Classification, diagnosis and treatment. *J. Ultrason.* **2018**, *18*, 148–151. [CrossRef] [PubMed] [PubMed Central]
6. Verde, F.; Fishman, E.K.; Johnson, P.T. Arterial pseudoaneurysms complicating pancreatitis: Literature review. *J. Comput. Assist. Tomogr.* **2015**, *39*, 7–12. [CrossRef] [PubMed]
7. Dávila Arias, C.; Ruiz-Rodríguez, A.J.; Cabrera Peña, Á. Hematochezia secondary to hemosuccus pancreaticus due to a pseudoaneurysm associated with a pancreatic pseudocyst. *Rev. Esp. Enfermedades Dig.* **2021**, *113*, 618. [CrossRef] [PubMed]
8. Branquinho, D.; Ramos-Andrade, D.; Elvas, L.; Amaro, P.; Ferreira, M.; Sofia, C. Drug-Induced Acute Pancreatitis and Pseudoaneurysms: An Ominous Combination. *GE Port. J. Gastroenterol.* **2016**, *23*, 309–313. [CrossRef] [PubMed] [PubMed Central]
9. Corvino, F.; Giurazza, F.; Ierardi, A.M.; Lucatelli, P.; Basile, A.; Corvino, A.; Niola, R. Splenic Artery Pseudoaneurysms: The Role of ce-CT for Diagnosis and Treatment Planning. *Diagnostics* **2022**, *12*, 1012. [CrossRef] [PubMed] [PubMed Central]
10. Okubo, R.; Kikuchi, S.; Otani, N.; Tsutsui, M.; Kamiya, H. Giant Superior Mesenteric Artery Aneurysm Treated by Endovascular Treatment in a Very Elderly Female. *Vasc. Spec. Int.* **2023**, *39*, 10. [CrossRef] [PubMed] [PubMed Central]
11. Saftoiu, A.; Iordache, S.; Ciurea, T.; Dumitrescu, D.; Popescu, M.; Stoica, Z. Pancreatic pseudoaneurysm of the superior mesenteric artery complicated with obstructive jaundice. A case report. *JOP* **2005**, *6*, 29–35. [PubMed]
12. Pulli, R.; Dorigo, W.; Troisi, N.; Pratesi, G.; Innocenti, A.A.; Pratesi, C. Surgical treatment of visceral artery aneurysms: A 25-year experience. *J. Vasc. Surg.* **2008**, *48*, 334–342. [CrossRef] [PubMed]
13. Mohan, I.V.; Stephen, M.S. Peripheral arterial aneurysms: Open or endovascular surgery? *Prog. Cardiovasc. Dis.* **2013**, *56*, 36–56. [CrossRef] [PubMed]
14. Thillai, M.; Sethi, P.; Narayana Menon, R.; Puthukudiyil Kader, N. Cystic artery pseudoaneurysm following acute necrotising pancreatitis. *BMJ Case Rep.* **2017**, *2017*, bcr2016218891. [CrossRef] [PubMed] [PubMed Central]
15. Wang, J.; Cao, D.; Tong, Q. Superior mesenteric artery branch pseudoaneurysm rupture mimicking acute pancreatitis in a patient with acute type B aortic dissection: A case report. *Medicine* **2019**, *98*, e16442. [CrossRef] [PubMed] [PubMed Central]

16. Sousa, J.; Costa, D.; Mansilha, A. Visceral artery aneurysms: Review on indications and current treatment strategies. *Int. Angiol.* **2019**, *38*, 381–394. [CrossRef] [PubMed]
17. Wang, L.; Shu, C.; Li, Q.; Jiang, X.; Li, X.; He, H.; Li, M. Experience of managing superior mesenteric artery aneurysm and its midterm follow-up results with 18 cases. *Vascular* **2021**, *29*, 516–526. [CrossRef] [PubMed]
18. Bouassida, M.; Benali, M.; Charrada, H.; Ghannouchi, M.; Chebbi, F.; Mighri, M.M.; Azzouz, M.M.; Touinsi, H.; Sassi, S. Gastrointestinal bleeding due to an erosion of the superior mesenteric artery: An exceptional fatal complication of pancreatic pseudocyst. *Pan Afr. Med. J.* **2012**, *12*, 62. [PubMed] [PubMed Central]
19. Ogino, H.; Banno, T.; Sato, Y.; Hara, M.; Shibamoto, Y. Superior mesenteric artery stent-graft placement in a patient with pseudoaneurysm developing from a pancreatic pseudocyst. *Cardiovasc. Interv. Radiol.* **2004**, *27*, 68–70. [CrossRef] [PubMed]
20. Stiru, O.; Gorduza, E.V.; Dorobantu, F.L.; Parasca, C.A.; Chioncel, O.; Bubenek Turconi, S.I.; Filipescu, D.C.; Iliescu, V.A. Surgical Management of Type A Acute Aortic Dissection in Patients with Marfan Syndrome: A Single Center Experience. *Med.-Surg. J.* **2016**, *120*, 611–618. [PubMed]
21. Geana, R.C.; Pavel, P.; Nayyerani, R.; Kulcsar, I.; Tulin, A.; Honciuc, O.; Balescu, I.; Bacalbasa, N.; Stiru, O.; Iliescu, V.A.; et al. Successfully superior mesenteric artery stenting in operated type A aortic dissection complicated with delayed mesenteric malperfusion. *SAGE Open Med. Case Rep.* **2021**, *9*, 2050313X211021184. [CrossRef] [PubMed] [PubMed Central]
22. Dumitrescu, C.I.; Ciobirca, C.; Popa, R.T.; Dumitrescu, D.; Tambura, C.G.; Ciobirca, D.M.; Stavaru, R.; Tiuca, M.F.; Maces, S.; Barbulescu, L.F.; et al. Preoperative Planning for Superior Mesenteric Artery Aneurysm. *Appl. Sci.* **2021**, *11*, 10311. [CrossRef]
23. Chaer, R.A.; Abularrage, C.J.; Coleman, D.M.; Eslami, M.H.; Kashyap, V.S.; Rockman, C.; Murad, M.H. The Society for Vascular Surgery clinical practice guidelines on the management of visceral aneurysms. *J. Vasc. Surg.* **2020**, *72*, 3S–39S. [CrossRef]
24. Guo, B.; Guo, D.; Xu, X.; Chen, B.; Shi, Z.; Luo, J.; Jiang, J.; Fu, W. Early and intermediate results of endovascular treatment of symptomatic and asymptomatic visceral artery aneurysms. *J. Vasc. Surg.* **2016**, *64*, 140–148. [CrossRef] [PubMed]
25. Venturini, M.; Marra, P.; Colombo, M.; Alparone, M.; Agostini, G.; Bertoglio, L.; Sallemi, B.C.; Salvioni, M.; Gusmini, S.; Balzano, G.; et al. Endovascular Treatment of Visceral Artery Aneurysms and Pseudoaneurysms in 100 Patients: Covered Stenting vs Transcatheter Embolization. *J. Endovasc. Ther.* **2017**, *24*, 709–717. [CrossRef]
26. Hemp, J.H.; Sabri, S.S. Endovascular management of visceral arterial aneurysms. *Tech. Vasc. Interv. Radiol.* **2015**, *18*, 14–23. [CrossRef] [PubMed]

life

Article

New Approaches Based on Inflammatory Indexes in the Evaluation of the Neoplastic Potential of Colon Polyps

Sedat Ciftel [1], Serpil Ciftel [2], Aleksandra Klisic [3,4] and Filiz Mercantepe [5,*]

1 Department of Gastroenterology and Hepatology, Erzurum Training and Research Hospital, 25100 Erzurum, Turkey; sedat.ciftel@saglik.gov.tr
2 Department of Endocrinology and Metabolism, Erzurum Training and Research Hospital, 25100 Erzurum, Turkey; serpil.ciftel@saglik.gov.tr
3 Faculty of Medicine, University of Montenegro, 81101 Podgorica, Montenegro; aleksandranklisic@gmail.com
4 Center for Laboratory Diagnostics, Primary Health Care Center, 81000 Podgorica, Montenegro
5 Department of Endocrinology and Metabolism, Faculty of Medicine, Recep Tayyip Erdogan University, 53010 Rize, Turkey
* Correspondence: filiz.mercantepe@saglik.gov.tr

Abstract: Colorectal polyps, precursors to colorectal cancer (CRC), require precise identification for appropriate diagnosis and therapy. This study aims to investigate the differences in hematological and inflammatory markers, specifically the CALLY index, HALP score, and immuno-inflammatory indexes, between neoplastic and nonneoplastic polyps. A retrospective cross-sectional study was conducted on 758 patients aged 61.0 ± 11.8 who underwent polypectomy between June 2021 and May 2024. Patients with colorectal adenocarcinoma ($n = 22$) were excluded. The polyps were classified into neoplastic and nonneoplastic categories based on histopathological evaluation. The study compared the CALLY index, HALP score, and various inflammatory indexes between neoplastic and nonneoplastic polyps. Out of 758 polyps analyzed, 514 were neoplastic, and 244 were nonneoplastic. Neoplastic polyps exhibited significantly lower CALLY and HALP scores ($p < 0.05$) and higher immuno-inflammatory indexes ($p < 0.05$) compared to nonneoplastic polyps. Dysplasia status, polyp diameter, and sigmoid colon localization were significant factors in determining neoplastic growth potential. No significant differences were observed in polyp localization in the proximal and distal colon segments or in solitary versus multiple polyps. The CALLY and HALP scores and immuno-inflammatory indexes can serve as valuable markers for distinguishing neoplastic from nonneoplastic polyps. These indexes reflect underlying inflammatory and immune responses, highlighting their potential utility in the early detection and risk stratification of colorectal polyps. Integrating these markers into clinical practice may enhance diagnostic accuracy and improve patient management, leading to timely interventions and better outcomes for individuals at risk of CRC.

Keywords: colorectal polyps; CALLY index; HALP score; immuno-inflammatory indexes

1. Introduction

Colorectal polyps are often-occurring lesions in the gastrointestinal tract that can serve as precursors to colorectal cancer (CRC). The CRC is widely recognized as a significant contributor to global cancer mortality. Hence, precise identification and categorizing of colon polyps is crucial in defining appropriate diagnostic and therapeutic approaches. Inflammation, dietary conditions, immunological function, and heredity may all have an impact on the development of CRC [1]. Colon polyps are classified into two primary categories based on their histological characteristics: neoplastic and nonneoplastic. Neoplastic polyps can develop into cancerous growths and are referred to as adenomatous polyps. On the other hand, nonneoplastic polyps are typically categorized as inflammatory, hyperplastic, or hamartomatous polyps. It is crucial to distinguish between these two types of polyps to provide proper therapeutic care and to effectively manage patients through early endoscopic therapies [2]. It is now known that colorectal carcinomas can arise not only from conventional adenomas but also from serrated polyps and hyperplastic polyps [3].

Recent research has focused on examining the predictive significance of different hematological and inflammatory markers in cancerous conditions. In this particular situation, additional factors such as the platelet–lymphocyte ratio (PLR); CALLY index; hemoglobin, albumin, lymphocyte, platelet score (HALP); and immunological inflammatory indexes may serve as valuable aids in distinguishing between neoplastic and nonneoplastic polyps. The CALLY and HALP scores can indicate cell proliferation and differentiation in polyps and their nutrition status. Current studies support the critical role of inflammatory and thrombotic processes in all stages of colorectal cancer development. The systemic immune-inflammatory index (SIII) and PLR can provide insights into the inflammatory response and the extent of immune cell infiltration. The pan-immune inflammation value (PIV) is a newly identified biomarker that can potentially reflect the body's immune response and systemic inflammatory status. It has been reported to have greater importance than the SIII in the prognosis of metastatic CRC [4].

The C-reactive protein (CRP) level in individuals with CRC is a clinical measure that indicates the extent of inflammation, according to reports [5]. The albumin level is a straightforward indicator of nutritional health. According to reports, low albumin and high CRP levels indicate inflammation and nutritional inadequacy [6]. The release of proinflammatory cytokines by the tumor can lead to chronic inflammation, which can disrupt the regeneration of lymphocytes by causing immunological dysregulation. Furthermore, tumor cells can exacerbate lymphocytopenia by attaching to lymphocyte receptors and triggering lymphocyte death through ligands. Additionally, it is believed that a reduction in the quantity of lymphocytes significantly influences the prognosis. A study examining systemic inflammatory markers for CRC risk discovered variations based on the cancer diagnosis and the timing of blood sampling. Elevated levels of the neutrophil–lymphocyte ratio (NLR), PLR, and SIII were associated with an increased risk, particularly in the year preceding cancer development [7]. The CALLY index, comprising CRP–albumin–lymphocyte parameters, was initially established by Hiroya Iida and colleagues to indicate postoperative prognosis in patients with hepatocellular carcinoma [8]. The CALLY index, a prognostic indicator, has also been linked with overall survival in patients with CRC [9].

The HALP score has emerged as a novel prognostic biomarker in recent years, with applications in predicting clinical prognosis in different types of neoplasms. HALP is an innovative immuno-nutritional marker that integrates commonly measured indicators of the immunological state, such as platelet and lymphocyte counts, with nutritional status markers including albumin, and hemoglobin as an indicator of anemia. Initially, Chen et al. [10] pioneered the development of this method to forecast the prognosis of gastric cancer. In contrast to the CALLY index, the HALP score incorporates hemoglobin, which serves as a marker for anemia, into its computation. Anemia is a common occurrence in all cancer patients, particularly those with gastrointestinal malignancies. It has been reported that the HALP score may also be useful as a clinical prognostic factor in patients with CRC [11]. The PLR is becoming more popular as a biomarker for predicting cancer prognosis. This is due to the fact that patients with chronic inflammatory solid carcinoma often have enhanced platelet production. Additionally, platelets have a strong connection to the growth of cancer [12]. While the predictive significance of these indexes is established in individuals with colon cancer, their potential relevance in detecting malignancy before cancer diagnosis has not been adequately investigated. The objective of this study is to examine potential variations in indexes between neoplastic and nonneoplastic polyps during the initial phases of malignancy progression. Additionally, it is crucial to investigate whether these characteristics vary based on the presence and forms of dysplasia and the localization and quantity of polyps. These examinations are the initial stage in detecting neoplastic polyps and identifying high-risk patients. They also contribute to the prevention, treatment, and early intervention of colorectal cancer.

2. Participants and Methods

This retrospective cross-sectional study included patients undergoing colonoscopy from June 2021 to May 2024 who had at least one eligible colorectal polyp resected with polypectomy by an expert gastroenterologist. Colorectal adenocarcinoma was initially detected in 22 of 780 patients, and patients with colorectal cancer were excluded from the study. A total of 758 patients, comprising 303 women and 455 men with an average age of 61.0 ± 11.8 years, were included in our study.

The patients were instructed to keep on a watery diet for three days and to discontinue using aspirin or anticoagulants five days before the colonoscopy. All patients were prepared with 3–4 L of polyethylene glycol solution until clear rectal fluid was evacuated. The hot snare polypectomy method was used for pedunculated polyps, and saline solution mixed with epinephrine was pre-injected for nonpedunculated polyp resection. The colonoscopy procedures were performed with the Olympus-H180 AL (Tokyo, Japan) video colonoscope system with deep sedation monitored by an anesthesiologist. Snares were inserted through the channel of the colonoscope. Resected polyps were placed in a formalin container by an expert pathologist for histopathological examination. The localization, size, number, and pathology of the polyps were recorded. Blood samples were obtained simultaneously with colonoscopy. Biochemical and hematological parameters of the patients were recorded.

The indexes we used in our study were calculated with the following formulas [4,8,10]:

$$
\begin{gathered}
\text{PLR} = \text{Platelet } (10^9/\text{L})/\text{Lymphocyte } (10^9/\text{L}) \\
\text{CALLY Index} = \text{Albumin } (\text{g/L}) \times \text{Lymphocyte } (10^9/\text{L})/\text{CRP } (\text{mg/dL}) \times 10^4 \\
\text{HALP score} = \text{Hemoglobin } (\text{g/L}) \times \text{Albumin } (\text{g/L}) \times \text{Lymphocyte } (10^9/\text{L})/\text{Platelet}(/\text{L}) \\
\text{PIV} = \text{Neutrophil } (10^9/\text{L}) \times \text{Platelet } (10^9/\text{L}) \times \text{Monocyte } (10^9/\text{L})/\text{Lymphocyte } (10^9/\text{L}) \\
\text{SIII} = \text{Neutrophil } (10^9/\text{L}) \times \text{Platelet } (10^9/\text{L})/\text{Lymphocyte } (10^9/\text{L}) \\
\text{SIRI} = \text{Neutrophil } (10^9/\text{L}) \times \text{Monocyte } (10^9/\text{L})/\text{Lymphocyte } (10^9/\text{L})
\end{gathered} \tag{1}
$$

We calculated the positive and negative predictive values (PPV, NPV) by using ROC analysis (Youden index calculation) with derived cut-off values for the new indexes.

The inclusion criteria were adult patients with colorectal polyps detected during colonoscopy who had undergone polypectomy and histopathological evaluation. The exclusion criteria were patients with cancer-detected polypectomy pathology, inflammatory bowel disease, polyposis syndromes, and rheumatological, hematological, infectious, liver, and malignant diseases that may have the potential to affect albumin and inflammatory parameters.

The study protocol received approval from the Ethics Committee of Erzurum Training and Research Hospital, with decision number 2022/15-153, dated 3 October 2022. The research was conducted in accordance with the ethical guidelines outlined in the Declaration of Helsinki.

Statistical Analysis

Statistical analyses were performed using IBM Statistical Package for Social Sciences software, version 22 (IBM Corp., Armonk, NY, USA). The Kolmogorov–Smirnov test and histograms were used to determine whether the variables were normally distributed or not. The Mann–Whitney U and Kruskal–Wallis tests were performed to compare with nonnormally distributed parameters. Student's *t*-test was used for normally distributed parameters. Comparisons between categorical variables were performed with the Chi-square test. The nonnormally distributed data are represented by medians and quartiles. The normally distributed data are expressed as the mean ± standard deviation. Spearman Correlation analyses were performed to evaluate continuous variables. A statistically significant p-value was considered as $p < 0.05$.

3. Results

Table 1 presents the results of the demographic analysis as well as the characteristics and localization of both neoplastic and nonneoplastic polyps. Out of the 780 polyps that were analyzed, 514 were found to be neoplastic, whereas 244 were nonneoplastic. The study excluded 22 patients whose pathology diagnosed colon adenocarcinoma. The prevalence of neoplastic polyps was 40.3% (207 individuals) among women and 59.7% (307 individuals) among men. The prevalence of nonneoplastic polyps was 39.3% (96 individuals) among women and 60.7% (148 individuals) among men. There was no statistically significant variation in the gender distribution across the groups ($p = 0.807$). Upon analyzing the dysplasia status of neoplastic polyps, it was found that 37.5% did not exhibit dysplasia, 49.0% had low-grade dysplasia, and 13.5% exhibited high-grade dysplasia. Nonneoplastic polyps showed no evidence of dysplasia in 95.1% of cases, whereas 4.5% exhibited low-grade dysplasia, and only 0.4% had high-grade dysplasia. There was a notable disparity between the groups regarding the occurrence of dysplasia ($p < 0.001$). A total of 81.1% of neoplastic polyps were pedunculated, whereas 18.9% were sessile. The percentages for nonneoplastic polyps were determined to be 75.0% and 25.0%, respectively. There was no statistically significant difference between the groups for the distribution of polyp pedunculation ($p = 0.052$). Among neoplastic polyps, 13.0% had diameters less than 5 mm, 40.3% between 5 and 10 mm, and 46.7% had diameters larger than 10 mm. In contrast, among nonneoplastic polyps, 21.7% had diameters less than 5 mm, 54.1% between 5 and 10 mm, and 24.2% had diameters greater than 10 mm. There was a notable disparity among the groups regarding the size of the polyp diameter ($p < 0.001$). Of all the neoplastic polyps, 20.8% were found in the proximal region, 67.1% in the distal region, and 12.1% in both the proximal and distal regions. On the other hand, 26.2% of the nonneoplastic polyps were located in the proximal region, 63.9% in the distal region, and 9.8% in both the proximal and distal regions. No statistically significant difference was observed between the groups regarding localization ($p = 0.210$). Rectum localization was observed in 26.5% of neoplastic polyps and 33.6% of nonneoplastic polyps. Furthermore, rectum localization was more prevalent in nonneoplastic polyps (n = 0.042). This study indicated that sigmoid localization was observed in 45.1% of neoplastic polyps and 33.6% of nonneoplastic polyps. Additionally, sigmoid localization was more frequently observed in neoplastic polyps compared to nonneoplastic polyps ($p = 0.003$). The locations of the descending colon, splenic flexure, transverse colon, hepatic flexure, ascending colon, and cecum did not show any significant differences between neoplastic and nonneoplastic colon polyps ($p \geq 0.05$). These data suggest that characteristics such as dysplasia status, polyp diameter, and sigmoid colon placement have a significant role in determining the likelihood of developing neoplastic growth.

Table 2 shows the allocation of cancerous and noncancerous growths. The distributions indicate that tubular adenomas are the predominant type of neoplastic polyps, whereas hyperplastic polyps are the most frequent nonneoplastic polyps. Furthermore, neoplastic polyps were also discovered to include less prevalent kinds, such as villous and serrated adenomas. A significant proportion of nonneoplastic polyps consisted of inflammatory polyps. Table 3 compares neoplastic and nonneoplastic polyps regarding age, diabetes mellitus, metabolic parameters, and lymphocyte indexes. The average age in the neoplastic polyp group was 61.6 ± 11.2 years, while the average age in the nonneoplastic polyp group was 59.8 ± 12.9 years. There was no significant difference in age between the two groups ($p = 0.070$). There was no difference in the frequency of diabetes between the neoplastic and nonneoplastic polyp groups (24.1% and 23.8%, respectively). No statistically significant differences were seen between the groups regarding glucose, total protein, neutrophil count, and platelet count ($p = 0.691$, $p = 0.170$, $p = 0.368$, and $p = 0.876$, respectively). Statistically significant differences were seen between the neoplastic and nonneoplastic polyp groups in terms of albumin, CRP, lymphocyte, PLR, CALLY index, HALP score, PIV, SIII, and SIRI ($p < 0.001$, $p < 0.001$, $p < 0.001$, $p < 0.001$, $p < 0.001$, $p = 0.013$, $p = 0.003$, and $p = 0.007$, respectively).

Table 1. Comparison of neoplastic and nonneoplastic polyp groups in terms of demographic findings, polyp characteristics, and localization.

	Neoplastic Polyps (n = 514)	Nonneoplastic Polyps (n = 244)	Total (n = 758)	*p*
Gender				
Female	207 (40.3)	96 (39.3)	303 (40.0)	0.807
Male	307 (59.7)	148 (60.7)	455 (60.0)	
Dysplasia				
No dysplasia	193 (37.5)	232 (95.1)	425 (56.1)	**0.001** *
Low-Grade Dysplasia	252 (49.0)	11 (4.5)	263 (34.7)	
High-Grade Dysplasia	69 (13.5)	1 (0.4)	70 (9.2)	
Polyp stalk				
Pedunculated polyps	417 (81.1)	183 (75.0)	600 (79.2)	0.052
Sessile polyps	97 (18.9)	61 (25.0)	158 (20.8)	
Polyp Diameter				
<5 mm	67 (13.0)	53 (21.7)	120 (15.8)	**0.001** *
5–10 mm	207 (40.3)	132 (54.1)	339 (44.7)	
≥10 mm	240 (46.7)	59 (24.2)	299 (39.5)	
Localization				
Proximal Colon	107 (20.8)	64 (26.2)	171 (22.6)	0.210
Distal Colon	345 (67.1)	156 (63.9)	501 (66.1)	
Proximal + Distal Colon	62 (12.1)	24 (9.8)	86 (11.3)	
Rectum	136 (26.5)	82 (33.6)	218 (28.8)	**0.042** *
Sigmoid colon	232 (45.1)	82 (33.6)	314 (41.4)	**0.003** *
Descending colon	69 (13.4)	33 (13.5)	102 (13.5)	0.970
Splenic flexure	39 (7.6)	15 (6.1)	54 (7.1)	0.471
Transvers colon	70 (13.6)	36 (14.8)	106 (14.0)	0.674
Hepatic flexure	31 (6.0)	9 (3.7)	40 (5.3)	0.178
Ascending colon	39 (7.6)	20 (8.2)	59 (7.8)	0.770
Cecum	33 (6.4)	17 (7.0)	50 (6.6)	0.777

* $p < 0.05$ is statically significant (bold).

Table 2. Distribution of neoplastic and nonneoplastic polyps.

Neoplastic Polyps	n (%)	Nonneoplastic Polyps	n (%)
Tubular adenoma	378 (73.6)	Hyperplastic polyps	165 (67.6)
Tubulovillous adenoma	116 (22.5)	Inflammatory polyps	71 (29.0)
Villous adenoma	18 (3.5)	Others (Ksantamatose, lymphoid, hamartomatous)	8 (3.4)
Serrated adenoma	2 (0.4)		
Total	**514**		**244**

The polyps were categorized into three groups based on the presence and severity of dysplasia: those without dysplasia, those with low-grade dysplasia, and those with high-grade dysplasia. These groups were then compared in terms of several clinical and biochemical markers. The findings of this comparison are displayed in Table 4. The mean ages did not differ significantly among the groups ($p = 0.182$), with mean ages of 60.8, 60.7, and 63.7 years, respectively. The levels of glucose, total protein, CRP, neutrophils, and platelets were comparable among all groups, and no statistically significant differences were detected ($p = 0.510$, $p = 0.343$, $p = 0.116$, $p = 0.311$, and $p = 0.670$, respectively). Nevertheless, there were notable variations between the three groups with respect to albumin, lymphocytes, PLR, CALLY index, HALP score, PIV, SIII, and SIRI ($p < 0.001$, $p < 0.001$, $p < 0.001$, $p = 0.003$, $p < 0.001$, $p = 0.017$, $p < 0.001$, and $p < 0.001$, respectively).

Table 3. Comparison of neoplastic and nonneoplastic polyp groups in terms of age, diabetes mellitus, biochemical parameters, and lymphocyte-based indexes.

	Neoplastic Polyps (n = 514)	Nonneoplastic Polyps (n = 244)	Total (n = 758)	*p*
Age (year)	61.6 ± 11.2	59.8 ± 12.9	61.0 ± 11.8	0.070
Glucose (mg/dL) (mean ± SD)	107 (±45)	108 (±44)	107 (±45)	0.691
DM n (%)	124 (24.1)	58 (23.8)	182 (24)	0.915
Total protein (g/L)	68 (36–84)	69 (46–89)	68 (36–89)	0.170
Albumin (g/L)	42 (19–52)	44 (26–53)	42 (19–53)	**0.001** *
CRP (mg/dl)	5.9 (0.1–161)	3.2 (0.0–138)	5 (0–161)	**0.001** *
Hemoglobin (g/dL), median (min-max)	14.2 (4.6–19.7)	14 (6.2–18.5)	14.1 (4.6–19.7)	0.989
Ferritin (ng/mL), median (min-max)	51 (1–1501)	54.4 (1.9–1650)	52 (1–1650)	0.823
Neutrophil (10^9/L)	4.46 (1.58–28)	4.32 (0.66–14.4)	4.42 (0.66–28.3)	0.368
Lymphocyte (10^9/L)	2.14 (0.19–6.80)	2.37 (0.49–6.68)	2.20 (0.19–6.80)	**0.001** *
Platelet (10^9/L)	271 (92–677)	270 (91–759)	270 (91–759)	0.876
PLR	128 (24–810)	115 (30–403)	124 (24–810)	**0.001** *
CALLY Index	0.16 (0.01–17.3)	0.29 (0.01–21.1)	0.18 (0.01–21.3)	**0.001** *
HALP Score	45.3 (3.91–218)	52.8 (11.2–189)	47.1 (3.91–218)	**0.001** *
PIV	333 (20–4167)	286 (19–5021)	316 (19–5021)	**0.013** *
SIII	564 (53–7063)	513 (55–5830)	554 (53–7063)	**0.003** *
SIRI	1.24 (0.13–16.2)	1.04 (0.1–18.6)	1.16 (0.10–18.6)	**0.007** *

DM, Diabetes mellitus; CRP, C-reactive protein; PLR, Platelet–lymphocyte ratio; PIV, Pan-immune inflammation value; SIII, Systemic immune-inflammation index; SIRI, Systemic Inflammation Response Index. * $p < 0.05$ is statically significant (bold).

Table 4. Comparison of parameters according to dysplasia.

	No-Dysplasia (ND), (n = 425)	Low-Grade Dysplasia (LGD), (n = 263)	High-Grade Dysplasia (HGD), (n = 70)	*p*
Age (year)	60.8 ± 12.4	60.7 ± 9.5	63.7 ± 9.5	0.182
Glucose (mg/dL), (mean ± SD)	109 (±48)	106 (±42)	102 (±34)	0.510
Total protein (g/L)	68 (36–89)	68 (41–81)	68 (43–76)	0.343
Albumin (g/L)	44 (19–53)	41 (24–49)	38 (26–47)	**0.001** *
CRP (mg/dL)	4.6 (0.0–161)	5.4 (0.1–106)	6.5 (0.1–147)	0.116
Neutrophil (10^9/L)	4.3 (0.6–28)	4.4 (1.6–21)	4.6 (1.6–23)	0.311
Lymphocyte (10^9/L)	2.3 (0.4–6.6)	2.1 (0.1–6.8)	1.8 (0.3–5.9)	**0.001** *
Platelet (10^9/L)	272 (91–759)	265 (113–563)	276 (109–575)	0.670
PLR	121 (24–406)	123 (34–727)	165 (67–810)	**0.001** *
CALLY Index	0.19 (0.0–21)	0.18 (0.0–20.8)	0.1 (0.01–7.3)	**0.003** *
HALP Score	49.9 (5.9–218)	46.5 (3.9–211)	30.7 (5.9–144)	**0.001** *
PIV	303 (19–4167)	316 (20–5021)	433 (46–3681)	**0.017** *
SIII	543 (53–7063)	527 (113–4256)	750 (105–5815)	**0.001** *
SIRI	1.09 (0.1–16)	1.2 (0.16–18)	1.48 (0.2–11.4)	**0.001** *

* $p < 0.05$ is statically significant (bold). CRP, C-reactive protein; PLR, Platelet–lymphocyte ratio; PIV, Pan-immune inflammation value; SIII, Systemic immune-inflammation index; SIRI, Systemic Inflammation Response Index. Albumin difference: HGD-LGD = 0.01, HGD-ND < 0.000, LGD-HGD < 0.000. Lymphocyte difference: HGD-LGD = 0.04, HGD-ND = 0.001, LGD-HGD = 0.003. PLR difference: HGD-ND < 0.001, HGD-LGD = 0.01. CALLY index difference: HGD-ND = 0.005. HALP score difference: HGD-LGD < 0.001, HGD-ND < 0.001. PIV index difference: HGD-NO dysplasia = 0.014. SIII difference: HGD-ND < 0.001, HGD-LGD < 0.001. SIRI difference: HGD-ND < 0.001, HGD-LGD = 0.048.

Table 5 shows the comparison of the PLR, CALLY index, HALP score, PIV, SIII, and SIRI parameters based on the location of polyps in the proximal colon, distal colon, and both colon segments. None of these analyzed indicators exhibited a noteworthy disparity across all three segments of the colon. Similarly, the data in Table 6 showed no significant differences in the PLR, CALLY index, HALP score, PIV, SIII, and SIRI parameters when comparing polyps based on whether they were solitary or multiple.

Table 5. Indexes according to localization of colon polyps.

	Proximal Colon (n = 171)	Distal Colon (n = 501)	Proximal + Distal Colon (n = 86)	*p*
PLR	127 (24–372)	121 (30–810)	139 (59–700)	0.235
CALLY index	0.16 (0.01–21)	0.19 (0.01–20)	0.20 (0.01–14)	0.994
HALP score	46 (9.5–211)	47 (5.9–218)	47 (3.9–131)	0.571
PIV	328 (30–3239)	310 (19–4099)	361 (20–5021)	0.688
SIII	582 (53–3339)	531 (55–5830)	554 (139–7063)	0.764
SIRI	1.13 (1.15–7.7)	1.15 (0.1–11.4)	1.31 (0.13–18.6)	0.309

PLR, Platelet–lymphocyte ratio; PIV, Pan-immune inflammation value; SIII, Systemic immune-inflammation index; SIRI, Systemic Inflammation Response Index.

Table 6. Indexes according to the number of polyps.

	Solitary (n = 580)	Multiple (n = 178)	*p*
PLR	122 (24–727)	132 (35–810)	0.339
CALLY index	0.19 (0.01–21)	0.16 (0.01–20)	0.257
HALP score	47.6 (6.4–211)	45.5 (3.9–218)	0.275
PIV	314 (19–4099)	336 (20–5021)	0.539
SIII	552 (53–5830)	557 (92–7063)	0.555
SIRI	1.13 (0.1–10.4)	1.25 (0.13–18.6)	0.150

PLR, Platelet–lymphocyte ratio; PIV, Pan-immune inflammation value; SIII, Systemic immune-inflammation index; SIRI, Systemic Inflammation Response Index.

To determine that polyp size is related to the inflammatory indexes utilized in our investigation, we established a cut-off value of 1 cm for polyp size. We compared the PLR, CALLY index, HALP score, PIV, SIII, and SIRI between polyps measuring ≥1 cm and those measuring <1 cm. The findings are presented in Table 7. The HALP score was considerably lower in colon polyps measuring ≥1 cm ($p = 0.036$). The CALLY index decreased in this group; however, no statistically significant difference was seen. The PIV, SIII, and SIRI levels increased in the ≥1 cm group, but no statistically significant difference was seen.

Table 7. Indexes according to the diameter of polyps.

	Polyp Size < 1 cm (n = 459)	Polyp Size ≥ 1 cm (n = 299)	*p*
CALLY index	0.18 (0.01–21)	0.17 (0.00–20)	0.256
HALP score	47.8 (8–218)	44.2 (3.9–211)	**0.036** *
PIV	312 (19–4167)	333 (20–5021)	0.547
SIII	544 (55–7063)	569 (53–5830)	0.313
SIRI	1.14 (0.1–16)	1.22 (0.13–18)	0.294

PIV, Pan-immune inflammation value; SIII, Systemic immune-inflammation index; SIRI, Systemic Inflammation Response Index. * $p < 0.05$ is statically significant (bold).

Logistic regression analysis evaluated the risk factors for developing neoplastic polyps (Table 8). In this study, bigger polyp diameter ($p < 0.001$, OR = 2.721, 95% CI 1.624–4.559), lower CALLY index ($p = 0.008$, OR = 0.927, 95% CI 0.876–0.980), and lower HALP score ($p = 0.035$, OR = 0.992, CI 0.986–0.999) all pointed to the growth of a neoplastic polyp. The PIV, SIII, and SIRI did not affect neoplastic polyp development ($p = 0.269$, $p = 0.413$, and $p = 0.870$, respectively). For every index analyzed in this current study, we calculated the PPV and NPV values (Table 9). Although the PPV for all indexes was above 70%, a small NPV was detected for all parameters (below 40%).

Table 8. Logistic regression analysis of risk factors for the development of neoplastic polyps.

Step 1	B	p	OR	95% CI for EXP(B)	
				Lower	Upper
Polyp diameter (≥1 cm)	1.001	0.000	2.721	1.624	4.559
CALLY index	−0.076	0.008	0.927	0.876	0.980
HALP score	−0.008	0.035	0.992	0.986	0.999
PIV	−0.001	0.269	0.999	0.998	1.000
SIII	0.000	0.413	1.000	1.000	1.001
SIRI	0.025	0.870	1.025	0.764	1.375

PIV, Pan-immune inflammation value; SIII, Systemic immune-inflammation index; SIRI, Systemic Inflammation Response Index.

Table 9. Positive and negative predictive values (PPV, NPV) of new indexes.

	PPV (%)	NPV (%)
PLR	71.5	36.3
CALLY Index	79.4	33.0
HALP Score	71.7	36.5
PIV	70.8	35.4
SIII	71.6	36.2
SIRI	72.6	37.3

PLR, Platelet–lymphocyte ratio; PIV, Pan-immune inflammation value; SIII, Systemic immune-inflammation index; SIRI, Systemic Inflammation Response Index.

4. Discussion

In the present study, the potential of using various indexes reflecting inflammation and immune status to assess colon polyps' neoplastic potential was investigated in addition to demographic and biochemical parameters. Significant differences were found between neoplastic and nonneoplastic polyps regarding hematological and biochemical parameters and lymphocyte indexes. In particular, inflammatory parameters such as CRP, albumin, PLR, CALLY index, HALP score, PIV, SIII, and SIRI were significantly different in neoplastic polyps compared to nonneoplastic polyps.

In the present study, both neoplastic and nonneoplastic polyps were found at similar rates in men and women, indicating that gender is not a significant risk factor in polyp characteristics. However, it was found that the frequency of polyps was generally higher in men. This finding, in line with data reported in previous studies, supports the effect of gender on the incidence of colon polyps while also highlighting the limited effect of gender on polyp characteristics. Colon polyps can be considered as precursor lesions of colon cancer. Gilbertson first suggested in the 1960s that colorectal cancer may arise from intermediate lesions in the colon [13]. In the late 1980s, Fearon and Vogelstein [14] described CRC as a genetic disease in which the progression from polyp to carcinoma is a sequence of specific genetic mutations.

The clinical importance of polyps is due to the fact that more than 95% of colon adenocarcinomas arise from polyps [15]. The vast majority of colorectal cancers develop from precancerous adenomatous or serrated polyps. It is the third most commonly diagnosed cancer in men in the United States. It is also the most common type of cancer diagnosed in men, with the most recent data in the United States showing an incidence rate of colorectal cancer in men of 42 cases per 100,000 men per year. This rate is lower in women, at 32 cases per 100,000 women. Beginning at age 50, the incidence is approximately 30% higher in men than women [16].

The prevalence of colon adenomas is higher in men. In a cross-sectional study, the risk of adenomas in screening colonoscopy was found to be 1.77 times higher in men than in women [17]. The same study reported that colon adenomas increased significantly in both genders with increasing age. In a multicenter study conducted in Turkey with 6508 patients, the frequency of colon polyps was found to be 37% in male patients and 27% in female patients. The frequency of CRC was found to be 3.8% in males and 1% in females [18]. Therefore, it is an expected finding that colon polyps are more frequently observed in men. Based on this information, we can conclude that neoplastic polyps, which have a higher malignant potential, should be more frequently seen in men. However, although both neoplastic and nonneoplastic polyps are more frequently seen in men when both sexes are evaluated within themselves, no gender-specific difference was found between them.

The findings of this study show that neoplastic polyps exhibit a greater proportion of high-grade dysplasia than nonneoplastic polyps. This is an expected finding. Most neoplastic polyps are adenomatous polyps. The significance of these polyps is that they undergo malignant degeneration. The size, histologic type, and degree of dysplasia of adenomas determine their malignant potential. Histologically, conventional adenomas are divided into tubular, tubulovillous, or villous histologic subtypes. As the degree of dysplasia and polyp size increase, the potential for malignant transformation of polyps also increases. Polyps smaller than 10 mm rarely and very slowly can become cancerous. Adenomas larger than 10 mm, villous in structure, or with high-grade dysplasia are at the highest risk of malignant transformation. A total of 1.7% of adenomas measuring 1–5 mm, 6.6% of adenomas measuring 6–9 mm, and 30.6% of adenomas measuring larger than 10 mm have advanced histologic features and have the potential to become cancerous [19]. Although nonneoplastic polyps generally have a low risk of becoming cancerous, this risk may increase under certain genetic conditions or in some exceptional cases. Therefore, correct identification of polyps and regular follow-up is essential. Hyperplastic polyps are the most common nonneoplastic polyps. The absence of atypia in the cells is an important point; therefore, they are considered not neoplastic. This is the point that is under debate. Today, it is reported that hyperplastic polyps carry a risk of cancer or indicate an increased risk of cancer in the presence of certain conditions [20]. Genetic studies have also shown that specific genetic changes (e.g., microsatellite instability—MSI) can be seen in hyperplastic polyps that are located in the right colon and reach diameters greater than 10 mm and that the risk of cancer development from such hyperplastic polyps will increase [21]. The results of our study show that neoplastic polyps have higher dysplasia degrees and larger sizes. In addition, no difference was found between neoplastic and nonneoplastic polyps regarding polyp stem and whether the polyps are located in the proximal or distal colon. However, nonneoplastic polyps are seen to be located in the rectum, while neoplastic polyps are more frequently located in the sigmoid region. In a study on the localization of colon polyps, generally, all types of polyps were found to be more frequent in the distal colon [22]. In another study, it was found that the most common location for polyps was the sigmoid colon region, but this study also showed that the pathology of the polyp was not related to the colon region [23]. In a study on determining high-malignant risk colorectal polyps, it was reported that the malignant potential was higher in the left colon (especially sigmoid and rectum) than in the right colon and that the risk of malignancy increased due to the risk of histological invasion when the polyp was sessile, in line with other studies [24]. In our study, neoplastic polyps were mainly located in the sigmoid colon.

Polyps are usually asymptomatic and are usually discovered incidentally during screening colonoscopies for CRC. However, patients may present with bright or dark red painless rectal bleeding, effacement, or mixed or dripping stools. Other presentations include diarrhea, constipation, abdominal pain, mucus in the stool, or symptoms and signs of iron deficiency anemia due to chronic bleeding [15]. In our study, hemoglobin and ferritin values were found to be similar among polyp types. In addition, these parameters were not associated with the degree of dysplasia. This finding demonstrates that although it is known that polyps can present with bleeding, their malignant potential is unrelated to anemia parameters.

In our study, it was found that glucose levels and DM incidence were not associated with the type of polyp and the presence of dysplasia. Literature studies have found that the risk of colorectal polyps in patients with type 2 DM increased by 1.23 times and that the incidence of colon polyps increased with the duration of diabetes [25]. However, to our knowledge, there is no study in the literature investigating the presence of DM in terms of polyp types.

However, a recent meta-analysis showed that patients with T2DM have a 30% higher risk of CRC than the general population [26]. Other studies have also shown that the risk of CRC is high in diabetic patients [27]. The difference may not have been found because our research was conducted in a single center, and both risk and protective factors such as smoking, alcohol, diet, medications, and NSAIDs (non-steroidal anti-inflammatory drugs) were not included in this study.

In this study, the use of inflammatory indexes in the evaluation of neoplastic and dysplastic potential of colon polyps was investigated. Our findings are consistent with the data in the current literature and support the role of inflammation in neoplastic processes. The fact that CRP, an important indicator of systemic inflammation, is found to be higher in neoplastic polyps suggests that they may be related to the inflammatory response. In addition, the low albumin levels in individuals with neoplastic polyps indicate that this parameter can also be used as a marker. Especially in the high-grade dysplasia group, the low albumin level may indicate an increase in inflammatory processes and protein catabolism. Indexes such as the PLR, CALLY index, HALP score, PIV, SIII, and SIRI are accepted as indicators of both inflammation and immune response. The fact that these indexes are higher in neoplastic polyps suggests that these polyps may be associated with inflammatory and immune responses. In particular, indexes such as the HALP score and CALLY index stand out as new parameters that may be important in evaluating neoplastic potential.

Many of the inflammation indexes we investigated were constructed on a lymphocyte basis. Lymphopenia can occur due to primary conditions such as congenital immunodeficiency disorders or acquired causes such as malnutrition, infectious diseases, sepsis, autoimmune and lymphoproliferative disorders, malignancies, drugs (steroids, chemotherapy), and protein-losing conditions such as severe burns, amyloidosis, and inflammatory bowel disease. Increasing evidence suggests that cancer progression is influenced by the systemic inflammatory response [28]. Immune modulators secreted by tumor cells, including TGF-β, IL-10, and CRP, impair lymphocyte action in systemic inflammation [29]. These cytokines and immunosuppressive factors released by the tumor can reduce the activity and number of lymphocytes. Chronic inflammation caused by malignancy can cause lymphocytes to be depleted and reduced by apoptotic processes. Tumor-infiltrating lymphocytes, such as natural killer and T helper type 1, are effective components against cancer growth and metastasis in various cancers through the production of interferon-gamma. The lymphocytic response is a key component of controlling cancer progression. Increased lymphocyte infiltration is considered an independent pretreatment neoadjuvant therapy response parameter in breast cancer [30]. CD8(+) T cells constitute the major effective cell group against cancer cells. To date, the prognostic importance of the presence of CD8(+) T lymphocytes in colorectal cancer has been demonstrated in many studies, with better survival outcomes demonstrated by more CD8(+) tumor-infiltrating lymphocytes [31]. The initial immune response to an early neoplasm is thought to reflect the response to acute tissue injury, with sequential infiltration by various myeloid populations leading to eventual infiltration by lymphocytes. Inflammation and the accompanying increase in stress may lead to increased cortisol levels, which may contribute to decreased lymphocyte numbers and function [32].

The relationship between inflammation and the development of neoplastic diseases continues to be the subject of many studies. The first evidence for this emerged in 1828 when the French surgeon Jean Nicholas Marjolin observed the development of squamous cell carcinoma around an open wound [33]. One of the closest relationships between chronic inflammation and cancer is observed in inflammatory bowel disease, where a 10-unit increase in the endoscopic inflammation score doubles the risk of colorectal cancer [33]. In the study conducted by Ruiya et al. [34], the preoperative CALLY index decreased significantly as the esophageal Ca stage increased. Moreover, patients with a decreased CALLY index had lower overall survival. A study conducted by Takeda et al. [35] on colorectal cancer reported that the CALLY index was an independent prognostic biomarker in these patients. In fact, in a study conducted by Furukawa et al. [9] on patients with colorectal cancer with liver metastases, there were more postoperative complications after metastasectomy in those with a low CALLY index. In a study conducted by Feng et al. [36], some parameters related to inflammation were reported as potential indicators that could help in the diagnosis of colorectal cancer. In their study, the early colorectal cancer group and the adenomatous polyp group were compared in terms of inflammatory parameters; the PLR and SIII were higher, hemoglobin and albumin were lower in the early colorectal cancer patients, and the average age of cancer patients was older than the other group, unlike in our study.

Colorectal cancers are more common in the elderly population. Approximately 80% of all new cases are diagnosed in individuals aged 55 years and older, and the median age at diagnosis in industrialized countries such as the United States is approximately 70 years. In our study, the age groups were similar regarding polyp type and dysplasia. This was probably because our patients did not have colorectal cancer. The transformation from adenomas to cancer occurs over a relatively long period.

The size of a polyp is regarded as a significant determinant in assessing the malignant potential of non-sessile polyps [2,37]. The increased prevalence of neoplastic polyps measuring $\geq$1 cm in our study results aligns with this information. Still, the fact that there was no link between polyp size and other indexes (PLR, CALLY index, PIV, SIII, and SIRI) shows that neoplastic potential is linked to the inflammatory indexes used in this study, no matter how big the polyp is. The relationship between the HALP score and polyp size was statistically very low in significance.

A study [38] reported an inflammatory polyp frequency of 2.9% among all polyps and 12% among nonneoplastic polyps, but our investigation revealed a frequency of 9.3% in all polyps and 29% in nonneoplastic polyps. Numerous variables contribute to the genesis of inflammatory polyps. In addition to inflammatory bowel disease, it may arise from chronic inflammation or tissue injury, environmental influences, dietary practices, tobacco and alcohol consumption, persistent intestinal infections, obesity, and the aging process. While we removed inflammatory bowel disease and other inflammatory rheumatological conditions from our investigation, additional factors were not excluded. In this community, encompassing the region where our study was performed, intestinal infections are prevalent due to smoking, obesity, and substandard living conditions, with a mean patient age of 61.0 $\pm$ 11.8 years. The explanations mentioned above may account for the elevated incidence of hyperplastic polyps observed. Moreover, our hospital is equipped with state-of-the-art facilities that provide a comprehensive view of the region, and the pathology reports at our center have been systematically reviewed by two pathologists. Nonetheless, no prior research exists in the literature with which we may compare the prevalence of polyps in our location. In this regard, our research is the inaugural investigation on this topic in our region.

The results of our study show that inflammatory indexes are useful for evaluating colon polyps' cancerous and precancerous potential. We posit that these indicators possess the potential to furnish valuable insights for the prompt identification, monitoring, and treatment of neoplastic and dysplastic polyps in clinical settings. It is important to consider the positive and negative aspects of our study while assessing its quality. The current study analyzed a total of 758 patients with polyps. This substantial sample size allowed for improved generalization of the results to the overall population and enhanced the reliability of the statistical analyses. The study assessed many inflammatory markers, including CRP, PLR, CALLY index, HALP score, PIV, SIII, and SIRI. This condition elucidated the correlation between inflammation and immune response in neoplastic polyps more thoroughly. An in-depth analysis of neoplastic and nonneoplastic polyps identified distinct biochemical and inflammatory disparities between these two categories. This led to the discovery of novel biomarkers for assessing the cancerous potential of polyps. Our study assessed the clinical use of novel indexes, namely, the HALP score and CALLY index, which have not been extensively investigated in the existing literature on colon polyps. An analysis of these indexes may offer novel strategies for clinical practice. The obtained data are derived from standard biochemical and hematological indicators and have the potential to provide therapeutically meaningful information for the early detection and treatment of neoplastic polyps. A significant advantage of investigating these inflammatory indexes in colon polyps is that they are simple, inexpensive, and accessible instruments. They can be used to determine the malignant potential of polyps and are easily integrated into clinical procedures. Furthermore, our study assessed inflammatory indicators and biochemical and demographic factors, including age and gender. This allowed us to conduct a comprehensive assessment of the cancerous potential of polyps. Although our study has numerous merits, it also possesses drawbacks. Our work is designed retrospectively, which introduces potential biases. For instance, certain inflammatory and immunological states could have influenced the relationship between the inflammatory indexes and neoplastic polyps, causing confounding effects. Nevertheless, as the anesthesiologist thoroughly assessed the patients who underwent colonoscopy before the operation, we believe that these factors did not substantially impact the study findings. This study was conducted in a single center, ensuring homogeneity in the study population. However, this may restrict the generalizability of the findings to other populations. A significant limitation of our study is the inability to assess the long-term impact of these indexes on predicting the probability of polyp malignant transformation, as there was a lack of long-term polyp follow-up. Furthermore, the precise threshold values of the inflammatory indexes employed in the study to predict the likelihood of malignancy have not been established. To our knowledge, the indexes examined in this study regarding colon polyps have not been previously addressed in the literature. This has hindered the complete comparison of our results with other similar research in the existing literature.

5. Conclusions

The use of the CALLY index, HALP score, and immuno-inflammatory indexes in clinical practice can contribute to risk stratification of colorectal polyps, potentially reducing the incidence of colorectal cancer (CRC) through timely interventions. When polyps are detected in patients undergoing endoscopic procedures, examining the inflammation indexes may be important in terms of providing an idea to the endoscopist about what kind of polypectomy method will be used for the polyp during the procedure and in planning the treatment and follow-up and in terms of giving a preliminary idea to the pathologists who will evaluate the polypectomy material in the process of differentiating the polyp from neoplastic or nonneoplastic. These markers improve diagnostic accuracy and offer a cost-effective method for identifying high-risk patients, promoting public health initiatives aimed at CRC prevention. This study also presents the impact of dysplasia, aging, and colon polyp localization on many measures of inflammatory and immunological responses. The involvement of inflammatory and immunological responses seems crucial in the progression of dysplasia and aging. Our study's results can offer significant insights for future investigations aiming to enhance comprehension of the impact of inflammation in clinical settings and for devising approaches for the prevention and treatment of disorders such as dysplasia.

Author Contributions: All authors take public responsibility for the content of the work submitted for review. The authors confirm their contribution to the paper as follows: S.C. (Sedat Ciftel), S.C. (Serpil Ciftel) and F.M. designed this study and were involved in the conceptualization, investigation, formal analysis, writing—original draft, and supervision. S.C. (Serpil Ciftel), F.M. and A.K. participated in the analysis and writing—original draft. The authors declare that all data were generated in-house, and no paper mill was used. All authors have read and agreed to the published version of the manuscript.

Funding: No financial resources were received at any stage of this study. In addition, The Recep Tayyip Erdogan University Development Foundation provided funding for the open-access publishing of this study.

Institutional Review Board Statement: Regional Erzurum Education and Training Hospital Clinical Research Ethical Committee (Erzurum, Turkey) (Approval Date: 3 October 2022, Approval Number: 2022/15–153).

Informed Consent Statement: An informed consent form is unnecessary as this is a retrospective study.

Data Availability Statement: All data generated or analyzed during this study are included in this article. The datasets in the current study are available from the corresponding author upon reasonable request.

Conflicts of Interest: The authors declare that they have no known competing financial interests or personal relationships that could have appeared to influence the work reported in this paper.

References

1. Sninsky, J.A.; Shore, B.M.; Lupu, G.V.; Crockett, S.D. Risk Factors for Colorectal Polyps and Cancer. *Gastrointest. Endosc. Clin. N. Am.* **2022**, *32*, 195–213. [CrossRef] [PubMed]
2. Johnson, G.G.R.J.; Helewa, R.; Moffatt, D.C.; Coneys, J.G.; Park, J.; Hyun, E. Colorectal Polyp Classification and Management of Complex Polyps for Surgeon Endoscopists. *Can. J. Surg.* **2023**, *66*, E491–E498. [CrossRef] [PubMed]
3. Pai, R.K.; Bettington, M.; Srivastava, A.; Rosty, C. An Update on the Morphology and Molecular Pathology of Serrated Colorectal Polyps and Associated Carcinomas. *Mod. Pathol.* **2019**, *32*, 1390–1415. [CrossRef] [PubMed]
4. Fucà, G.; Guarini, V.; Antoniotti, C.; Morano, F.; Moretto, R.; Corallo, S.; Marmorino, F.; Lonardi, S.; Rimassa, L.; Sartore-Bianchi, A.; et al. The Pan-Immune-Inflammation Value Is a New Prognostic Biomarker in Metastatic Colorectal Cancer: Results from a Pooled-Analysis of the Valentino and TRIBE First-Line Trials. *Br. J. Cancer* **2020**, *123*, 403–409. [CrossRef]
5. Nimptsch, K.; Aleksandrova, K.; Boeing, H.; Janke, J.; Lee, Y.; Jenab, M.; Bueno-de-Mesquita, H.B.; Jansen, E.H.; Tsilidis, K.K.; Trichopoulou, A.; et al. Association of *CRP* Genetic Variants with Blood Concentrations of C-reactive Protein and Colorectal Cancer Risk. *Int. J. Cancer* **2015**, *136*, 1181–1192. [CrossRef]
6. Eckart, A.; Struja, T.; Kutz, A.; Baumgartner, A.; Baumgartner, T.; Zurfluh, S.; Neeser, O.; Huber, A.; Stanga, Z.; Mueller, B.; et al. Relationship of Nutritional Status, Inflammation, and Serum Albumin Levels During Acute Illness: A Prospective Study. *Am. J. Med.* **2020**, *133*, 713–722.e7. [CrossRef]
7. Nøst, T.H.; Alcala, K.; Urbarova, I.; Byrne, K.S.; Guida, F.; Sandanger, T.M.; Johansson, M. Systemic Inflammation Markers and Cancer Incidence in the UK Biobank. *Eur. J. Epidemiol.* **2021**, *36*, 841–848. [CrossRef]
8. Iida, H.; Tani, M.; Komeda, K.; Nomi, T.; Matsushima, H.; Tanaka, S.; Ueno, M.; Nakai, T.; Maehira, H.; Mori, H.; et al. The superiority of CRP-Albumin-Lymphocyte Index (CALLY Index) as a Non-Invasive Prognostic Biomarker after Hepatectomy for Hepatocellular Carcinoma. *HPB* **2022**, *24*, 101–115. [CrossRef]
9. Furukawa, K.; Tsunematsu, M.; Tanji, Y.; Ishizaki, S.; Akaoka, M.; Haruki, K.; Uwagawa, T.; Onda, S.; Matsumoto, M.; Ikegami, T. Impact of C-Reactive Protein–Albumin–Lymphocyte (CALLY) Index on Prognosis after Hepatectomy for Colorectal Liver Metastasis. *Surg. Oncol.* **2023**, *47*, 101911. [CrossRef]
10. Chen, X.-L.; Xue, L.; Wang, W.; Chen, H.-N.; Zhang, W.-H.; Liu, K.; Chen, X.-Z.; Yang, K.; Zhang, B.; Chen, Z.-X.; et al. Prognostic Significance of the Combination of Preoperative Hemoglobin, Albumin, Lymphocyte and Platelet in Patients with Gastric Carcinoma: A Retrospective Cohort Study. *Oncotarget* **2015**, *6*, 41370–41382. [CrossRef]
11. Jiang, H.; Li, H.; Li, A.; Tang, E.; Xu, D.; Chen, Y.; Zhang, Y.; Tang, M.; Zhang, Z.; Deng, X.; et al. Preoperative Combined Hemoglobin, Albumin, Lymphocyte and Platelet Levels Predict Survival in Patients with Locally Advanced Colorectal Cancer. *Oncotarget* **2016**, *7*, 72076–72083. [CrossRef] [PubMed]

12. Zhao, Y.; Si, G.; Zhu, F.; Hui, J.; Cai, S.; Huang, C.; Cheng, S.; Fathy, A.H.; Xiang, Y.; Li, J. Prognostic Role of Platelet to Lymphocyte Ratio in Hepatocellular Carcinoma: A Systematic Review and Meta-Analysis. *Oncotarget* **2017**, *8*, 22854–22862. [CrossRef] [PubMed]
13. Va, G.; Gl, K.; Ph, L.; Oh, W. Invasive carcinoma of the large intestine: A preventable disease? *Surgery* **1965**, *57*, 363–365.
14. Vogelstein, B.; Fearon, E.R.; Hamilton, S.R.; Kern, S.E.; Preisinger, A.C.; Leppert, M.; Smits, A.M.M.; Bos, J.L. Genetic Alterations during Colorectal-Tumor Development. *N. Engl. J. Med.* **1988**, *319*, 525–532. [CrossRef] [PubMed]
15. Meseeha, M.; Attia, M. Colon Polyps. In *StatPearls [Internet]*; StatPearls Publishing: Treasure Island, FL, USA, 2023.
16. JF, E.J.; Lam, F.; Colombet, M.; Mery, L.; Piñeros, M. *Global Cancer Observatory: Cancer Today*; International Agency for Research on Cancer: Lyon, France, 2022.
17. Corley, D.A.; Jensen, C.D.; Marks, A.R.; Zhao, W.K.; De Boer, J.; Levin, T.R.; Doubeni, C.; Fireman, B.H.; Quesenberry, C.P. Variation of Adenoma Prevalence by Age, Sex, Race, and Colon Location in a Large Population: Implications for Screening and Quality Programs. *Clin. Gastroenterol. Hepatol.* **2013**, *11*, 172–180. [CrossRef]
18. Erdem, L.; Akbal, E.; Koçak, E.; Tucer, D.; Üçbilek, E.; Uyanıkoğlu, A.; Dolapçıoğlu, C.; Erim, E.A.; Şirin, G.; Alkım, H.; et al. A New Risk-Scoring System for Colorectal Cancer and Polyp Screening by Turkish Colorectal Cancer and Polyp Study Group. *Turk. J. Gastroenterol.* **2022**, *33*, 286–293. [CrossRef]
19. Salmo, E.; Haboubi, N. Adenoma and Malignant Colorectal Polyp: Pathological Considerations and Clinical Applications. *EMJ Gastroenterol.* **2018**, *7*, 92–102. [CrossRef]
20. Schreiner, M.A.; Weiss, D.G.; Lieberman, D.A. Proximal and Large Hyperplastic and Nondysplastic Serrated Polyps Detected by Colonoscopy Are Associated With Neoplasia. *Gastroenterology* **2010**, *139*, 1497–1502. [CrossRef]
21. Jass, J.R. Hyperplastic polyps of the colorectum-innocent or guilty? *Dis. Colon. Rectum.* **2001**, *44*, 163–166. [CrossRef] [PubMed]
22. Almadi, M.A.; Alharbi, O.; Azzam, N.; Wadera, J.; Sadaf, N.; Aljebreen, A.M. Prevalence and Characteristics of Colonic Polyps and Adenomas in 2654 Colonoscopies in Saudi Arabia. *Saudi J. Gastroenterol.* **2014**, *20*, 154. [CrossRef]
23. Kazem Shahmoradi, M.; Soleimaninejad, M.; Sharifian, M. Evaluation of Colonoscopy Data for Colorectal Polyps and Associated Histopathological Findings. *Ann. Med. Surg.* **2020**, *57*, 7–10. [CrossRef] [PubMed]
24. Di Gregorio, C.; Bonetti, L.R.; De Gaetani, C.; Pedroni, M.; Kaleci, S.; Ponz De Leon, M. Clinical Outcome of Low- and High-Risk Malignant Colorectal Polyps: Results of a Population-Based Study and Meta-Analysis of the Available Literature. *Intern. Emerg. Med.* **2014**, *9*, 151–160. [CrossRef] [PubMed]
25. Hsu, P.-K.; Huang, J.-Y.; Su, W.-W.; Wei, J.C.-C. Type 2 Diabetes and the Risk of Colorectal Polyps: A Retrospective Nationwide Population-Based Study. *Medicine* **2021**, *100*, e25933. [CrossRef] [PubMed]
26. Larsson, S.C.; Orsini, N.; Wolk, A. Diabetes Mellitus and Risk of Colorectal Cancer: A Meta-Analysis. *JNCI J. Natl. Cancer Inst.* **2005**, *97*, 1679–1687. [CrossRef] [PubMed]
27. Guraya, S.Y. Association of Type 2 Diabetes Mellitus and the Risk of Colorectal Cancer: A Meta-Analysis and Systematic Review. *World J. Gastroenterol.* **2015**, *21*, 6026–6031. [CrossRef]
28. Balkwill, F.; Mantovani, A. Inflammation and Cancer: Back to Virchow? *Lancet* **2001**, *357*, 539–545. [CrossRef]
29. Ubukata, H.; Motohashi, G.; Tabuchi, T.; Nagata, H.; Konishi, S.; Tabuchi, T. Evaluations of Interferon-γ/Interleukin-4 Ratio and Neutrophil/Lymphocyte Ratio as Prognostic Indicators in Gastric Cancer Patients. *J. Surg. Oncol.* **2010**, *102*, 742–747. [CrossRef]
30. Chen, Y.; Chen, K.; Xiao, X.; Nie, Y.; Qu, S.; Gong, C.; Su, F.; Song, E. Pretreatment Neutrophil-to-Lymphocyte Ratio Is Correlated with Response to Neoadjuvant Chemotherapy as an Independent Prognostic Indicator in Breast Cancer Patients: A Retrospective Study. *BMC Cancer* **2016**, *16*, 320. [CrossRef]
31. Efil, S.C.; Guner, G.; Guven, D.C.; Celikten, B.; Celebiyev, E.; Taban, H.; Akyol, A.; Isik, A.; Kilickap, S.; Yalcin, S.; et al. Prognostic and Predictive Value of Tumor Infiltrating Lymphocytes in Combination with Systemic Inflammatory Markers in Colon Cancer. *Clin. Res. Hepatol. Gastroenterol.* **2023**, *47*, 102171. [CrossRef]
32. Deitch, E.A.; Bridges, R.M. Stress Hormones Modulate Neutrophil and Lymphocyte Activity in Vitro. *J. Trauma Acute Care Surg.* **1987**, *27*, 1146–1154. [CrossRef]
33. Faye, A.S.; Holmer, A.K.; Axelrad, J.E. Cancer in Inflammatory Bowel Disease. *Gastroenterol. Clin. N. Am.* **2022**, *51*, 649–666. [CrossRef] [PubMed]
34. Ma, R.; Okugawa, Y.; Shimura, T.; Yamashita, S.; Sato, Y.; Yin, C.; Uratani, R.; Kitajima, T.; Imaoka, H.; Kawamura, M.; et al. Clinical Implications of C-Reactive Protein–Albumin–Lymphocyte (CALLY) Index in Patients with Esophageal Cancer. *Surg. Oncol.* **2024**, *53*, 102044. [CrossRef] [PubMed]
35. Takeda, Y.; Sugano, H.; Okamoto, A.; Nakano, T.; Shimoyama, Y.; Takada, N.; Imaizumi, Y.; Ohkuma, M.; Kosuge, M.; Eto, K. Prognostic Usefulness of the C-Reactive Protein-Albumin-Lymphocyte (CALLY) Index as a Novel Biomarker in Patients Undergoing Colorectal Cancer Surgery. *Asian J. Surg.* **2024**, *47*, 3492–3498. [CrossRef] [PubMed]
36. Feng, Z.; Lin, H.; Yang, X.; Cao, S.; Gu, X.; Zhang, Z.; Deng, W. Diagnostic Value of Inflammation-Related Indicators in Distinguishing Early Colon Cancer and Adenomatous Polyps. *Cancer Control* **2023**, *30*, 10732748231180745. [CrossRef] [PubMed]

37. Wieszczy, P.; Kaminski, M.F.; Franczyk, R.; Loberg, M.; Kobiela, J.; Rupinska, M.; Kocot, B.; Rupinski, M.; Holme, O.; Wojciechowska, U.; et al. Colorectal Cancer Incidence and Mortality After Removal of Adenomas During Screening Colonoscopies. *Gastroenterology* **2020**, *158*, 875–883.e5. [CrossRef]
38. Koyuncuer, A.; Zenginkinet, T. New Classification of Benign Epithelial Tumors: Colorectal Polyps and Synchronous Neoplasms: An Update and Critical Assessment: An Analysis of 678 Consecutive Cases and 1137 Polyps. *Medeni. Med. J.* **2023**, *38*, 39–44. [CrossRef]

life

MDPI

Article

Metabolic Dysfunction-Associated Steatotic Liver Disease in Patients with Inflammatory Bowel Diseases: A Pilot Study

Ludovico Abenavoli [1,*], Rocco Spagnuolo [1], Giuseppe Guido Maria Scarlata [1], Maria Luisa Gambardella [1], Luigi Boccuto [2], Nahum Méndez-Sánchez [3] and Francesco Luzza [1]

[1] Department of Health Sciences, University "Magna Græcia", Viale Europa, 88100 Catanzaro, Italy; spagnuolo@unicz.it (R.S.); giuseppeguidomaria.scarlata@unicz.it (G.G.M.S.); marialuisa.gambardella@studenti.unicz.it (M.L.G.); luzza@unicz.it (F.L.)

[2] Healthcare Genetics and Genomics Doctoral Program, School of Nursing, College of Behavioral, Social and Health Sciences, Clemson University, Clemson, SC 29634, USA; lboccut@clemson.edu

[3] Faculty of Medicine, National Autonomous University of Mexico, Mexico City 04510, Mexico; nmendez@medicasur.org.mx

* Correspondence: l.abenavoli@unicz.it; Tel.: +39-0961-3694-387

Abstract: Background: Inflammatory bowel disease (IBD) is characterized by persistent inflammation and is often associated with metabolic dysfunction-associated steatotic liver disease (MASLD). IBD patients are at risk of developing MASLD due to shared risk factors such as gut dysbiosis and systemic inflammation. The new MASLD nomenclature emphasizes the link between liver steatosis and cardiometabolic comorbidities. However, the prevalence of MASLD in IBD patients remains poorly explored. The main aim of this cross-sectional study is to assess the prevalence of ultrasound (US) and the clinical features of MASLD in patients with IBDs. Materials and Methods: We conducted a retrospective study enrolling 272 Italian IBD patients attending Renato Dulbecco Teaching Hospital in a period between 1 January 2021 and 31 December 2023. MASLD was diagnosed based on the presence of liver steatosis with cardiometabolic risk factors, using established guidelines. Demographic, clinical, and laboratory data were collected and analyzed. Statistical significance was determined at a p-value < 0.05. Results: Of the 272 IBD patients, 6% had non-alcoholic fatty liver disease (NAFLD), while 18% had MASLD. Patients with IBD-MASLD were significantly older, had higher body mass index, waist circumference, and triglyceride levels, and were more likely to have type 2 diabetes mellitus and hypertension compared to those with IBD-NAFLD. IBD-MASLD patients also showed higher disease activity scores and required more frequent surgical interventions. Bivariate logistic regression revealed triglyceride levels as a significant predictor of MASLD in IBD patients. Conclusions: MASLD is more prevalent in IBD patients, highlighting the importance of early detection of liver steatosis in this at-risk population. The association between MASLD and cardiometabolic risk factors underscores the need for a multidisciplinary approach to manage these patients effectively. Further studies in larger cohorts are necessary to confirm these findings and explore the pathophysiological mechanisms involved.

Keywords: Crohn's disease; ulcerative colitis; liver ultrasound; metabolic dysfunction-associated fatty liver disease

1. Introduction

Inflammatory bowel disease (IBD) includes two different conditions, ulcerative colitis (UC) and Crohn's disease (CD), characterized by persistent inflammation and subsequent gastrointestinal tract damage [1,2]. IBDs pose a significant public health challenge due to their global prevalence. In Europe, the prevalence of CD ranges from 1.5 to 213 cases per 100,000 people, while UC occurs at a rate of 2.4 to 294 cases per 100,000 individuals [3]. The typical symptoms of IBD, such as abdominal pain, bloating, and altered bowel habits, often overlap with irritable bowel syndrome (IBS), which, despite being a distinct pathological entity, requires a differential diagnosis. Indeed, a recent meta-analysis based on 27 studies showed that IBS symptoms were present in 32% of cases of IBD patients in remission [4]. Additionally, IBS and IBD predominantly affect young adults and have a higher prevalence in females, indicating a demographic similarity [5]. In an observational study, the Authors found a significantly higher incidence of IBD among patients with IBS. The incidence rate of IBD was 8.6 times higher ($p < 0.0001$) in individuals with IBS, at 238.1 per 100,000 person-years, compared to 27.8 per 100,000 person-years in the general population. At the same time, in IBS cases, the risk of developing IBD was higher, with a 15-fold increase compared to subjects without IBS [6]. Furthermore, several additional manifestations beyond the intestine may affect IBD patients, including joint pain, skin conditions, oral ulcers, and non-alcoholic fatty liver disease (NAFLD) [7]. This condition results from the triglyceride accumulation in over 5% of hepatocytes without excessive alcohol consumption [8]. Failure to diagnose NAFLD early can result in steatohepatitis, cirrhosis, and hepatocellular carcinoma [9]. Common pathophysiological mechanisms are involved in the clinical presentation of NAFLD and IBS [10]. Both conditions are associated with microbial dysbiosis, where an imbalance in the gut microbiota composition contributes to disease progression. This event can lead to an impaired intestinal barrier, resulting in increased gut permeability, known as leaky gut, and subsequent systemic inflammation [11]. In this context, several studies have shown the prevalence of IBS in NAFLD patients to be around 29%, with a 13% increased risk associated with female gender. However, the prevalence of IBS rises significantly with the severity of NAFLD: 11.3% in mild cases, 27.7% in moderate cases, and 58.3% in severe cases [12–14]. Furthermore, NAFLD is often related to dysmetabolic features such as type 2 diabetes mellitus (T2DM), hypertension, obesity, and dyslipidemia, which complicates patient management by requiring a multi-disciplinary and highly specialized approach [15]. Hence, in recent years, the terminology NAFLD has been substituted with metabolic dysfunction-associated fatty liver disease (MAFLD) and later with metabolic dysfunction-associated steatotic liver disease (MASLD) [16,17]. The literature reports that IBD is a risk factor for NAFLD development due to a yet poorly elucidated interplay that involves lifestyle, genetic, and epigenetic factors as well as gut microbiota dysbiosis [18–21]. NAFLD prevalence in patients with IBD is quite heterogeneous due to the different diagnostic techniques used, ranging from 20 to 30% of cases detected by liver ultrasound (US) to around 70% with transient elastography [22,23]. In this regard, its prevalence is higher than in the general population (25%) [24]. Recently, we evaluated the prevalence of US and the clinical features of IBD patients with NAFLD and MAFLD [25,26]. However, there is a lack of observational studies about the prevalence of MASLD in patients with IBD in a real-life setting. Indeed, the application of the new MASLD nomenclature requires further investigation, as, according to recent surveys of a randomly selected cohort of 1016 patients, the prevalence of liver steatosis was 27% (261/1016). However, 247/261 patients (89.2%) overlapped with the new definitions for fatty liver disease. In contrast, the population represented exclusively by the presence of fatty liver and not falling under any of the new definitions was represented by only 2.2% (6/277) of the investigated subjects [27]. This suggests that the new definition of MASLD is more inclusive, capturing that portion of patients with fatty liver who carry cardiometabolic comorbidities [28]. While considering both issues, we focused on the fatty liver condition, mainly evaluating the application of the new MASLD nomenclature to an at-risk and still-not-fully studied population such as that of IBD patients. By doing this, it will be possible to assess other potential causes of fatty liver disease in the IBD population besides metabolic risk. For this reason, the main aim of this cross-sectional study is to assess the US prevalence and the clinical features of MASLD in patients with IBDs.

2. Materials and Methods

2.1. Patients

We conducted a retrospective study involving Italian patients of both genera attending Renato Dulbecco Teaching Hospital of Catanzaro (Italy) in a period between 1 January 2021 and 31 December 2023, diagnosed with IBD in accordance with international guidelines [29]. To be included, participants had to be (i) aged 18 years or older, and (ii) have undergone a liver US at the time of hospital admission. Exclusion criteria included the following: (i) a history of alcohol or drug abuse, (ii) current or past viral hepatitis infection, (iii) a diagnosis of autoimmune liver diseases, (iv) liver cirrhosis, (v) any cancer diagnosis, and (vi) pregnancy or breastfeeding. Data collected from each patient included the following: (i) demographic and anthropometric information, (ii) details about their IBD condition, (iii) disease phenotype and location, (iv) metabolic features, (v) laboratory test results, and (vi) current medications. Among the 3325 patients screened, 272 had IBD and, for this reason, were enrolled in the study.

2.2. Diagnosis of NAFLD and MASLD

All patients underwent liver assessment using US, adhering to the protocols from our previous investigations [25,26]. The US was performed by an experienced operator using the LOGIQ S8 XDclear 2.0+ (GE HealthCare, Milan, Italy) with a 3.5 MHz convex transducer for B-mode imaging. Participants fasted for at least 4 h prior to the exam and followed a low-fiber diet while taking 80 mg of simethicone three times daily for three days before the procedure. Liver steatosis was graded as mild (S1), moderate (S2), or severe (S3). S1 was identified by a slight increase in liver echogenicity and minimal contrast between liver and kidney echoes, S2 exhibited higher liver echogenicity, reduced portal vein wall echoes, noticeable posterior beam attenuation, and greater contrast between liver and kidney echoes, while S3 involved marked beam penetration reduction, the absence of echoes from much of the portal vein wall, and a substantial difference in hepatic and renal echoes. A liver steatosis grade of S1 or higher was used for diagnosis [30]. For NAFLD evaluation, alcohol consumption was defined as less than 210 g per week for men and 140 g per week for women (equivalent to 30 g/day for men and 20 g/day for women) [31]. Diagnostic criteria for MASLD were applied based on Rinella et al.'s guidelines, requiring the presence of liver steatosis alongside at least one of five cardiometabolic risk factors: (i) body mass index (BMI) $\geq$ 25 kg/m^2 or waist circumference >94 cm for men and >80 cm for women; (ii) fasting blood glucose $\geq$ 100 mg/dL or a diagnosis and/or treatment for T2DM; (iii) blood pressure $\geq$ 135/85 mmHg or the use of antihypertensive medications; (iv) triglycerides $\geq$ 150 mg/dL or use of lipid-lowering medication; and (v) high-density lipoproteins (HDL) $\leq$ 40 mg/dL in men and $\leq$50 mg/dL in women, or treatment with lipid-lowering drugs [17]. Information on past medical history, laboratory results, and endoscopic findings was gathered, and if laboratory and endoscopy data were missing, results from tests performed within 15 days before or after the liver US were used.

2.3. Statistical Analysis

We presented numerical variables as mean $\pm$ standard deviation (SD) and nominal variables as absolute counts and percentages. Continuous variables were compared using the Mann–Whitney U test after confirming normality with the Shapiro–Wilk test. Categorical variables were analyzed using the chi-square (χ^2) test. Bivariate logistic regression was performed to identify independent variables. Statistical significance was determined at a p-value < 0.05. Data analysis was conducted using SPSS 26.0 software (IBM Corp., Armonk, NY, USA).

3. Results

3.1. Characteristics of Participants

Table 1 outlines the principal clinical and laboratory features of the individuals included in our investigation. Most IBD patients enrolled were females (n = 218, 80%) with a BMI of 24 $\pm$ 4 Kg/m^2 and a waist circumference of 91 $\pm$ 12 cm. Only n = 19 (7%) were active smokers. Most of these had UC (n = 178, 65%), with pancolitis (n = 91; 51%) and a full Mayo Score of 2 $\pm$ 1. Disease duration was 13 $\pm$ 11 years, and the age at onset was 26 $\pm$ 15 years, while n = 68 (25%) and n = 29 (11%) of IBD patients showed an active disease and extraintestinal manifestations, respectively. As for dysmetabolic comorbidities, *n* = 17 (6%), *n* = 41 (15%), and *n* = 21 (7%) of enrolled patients showed T2DM, hypertension, and dyslipidemia, respectively. Most IBD patients were treated with salicylates (*n* = 129, 47%) and biological therapy (*n* = 122, 45%). Surgical treatment was reported in *n* = 49 of patients (18%).

Table 1. Clinical and laboratory features of enrolled IBD patients.

	IBD (N = 272)
Demographic and anthropometric	
Age (years)	46 ± 16
Male gender, *n* (%)	54 (20)
Female gender, *n* (%)	218 (80)
Active smokers, *n* (%)	19 (7)
BMI (Kg/m^2)	24 ± 4
Waist circumference (cm)	91 ± 12
Disease characteristics	
Disease duration (years)	13 ± 11
Age at onset (years)	26 ± 15
Crohn's Disease, *n* (%)	94 (35)
CD (Harvey Bradshaw index)	6 ± 3
Ulcerative Colitis, *n* (%)	178 (65)
UC (full Mayo Score)	2 ± 1
Active disease, *n* (%)	68 (25)
Extraintestinal manifestations, *n* (%)	29 (11)
Surgery, *n* (%)	49 (18)
CD disease location and phenotype	
Ileal, *n* (%) *	46 (49)
Colonic, *n* (%) *	14 (15)
Ileo-Colonic, *n* (%) *	33 (35)
Upper GI, *n* (%) *	1 (1)
Inflammatory, *n* (%) *	37 (39)
Fistulizing, *n* (%) *	26 (28)
Stenosing, *n* (%) *	31 (33)
UC disease location	
Proctitis, *n* (%) *	10 (6)
Proctosigmoiditis, *n* (%) *	40 (22)
Left-side, *n* (%) *	37 (21)
Pancolitis, *n* (%) *	91 (51)
Dysmetabolic comorbidities	
T2DM, *n* (%)	17 (6)
Hypertension, *n* (%)	41 (15)
Dyslipidemia, *n* (%)	21 (7)
Laboratory parameters (mean ± SD)	
ALT (UI/L)	19 ± 10
AST (UI/L)	19 ± 8
Total cholesterol (mg/dL)	168 ± 39
LDL (mg/dL)	102 ± 33
HDL (mg/dL)	56 ± 15
Triglycerides (mg/dL)	98 ± 45
Fasting blood glucose (mg/dL)	87 ± 17
Fasting insulinemia (mg/dL)	9 ± 6
HOMA-IR	2 ± 2
CRP (mg/L)	6 ± 10
Fecal calprotectin (mcg/gr)	591 ± 1296

Table 1. *Cont.*

	IBD (N = 272)
Medications	
Salicylates, *n* (%)	129 (47)
Azathioprine, *n* (%)	40 (15)
>3 cycles of steroids, *n* (%)	20 (7)
Biological therapy, *n* (%)	122 (45)
Anti-TNF-α, *n* (%)	81 (30)
Vedolizumab, *n* (%)	27 (10)
Ustekinumab, *n* (%)	15 (5)
>1 Biological drug, *n* (%)	26 (9)
Current biological therapy duration (years)	3 ± 2
Total biological therapy duration (years)	4 ± 4

Abbreviations: IBD, inflammatory bowel disease; BMI, body mass index; CD, Crohn's disease; UC, ulcerative colitis; T2DM, type 2 diabetes mellitus; ALT, alanine aminotransferase; AST, aspartate aminotransferase; LDL, low-density lipoprotein; HDL, high-density lipoprotein; HOMA-IR, homeostasis model assessment of insulin resistance; CRP, C-reactive protein; TNF-α, tumor necrosis factor-alfa. * *n*, (%) was evaluated with regard to CD and UC patients, respectively.

3.2. NAFLD and MASLD Prevalence in Patients with IBD

The US prevalence of NAFLD and MASLD among individuals with IBD was 6% and 18%, respectively.

3.3. Comparison and Bivariate Logistic Regression Analysis between Study Cohorts

As outlined in Table 2, participants with IBD were categorized based on the presence of NAFLD and MASLD, respectively.

Table 2. Comparison of IBD patients according to NAFLD and MASLD diagnosis.

	IBD-NAFLD (N = 18)	IBD-MASLD (N = 48)	*p*-Value
Demographic and anthropometric			
Age (years)	43 ± 15	53 ± 13	0.020
Male gender, *n* (%)	18 (100)	34 (71)	0.006
Female gender, *n* (%)	0	14 (29)	
Active smokers, *n* (%)	0	2 (4)	0.526
BMI (Kg/m^2)	23 ± 1	27 ± 5	<0.001
Waist circumference (cm)	86 ± 1	101 ± 11	<0.001
Disease characteristics			
Disease duration (years)	17 ± 11	15 ± 11	0.267
Age at onset (years)	26 ± 15	39 ± 15	0.004
Crohn's Disease, *n* (%)	6 (33)	18 (37.5)	0.495
CD (Harvey Bradshaw index)	3 ± 3	5 ± 2	0.003
Ulcerative Colitis, *n* (%)	12 (67)	30 (62.5)	0.495
UC (full Mayo Score)	1.7 ± 1	2.3 ± 1	0.003
Active disease, *n* (%)	4 (22)	11 (23)	0.616
Extraintestinal manifestations, *n* (%)	2 (11)	7 (15)	0.533
Mild steatosis, *n* (%)	10 (55)	28 (58)	
Moderate steatosis, *n* (%)	6 (33)	16 (33)	0.761
Severe steatosis, *n* (%)	2 (12)	4 (9)	
Surgery, *n* (%)	0	13 (27)	0.009
CD disease location and phenotype			
Ileal, *n* (%) *	6 (100)	8 (45)	
Colonic, *n* (%) *	0	3 (17)	0.027
Ileo-Colonic, *n* (%) *	0	6 (33)	

Table 2. *Cont.*

	IBD-NAFLD (N = 18)	IBD-MASLD (N = 48)	*p*-Value
Upper GI, *n* (%) *	0	1 (5)	
Inflammatory, *n* (%) *	6 (100)	5 (28)	
Fistulizing, *n* (%) *	0	4 (22)	0.005
Stenosing, *n* (%) *	0	9 (50)	
UC disease location			
Proctitis, *n* (%) *	1 (8)	2 (7)	
Proctosigmoiditis, *n* (%) *	2 (17)	7 (23)	
Left-side, *n* (%) *	4 (33)	7 (23)	0.770
Pancolitis, *n* (%) *	5 (42)	14 (47)	
Dysmetabolic comorbidities			
T2DM, *n* (%)	0	9 (19)	0.045
Hypertension, *n* (%)	0	18 (37)	0.012
Dyslipidemia, *n* (%)	1 (9)	5 (10)	0.622
Laboratory parameters (mean ± SD)			
ALT (UI/L)	24 ± 7	23 ± 12	0.395
AST (UI/L)	25 ± 9	22 ± 9	0.170
Total cholesterol (mg/dL)	175 ± 17	169 ± 45	0.255
LDL (mg/dL)	106 ± 21	105 ± 37	0.594
HDL (mg/dL)	56 ± 8	49 ± 15	0.031
Triglycerides (mg/dL)	81 ± 17	121 ± 55	0.001
Fasting blood glucose (mg/dL)	83 ± 8	94 ± 23	0.019
Fasting insulinemia (mg/dL)	7 ± 2	12 ± 9	0.001
HOMA-IR	1.5 ± 0.45	3 ± 2	0.002
CRP (mg/L)	5 ± 3	7 ± 13	0.324
Fecal calprotectin (mcg/gr)	215 ± 378	464 ± 929	0.594
Medications			
Salicylates, *n* (%)	8 (44)	23 (48)	0.511
Azathioprine, *n* (%)	2 (11)	3 (6)	0.416
>3 cycles of steroids, *n* (%)	2 (11)	3 (6)	0.416
Biological therapy, *n* (%)	8 (44)	24 (50)	0.511
Anti-TNF-α, *n* (%)	6 (33)	16 (32)	0.610
Vedolizumab, *n* (%)	2 (11)	3 (6)	0.367
Ustekinumab, *n* (%)	0	5 (11)	0.192
>1 Biological drug, *n* (%)	0	6 (12)	0.135
Current biological therapy duration (years)	4 ± 3	3 ± 3	0.724
Total biological therapy duration (years)	6 ± 3	5 ± 3	0.287

Abbreviations: IBD, inflammatory bowel disease; BMI, body mass index; CD, Crohn's disease; UC, ulcerative colitis; T2DM, type 2 diabetes mellitus; ALT, alanine aminotransferase; AST, aspartate aminotransferase; LDL, low-density lipoprotein; HDL, high-density lipoprotein; HOMA-IR, homeostasis model assessment of insulin resistance; CRP, C-reactive protein; TNF-α, tumor necrosis factor-alfa. * The *p*-value was evaluated with regard to CD and UC patients, respectively.

When comparing IBD-MASLD patients to those with IBD-NAFLD, all male patients in the IBD-NAFLD group [n = 18 (100%) vs. n = 34 (71%), p = 0.006] were significantly younger (43 ± 15 vs. 53 ± 13 years, p = 0.020) and had lower BMI (23 ± 1 vs. 27 ± 5 kg/m^2, $p < 0.001$) and waist circumference (86 ± 1 vs. 101 ± 11 cm, $p < 0.001$). None of the IBD-NAFLD patients were active smokers [n = 0 vs. n = 2 (4%), p = 0.526]. In contrast, a significant proportion of IBD-MASLD patients had T2DM [n = 9 (19%) vs. 0, p = 0.045] and hypertension [n = 18 (37%) vs. 0, p = 0.012], while there was no significant difference in dyslipidemia between the two groups [n = 5 (10%) vs. n = 1 (9%), p = 0.622]. In terms of laboratory results, IBD-MASLD patients showed higher triglyceride levels (121 ± 55 vs. 81 ± 17 mg/dL, p = 0.001), fasting blood glucose (94 ± 23 vs. 83 ± 8 mg/dL, p = 0.019), fasting insulin (12 ± 9 vs. 7 ± 2 mg/dL, p = 0.001), and homeostasis model assessment of insulin resistance (HOMA-IR; 3 ± 2 vs. 1.5 ± 0.45 mg/dL, $p = 0.002$). They also had lower HDL cholesterol levels (49 ± 15 vs. 56 ± 8 mg/dL, $p = 0.031$). Other laboratory results showed no significant differences between the two groups. Most IBD-NAFLD patients had UC [$n = 12$ (67%) vs. $n = 30$ (62.5%), $p = 0.495$], but CD showed a significantly more frequent ileal involvement [$n = 6$ (100%) vs. $n = 8$ (45%), $p = 0.027$] and an inflammatory disease phenotype [$n = 6$ (100%) vs. $n = 5$ (28%), $p = 0.005$]. IBD-MASLD patients had higher disease activity scores, including the Harvey–Bradshaw Index (5 ± 2 vs. 3 ± 3, $p = 0.003$) and Full Mayo Score (2.3 ± 1 vs. 1.7 ± 1, $p = 0.003$). Additionally, more IBD-MASLD patients required surgery [$n = 13$ (27%), $p = 0.009$]. Regarding treatment, most IBD-MASLD patients were treated with salicylates [$n = 23$ (48%) vs. $n = 8$ (44%), $p = 0.511$] and biological therapies [$n = 24$ (50%) vs. $n = 8$ (44%), $p = 0.511$], with no significant differences between groups. Lastly, bivariate logistic regression revealed that elevated triglyceride levels were significantly associated with IBD-MASLD after adjusting for age (odds ratio [OR] = 1.033, 95% confidence interval [CI] 1.007–1.059, $p = 0.012$).

4. Discussion

Liver steatosis is a frequent hepatobiliary manifestation in patients with IBD [32]. Fatty deposition in the hepatocytes and the possible subsequent inflammation can be directly related to the severity of the IBDs as well as to nutritional status and corticosteroid use [33]. Considering the recent change in the nomenclature definition of fatty liver disease from NAFLD to MASLD, we have studied their relationship and a possible pathogenetic way with IBDs. In this context, our analysis shows a US prevalence of NAFLD and MASLD among IBD patients of 6% and 18%, respectively. On the one hand, these findings are in line with our preliminary results, reporting a US prevalence of fatty liver disease associated with dysmetabolic comorbidities of 23% in another cohort of IBD patients [25,26]. On the other hand, we were able to identify a cohort of IBD patients who have fatty liver disease that is not related to cardiometabolic comorbidities and, therefore, does not fall under the new MASLD nomenclature. The prevalence of 6% shown in our IBD-NAFLD cohort is three times more than the prevalence of 2.2% shown by Song et al., although the survey was performed in the general population [27]. This finding confirms that IBDs are a risk factor for fatty liver disease, allowing us to hypothesize how localized inflammatory events in the gut–liver axis may be a prompter for the establishment of liver steatosis. Accordingly, IBD-NAFLD patients show gut dysbiosis that could support this evidence [34]. Currently, the only epidemiological data on this association reported a US prevalence of MASLD among IBD-lean patients of 21% [35]. At the same time, MASLD is an independent predictor of extra-hepatic comorbidities in IBD patients [36]. However, more investigations are needed to better define the exact prevalence of fatty liver disease in IBDs. Indeed, few studies have been performed in the general population, with an extensive range of results (among 10–84%) due to the variability of the diagnostic tools used and the different characteristics of selected patients [27,37–40]. When compared to the IBD-NAFLD group, most of the patients with IBD-MASLD included in our analysis were males who were older and had a later onset. Recent epidemiological studies demonstrated how IBD homogeneously affects women and men between the second and third decades of life [41,42]. Indeed, when considering the aggregated data of all our IBD patients, the female gender is more prevalent than the male gender (80% vs. 20%). However, liver steatosis and the associated cardiometabolic comorbidities are more frequent in males after the fifth decade of life [43]. This evidence confirms our previous data, in which the IBD-NAFLD group is exclusively represented by males, while the IBD-MASLD group shows a higher prevalence of males than females (71% vs. 29%). Patients with CD and MASLD showed significantly higher disease index based on the Harvey–Bradshaw Index than patients with CD and NAFLD. Likewise, patients with UC and MASLD had a significantly higher disease index, considering the Full Mayo Score, than patients with UC and NAFLD [29]. These results may be related to the mutual relationship between disease activity, extent of disease, and cardiometabolic comorbidities [21]. For this reason, a significantly higher percentage of IBD-MASLD patients were undergoing surgery [44]. As reported in Table 2, our IBD-MASLD patients had significantly higher levels of anthropometric parameters than the IBD-NAFLD group, especially BMI and waist circumference. On the contrary, in the study by Martínez-Domínguez et al., IBD was an independent risk factor related to MASLD in lean patients [35]. The new MASLD nomenclature requires lower waist circumference values to be diagnosed than MAFLD (94/80 cm for the diagnosis of MASLD vs. 102/88 cm for the diagnosis of MAFLD) [16,17]. In a recent study, it was noted that the distinction between MAFLD and MASLD primarily lies in the categorization of lean individuals. While MASLD requires patients to exhibit one metabolic risk abnormality, MAFLD necessitates two. This discrepancy can result in overdiagnosis or misclassification of individuals who do not possess a high metabolic risk as per the MASLD criteria [45]. Moreover, besides higher BMI and waist circumference levels, our IBD-MASLD patients showed changes in glucose and lipid profile and, in particular, significantly higher levels of triglycerides, fasting blood glucose, fasting insulinemia, HOMA-IR, and significantly lower levels of HDL than IBD-NAFLD group, according to recent studies [37,39]. However, although insulin resistance is often associated with several inflammatory conditions, this parameter is not always detectable for IBD patients, especially those with less disease activity. Indeed, Carrillo-Palau et al. highlighted that NAFLD is related to the dysfunction of the beta cells in patients affected by IBD, promoting the development of insulin resistance [46]. Furthermore, our IBD-MASLD group showed a significantly higher percentage of cardiometabolic comorbidities, while De A et al. reported a lower prevalence of T2DM and hypertension (15% and 11%, respectively) in their MASLD-lean patients [40]. According to He et al., the updated nomenclature provides a more precise identification of individuals at higher risk for T2DM [38]. Finally, triglyceride levels were significantly associated with the presence of IBD-MASLD after bivariate logistic regression. Similar data are reported in the literature, but in patients with NAFLD and incident NAFLD after a four-year follow-up [47,48]. The primary limitations of our study include its small sample size, retrospective design, and the absence of a control group of healthy individuals. At the same time, the decision not to include IBD alone as a control group is motivated by the intention to compare two different nomenclatures in an at-risk population such as that of IBD patients. Furthermore, as a cross-sectional study, we cannot identify an etiologic hypothesis attributable to cardiometabolic factors. Finally, the possibility of a genetic predisposition to fatty liver disease, other than transient elastography, could not be assessed. The new MASLD nomenclature has been proposed by the Delphi consensus statement signed by 236 experts on steatotic liver disease from 56 countries and supported by national and international hepatological societies. It includes the presence of cardiometabolic comorbidities, thus increasing the knowledge of the pathophysiological mechanisms concomitant to hepatic steatosis and promoting a multidisciplinary approach to patient management [17,49]. Indeed, patients with both fatty liver disease and IBD have a worse prognosis in terms of mortality than patients with IBD alone [50]. However, there are still few studies in the literature addressing this issue because it was only recently proposed by the scientific community. For this reason, applying this new nomenclature to fatty liver disease in the clinical setting of IBDs can improve their management.

5. Conclusions

Our study shows how patients with liver steatosis have cardiometabolic comorbidities ascribable to the new definition of MASLD. In addition, the high prevalence of MASLD in the clinical setting of IBDs indicates a pivotal role in the early diagnosis of hepatic fat accumulation in patients with IBDs, and therefore at risk. At the same time, it is necessary to identify new potential biomarkers as predictors of MASLD risk in IBD patients. New studies in larger population cohorts are needed to confirm our data and evaluate the role of IBDs as a risk factor for MASLD onset and progression.

Author Contributions: Conceptualization: L.A.; formal analysis: R.S. and G.G.M.S.; data curation: G.G.M.S. and M.L.G.; original draft preparation: L.A., R.S. and G.G.M.S.; manuscript review and editing: L.B. and N.M.-S.; supervision: F.L. All authors have read and agreed to the published version of the manuscript.

Funding: This study did not receive any external funding.

Institutional Review Board Statement: The study was approved by the ethics committee of the Magna Graecia University of Catanzaro (protocol number 150, approval date 22 April 2021). This research adhered to the principles set forth in the Declaration of Helsinki.

Informed Consent Statement: Informed consent was waived due to the study's retrospective design.

Data Availability Statement: The original contributions presented in the study are included in the article, further inquiries can be directed to the corresponding author.

Conflicts of Interest: The authors declare no conflicts of interest.

Abbreviations

ALT	alanine aminotransferase
AST	aspartate aminotransferase
BMI	body mass index
CD	Crohn's disease
CI	confidence interval
CRP	C-reactive protein
HDL	high-density lipoprotein
HOMA-IR	homeostasis model assessment of insulin resistance
IBD	inflammatory bowel disease
IBS	irritable bowel syndrome
LDL	low-density lipoprotein
MAFLD	metabolic dysfunction-associated fatty liver disease
MASLD	metabolic dysfunction-associated steatotic liver disease
NAFLD	non-alcoholic fatty liver disease
OR	odds ratio
S1	mild liver steatosis
S2	moderate liver steatosis
S3	severe liver steatosis
SD	standard deviation
T2DM	type 2 diabetes mellitus
TNF-α	tumor necrosis factor-alfa
UC	ulcerative colitis
US	ultrasound
χ^2	chi-square

References

1. Tavakoli, P.; Vollmer-Conna, U.; Hadzi-Pavlovic, D.; Grimm, M.C. A Review of Inflammatory Bowel Disease: A Model of Microbial, Immune and Neuropsychological Integration. *Public Health Rev.* **2021**, *42*, 1603990. [CrossRef] [PubMed]
2. Le Berre, C.; Danese, S.; Peyrin-Biroulet, L. Can we change the natural course of inflammatory bowel disease? *Ther. Adv. Gastroenterol.* **2023**, *16*, 17562848231163118. [CrossRef] [PubMed]
3. Mak, W.Y.; Zhao, M.; Ng, S.C.; Burisch, J. The epidemiology of inflammatory bowel disease: East meets west. *J. Gastroenterol. Hepatol.* **2020**, *35*, 380–389. [CrossRef] [PubMed]
4. Fairbrass, K.M.; Costantino, S.J.; Gracie, D.J.; Ford, A.C. Prevalence of irritable bowel syndrome-type symptoms in patients with inflammatory bowel disease in remission: A systematic review and meta-analysis. *Lancet Gastroenterol. Hepatol.* **2020**, *5*, 1053–1062. [CrossRef] [PubMed]
5. Quigley, E.M. Overlapping irritable bowel syndrome and inflammatory bowel disease: Less to this than meets the eye? *Ther. Adv. Gastroenterol.* **2016**, *9*, 199–212. [CrossRef]
6. Porter, C.K.; Cash, B.D.; Pimentel, M.; Akinseye, A.; Riddle, M.S. Risk of inflammatory bowel disease following a diagnosis of irritable bowel syndrome. *BMC Gastroenterol.* **2012**, *12*, 55. [CrossRef]

7. Perler, B.K.; Ungaro, R.; Baird, G.; Mallette, M.; Bright, R.; Shah, S.; Shapiro, J.; Sands, B.E. Presenting symptoms in inflammatory bowel disease: Descriptive analysis of a community-based inception cohort. *BMC Gastroenterol.* **2019**, *19*, 47. [CrossRef]
8. Pouwels, S.; Sakran, N.; Graham, Y.; Leal, A.; Pintar, T.; Yang, W.; Kassir, R.; Singhal, R.; Mahawar, K.; Ramnarain, D. Non-alcoholic fatty liver disease (NAFLD): A review of pathophysiology, clinical management and effects of weight loss. *BMC Endocr. Disord.* **2022**, *22*, 63. [CrossRef]
9. Simon, T.G.; Roelstraete, B.; Hagström, H.; Loomba, R.; Ludvigsson, J.F. Progression of non-alcoholic fatty liver disease and long-term outcomes: A nationwide paired liver biopsy cohort study. *J. Hepatol.* **2023**, *79*, 1366–1373. [CrossRef]
10. Purssell, H.; Whorwell, P.J.; Athwal, V.S.; Vasant, D.H. Non-alcoholic fatty liver disease in irritable bowel syndrome: More than a coincidence? *World J. Hepatol.* **2021**, *13*, 1816–1827. [CrossRef]
11. Scalera, A.; Di Minno, M.N.; Tarantino, G. What does irritable bowel syndrome share with non-alcoholic fatty liver disease? *World J. Gastroenterol.* **2013**, *19*, 5402–5420. [CrossRef] [PubMed]
12. Franco, L.; Jones-Pauley, M.; Tamimi, O.; Neshatian, L.; Nguyen, D.; Graviss, E.; Quigley, E.M.; Victor, D., 3rd. Irritable Bowel Syndrome Symptoms in Nonalcoholic Fatty Liver Disease Patients Are an Indicator of Depression and Anxiety. *J. Clin. Gastroenterol.* **2023**, *57*, 1016–1023. [CrossRef] [PubMed]
13. Wu, S.; Yuan, C.; Yang, Z.; Liu, S.; Zhang, Q.; Zhang, S.; Zhu, S. Non-alcoholic fatty liver is associated with increased risk of irritable bowel syndrome: A prospective cohort study. *BMC Med.* **2022**, *20*, 262. [CrossRef] [PubMed]
14. Singh, S.P.; Kar, S.K.; Panigrahi, M.K.; Misra, B.; Pattnaik, K.; Bhuyan, P.; Meher, C.; Agrawal, O.; Rout, N.; Swain, M. Profile of patients with incidentally detected nonalcoholic fatty liver disease (IDNAFLD) in coastal eastern India. *Trop. Gastroenterol.* **2013**, *34*, 144–152. [CrossRef]
15. Labenz, C.; Kostev, K.; Alqahtani, S.A.; Galle, P.R.; Schattenberg, J.M. Impact of Non-Alcoholic Fatty Liver Disease on Metabolic Comorbidities in Type 2 Diabetes Mellitus. *Exp. Clin. Endocrinol. Diabetes* **2022**, *130*, 172–177. [CrossRef]
16. Eslam, M.; Sanyal, A.J.; George, J.; International Consensus Panel. MAFLD: A Consensus-Driven Proposed Nomenclature for Metabolic Associated Fatty Liver Disease. *Gastroenterology* **2020**, *158*, 1999–2014.e1. [CrossRef]
17. Rinella, M.E.; Lazarus, J.V.; Ratziu, V.; Francque, S.M.; Sanyal, A.J.; Kanwal, F.; Romero, D.; Abdelmalek, M.F.; Anstee, Q.M.; Arab, J.P.; et al. A multisociety Delphi consensus statement on new fatty liver disease nomenclature. *J. Hepatol.* **2023**, *79*, 1542–1556. [CrossRef] [PubMed]
18. Rodriguez-Duque, J.C.; Calleja, J.L.; Iruzubieta, P.; Hernández-Conde, M.; Rivas-Rivas, C.; Vera, M.I.; Garcia, M.J.; Pascual, M.; Castro, B.; García-Blanco, A.; et al. Increased risk of MAFLD and Liver Fibrosis in Inflammatory Bowel Disease Independent of Classic Metabolic Risk Factors. *Clin. Gastroenterol. Hepatol.* **2023**, *21*, 406–414.e7. [CrossRef]
19. Maresca, R.; Mignini, I.; Varca, S.; Calvez, V.; Termite, F.; Esposto, G.; Laterza, L.; Scaldaferri, F.; Ainora, M.E.; Gasbarrini, A.; et al. Inflammatory Bowel Diseases and Non-Alcoholic Fatty Liver Disease: Piecing a Complex Puzzle Together. *Int. J. Mol. Sci.* **2024**, *25*, 3278. [CrossRef] [PubMed]
20. Mancina, R.M.; Spagnuolo, R.; Milano, M.; Brogneri, S.; Morrone, A.; Cosco, C.; Lazzaro, V.; Russo, C.; Ferro, Y.; Pingitore, P.; et al. PNPLA3 148M Carriers with Inflammatory Bowel Diseases Have Higher Susceptibility to Hepatic Steatosis and Higher Liver Enzymes. *Inflamm. Bowel Dis.* **2016**, *22*, 134–140. [CrossRef]
21. Chao, C.Y.; Battat, R.; Al Khoury, A.; Restellini, S.; Sebastiani, G.; Bessissow, T. Co-existence of non-alcoholic fatty liver disease and inflammatory bowel disease: A review article. *World J. Gastroenterol.* **2016**, *22*, 7727–7734. [CrossRef] [PubMed]
22. Principi, M.; Iannone, A.; Losurdo, G.; Mangia, M.; Shahini, E.; Albano, F.; Rizzi, S.F.; La Fortezza, R.F.; Lovero, R.; Contaldo, A.; et al. Nonalcoholic Fatty Liver Disease in Inflammatory Bowel Disease: Prevalence and Risk Factors. *Inflamm. Bowel Dis.* **2018**, *24*, 1589–1596. [CrossRef] [PubMed]
23. Navarro, P.; Gutiérrez-Ramírez, L.; Tejera-Muñoz, A.; Arias, Á.; Lucendo, A.J. Systematic Review and Meta-Analysis: Prevalence of Non-Alcoholic Fatty Liver Disease and Liver Fibrosis in Patients with Inflammatory Bowel Disease. *Nutrients* **2023**, *15*, 4507. [CrossRef] [PubMed]
24. Riazi, K.; Azhari, H.; Charette, J.H.; Underwood, F.E.; King, J.A.; Afshar, E.E.; Swain, M.G.; Congly, S.E.; Kaplan, G.G.; Shaheen, A.A. The prevalence and incidence of NAFLD worldwide: A systematic review and meta-analysis. *Lancet Gastroenterol. Hepatol.* **2022**, *7*, 851–861. [CrossRef]
25. Abenavoli, L.; Spagnuolo, R.; Scarlata, G.G.M.; Scarpellini, E.; Boccuto, L.; Luzza, F. Ultrasound Prevalence and Clinical Features of Nonalcoholic Fatty Liver Disease in Patients with Inflammatory Bowel Diseases: A Real-Life Cross-Sectional Study. *Medicina* **2023**, *59*, 1935. [CrossRef]
26. Abenavoli, L.; Scarlata, G.G.; Spagnuolo, R.; Luzza, F. Can dysmetabolic comorbidities carry hepatic fat accumulation in patients with inflammatory bowel diseases? *Minerva Gastroenterol* **2024**. *Epub ahead of print*. [CrossRef]
27. Song, S.J.; Lai, J.C.; Wong, G.L.; Wong, V.W.; Yip, T.C. Can we use old NAFLD data under the new MASLD definition? *J. Hepatol.* **2024**, *80*, e54–e56. [CrossRef]
28. Colaci, C.; Gambardella, M.L.; Scarlata, G.G.M.; Boccuto, L.; Colica, C.; Luzza, F.; Scarpellini, E.; Mendez-Sanchez, N.; Abenavoli, L. Dysmetabolic comorbidities and non-alcoholic fatty liver disease: A stairway to metabolic dysfunction-associated steatotic liver disease. *Hepatoma Res.* **2024**, *10*, 16. [CrossRef]
29. Maaser, C.; Sturm, A.; Vavricka, S.R.; Kucharzik, T.; Fiorino, G.; Annese, V.; Calabrese, E.; Baumgart, D.C.; Bettenworth, D.; Borralho Nunes, P.; et al. ECCO-ESGAR Guideline for Diagnostic Assessment in IBD Part 1: Initial diagnosis, monitoring of known IBD, detection of complications. *J. Crohns Colitis* **2019**, *13*, 144–164. [CrossRef]

30. European Association for the Study of the Liver (EASL); European Association for the Study of Diabetes (EASD); European Association for the Study of Obesity (EASO). EASL-EASD-EASO Clinical Practice Guidelines for the management of non-alcoholic fatty liver disease. *J. Hepatol.* **2016**, *64*, 1388–1402. [CrossRef]
31. Choi, J.H.; Sohn, W.; Cho, Y.K. The effect of moderate alcohol drinking in nonalcoholic fatty liver disease. *Clin. Mol. Hepatol.* **2020**, *26*, 662–669. [CrossRef] [PubMed]
32. Lu, S.; Yao, J.; Zhi, M. Therapeutic effect of ustekinumab on patients with extra-intestinal manifestations of Crohn's disease. *Expert. Rev. Gastroenterol. Hepatol.* **2023**, *17*, 379–384. [CrossRef] [PubMed]
33. Magen-Rimon, R.; Day, A.S.; Shaoul, R. Nutritional aspects of inflammatory bowel disease. *Expert. Rev. Gastroenterol. Hepatol.* **2023**, *17*, 731–740. [CrossRef] [PubMed]
34. De Caro, C.; Spagnuolo, R.; Quirino, A.; Mazza, E.; Carrabetta, F.; Maurotti, S.; Cosco, C.; Bennardo, F.; Roberti, R.; Russo, E.; et al. Gut Microbiota Profile Changes in Patients with Inflammatory Bowel Disease and Non-Alcoholic Fatty Liver Disease: A Metagenomic Study. *Int. J. Mol. Sci.* **2024**, *25*, 5453. [CrossRef]
35. Martínez-Domínguez, S.J.; García-Mateo, S.; Gargallo-Puyuelo, C.J.; Gallego-Llera, B.; Callau, P.; Mendi, C.; Arroyo-Villarino, M.T.; Simón-Marco, M.Á.; Ampuero, J.; Gomollón, F. Inflammatory Bowel Disease Is an Independent Risk Factor for Metabolic Dysfunction-Associated Steatotic Liver Disease in Lean Individuals. *Inflamm. Bowel Dis.* **2024**, *30*, 1274–1283. [CrossRef]
36. Kablawi, D.; Sasson, S.; Aljohani, F.; Palumbo, C.S.; Bitton, A.; Afif, W.L.; Lakatos, P.; Wild, G.; Bessissow, T.; Sebastiani, G. A259 Metabolic Dysfunction-Associated Steatotic Liver Disease Is Associated With Multi-Organ Comorbidities And Fibrosis Progression In Patients With Inflammatory Bowel Disease (IBD). *J. Can. Assoc. Gastroenterol.* **2024**, *7*, 208–209. [CrossRef]
37. Perazzo, H.; Pacheco, A.G.; Griep, R.H.; Gracindo, R.; Goulart, A.C.; da Fonseca, M.D.J.M. Changing from NAFLD through MAFLD to MASLD: Similar prevalence and risk factors in a large Brazilian cohort. *J. Hepatol.* **2024**, *80*, e72–e74. [CrossRef]
38. He, L.; Zheng, W.; Qiu, K.; Kong, W.; Zeng, T. Changing from NAFLD to MASLD: The new definition can more accurately identify individuals at higher risk for diabetes. *J. Hepatol.* **2024**, *80*, e85–e87. [CrossRef]
39. Yang, A.; Zhu, X.; Zhang, L.; Ding, Y. Transitioning from NAFLD to MAFLD and MASLD: Consistent prevalence and risk factors in a Chinese cohort. *J. Hepatol.* **2024**, *80*, e154–e155. [CrossRef]
40. De, A.; Bhagat, N.; Mehta, M.; Taneja, S.; Duseja, A. Metabolic dysfunction-associated steatotic liver disease (MASLD) definition is better than MAFLD criteria for lean patients with NAFLD. *J. Hepatol.* **2024**, *80*, e61–e62. [CrossRef]
41. Crocetti, E.; Bergamaschi, W.; Russo, A.G. Population-based incidence and prevalence of inflammatory bowel diseases in Milan (Northern Italy), and estimates for Italy. *Eur. J. Gastroenterol. Hepatol.* **2021**, *33*, e383–e389. [CrossRef] [PubMed]
42. Fornari, C.; Madotto, F.; Fiorino, G.; Ardizzone, S.; Bortoli, A.; Cestari, R.; Conti, S.; Cortellezzi, C.; Mantovani, L.G.; Massari, A.; et al. Inflammatory bowel diseases in Italy: Incidence trends and patients' characteristics. *Value Health* **2013**, *16*, 7. [CrossRef]
43. Lin, Y.; Feng, X.; Cao, X.; Miao, R.; Sun, Y.; Li, R.; Ye, J.; Zhong, B. Age patterns of nonalcoholic fatty liver disease incidence: Heterogeneous associations with metabolic changes. *Diabetol. Metab. Syndr.* **2022**, *14*, 181. [CrossRef] [PubMed]
44. Pavel, C.; Diculescu, M.; Constantinescu, G.; Plotogea, O.-M.; Sandru, V.; Meianu, C.; Dina, I.; Pop, I.; Butuc, A.; Mihaila, M.; et al. Surgery for Inflammatory Bowel Disease in the Era of Biologic Therapy: A Multicenter Experience from Romania. *Medicina* **2023**, *59*, 337. [CrossRef] [PubMed]
45. Ramírez-Mejía, M.M.; Jiménez-Gutiérrez, C.; Eslam, M.; George, J.; Méndez-Sánchez, N. Breaking new ground: MASLD vs. MAFLD-which holds the key for risk stratification? *Hepatol. Int.* **2024**, *18*, 168–178. [CrossRef]
46. Carrillo-Palau, M.; Hernández-Camba, A.; Hernández Alvarez-Buylla, N.; Ramos, L.; Alonso-Abreu, I.; Hernández-Pérez, A.; Vela, M.; Arranz, L.; Hernández-Guerra, M.; González-Gay, M.Á.; et al. Insulin Resistance Is Not Increased in Inflammatory Bowel Disease Patients but Is Related to Non-Alcoholic Fatty Liver Disease. *J. Clin. Med.* **2021**, *10*, 3062. [CrossRef]
47. Tomizawa, M.; Kawanabe, Y.; Shinozaki, F.; Sato, S.; Motoyoshi, Y.; Sugiyama, T.; Yamamoto, S.; Sueishi, M. Triglyceride is strongly associated with nonalcoholic fatty liver disease among markers of hyperlipidemia and diabetes. *Biomed. Rep.* **2014**, *2*, 633–636. [CrossRef]
48. Sung, K.C.; Kim, B.S.; Cho, Y.K.; Park, D.I.; Woo, S.; Kim, S.; Wild, S.H.; Byrne, C.D. Predicting incident fatty liver using simple cardio-metabolic risk factors at baseline. *BMC Gastroenterol.* **2012**, *12*, 84. [CrossRef]
49. Semmler, G.; Wernly, B.; Datz, C. What's in a name? New nomenclature for steatotic liver disease—To be or not to be? *J. Hepatol.* **2024**, *80*, e56–e58. [CrossRef]
50. Boustany, A.; Rahhal, R.; Mitri, J.; Onwuzo, S.; Abou Zeid, H.K.; Baffy, G.; Martel, M.; Barkun, A.N.; Asaad, I. The impact of nonalcoholic fatty liver disease on inflammatory bowel disease-related hospitalization outcomes: A systematic review. *Eur. J. Gastroenterol. Hepatol.* **2023**, *35*, 1067–1074. [CrossRef]

life

Article

The Hepatoprotective Effects of *Camellia sinensis* on Cisplatin-Induced Acute Liver Injury

Adnan Yilmaz [1,*], Fatih Dizman [2], Kerimali Akyildiz [1], Sibel Mataraci Karakas [1], Tolga Mercantepe [3], Huseyin Avni Uydu [4], Levent Tumkaya [5] and Koksal Ozturk [2]

1 Department of Biochemistry, Faculty of Medicine, Recep Tayyip Erdogan University, 53010 Rize, Turkey; kerimali.akyildiz@erdogan.edu.tr (K.A.); sibel.karakas@erdogan.edu.tr (S.M.K.)
2 Recep Tayyip Erdogan University Research and Training Hospital, 53010 Rize, Turkey; fatihdizman0653@gmail.com (F.D.); koksal6161.5@gmail.com (K.O.)
3 Department of Histology and Embryology, Faculty of Medicine, Recep Tayyip Erdogan University, 53010 Rize, Turkey; tolga.mercantepe@erdogan.edu.tr
4 Department of Biochemistry, Faculty of Medicine, Samsun University, 55000 Samsun, Turkey; huseyinavni.uydu@samsun.edu.tr
5 Department of Histology and Embryology, Faculty of Medicine, Ondokuz Mayis University, 55000 Samsun, Turkey; levent.tumkaya@erdogan.edu.tr
* Correspondence: adnan.yilmaz@erdogan.edu.tr; Tel.: +90-532-708-87-24

Abstract: Acute liver injury is an increasing global health problem. It is a widespread side effect of cisplatin treatment in the clinic and can lead to liver failure if not treated promptly. Previous studies have revealed that green tea can protect some organs from treatments. However, the potential of white tea to prevent the negative effects of acute liver injury has not been addressed so far. The purpose of this study was to investigate the reduction in cisplatin-induced liver injury in rats receiving white tea. Female Sprague Dawley rats with similar weight were selected in this study. Twenty-four rats were divided into three groups of eight animals each and ad libitum nutrition was provided. The control and cisplatin groups were given tap water only, while the white tea + cisplatin group received white tea at a 0.5% weight/volume concentration for four weeks. At the end of the fourth week, the white tea + cisplatin group and the cisplatin group received a single dose of cisplatin (7 mg/kg) via the intraperitoneal route. Five days after that procedure, the rats were anesthetized. Liver tissues and blood samples were collected, which were used for biochemical and histopathological analyses. According to biochemical results, liver tissue MDA and GSH, serum ALT, and AST levels significantly increased in the cisplatin group compared to the control group. Compared with the cisplatin group, although MDA, AST, ALT, and GSH levels were lower in the white tea + cisplatin group, only GSH levels were statistically different. The examination of histopathological and immunohistochemical findings revealed apoptotic cells, vascular congestion, and sinusoidal dilatation in the cisplatin group compared to the control group. This adverse event decreased in the white tea + cisplatin group compared to the cisplatin group. In conclusion, white tea exhibits an ameliorating effect on cisplatin-induced liver injury.

Keywords: cisplatin; white tea; liver; oxidative stress; rat

1. Introduction

The *Globocan* 2022 report published by the International Agency for Research on Cancer (IARC) stated that 19.96 million new cases had been diagnosed in that year and that cancer was responsible for 9.74 million deaths [1]. There are more than 100 forms of cancer treatment, but chemotherapy, radiotherapy, and surgery, either alone or in combination when necessary, are some of the most frequently employed therapeutic methods. Chemotherapy aims to kill tumor cells through the oral and/or intravenous administration of cytotoxic or antineoplastic chemotherapeutic chemical agents [2]. However, antineoplastic drugs also damage healthy cells in addition to the tumor cells they destroy, either through their direct effect on DNA or by halting cell division [3,4].

Cisplatin (*cis-diamminedichloroplatinum (II)*), an anti-tumoral drug, is an organic platinum derivative and the best known and most frequently used chemotherapeutic agent in the treatment of cancer [5,6]. It is employed in the treatment of several cancer types, including those of the bladder, head, neck, lung, ovary, and testis [7–9]. However, hepatotoxicity occurs after nephrotoxicity in a dose-dependent manner following cisplatin use [10].

Cisplatin results in the production of hydroxyl, hydrogen peroxide, and superoxide radicals in tissues. These radicals react with various cellular components such as DNA, protein, and membrane lipids [11]. Moreover, cisplatin exposure induces oxidative stress; increases protein oxidation, malondialdehyde (MDA), and 8-hydroxy-2′-deoxyguanosine (8-OHdG) levels; and decreases GSH content, SOD, GPx, CAT, glutathione-S-transferase (GST), and glutathione reductase (GR) levels [12]. MDA levels are currently measured as a biomarker of lipid peroxidation in living tissues [13]. In addition, GSH, which contains the greatest total thiol group, is the most prominent among the antioxidant enzymes that prevent oxidative stress [14].

Tea is produced from the leaves of the *Camellia sinensis* plant, which belongs to the Theaceae family, and is one of the most popular and consumed beverages worldwide [15]. Depending on the processing technique, tea is most commonly classified as green, black, oolong, or white tea (WT) [16]. WT differs from other teas in that it uses only young leaves of the *C. sinensis* plant. WT has important benefits due to its natural antioxidants with biological effects on human health and its high content of catechins and derivatives, as well as other tea components [17].

With its rich catechin and flavonoid content, particularly epigallocatechin gallate (EGCG), *C. sinensis* has been described as one of a thousand promising phytotherapeutic agents [14]. EGCG is the most abundant, with strong antioxidant activity in white tea, and is responsible for the most cancer chemoprevention [18]. Moreover, recent studies on *C. sinensis* have reported that EGCG, EG, and flavonoids in particular prevent lipid accumulation in liver and liver cancer [19,20].

In the literature, no research has been found on the effects of WT on liver damage, which is richer than other teas in terms of contents and produced with less processing [20–24]. The purpose of the present study was to investigate the level of liver damage caused by cisplatin used in chemotherapy and to determine whether chronic white tea consumption can reduce or eliminate that injury. Another aim of this study was to describe different perspectives aimed at treatment or prevention for scientists and physicians working in this field through the results obtained.

2. Materials and Methods

Our study is an experimental animal study and is written according to the ARRIVE 3.0 guideline.

2.1. Chemicals

Cisplatin was obtained from Faulding Pharmaceuticals PLC (Lemington Spa, Warwickshire, UK), and the other chemicals employed in the study were procured from Sigma (Sigma Chemicals Co., St. Louis, MO, USA).

2.2. The Experimental Animals and Study Groups

For the animal selection in our study, Sprague Dawley rats were selected depending on the type of research, applicability, and possibilities. The sample size of our study was calculated in accordance with the studies of Arifin et al. Twenty-four female Sprague Dawley rats (age: 12–14 weeks; weight: 250–300 g) were obtained from the Recep Tayyip Erdoğan University Experimental Animals Research Center, Turkey. Approval for the study was granted by the Recep Tayyip Erdoğan University Laboratory Animals Local Ethical

Committee (no. 2019/12). The rats were housed in transparent polyethylene cages, each containing eight animals, and were allowed ad libitum access to chow and tap water. The rats were placed into artificially controlled rooms at 23 ± 2 °C in a 12 h light/dark cycle and 55 ± 5% humidity one week before the commencement of the study for adaptation. Following the adaptation stage, the rats were divided into three groups, with eight subjects in each group: control, cisplatin (CP), and cisplatin + white tea (CP + WT).

The control and CP groups were given only tap water, while the CP + WT group received 0.5% (*w*/*v*) white tea added to tap water daily for four weeks. Following this, both the CP + WT and CP groups received a single intraperitoneal (i.p.) dose of 7 mg/kg cisplatin. After that procedure, the rats were anesthetized with ketamine-xylazine, and blood and liver tissue samples were collected.

2.3. The Procurement and Preparation of White Tea

The white tea was obtained from a producer (General Directorate of Tea Enterprises, Rize, Turkey). Appropriate amounts of tea leaves were weighed. The tea was added to boiled water (0.5 g/100 mL) and steeped for 3 min [5]. The content of white tea used in the study was determined by high performance liquid chromatography (HPLC) (Table 1).

Table 1. The catechin and mineral HPLC analysis results of the white tea used in the study.

Component	Amount in Dry Weight
Gallic acid	0.13 (%)
Caffeine	5.62 (%)
EGC (epigallocatechin)	2.54 (%)
EC (epicatechin)	0.91 (%)
EGCG (epigallocatechin gallate)	10.39 (%)
ECG (epicatechin gallate)	3.58 (%)
Copper	0.08 (ppm)
Iron	0.12 (ppm)
Zinc	0.54 (ppm)
Sodium	2.87 (ppm)
Potassium	283.00 (ppm)
Calcium	6.12 (ppm)
Magnesium	26.88 (ppm)
Aluminum	0.98 (ppm)

2.4. Blood and Liver Tissues Collection

Rat blood samples were collected from the left ventricle under general anesthesia after 12 h of fasting. The samples were placed into tubes with no anticoagulant and left at room temperature for a few minutes, after which they were centrifuged at +4 °C for 5 min at 3500 rpm and stored at −80 °C until the alanine amino transaminase (ALT) and aspartate amino transaminase (AST) analyses.

The liver tissues were washed three times in cold (4 °C) 0.9% sodium chloride. A pH 7.4 homogenization solution was prepared, consisting of 20 mM 1 L sodium phosphate + 140 mM potassium chloride [18]. Homogenization solution was added to 0.1 g of liver tissue in the amount of 1 mL. Following homogenization at 30 Hertz for 3 min, the homogenates were centrifuged at 800 g for 10 min at 4 °C, and the resulting supernatants were employed in GSH and MDA analyses.

Liver tissues set aside for histopathological examination were placed into 10% formaldehyde. All tissues were stored at −80 °C until analysis. Caspase-3 activities in liver tissues were determined immunohistochemically.

2.5. Biochemical Analysis

2.5.1. Determination of Serum ALT and AST Levels

Serum AST and ALT levels were measured on an Abbott Architect®c16000 device (Abbott Diagnostics, Abbott Park, IL, USA).

2.5.2. Determination of Tissue MDA and GSH Levels

The levels of MDA were measured according to the method of Draper and Hadley. MDA, the end product of lipid peroxidation, was measured with the results being expressed as nmol/g tissue [21].

The GSH levels were determined by the Ellman method. In the measurement of GSH levels, the free sulfhydryl groups in the homogenate were determined by a spectrophotometric reading of the color formed, and the data were expressed as nmol/g tissue [22].

2.6. Histopathological Analysis

The rat liver tissues were quickly trimmed and fixed for 36 h in a 10% formalin solution (Sigma Aldrich, St. Louis, MO, USA). Following routine procedures, the tissues were passed through an increasing alcohol series and rendered transparent before being embedded in paraffin blocks (Merck, Darmstadt, Germany). Sections 4–5 µm in thickness were then obtained from these blocks using a microtome (Leica, RM2125RT, Nußloch, Germany). These were then stained with hematoxylin (Harris hematoxylin, Merck, Germany) and eosin (H&E) (Eosin G, Merck, Germany) and Goldner's Masson trichrome (Merck, Darmstadt, Germany). After staining, the tissues were examined under a light microscope (Olympus BX51, Olympus Corporation, Tokyo, Japan) and photographed with an Olympus DP71 camera (Olympus Corporation, Tokyo, Japan).

2.7. Immunohistochemical Analysis (IHC)

The avidin–biotin peroxidase complex method was employed to determine the immunoreactivity of the caspase-3 primary antibody used to assay apoptotic hepatocytes. Sections 2–3 µm in thickness taken from the paraffin blocks were placed onto positively charged slides and subjected to deparaffinization. They were next incubated with 3% H_2O_2 solution to block endogenous peroxidase activity. Following a 20 min application of a blocking solution to prevent background staining, they were incubated with primary antibodies (Caspase-3, Rabbit polyclonal, Abcam, UK) for 60 min. Following the application of the primary antibody, the tissues were incubated with a secondary antibody (Goat Anti-Rabbit IgG H&L (HRP) ab205718, Abcam, UK). Diaminobenzidine chromogen (DAB Chromogen, Abcam, UK) was then dropped onto the tissues, and an image signal was obtained under a light microscope. Counterstaining was applied with Harris hematoxylin (Merck, Darmstadt, Germany), and the tissues were finally covered with an appropriate closing solution.

2.8. Statistical Analysis

For data analysis, the Statistical Package for Social Sciences (SPSS; version 18 for Windows, IBM, Chicago, Illinois, USA) was used. The data obtained as a result of the analyses were evaluated to determine whether they conformed to a normal distribution by using the Shapiro–Wilk test, a QQ plot, kurtosis and skewness values, and Levene's test. The parametric data were presented as mean ± SD. Differences among groups were analyzed by one-way analysis of variance (ANOVA), and post hoc LSD tests were performed. A p value of less than 0.05 was regarded to be statistically significant.

The data obtained from the immunohistochemical analyses were calculated as a median and standard deviation (maximum, minimum) for non-parametric data using SPSS 18.00 software, and intergroup comparisons were performed using the Kruskal–Wallis and Tamhane T2 tests. p values < 0.05 were regarded as significant.

3. Results

3.1. Biochemical Results

Hepatic tissue GSH and MDA levels showed a significant difference in the cisplatin group compared to the control group. Moreover, in the cisplatin + white tea group, MDA and GSH levels decreased compared to the cisplatin group (Table 2).

Table 2. MDA and GSH levels in rat liver tissues.

	MDA (nmol/g Tissue)	GSH (μmol/g Tissue)
Control	1.17 ± 0.11	14.90 ± 2.04
Cisplatin	1.56 ± 0.26 ^{a,*}	16.74 ± 2.00 ^{a,**}
Cisplatin + White Tea	1.39 ± 0.39	15.08 ± 1.38 ^{b,*}

*: $p < 0.05$; **: $p < 0.01$; ^{a}: Significantly different compared with the control group; ^{b}: Significantly different compared with the CP group.

Serum ALT and AST levels significantly decreased in the cisplatin group compared to the control group and decreased in the cisplatin + white tea group compared to the cisplatin group (Table 3).

Table 3. Serum AST and ALT levels.

	AST (U/L)	ALT (U/L)
Control	71.13 ± 4.49	35.25 ± 4.89
Cisplatin	97.88 ± 7.20 ^{a,**}	43.75 ± 7.61 ^{a,*}
Cisplatin + White Tea	77.00 ± 6.21	40.38 ± 3.89

*: $p < 0.05$; **: $p < 0.01$; ^{a}: Significantly different compared with the control group.

3.2. Histopathological and Immunohistochemical Results

The examination of the sections stained with hematoxylin–eosin (H&E) under light microscopy revealed a normal structure in the Remark cordons and sinusoids consisting of hepatocytes around the central vein, where the liver tissue exhibited a normal structure (Figure 1A–C).

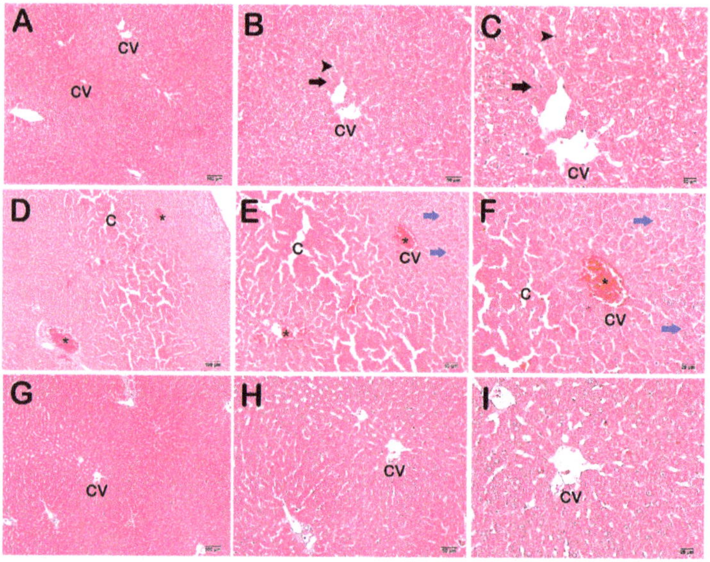

Figure 1. Light microscopic images of liver tissue sections from the control group stained with H&E. (**A**) (×10), (**B**) (×20), (**C**) (×40) Control Group: Normally structured cells are observed in the hepatocytes (arrow) and sinusoids (arrowhead), with a normal central vein (CV) in the healthy liver tissue. (**D**) (×10), (**E**) (×20), (**F**) (×40) CP Group: Diffuse vascular congestion (asterisk) and sinusoidal dilatations (c) observed in the liver parenchyma. In addition, diffuse vacuolization in the necrotic hepatocytes (blue arrow) observed in the hepatic cords. (**G**) (×10), (**H**) (×20), (**I**) (×40) CP + WT Group: A decrease in diffuse vascular congestion and sinusoidal dilatations is observed.

Widespread vascular congestion, sinusoidal dilatations, and numerous necrotic hepatocytes were observed in the section from the CP group (Figure 1A–C).

A decrease in vascular congestion and sinusoidal dilatations was observed in the CP + WT group (Figure 1A–C)

Microscopic images of the control group sections stained with Goldner's Masson trichrome exhibited a normal structure in the Remark cordons and sinusoids consisting of normal hepatocytes (Figure 2A,B). Diffuse vascular congestion, sinusoidal dilatations, and numerous necrotic hepatocytes were observed in sections from the CP group (Figure 2A,B). A decrease in vascular congestion and sinusoidal dilatations was observed in the CP + WT group (Figure 2A,B).

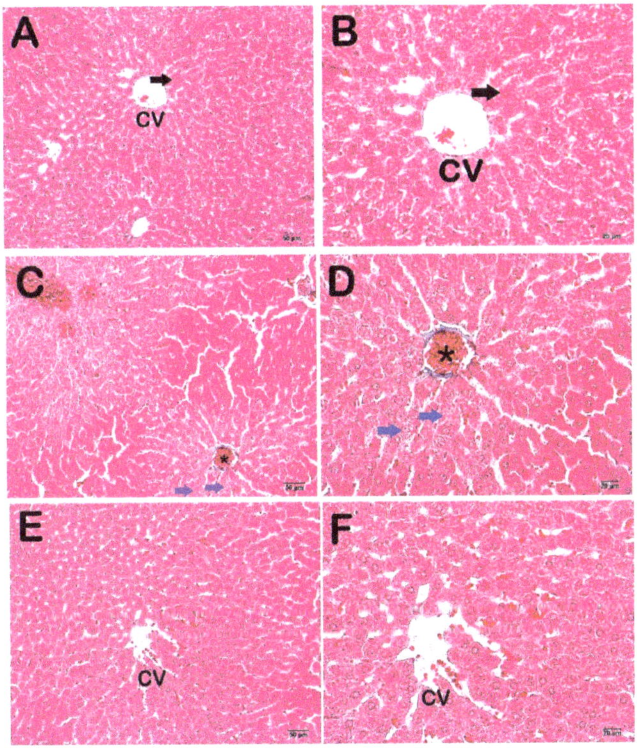

Figure 2. Light microscopic images of liver tissue sections from the control group stained with Masson's trichrome. (**A**) (×20), (**B**) (×40) Control Group: In the sections of the control group, normal structure hepatocytes (arrow) and central vein (CV) are observed in the hepatic cords. (**C**) (×20), (**D**) (×40) CP Group: The light microscopic examination of sections from the CP group shows a decrease in necrotic hepatocytes (blue arrow) and diffuse vascular congestion (asterisk). (**E**) (×20), (**F**) (×40) CP + WT Group: Light microscopic examination of sections from the CP + WT group shows a decrease in diffuse vascular congestion and sinusoidal dilatations.

Light microscopic images of liver tissues stained with the caspase-3 primary antibody from the control group exhibited hepatocytes with a normal appearance (Figure 3A,B), while apoptotic hepatocytes were observed in the CP group (blue arrow) (Figure 3A,B), and the numbers of apoptotic hepatocytes decreased in the CP + WT group (Figure 3A,B).

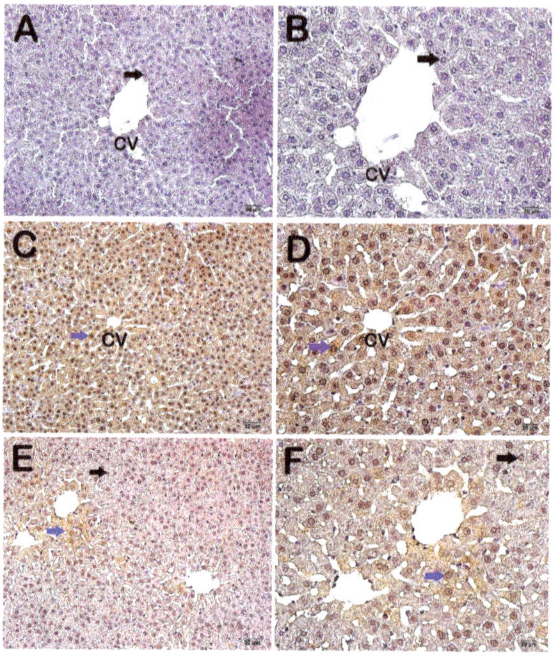

Figure 3. The light microscopic images of the liver tissue sections from the control group stained with the caspase-3 primary antibody. (**A**) (×20), (**B**) (×40) Control Group: It is observed that the normal hepatocytes (black arrow) are immunonegative in terms of Caspase primary antibody (caspase-3 positivity score: 0.00 ± 0.35). (**C**) (×20), (**D**) (×40) CP Group: It is observed that the number of apoptotic hepatocytes (blue arrow) showing intense Caspase-3 immunopositivity is increased (caspase-3 positivity score: 3.00 ± 0.46). (**E**) (×20), (**F**) (×40) CP + WT: It is observed that the number of hepatocytes showing intense Caspase-3 immunopositivity is decreased (caspase-3 positivity score: 1.00 ± 0.46).

Caspase-3 positivity evaluation is made in Tables 4 and 5. The caspase-3 positivity score of 0.00 ± 0.35 in the control group increased to 3.00 ± 0.46 following cisplatin administration ($p = 0.00$; Table 5). The caspase-3 positivity score of 3.00 ± 0.46 in the CP group decreased to 1.00 ± 0.46 in the CP + WT group ($p = 0.00$; Table 5).

Table 4. Caspase-3 positivity scoring table.

Score	Finding
0	Less than 5% caspase-3 positive hepatocytes
1	Less than 25% caspase-3 positive hepatocytes
2	Less than 50% caspase-3 positive hepatocytes
3	More than 50% caspase-3 positive hepatocytes

Table 5. Semi-quantitative analysis results (median ± standard deviation).

Group	Caspase-3 Positivity Score
Control	0.00 ± 0.35
Cisplatin	3.00 ± 0.46 [a]
Cisplatin+ White tea	1.00 ± 0.46 [b]

[a]: $p = 0.00$, compared with the control group; [b]: $p = 0.00$, compared with the CP group. Kruskal–Wallis, Tamhane's T2 test.

4. Discussion

Although chemotherapy is a very effective method in the treatment of cancer and one that can be applied irrespective of the type of cancer or the stage of the disease [23], the side effects of the chemotherapeutic agents and resistant cells represent a limiting factor in the administration of anti-cancer chemotherapy [24]. Cisplatin, one of the most frequently employed chemotherapeutic agents, may result in side effects including nephrotoxicity, hepatotoxicity, ototoxicity, neurotoxicity, myelosuppression, nausea, and vomiting [25]. The kidneys function together with the hepatobiliary system in the expulsion of organic platinum cisplatin-derived metabolites from the body, and accumulation mostly occurs in the kidneys [26].

Cisplatin nephrotoxicity is one of the most common side effects at the doses used in clinical practice. Hepatotoxicity is less common, although it can also occur in the case of exposure to high-dose cisplatin. Liver toxicity derives from the liver representing the main site of the metabolism of numerous drugs and chemical substances. After the kidneys, most cisplatin accumulation occurs in the liver, and this gives rise to hepatotoxicity with high-dose use. Hepatic necrosis may develop as a result, and apoptotic lesions can be seen in the liver. Studies concerning cisplatin hepatotoxicity are limited, and the mechanism has not yet been fully explained [27–29].

Drugs are given concurrently with cisplatin for the purpose of reducing or eliminating cisplatin toxicity [30]. Several studies have also investigated the use of food supplements in addition to drugs for reducing this toxicity [31–33].

Various parameters are used to evaluate the severity of oxidative stress. The measurement of MDA, a marker of lipid peroxidation resulting from the effects of oxidative damage on cell membrane lipids, and GSH, a highly important non-enzymatic antioxidant found in antioxidant systems that protect cells against the adverse effects of oxidative damage, yields some information and predictions concerning liver tissue damage [34,35].

Studies have shown that cisplatin and toxic substances with effects similar to those of cisplatin increase tissue MDA levels, although tissue GSH levels and antioxidant activities are still controversial [29,31,33,36]. Some studies have reported that cisplatin reduces GSH levels and antioxidant enzyme activities [29,37–39], while others have reported no change or even an increase [33,40–42].

Almost all studies of the oxidative stress caused by cisplatin have reported that it raises tissue MDA levels, and experimental research such as that by Karahan et al. [33], Tarladaçalışır et al. [28], and Greggi et al. [40] has reported positive findings with some food supplements to eliminate this negativity caused by cisplatin. In the present study, liver tissue MDA levels, which increased in parallel with the use of cisplatin, and liver tissue GSH levels, which rose with the stimulation of antioxidant systems in response to this toxic effect, decreased with the therapeutic use of white tea. The increase in GSH levels in the groups receiving cisplatin and the partial decrease in the white tea group suggest that the antioxidant systems are stimulated to eliminate the adverse situation in the cells resulting from the use of cisplatin.

ALT is highly expressed in hepatocytes, and thus abnormal levels of ALT tend to be more specific to liver damage. Moreover, AST is found in several tissues, such as liver, kidney, and lung. Elevated levels of ALT and AST in the bloodstream are generally considered to be a sign of liver tissue damage [43,44].

In our study, rat serum AST and ALT levels increased in the CP group compared to the control group, but decreased in the CP + WT group. The AST and ALT levels were parallel in the rat liver tissue and serum. This supports the idea of the liver damage being caused by cisplatin and the improvement in this damage resulting from white tea. In their rat study on cisplatin, Martins et al. administered a single 10 mg/kg dose of cisplatin and sacrificed the animals after 72 h. The rats' serum AST and ALT values increased significantly in the cisplatin group compared to the control group. We ascribe the difference between our hepatotoxicity findings and those of Martin et al. to the differences in the cisplatin doses applied and the life spans of the experimental subjects (acute and chronic) [29].

This also shows the vital importance of effective dose limitation in individuals due to receive cisplatin.

Among the types of tea, EGCG is most commonly found in white tea. It is considered the most bioactive component of tea and is thought to play an important role in preventing liver damage and cancer. There are no studies on white tea and the effects of white tea on liver damage in the literature. Unlike white tea, the literature has a few studies using other teas. In a study with pu-erh tea, there was a significant decrease in the levels of ALT, AST, and MDA; the opposite was true for GSH in the pu-erh tea group contrary to the cisplatin groups [45]. In another study, Amidi et al. investigated the effects of green tea on cisplatin-induced experimental liver function. According to the results, there was a significant difference in ALT and AST levels in the green tea group compared to the cisplatin group [46]. In other studies, analyses of the oxidative stress parameters (MDA, GSH, etc.) and the liver enzyme levels showed more significant differences in the WT groups. The reason for this is that WT has richer content than other teas [47–50].

The histopathological findings of the present study revealed a decrease in vascular congestion and sinusoidal dilatations in the liver tissue sections from the CP + WT group compared to the cisplatin group, while the immunohistochemical findings revealed a decrease in apoptotic hepatocytes compared to the CP group. When the biochemical results are evaluated together with the histological findings, the decreases in the biochemical analysis findings in the CP + WT group compared to the CP group strengthen the idea that the use of white tea supports antioxidant defense systems.

In their histological examination of the effects of vitamins E and C on cisplatin hepatotoxicity, Kanter et al. [42] reported that antioxidants with differing characteristics assisted with reducing cisplatin-derived hepatotoxicity. Our histological findings also revealed a decrease in cisplatin-induced apoptotic hepatocytes in the rats that were administered white tea extracts, similar to the therapeutic findings observed with vitamin E and C antioxidants. This also reinforces the idea that the antioxidant properties of white tea can be as valuable as enzymatic or non-enzymatic antioxidants.

Secondary organ damage due to chemotherapy has always attracted increasing interest in the scientific community. Plant extracts and bioactive dietary components play an important role in protecting human health and well-being. In addition, they have the potential to regulate risk factors and manage symptoms in many pathologies, such as various organ toxicities, obesity, respiratory diseases, and metabolic disorders. In this context, white tea is a powerful antioxidant due to its high catechin and flavonoid content, and it might contribute to reducing the number of patients applying to clinics due to the side effects of chemotherapy with its effect of reducing secondary organ toxicity resulting from chemotherapy.

However, despite all these findings, there are several limitations to this research. First of all, this is an animal model study. Although it represents a pilot study concerning the hepatoprotective effect of *C. sinensis*, our study did not include biochemical, histopathological, and immunohistochemical analyses. Oxidative stress was assessed by measuring MDA and GSH levels in biochemical analyses. The evaluation of oxidative stress should be supported by studies addressing the analyses of other oxidant/antioxidant enzymes and/or proteins. Again, apoptosis was assessed using immunohistochemical analyses in our study. Apoptosis should be supported by studies addressing the Tunel method, as well as intracellular calcium and mitochondrial calcium levels. It now needs to be supported by further research considering oxidant/antioxidant molecules and enzymes to elucidate the cellular damage caused by cisplatin.

5. Conclusions

In conclusion, we think that drug and nutrition supplements intended to minimize oxidative injury and eliminate cisplatin-derived side effects also need to be very carefully selected. Although we think that white tea has a positive effect on cisplatin-induced liver damage, we also believe that further studies are now needed for a fuller understanding of its antioxidant properties.

Author Contributions: A.Y., F.D., and K.A.: Conceptualization, Methodology, Formal Analysis, Investigation, Writing—Original Draft. F.D., A.Y., S.M.K., T.M., H.A.U., L.T., and K.O.: Conceptualization, Methodology, Investigation, Data Curation, Writing—Original Draft. F.D., A.Y., S.M.K., and T.M.: Methodology, Software, Investigation, Writing—Original Draft, Writing—Review and Editing. All authors have read and agreed to the published version of the manuscript.

Funding: This study has been supported by the Recep Tayyip Erdoğan University Development Foundation (Grant number: 02024007031027).

Institutional Review Board Statement: The study was conducted in accordance with the Declaration of Helsinki, and approved by the Laboratory Animals Institutional Ethical Committee of Recep Tayyip Erdoğan University (Protocol Code: 12/2019, Date of approval: 27 February 2019).

Informed Consent Statement: Not applicable.

Data Availability Statement: All data generated for the manuscript are included in the study and are available upon request.

Conflicts of Interest: The authors declare that there are no conflicts of interest.

References

1. Bray, F.; Laversanne, M.; Sung, H.; Ferlay, J.; Siegel, R.L.; Soerjomataram, I.; Jemal, A. Global cancer statistics 2022: GLOBOCAN estimates of incidence and mortality worldwide for 36 cancers in 185 countries. *CA Cancer J. Clin.* **2024**, *74*, 229–263. [CrossRef] [PubMed]
2. Baykara, O. Current Modalities in Treatment of Cancer. *Balikesir Health Sci. J.* **2016**, *5*, 154–165. [CrossRef]
3. Aynacıoglu, A.; Ozkur, M.; Nacak, M.; Saracaloglu, A. *Farmabul*, 1st ed.; Çukurova Nobel Tip Kitabevi: Adana, Turkey, 2014.
4. Huang, X.; Gao, C.; Cai, W.; Tao, Y.; Zhong, X.; Liu, H.; Hong, X.; Ding, X.; Lu, H.; Lai, W.; et al. Effect of occupational exposure to antineoplastic drugs on DNA damage in nurses: A cross-sectional study. *Occup. Environ. Med.* **2022**, *79*, 253–258. [CrossRef]
5. Saral, S.; Dokumacioglu, E.; Mercantepe, T.; Atak, M.; Cinar, S.; Saral, O.; Yildiz, L.; Iskender, H.; Tumkaya, L. The effect of white tea on serum TNF-α/NF-κB and immunohistochemical parameters in cisplatin-related renal dysfunction in female rats. *Biomed. Pharmacother.* **2019**, *112*, 108604. [CrossRef] [PubMed]
6. Lebaschi, S.; Hekmati, M.; Veisi, H. Green synthesis of palladium nanoparticles mediated by black tea leaves (*Camellia sinensis*) extract: Catalytic activity in the reduction of 4-nitrophenol and Suzuki-Miyaura coupling reaction under ligand-free conditions. *J. Colloid. Interface Sci.* **2017**, *485*, 223–231. [CrossRef] [PubMed]
7. Tang, C.; Livingston, M.J.; Safirstein, R.; Dong, Z. Cisplatin nephrotoxicity: New insights and therapeutic implications. *Nat. Rev. Nephrol.* **2023**, *19*, 53–72. [CrossRef]
8. Manohar, S.; Leung, N. Cisplatin nephrotoxicity: A review of the literature. *J. Nephrol.* **2018**, *31*, 15–25. [CrossRef]
9. Mercantepe, T.; Unal, D.; Tümkaya, L.; Yazici, Z.A. Protective effects of amifostine, curcumin and caffeic acid phenethyl ester against cisplatin-induced testis tissue damage in rats. *Exp. Ther. Med.* **2018**, *15*, 3404–3412. [CrossRef]
10. Mercantepe, F.; Mercantepe, T.; Topcu, A.; Yılmaz, A.; Tumkaya, L. Protective effects of amifostine, curcumin, and melatonin against cisplatin-induced acute kidney injury. *Naunyn Schmiedebergs Arch. Pharmacol.* **2018**, *391*, 915–931. [CrossRef]
11. Alibakhshi, T.; Khodayar, M.J.; Khorsandi, L.; Rashno, M.; Zeidooni, L. Protective effects of zingerone on oxidative stress and inflammation in cisplatin-induced rat nephrotoxicity. *Biomed. Pharmacother.* **2018**, *105*, 225–232. [CrossRef]
12. Liu, H.M.; Cheng, M.Y.; Xun, M.H.; Zhao, Z.W.; Zhang, Y.; Tang, W.; Cheng, J.; Ni, J.; Wang, W. Possible Mechanisms of Oxidative Stress-Induced Skin Cellular Senescence, Inflammation, and Cancer and the Therapeutic Potential of Plant Polyphenols. *Int. J. Mol. Sci.* **2023**, *24*, 3755. [CrossRef] [PubMed]
13. Tsikas, D. Assessment of lipid peroxidation by measuring malondialdehyde (MDA) and relatives in biological samples: Analytical and biological challenges. *Anal. Biochem.* **2017**, *524*, 13–30. [CrossRef] [PubMed]
14. Taghizadeh, F.; Hosseinimehr, S.J.; Zargari, M.; Karimpour Malekshah, A.; Mirzaei, M.; Talebpour Amiri, F. Alleviation of cisplatin-induced hepatotoxicity by gliclazide: Involvement of oxidative stress and caspase-3 activity. *Pharmacol. Res. Perspect.* **2021**, *9*, e00788. [CrossRef] [PubMed]
15. Akbulut, A.; Kar, S.M.; Ozcan, A. Comparison of black, green and white teas in terms of quality criteria, mineral contents, antioxidant and antimicrobial activity. *Acad. J. Agric.* **2020**, *9*, 279–288.
16. Wong, M.; Sirisena, S.; Ng, K. Phytochemical profile of differently processed tea: A review. *J. Food Sci.* **2022**, *5*, 1925–1942. [CrossRef]
17. Gabr, G.A.; Hassan, H.M.M.; Seshadri, V.D.; Hassan, N.M.M. Comparative study of phenolic profile, antioxidant and antimicrobial activities of aqueous extract of white and green tea. *Z. Naturforsch. C J. Biosci.* **2022**, *77*, 483–492. [CrossRef]

18. Haghparasti, Z.; Mahdavi Shahri, M. Green synthesis of water-soluble nontoxic inorganic polymer nanocomposites containing silver nanoparticles using white tea extract and assessment of their in vitro antioxidant and cytotoxicity activities. *Mater. Sci. Eng. C Mater. Biol. Appl.* **2018**, *87*, 139–148. [CrossRef]
19. Liu, Q.; Ding, X.; Xu, X.; Lai, H.; Zeng, Z.; Shan, T.; Zhang, T.; Chen, M.; Huang, Y.; Huang, Z.; et al. Tumor-targeted hyaluronic acid-based oxidative stress nanoamplifier with ROS generation and GSH depletion for antitumor therapy. *Int. J. Biol. Macromol.* **2022**, *207*, 771–783. [CrossRef]
20. Cravotto, G.; Boffa, L.; Genzini, L.; Garella, D. Phytotherapeutics: An evaluation of the potential of 1000 plants. *J. Clin. Pharm. Ther.* **2010**, *35*, 11–48. [CrossRef]
21. Draper, H.H.; Hadley, M. Malondialdehyde determination as index of lipid Peroxidation. *Methods Enzymol.* **1990**, *186*, 421–431.
22. Ellman, G.L. Tissue sulfhydryl groups. *Arch. Biochem. Biophys.* **1959**, *82*, 70–77. [CrossRef] [PubMed]
23. Matsuyama, R.; Reddy, S.; Smith, T.J. Why do patients choose chemotherapy near the end of life? A review of the perspective of those facing death from cancer. *J. Clin. Oncol.* **2006**, *24*, 3490–3496. [CrossRef] [PubMed]
24. Bartelink, H.; Schellens, J.H.M.; Verheij, M. The combined use of radiotherapy and chemotherapy in the treatment of solid tumours. *Eur. J. Cancer* **2002**, *38*, 216–222. [CrossRef]
25. Arifin, W.N.; Zahiruddin, W.M. Sample Size Calculation in Animal Studies Using Resource Equation Approach. *Malays. J. Med. Sci.* **2017**, *24*, 101–105.
26. Motwani, S.S.; Kaur, S.S.; Kitchlu, A. Cisplatin Nephrotoxicity: Novel Insights into Mechanisms and Preventative Strategies. *Semin. Nephrol.* **2022**, *42*, 151341. [CrossRef]
27. Pezeshki, Z.; Khosravi, A.; Nekuei, M.; Khoshnood, S.; Zandi, E.; Eslamian, M.; Talebi, A.; Emami, S.N.; Nematbakhsh, M. Time course of cisplatin-induced nephrotoxicity and hepatotoxicity. *J. Nephropathol.* **2017**, *6*, 163–167. [CrossRef] [PubMed]
28. Tarladacalisir, Y.T.; Uygun, M.; Akpolat, M.; Uz, Y.H. Histological Examination of the Effects of Vitamins on Preventing Cisplatin Hepatotoxicity. *Balkan Med. J.* **2005**, *22*, 124–131.
29. Martins, N.; Santos, N.; Curti, C.; Bianchi, L.; Santos, A. Thimerosal distribution and metabolism in neonatal mice. *J. Appl. Toxicol.* **2008**, *28*, 337–344. [CrossRef]
30. Dasari, S.; Bernard Tchounwou, P. Cisplatin in cancer therapy: Molecular mechanisms of action. *Eur. J. Pharmacol.* **2014**, *740*, 364–378. [CrossRef]
31. Nazıroğlu, M.; Yürekli, V.A. Effects of antiepileptic drugs on antioxidant and oxidant molecular pathways: Focus on trace elements. *Cell. Mol. Neurobiol.* **2013**, *33*, 589–599. [CrossRef]
32. Hockenberry, M.J.; Hooke, M.C.; Gregurich, M.; McCarthy, K. Carnitine plasma levels and fatigue in children/adolescents receiving cisplatin, ifosfamide, or doxorubicin. *J. Pediatr. Hematol. Oncol.* **2009**, *31*, 664–669. [CrossRef]
33. Karahan, I.; Yilmaz, S.; Atessahin, A. Effects of lycopene on cisplatin and gentamicin induced oxidative stres in blood and liver in rats. *Fırat. Univ. Med. J. Health Sci.* **2006**, *20*, 39–43.
34. Blumberg, J. Use of biomarkers of oxidative stress in research studies. *J. Nutr. Am. Soc. Nutr.* **2004**, *134*, 3188S–3189S. [CrossRef] [PubMed]
35. Tüközan, N.; Erdamar, H.; Seven, I. Measurement of Total Malondialdehyde in Plasma and Tissues by High-Performance Liquid Chromatography and Thiobarbituric Acid Assay. *Firat Tip Derg.* **2006**, *11*, 88–92.
36. Ateşşahin, A.; Şanna, E.; Türk, G.; Çeribaşi, A.O.; Yilmaz, S.; Yüce, A.; Bulmuş, Ö. Chemoprotective effect of melatonin against cisplatin-induced testicular toxicity in rats. *J. Pineal. Res.* **2006**, *41*, 21–27. [CrossRef]
37. Iraz, M.; Ozerol, E.; Gulec, M.; Tasdemir, S.; Idiz, N.; Fadillioglu, E.; Naziroglu, M.; Akyol, O. Protective effect of caffeic acid phenethyl ester (CAPE) administration on cisplatin-induced oxidative damage to liver in rat. *Cell Biochem. Func.* **2006**, *24*, 357–361. [CrossRef]
38. Sugiyama, S.; Hayakawa, M.; Kato, T.; Hanaki, Y.; Shimizu, K.; Ozawa, T. Adverse effect of anti-tumor drug, cisplatin, on rat kidney mitochondria: Disturbances in glutathione peroxidase activity. *Biochem. Biophys. Res. Commun.* **1989**, *159*, 1121–1127. [CrossRef]
39. Işeri, S.; Ercan, F.; Gedik, N.; Yüksel, M.; Alican, I. Simvastatin attenuates cisplatin-induced kidney and liver damage in rats. *Toxicology* **2007**, *230*, 256–264. [CrossRef]
40. Greggi, L.M.; D'arc, C.; Darin, J.; Bianchi, M.D.L.P. Protective effects of vitamin C against cisplatin-induced nephrotoxicity and lipid peroxidation in adult rats: A dose-dependent study. *Pharmacol. Res.* **2000**, *41*, 405–441. [CrossRef]
41. Mora, L.; De, O.; Antunes, L.M.G.; Francescato, H.D.C.; Bianchi, M.L.P. The effects of oral glutamine on cisplatin-induced nephrotoxicity in rats. *Pharmacol. Res.* **2003**, *47*, 517–522. [CrossRef]
42. Naziroğlu, M.; Karaoğlu, A.; Aksoy, A.O. Selenium and high dose vitamin E administration protects cisplatin-induced oxidative damage to renal, liver and lens tissues in rats. *Toxicology* **2004**, *195*, 221–230. [CrossRef] [PubMed]
43. Alshuweishi, Y.; Alfaifi, M.; Almoghrabi, Y.; Alfhili, M.A. AST and ALT APRI Scores and Dysglycemia in Saudi Arabia: A Retrospective Population Study. *Life* **2023**, *13*, 1881. [CrossRef]
44. Tamber, S.S.; Bansal, P.; Sharma, S.; Singh, R.B.; Sharma, R. Biomarkers of liver diseases. *Mol. Biol. Rep.* **2023**, *50*, 7815–7823. [CrossRef]
45. Zheng, X.N.; Wang, X.W.; Li, L.Y.; Xu, Z.W.; Huang, H.Y.; Zhao, J.S.; Zhang, D.; Yin, X.; Sheng, J.; Tang, J.T. Pu-erh tea powder preventive effects on cisplatin-induced liver oxidative damage in Wistar rats. *Asian Pac. J. Cancer Prev.* **2014**, *15*, 7389–7394. [CrossRef]

46. Amidi, N.; Moradkhani, S.; Sedaghat, M.; Khiripour, N.; Larki-Harchegani, A.; Zadkhosh, N.; Ranjbar, A. Effect of green tea on inflammation and oxidative stress in cisplatin-induced experimental liver function. *J. Herbmed Pharmacol.* **2016**, *5*, 99–102.
47. Ani, F.I.; Nabofa, E.E.W.; Omobowale, T.O.; Ajuzie, N.C.; Ajemigbitse, J.; Oyagbemi, A.A.; Attah, A.F.; Adeoye, B.K.; Azubuike-Osu, S.O.; Adedapo, A.A.; et al. Infused aqueous curry tea extracts ameliorate Nω -Nitro-L-Arginine Methyl Ester-induced liver dysfunction in male albino Wistar rats. *J. Food Biochem.* **2022**, *46*, e14198. [CrossRef]
48. Tang, Z.; Zhan, L.; He, R.; Zhou, Y.; Tang, Q.; Liu, Z.; Zhang, S.; Liu, A. Hepatoprotective Effect of Tea Composite Solid Beverage on Alcohol-Caused Rat Liver Injury. *Foods* **2023**, *12*, 4126. [CrossRef]
49. Wang, R.; Yang, Z.; Zhang, J.; Mu, J.; Zhou, X.; Zhao, X. Liver Injury Induced by Carbon Tetrachloride in Mice Is Prevented by the Antioxidant Capacity of Anji White Tea Polyphenols. *Antioxidants* **2019**, *8*, 64. [CrossRef]
50. Mostafa-Hedeab, G.; Ewaiss Hassan, M.; Halawa, T.F.; Ahmed Wani, F. Epigallocatechin gallate ameliorates tetrahydrochloride-induced liver toxicity in rats via inhibition of TGFβ/p-ERK/p-Smad1/2 signaling, antioxidant, anti-inflammatory activity. *Saudi Pharm J.* **2022**, *30*, 1293–1300. [CrossRef]

life

MDPI

Case Report

Application of Functional Neurology Therapy in a Lactose-Intolerant Patient

Jorge Rey-Mota [1], Guillermo Escribano-Colmena [1], David Martín-Caro Álvarez [2], Jhulliana Vasquez Perez [3], Eduardo Navarro-Jimenez [3] and Vicente Javier Clemente-Suárez [4,5,*]

1 Independent Researcher, 28660 Boadilla del Monte, Spain; jreymota@gmail.com (J.R.-M.); escribanocolmenaguillermo@gmail.com (G.E.-C.)
2 Toledo Physiotherapy Research Group (GIFTO), Faculty of Physiotherapy and Nursing of Toledo, Universidad de Castilla-La Mancha, 45071 Toledo, Spain; david.martincaro@uclm.es
3 Facultad de Ciencias de la Salud, Universidad Simón Bolívar, Barranquilla 080005, Colombia; jhulliana.vasquez@unisimon.edu.co (J.V.P.); eduardo.navarro@unisimon.edu.co (E.N.-J.)
4 Faculty of Sports Sciences, Universidad Europea de Madrid, Tajo Street, s/n, 28670 Madrid, Spain
5 Grupo de Investigación en Cultura, Educación y Sociedad, Universidad de la Costa, Barranquilla 080002, Colombia
* Correspondence: vctxente@yahoo.es; Tel.: +34-902232350; Fax: +34-911-413-585

Abstract: This case report examines the impact of a single session of functional neurology on a 35-year-old female patient diagnosed with lactose intolerance. The patient presented with severe gastrointestinal symptoms, including frequent diarrhea, bloating, and vomiting upon dairy consumption. The intervention aimed to reset dysfunctional neurological programs believed to contribute to her condition. The study utilized a standardized lactose intolerance breath test to measure the hydrogen and methane levels at various intervals before and after treatment. Post-treatment results showed symptomatic relief with the patient reporting normalized bowel movements and the absence of previous symptoms. Despite these improvements, the biochemical markers at higher time points (150 and 175 min) post-treatment remained similar to the pre-treatment values, indicating persistent lactose malabsorption and highlighting the variability of hydrogen measurements. This case report suggests that a single session of functional neurology can significantly alleviate the symptoms of lactose intolerance. However, the preliminary nature of these results underscores the need for further research involving larger sample sizes and long-term follow-up to fully understand the treatment's efficacy and underlying mechanisms.

Keywords: functional neurology; lactose intolerance; gastrointestinal symptoms; neurological dysfunction; biochemical markers; breath test

1. Introduction

The prevalence of food intolerances and allergies has been rising significantly in recent years, affecting millions globally. This trend has been observed across various populations and age groups, with children being particularly susceptible. A study by Sicherer and Sampson [1] highlights that food allergies impact approximately 8% of children and 5% of adults in the United States, with similar patterns reported worldwide. These conditions can manifest through a range of symptoms, including gastrointestinal distress, dermatological reactions, and respiratory issues, significantly impairing the quality of life and posing substantial public health concerns [1,2]. Furthermore, food intolerances, often confused with allergies, also show a significant prevalence. These intolerances, which include non-IgE-mediated reactions like lactose intolerance, fructose malabsorption, and histamine intolerance, can lead to chronic gastrointestinal symptoms and are increasingly recognized as important contributors to functional abdominal pain syndromes [3]. The differentiation between food allergies, sensitivities, and intolerances is crucial for accurate diagnosis and management, which requires tailored approaches to each condition [4]. Effective management strategies are essential to mitigate the impact on patients' daily lives and to prevent complications associated with these conditions. In this line, food allergies involve immune responses, typically IgE-mediated, leading to reactions like anaphylaxis. Sensitivities may not involve the immune system and can cause various symptoms. Intolerances, like lactose intolerance, involve digestive system issues due to enzyme deficiencies.

Specifically, lactose intolerance is a prevalent condition characterized by the inability to fully digest lactose, a sugar found in milk and dairy products, due to insufficient levels of lactase, the enzyme responsible for breaking down lactose in the small intestine. This condition leads to symptoms such as abdominal pain, bloating, gas, and diarrhea following the consumption of lactose-containing foods [5]. The primary cause of lactose intolerance is lactase non-persistence, a genetic condition in which the activity of lactase decreases significantly after weaning, a trait that affects the majority of the world's population. In contrast, lactase persistence, where high levels of lactase activity continue into adulthood, is primarily seen in populations with a long history of dairy consumption, such as those of Northern European descent [6]. Recent studies indicate an increasing prevalence of lactose intolerance globally, with significant variations across different regions and populations. This rise may be attributed to better diagnostic tools and increased awareness, along with changes in dietary habits and possibly environmental factors affecting gut microbiota composition [7]. Mechanistically, undigested lactose in the small intestine undergoes fermentation by gut bacteria, producing gases like hydrogen, methane, and short-chain fatty acids. This process not only leads to gastrointestinal symptoms but can also influence gut motility and water absorption, exacerbating symptoms like diarrhea. Additionally, factors such as the amount of lactose ingested, the rate of intestinal transit, and the presence of other gastrointestinal disorders can modulate symptom severity [7]. The increase in diagnosed cases of lactose intolerance can also be linked to advancements in diagnostic methods, such as the hydrogen breath test, which measures hydrogen production after lactose ingestion, and genetic tests that identify polymorphisms associated with lactase non-persistence [8].

Functional neurology is emerging as a promising field in addressing various pathologies, including food intolerances. This discipline integrates principles from traditional neurology with functional medicine, focusing on the interconnectedness of neurological and systemic health. Functional neurology emphasizes individualized treatment plans based on a comprehensive assessment of a patient's neurological function, aiming to restore balance and improve overall health outcomes [9,10]. Recent advancements in this field have shown potential in treating conditions that are not adequately managed by conventional approaches, offering new hope for patients with chronic and complex health issues [11]. Previous authors have highlighted the possible areas of treatment of functional neurology, proposing that this treatment could alleviate symptoms associated with food intolerances, leading to improved quality of life for patients [10]. Functional neurology focuses on the interplay between neurological function and systemic health. Previous studies have shown potential benefits in addressing gastrointestinal symptoms by resetting dysfunctional neurological pathways [10,11].

The objective of this case report was to analyze the effect of a single session of functional neurology on the symptoms and biochemical parameters of a breath test for lactose intolerance in a female patient with lactose intolerance. We hypothesized that a single session of functional neurology would significantly improve the symptoms and biochemical parameters of a breath test in a female patient with lactose intolerance.

2. Materials and Methods

2.1. Participant

A 35-year-old female patient with a height of 160 cm and a weight of 58 kg, diagnosed with lactose intolerance seven years ago, was analyzed in this case report. Prior to the treatment, she experienced frequent diarrhea, typically having bowel movements 3 to 5 times a day, often with a very foul odor. She also reported abdominal bloating and a bad taste in her mouth. Upon consuming large amounts of dairy, she would suffer from severe symptoms, including vomiting (with curdled milk present), fever, and intense diarrhea, indicating her intestines' inability to process lactose. The diagnosis of lactose intolerance was confirmed through a hydrogen breath test, which showed elevated hydrogen and methane levels post-lactose ingestion. Other gastrointestinal disorders, such as celiac disease and inflammatory bowel disease, were ruled out based on the patient's history and the relevant tests. The patient's medical history included previous treatments such as dietary modifications and over-the-counter enzyme supplements, which provided limited relief. Laboratory parameters like complete blood count and inflammatory markers were within normal ranges. The study's procedures complied with the Helsinki Declaration, ensuring ethical standards were met, with ethical approval granted by the European University's Bioethics Committee under code 2024-738.

2.2. Lactose Intolerance Test

The lactose intolerance breath test was conducted following the standard methodology as outlined in the literature [12]. The test involved measuring the levels of hydrogen and methane in the patient's breath at baseline and at various intervals after lactose ingestion. The patient first provided a baseline breath sample, which was then analyzed for hydrogen and methane concentrations. Subsequently, the patient ingested a lactose solution, and breath samples were collected at 25 min intervals for up to 175 min. The levels of hydrogen and methane in the breath samples were measured and recorded at each interval. The interpretation of the results was based on established criteria: an increase in hydrogen levels of more than 20 parts per million (ppm) or an increase in methane levels of more than 12 ppm from the baseline indicated lactose malabsorption. If both gases showed elevated levels, it confirmed lactose intolerance. Controls included a baseline breath test and a standardized lactose solution ingestion. The test was conducted using the QuinTron Model SC BreathTracker (Serial No. XYZ123, QuinTron Instrument Company, Inc., Milwaukee, WI, USA). The patient adhered to a lactose-free diet for 24 h before the test to ensure accurate baseline measurements. In addition, happiness and enjoyment of life were measured using a 0–100 scale.

2.3. Functional Neurology Intervention

The patient underwent a treatment with functional neurology targeting several dysfunctional nociceptors causing her lactose intolerance. To standardize the protocol, the methodology described by ®NeuroReEvolution (http://nre-therapy.com/, accessed on 1 August 2024), was followed, involving a comprehensive clinical diagnosis that included oral and visual assessments, functional neurology tests on joints, and a tailored intervention based on the identified neurological disorders. The practitioner, certified with a Level III in the Functional Neurology Manual Muscle Test from ®NeuroReEvolution, ensured a high degree of expertise in diagnosing and addressing specific nervous system disorders. The intervention involved techniques such as proprioceptive reflex correction, desensitization of trigger points, and systemic integration through blink reflex. Each session lasted approximately 45 min, with follow-up assessments conducted one week post-intervention. Proprioceptive reflexes were corrected to improve posture, balance, and movement, while trigger points were desensitized to normalize reflex responses and restore function [10].

3. Results and Discussion

After the treatment, the patient experienced a significant improvement in intestinal transit, being pleasantly surprised by having only one normal bowel movement per day. She reported the complete absence of all previous symptoms and expressed increased happiness and enjoyment of life. The patient's score improved from 45 pre-treatment to 85 post-treatment, indicating a substantial enhancement in overall well-being and daily functioning.

Before the functional neurology treatment, the patient's breath test results showed elevated levels of hydrogen and methane, indicating lactose malabsorption. At baseline (0 min), the hydrogen and methane levels were 4 ppm and 8 ppm, respectively (Figure 1). These levels increased over time, reaching peaks of 70 ppm for hydrogen and 16 ppm for methane at 100 min and 150 min, respectively. After the treatment, there was a reduction in the combined levels of hydrogen and methane. At baseline, the combined level was 2 ppm, and although there were increases at subsequent time points, the levels were generally lower compared to the pre-treatment results. For instance, at 50 min, the combined level was 3 ppm, and at 100 min, it was 36 ppm, but, at 150 and 175 min the values were similar in the pre- and post-evaluations (Table 1).

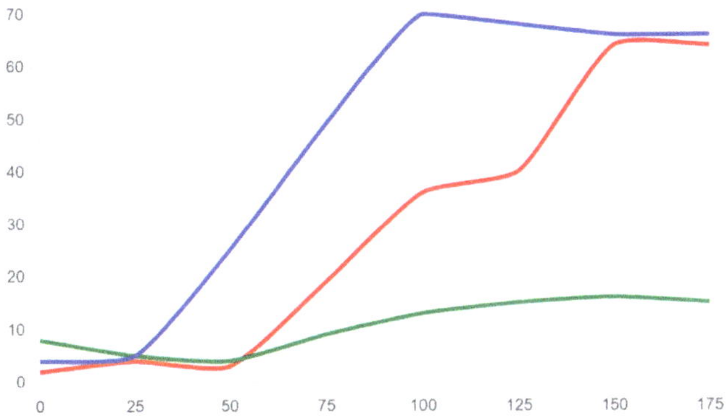

Figure 1. Changes in hydrogen and methane levels over time. X: gas levels (ppm); Y: time (minutes); The blue line represents the pre-treatment hydrogen levels, the green line represents the pre-treatment methane levels, and the red line represents the post-treatment combined hydrogen and methane levels.

Table 1. Hydrogen and Methane Levels Before and After Functional Neurology Treatment.

Time (Minutes)	Pre-Treatment Hydrogen (ppm)	Pre-Treatment Methane (ppm)	Post-Treatment Hydrogen + Methane (ppm)
0	4	8	2
25	5	5	4
50	25	4	3
75	49	9	19
100	70	13	36
125	68	15	40
150	66	16	64
175	66	15	64

Lactose intolerance may originate from the activation of nociceptors triggered by a traumatic event that overwhelms the central nervous system (CNS). This response aims to allocate energy to manage the stressor, potentially inhibiting hormone release, including lactase production. Consequently, energy is redirected to address the primary traumatic stressor, deeming lactase production less critical for immediate survival. The problem arises when this adaptive program remains active long-term, inhibiting lactase production persistently. Then, traumatic experiences can lead to prolonged activation of the CNS, as it prioritizes immediate survival over other bodily functions. This can result in the suppression of lactase production, as energy and resources are diverted to cope with the stressor. The prolonged stress response and the resulting energy reallocation may inhibit the production of lactase, the enzyme required to digest lactose, thereby leading to lactose intolerance [6].

Nociceptors, specialized sensory receptors that detect tissue damage, can initiate a cascade of events in the CNS, leading to various physiological responses. These responses are aimed at survival and immediate energy allocation to cope with the traumatic event [13]. The sustained activation of these nociceptive pathways can lead to the prolonged suppression of functions not critical for immediate survival, such as lactase production [14]. In the context of lactose intolerance, this mechanism can explain why some individuals experience persistent symptoms long after the initial traumatic event has passed. Functional neurology interventions may help reset these dysfunctional neurological programs, thereby restoring normal lactase production and alleviating symptoms of lactose intolerance [15].

The functional neurology intervention successfully eliminated the patient's symptoms of lactose intolerance, such as frequent diarrhea, bloating, and severe gastrointestinal distress upon consuming dairy products. Despite these improvements, biochemical markers at higher time points (150 and 175 min) post-treatment remained similar to pre-treatment values, indicating persistent lactose malabsorption and highlighting the variability of the hydrogen measurements. This underscores the necessity for further research involving multiple tests or subjects to validate these preliminary findings. This discrepancy suggests that while functional neurology may effectively reset dysfunctional neurological programs and alleviate symptoms, the underlying biochemical response to lactose ingestion may remain unchanged. Then, the persistence of high hydrogen and methane levels at 150 and 175 min indicates that the biochemical processes underlying lactose malabsorption were not fully normalized. This observation aligns with the understanding that while functional neurology can modify neural pathways and alleviate symptoms, it may not directly impact the gut microbiota's role in fermenting undigested lactose [16]. The sustained high levels of these gases suggest that the gut bacteria continued to ferment lactose, producing hydrogen and methane, even after the neurological symptoms were addressed. This points to the complex interplay between the nervous system and gut microbiota in lactose intolerance. The findings highlight the need for a comprehensive treatment approach that includes both neurological and dietary interventions to fully address the condition [17]. Despite significant symptomatic relief, the persistence of elevated biochemical markers suggests that functional neurology may not fully normalize lactose metabolism. This discrepancy highlights the complexity of lactose intolerance, which may involve both neurological and gut microbiota factors. The literature supports the idea that CNS trauma can affect digestive enzyme production [18–20]. Further studies are needed to explore this relationship and validate the findings of this case report.

This study has several limitations that should be acknowledged. Firstly, it is a single case report, which limits the generalizability of the findings. Further studies involving larger sample sizes are necessary to validate the results and determine the broader applicability of functional neurology interventions for lactose intolerance. Also, the breath test used for lactose intolerance is not very specific, which may limit the accuracy of the diagnosis and interpretation of results. Additionally, the study lacked a long-term follow-up to assess the sustainability of the symptomatic relief provided by the intervention. Future research should include longitudinal studies to monitor the persistence of treatment effects over time. Moreover, the biochemical tests indicated that while symptoms were alleviated, the underlying lactose malabsorption persisted, suggesting the need for a multifaceted treatment approach that also addresses gut microbiota.

Case reports play a crucial role in the medical literature, as they provide valuable insights into new or rare conditions, therapeutic effects, and potential adverse events, thus paving the way for further research and advancements in clinical practice [21–24]. The findings from this case report suggest that functional neurology can be a valuable complementary therapy for managing symptoms of lactose intolerance. However, it is crucial to recognize that the observed improvements might include placebo effects, and further research with larger sample sizes and multiple tests is essential to substantiate these findings. This approach may be particularly beneficial for patients who do not respond adequately to dietary modifications alone. Practitioners could consider integrating functional neurology techniques to address the neurological aspects of food intolerances, potentially improving patient outcomes. Additionally, this study highlights the importance of personalized treatment plans that consider both neurological and gastrointestinal factors.

In conclusion, this case report demonstrates that a single session of functional neurology can significantly alleviate the symptoms of lactose intolerance in the observed case. However, the persistence of elevated biochemical markers and the potential for placebo effects underscore the need for comprehensive treatment strategies and further research involving larger sample sizes and multiple tests. These findings underscore the need for a comprehensive treatment strategy that includes both neurological and dietary interventions. Further research with larger sample sizes and long-term follow-up is essential to fully understand the potential of functional neurology in treating lactose intolerance and to develop integrated treatment protocols that address both symptomatic relief and underlying biochemical imbalances.

Author Contributions: Conceptualization, J.R.-M. and D.M.-C.Á.; investigation, J.R.-M.; writing—original draft preparation, all authors; writing—review and editing, all authors; supervision J.R.-M., V.J.C.-S. and D.M.-C.Á. All authors have read and agreed to the published version of the manuscript.

Funding: This research received no external funding.

Institutional Review Board Statement: The study was conducted in accordance with the Declaration of Helsinki and approved by the university's ethics Committee of Universidad Europea de Madrid, assigning it an internal code 2024-738.

Informed Consent Statement: Informed consent was obtained from all subjects involved in the study.

Data Availability Statement: Data are contained within the article.

Conflicts of Interest: The authors declare no conflict of interest. Guillermo Escribano-Colmena and Jorge Rey-Mota are affiliated with ®NeuroReEvolution.

References

1. Sicherer, S.H.; Sampson, H.A. Food allergy: Epidemiology, pathogenesis, diagnosis, and treatment. *J. Allergy Clin. Immunol.* **2014**, *133*, 291–307. [CrossRef] [PubMed]
2. Nwaru, B.I.; Hickstein, L.; Panesar, S.S.; Roberts, G.; Muraro, A.; Sheikh, A. Prevalence of common food allergies in Europe: A systematic review and meta-analysis. *Allergy* **2014**, *69*, 992–1007. [CrossRef] [PubMed]
3. Gjini, B.; Melchior, I.; Euler, P.; Kreysel, C.; Kalde, S.; Krummen, B.; Kiesslich, R.; Hemmerlein, B.; Frieling, T. Food intolerance in patients with functional abdominal pain: Evaluation through endoscopic confocal laser endomicroscopy. *Endosc. Int. Open* **2023**, *11*, E67–E71. [CrossRef]
4. Holscher, H.D.; Chumpitazi, B.P.; Dahl, W.J.; Fahey, G.C.; Liska, D.J.; Slavin, J.L.; Verbeke, K. Perspective: Assessing Tolerance to Nondigestible Carbohydrate Consumption. *Adv. Nutr.* **2022**, *13*, 2084–2097. [CrossRef] [PubMed]
5. Ugidos-Rodríguez, S.; Matallana-González, M.C.; Sánchez-Mata, M.C. Lactose malabsorption and intolerance: A review. *Food Funct.* **2018**, *9*, 4056–4068. [CrossRef] [PubMed]
6. Misselwitz, B.; Butter, M.; Verbeke, K.; Fox, M.R. Update on lactose malabsorption and intolerance: Pathogenesis, diagnosis and clinical management. *Gut* **2019**, *68*, 2080–2091. [CrossRef] [PubMed]
7. Catanzaro, R.; Sciuto, M.; Marotta, F. Lactose Intolerance—Old and New Knowledge on Pathophysiological Mechanisms, Diagnosis, and Treatment. *SN Compr. Clin. Med.* **2021**, *3*, 499–509. [CrossRef]
8. Bayless, T.M.; Brown, E.; Paige, D.M. Lactase Non-persistence and Lactose Intolerance. *Curr. Gastroenterol. Rep.* **2017**, *19*, 23. [CrossRef] [PubMed]
9. Meyer, A.-L.; Leboeuf-Yde, C. Unravelling functional neurology: A critical review of clinical research articles on the effect or benefit of the functional neurology approach. *Chiropr. Man. Therap.* **2018**, *26*, 30. [CrossRef]
10. Rey-Mota, J.; Escribano-Colmena, G.; Fernández-Lucas, J.; Parraca, J.A.; Clemente-Suárez, V.J. Impact of professional experience on clinical judgment and muscular response in various neuromuscular tests. *Physiol. Behav.* **2024**, *283*, 114602. [CrossRef]
11. Møller, A.R. *Neural Plasticity and Disorders of the Nervous System*; Cambridge University Press: Cambridge, UK, 2006.
12. Robles, L.; Priefer, R. Lactose Intolerance: What Your Breath Can Tell You. *Diagnostics* **2020**, *10*, 412. [CrossRef] [PubMed]

13. Pinho-Ribeiro, F.A.; Verri, W.A.; Chiu, I.M. Nociceptor Sensory Neuron–Immune Interactions in Pain and Inflammation. *Trends Immunol.* **2017**, *38*, 5–19. [CrossRef] [PubMed]
14. Shulpekova, Y.O.; Nechaev, V.M.; Popova, I.R.; Deeva, T.A.; Kopylov, A.T.; Malsagova, K.A.; Kaysheva, A.L.; Ivashkin, V.T. Food Intolerance: The Role of Histamine. *Nutrients* **2021**, *13*, 3207. [CrossRef] [PubMed]
15. Li, A.; Zheng, J.; Han, X.; Yang, S.; Cheng, S.; Zhao, J.; Zhou, W.; Lu, Y. Advances in Low-Lactose/Lactose-Free Dairy Products and Their Production. *Foods* **2023**, *12*, 2553. [CrossRef] [PubMed]
16. Shaukat, A. Systematic Review: Effective Management Strategies for Lactose Intolerance. *Ann. Intern. Med.* **2010**, *152*, 797–803. [CrossRef] [PubMed]
17. Lange, K.W.; Lange, K.M.; Nakamura, Y.; Reissmann, A. Nutrition in the Management of ADHD: A Review of Recent Research. *Curr. Nutr. Rep.* **2023**, *12*, 383–394. [CrossRef] [PubMed]
18. Furness, J.B. Integrated neural and endocrine control of gastrointestinal function. In *The Enteric Nervous System: 30 Years Later*; Springer: Berlin/Heidelberg, Germany, 2016; pp. 159–173.
19. Morys, J.; Malecki, A.; Nowacka-Chmielewska, M.M. Stress and the gut-brain axis: An inflammatory perspective. *Front. Mol. Neurosci.* **2024**, *17*, 1415567. [CrossRef] [PubMed]
20. Zheng, Y.; Bonfili, L.; Wei, T.; Eleuteri, A.M. Understanding the gut–brain axis and its therapeutic implications for neurodegenerative disorders. *Nutrients* **2023**, *15*, 4631. [CrossRef] [PubMed]
21. Clemente-Suárez, V.J. Multidisciplinary intervention in the treatment of mixed anxiety and depression disorder. *Physiol. Behav.* **2020**, *219*, 112858. [CrossRef]
22. Belinchón-deMiguel, P.; Navarro-Jiménez, E.; Laborde-Cárdenas, C.C.; Clemente-Suárez, V.J. Evolutionary Echoes: A Four-Day Fasting and Low-Caloric Intake Study on Autonomic Modulation and Physiological Adaptations in Humans. *Life* **2024**, *14*, 456. [CrossRef]
23. Gonçalves, C.; Parraca, J.A.; Bravo, J.; Abreu, A.; Pais, J.; Raimundo, A.; Clemente-Suárez, V.J. Influence of two exercise programs on heart rate variability, body temperature, central nervous system fatigue, and cortical arousal after a heart attack. *Int. J. Environ. Res. Public Health* **2022**, *20*, 199. [CrossRef] [PubMed]
24. Ortega-Loubon, C.; Culquichicón, C.; Correa, R. The importance of writing and publishing case reports during medical training. *Cureus* **2017**, *9*, e1964. [CrossRef] [PubMed]

MDPI AG
Grosspeteranlage 5
4052 Basel
Switzerland
Tel.: +41 61 683 77 34

Life Editorial Office
E-mail: life@mdpi.com
www.mdpi.com/journal/life

www.ingramcontent.com/pod-product-compliance
Lightning Source LLC
Chambersburg PA
CBHW061600220926
51850CB00005B/386
* 9 7 8 3 7 2 5 8 7 8 6 7 3 *